High Altitude: Human Adaptation to Hypoxia

High Altitude: Human Adaptation to Hypoxia

Editor: Stephan Blackwood

AMERICAN
MEDICAL PUBLISHERS
www.americanmedicalpublishers.com

AMERICAN
MEDICAL PUBLISHERS
www.americanmedicalpublishers.com

Cataloging-in-Publication Data

High altitude : human adaptation to hypoxia / edited by Stephan Blackwood.
p. cm.
Includes bibliographical references and index.
ISBN 979-8-88740-182-9
1. Anoxemia. 2. Adaptation (Physiology). 3. Altitude, Influence of.
4. Altitudes. I. Blackwood, Stephan.
RC103.A4 H54 2023
616.989 3--dc23

American Medical Publishers,
41 Flatbush Avenue,
1st Floor, New York,
NY 11217, USA

ISBN 979-8-88740-182-9 (Hardback)

Contents

Preface

This book has been an outcome of determined endeavour from a group of educationists in the field. The primary objective was to involve a broad spectrum of professionals from diverse cultural background involved in the field for developing new researches. The book not only targets students but also scholars pursuing higher research for further enhancement of the theoretical and practical applications of the subject.

Hypoxia is referred to as the condition of low oxygen level and it occurs naturally in high altitudes. As the altitude rises, total atmospheric pressure falls down and causes a lower partial pressure of oxygen causing hypobaric hypoxia. The humans have adjusted themselves to hypoxia that occurs at high altitude in various locations, which is possible due to genetic basis. The genetic signatures of certain populations are recognized in the hypoxia-inducible factor (HIF) pathway, responsible for the organization of transcriptional response to hypoxia. These genetic signatures are found in the HIF2A gene in Tibetans, which encodes for the prolyl hydroxylase domain protein 2 and HIF-2α gene. Adaptation to high altitude is the result of various genes that act in coordination with each other. Novel therapeutic approaches can be identified by unraveling the mechanisms of these genes. This book provides comprehensive insights on hypoxia. It will help the readers in keeping pace with the rapid developments in the study of human adaptation to hypoxia.

It was an honour to edit such a profound book and also a challenging task to compile and examine all the relevant data for accuracy and originality. I wish to acknowledge the efforts of the contributors for submitting such brilliant and diverse chapters in the field and for endlessly working for the completion of the book. Last, but not the least; I thank my family for being a constant source of support in all my research endeavours.

Editor

1

Hematological Risk Factors for High-Altitude Headache in Chinese Men Following Acute Exposure at 3,700 m

He Huang[1,2,3†], Bao Liu[1,2,3,4†], Gang Wu[1,2,3], Gang Xu[1,2,3], Bing-Da Sun[1,2,3] and Yu-Qi Gao[1,2,3]*

[1] Institute of Medicine and Hygienic Equipment for High Altitude Region, College of High Altitude Military Medicine, Third Military Medical University, Chongqing, China, [2] Key Laboratory of High Altitude Environmental Medicine, Third Military Medical University, Ministry of Education, Chongqing, China, [3] Key Laboratory of High Altitude Medicine, Chinese People's Liberation Army, Chongqing, China, [4] The 12th Hospital of Chinese People's Liberation Army, Kashi Xinjiang, China

***Correspondence:**
Yu-Qi Gao
gaoy66@yahoo.com

[†] These authors have contributed equally to this work.

Background: High-altitude headache (HAH) is a notably common disorder affecting the daily life of travelers ascending to high altitude. Hematological parameters are important clinical examinations for various diseases. Today, hematological characteristics of HAH remain unrevealed. Above all, we aimed to ascertain hematological characteristics and independent risk factors/predictors associated with HAH before and after exposure at 3,700 m.

Methods: Forty five healthy men were enrolled in present study. Demographic and clinical data, physiological and hematological parameters were collected 3 days before the ascent and after acute exposure at 3,700 m.

Results: HAH patients featured significantly lower white blood cell count (WBC), neutrophil count (NEU#) and percentage (NEU%), and higher percentage of lymphocyte (LYM%) at 3,700 m and significantly lower NEU#, reticulocyte count (RET#) and percentage (RET%) at sea level (all $P < 0.05$). HAH severity was significantly and negatively associated with WBC, NEU#, and NEU% at 3,700 m and RET# at sea level, whereas was positively associated with LYM% at 3,700 m (all $P < 0.05$). Moreover, we have found that RET# at sea level and NEU% at 3,700 m was an independent predictor and risk factor for HAH, respectively.

Conclusion: The present study is the first to examine the hematological characteristics of HAH. Furthermore, lower RET# at sea level and lower NEU% at 3,700 m is a novel independent predictor and risk factor for HAH, respectively.

Keywords: headache, high-altitude headache, acute mountain sickness, hematological parameters, risk factor

---

Abbreviations: AMS, Acute mountain sickness; CCL8, C-C Motif Chemokine Ligand 8; CI, confidence interval; DBP, diastolic blood pressure; HAH, high-altitude headache; HAH+, participants with HAH; HAH−, participants without HAH; HR, heart rate; IL-1β, interleukin-1β; IL-6, interleukin-6; IL-10, interleukin-10; SBP, systolic blood pressure; SpO_2, pulse oxygen saturation; TNF-α, tumor necrosis factor-α.

INTRODUCTION

Headache is the fundamental symptom for a diagnosis of acute mountain sickness (AMS) according to the Lake Louise Scoring System (Imray et al., 2010; Bartsch and Swenson, 2013; Davis and Hackett, 2017). In this context, high-altitude headache (HAH) is a defined and recognized headache disorder, which occurs within 24 h after ascending to an altitude of >2,500 m, based on the International Classification of Headache Disorders 3β criteria (Marmura and Hernandez, 2015; Kim et al., 2016). Approximately 80% of people are thought to experience headache after rapidly ascending to high altitudes, which is associated with disturbances in their daily life and work that create an important public health problem (Carod-Artal, 2014).

During recent decades, numerous researchers have systematically investigated the epidemiology, clinical manifestations, pathophysiological mechanisms, risk factors, prevention, and treatment of HAH (Wilson et al., 2009; Carod-Artal, 2014; Marmura and Hernandez, 2015). Clinical studies have demonstrated that HAH ordinarily presents as a sudden attack and partially mimics the features of migraine (Silber et al., 2003; Broessner et al., 2016). Current studies regarding the pathophysiological etiology of HAH have suggested that HAH can be induced by hypobaric hypoxia causing overperfusion of the microvascular beds, brain swelling, activation of the trigeminal vascular system, and sensitization of intracranial pain receptors (Burtscher et al., 2011). Furthermore, the known independent risk factors for HAH include increased heart rate (HR), posterior cerebral circulation, vertebral artery diastolic velocity, and anxiety; decreased pulse oxygen saturation (SpO_2) and vigor; and a history of migraine or microRNA dysregulation (Silber et al., 2003; Lawley, 2011; Alizadeh et al., 2012; Bian et al., 2013, 2015; Liu et al., 2016; Dong et al., 2017; Guo et al., 2017). However, the actual underlying mechanisms, clinical manifestations and risk factors/predictors remain not entirely clear, despite accumulating evidence regarding HAH (Marmura and Hernandez, 2015).

Hematological parameters are important clinical markers and can be analyzed using simple, rapid, and inexpensive techniques (Devasena, 2017). Numerous researchers have suggested that hematological changes are closely associated with various diseases, including myelodysplastic syndrome, laryngeal squamous cell cancer, stable coronary artery disease, stroke, and acute pulmonary embolism (Nayak et al., 2011; List et al., 2012; Zorlu et al., 2012; Ayhan et al., 2013; Sahin et al., 2015; Soderholm et al., 2015; Hsueh et al., 2017). Moreover, recent studies have indicated that migraine conditions may be related to some hematological parameters, especially high hemoglobin levels and broad red blood cell distribution width (Celikbilek et al., 2013; Lippi et al., 2014). Thus, hematological changes are an attractive area for improving our understanding of HAH, although we are not aware of any studies that have examined this issue.

The present study was based on the hypothesis that hematological parameters would be closely related to HAH. Therefore, we evaluated the hematological characteristics of participants before and after exposure to high altitude, which may provide useful information regarding HAH-specific hematological phenotypes, independent risk factors, and predictors.

METHODS

Participants

The inclusion criteria were healthy 18–60-year-old Chinese men whose primary residence was at an altitude of ≤1,000 m. The exclusion criteria were cardio-cerebrovascular diseases, respiratory diseases, neuropsychological diseases, kidney disorders, liver disorders, migraine or other headaches, history of travel to an altitude of >2,500 m during the last 2 years, and regularly drinking coffee or tea. Based on these criteria, we successfully recruited and enrolled 45 Chinese men who were healthy and 18–35 years old. The study's protocol was approved by the Third Military Medical University Ethics Committee (China), and complied with the requirements of the Declaration of Helsinki. All participants signed informed consent forms before their enrollment.

Procedures

During the study, all participants rapidly ascended from Chongqing (sea level, altitude of 200 m) to Lhasa (altitude of 3,700 m) by train within 48 h. Three days before the ascent, the participants provided demographic data and underwent measurements of physiological and hematological parameters at sea level. Within 24 h after their arrival at 3,700 m, the participants underwent assessments of their physiological and hematological parameters, as well as HAH. During the study, the participants maintained the same diet (no coffee, tea, or alcoholic drinks) and avoided strenuous activity to ensure a similar level of physical activity. The participants were monitored by physicians for any signs of high-altitude cerebral or pulmonary edema (Hackett and Roach, 2004; Pennardt, 2013). The possibility of emergent cases of these conditions was addressed by planning for immediate evacuation and treatment using oxygen supplementation and medication.

Demographic and Clinical Data Collection

Three days before their ascent, the participants completed self-administered questionnaires to obtain their demographic data (body mass index [BMI], age, smoking history, and drinking history). After the acute exposure at 3,700 m, the physicians scored the participants based on the clinical features of HAH: headache (0 = none, 1 = mild, 2 = moderate, 3 = severe), the location of the headache (bilateral, frontal, frontal-temporal, or other), and factors that worsened the headache (exertion, movement, straining, coughing, or other). The diagnosis of HAH was based on fulfilling at least two of the International Classification of Headache Disorders 3β criteria (Marmura and Hernandez, 2015): mild or moderate severity; bilateral location; and aggravation caused by exertion, movement, straining, coughing, and/or bending.

Measurement of Physiological Parameters

During the pre-exposure and post-exposure examinations, physicians measured the participants' physiological parameters, including HR, SpO_2, diastolic blood pressure (DBP), and systolic blood pressure (SBP). The participants rested for 30 min before being evaluated using a sphygmomanometer (HEM-6200; OMRON, China) and a pulse oximeter (NONIN-9550; Nonin Onyx, USA).

Blood Collection and Hematological Parameter Measurements

Pre-exposure and post-exposure venous blood samples were collected from the participants by qualified nurses using EDTA-coated tubes and standard procedures. The blood samples were stored at 4°C until the testing using the AU-2700 analyzers (Olympus, Tokyo, Japan) and commercial reagents. The hematological parameters were white blood cell count (WBC), red blood cell count (RBC), hematocrit (HCT), mean corpuscular volume, red cell distribution width and its coefficient of variation, platelet count, mean platelet volume, plateletcrit, platelet distribution width, platelet-large cell ratio, hemoglobin (HGB), mean corpuscular hemoglobin and concentration, neutrophil count (NEU#), reticulocyte count (RET#), lymphocyte count (LYM#), eosinophil count (EOS#), monocyte count (MON#), neutrophil percentage (NEU%), reticulocyte percentage (RET%), lymphocyte percentage (LYM%), eosinophil percentage (EOS%), and monocyte percentage (MON%) (Supplementary Table 1).

Statistical Analysis

The parameters' normality was assessed using the Shapiro-Wilk's test. Normally distributed data were presented as mean ± standard deviation, non-normally distributed data were presented as median (interquartile range), and categorical data were presented as number (percentage). Differences between the groups with and without HAH (HAH+/HAH−) were compared using the independent *t*-test for normally distributed data and the Mann-Whitney *U*-test for non-normally distributed data. Spearman correlation coefficients were evaluated for the relationships between the parameters and HAH severity scores. Univariate logistic regression was used to identify risk factors and predictors, and significant factors from the aforementioned analyses were included in adjusted logistic regression (**Figure 1**). All analyses were performed using IBM SPSS software (version 19; IBM Corp, Armonk, NY, USA), and differences were

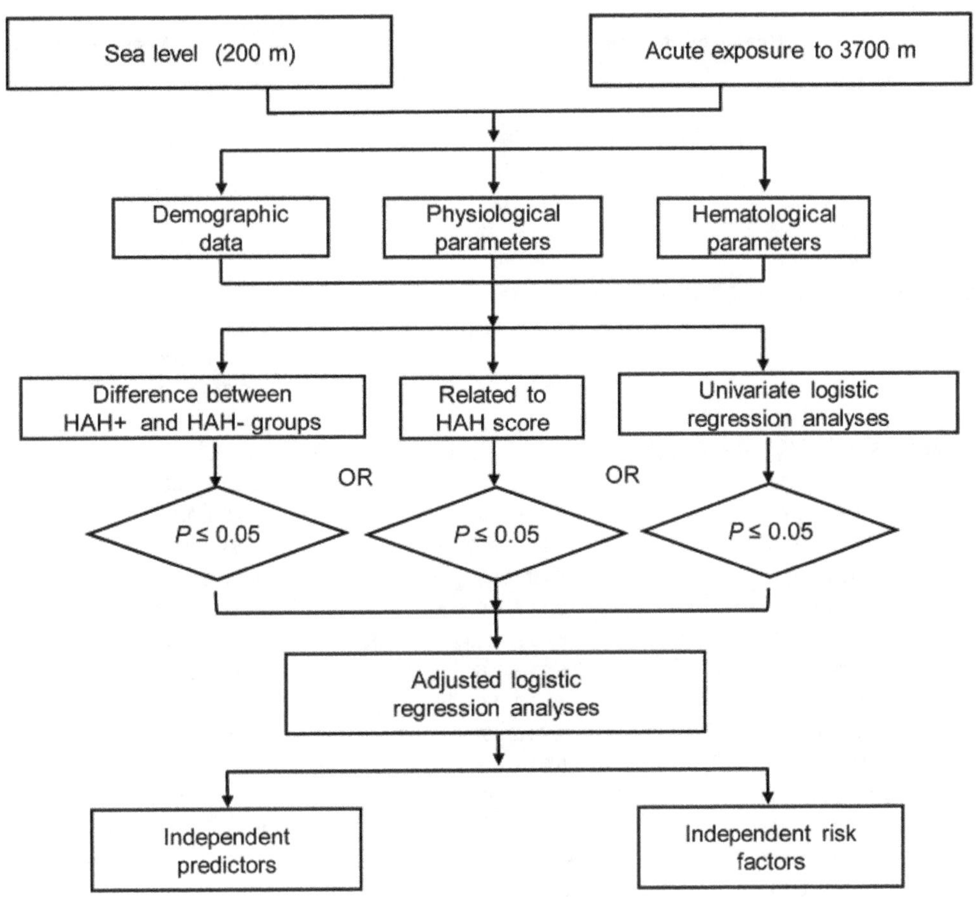

FIGURE 1 | The flow diagram of this study. HAH+, participants with high-altitude headache (HAH); HAH−, participants without HAH.

considered statistically significant at a P-value of < 0.05. All statistical methods and results were discussed with and guided by statisticians from the Third Military Medical University.

RESULTS

Demographic and Clinical Characteristics

All 45 participants completed the pre-exposure and post-exposure assessments, and had complete data regarding their physiological and hematological parameters. The incidence of HAH was 51.1%, although no significant differences were observed between the HAH+ and HAH− groups for age, BMI, drinking, and smoking (all $P > 0.05$, **Table 1**).

HAH-Related Parameters at Sea Level

Compared to the HAH− group, the HAH+ group had significantly lower pre-exposure values for RET% (0.76 ± 0.25% vs. 0.89 ± 0.22%), RET# (37.93 ± 12.25 10^9/L vs. 45.41 ± 9.52 10^9/L), and NEU# (2.94 ± 0.77 10^9/L vs. 3.62 ± 1.35 10^9/L) (all $P < 0.05$). There were no significant differences in the pre-exposure physiological parameters (all $P > 0.05$, **Table 1**, Supplementary Table 2A).

HAH-Related Parameters at 3,700 m

Compared to the HAH− group, the HAH+ group had significantly lower post-exposure values for NEU# (51.04 ± 6.75 10^9/L vs. 56.70 ± 6.59 10^9/L), NEU% (3.26 ± 0.77% vs. 4.16 ± 1.31%), and WBC (6.33 ± 1.09 10^9/L vs. 7.22 ± 1.62 10^9/L), as well as significantly higher LYM% (37.70 ± 6.45% vs. 32.82 ± 6.13%) (all $P < 0.05$). Similar to the pre-exposure, there were no significant differences in the post-exposure physiological parameters (all $P > 0.05$, **Table 1**, Supplementary Table 2A).

Associations between HAH Severity and the Pre-/Post-exposure Parameters

Among the pre-exposure parameters, only RET# was significantly associated with HAH severity ($r = -0.315$, $P = 0.035$). Among the post-exposure parameters, HAH severity was significantly and negatively associated with WBC ($r = -0.319$, $P = 0.032$), NEU# ($r = -0.315$, $P = 0.035$), and NEU% ($r = -0.383$, $P = 0.009$). Furthermore, HAH severity was positively associated with post-exposure LYM% ($r = 0.348$, $P = 0.019$). No other significant associations were observed between the remaining demographic or physiological parameters and HAH severity (all $P > 0.05$, **Table 2**, Supplementary Table 2B).

TABLE 1 | Differences of each variable between HAH+ and HAH− groups.

	Measurements at sea level		Measurements at 3,700 m	
	HAH+ (23)	**HAH− (22)**	**HAH+ (23)**	**HAH− (22)**
DEMOGRAPHIC DATA				
Age (year)	26.1 (3.0)	24.4 (9.0)	The same as sea level	
BMI (kg/m^2)	20.8 (3.0)	22.2 (1.5)	The same as sea level	
Smoking	2 (8.70%)	3 (13.6%)	The same as sea level	
Drinking	7 (30.4%)	5 (22.7%)	The same as sea level	
PHYSIOLOGICAL PARAMETERS				
SBP (mmHg)	110.6 ± 8.2	110.1 ± 6.7	122.6 ± 13.7	123.3 ± 10.8
DBP (mmHg)	67.0 ± 7.4	67.2 ± 5.2	73.5 ± 10.3	71.7 ± 9.0
HR (beats/min)	65.3 ± 10.8	68.5 ± 8.4	83.3 ± 12.9	88.3 ± 8.8
SpO_2 (%)	98.0 (1.0)	98.0 (1.0)	88.5 ± 2.6	87.2 ± 3.1
HEMATOLOGICAL PARAMETERS				
WBC (10^9/L)	5.61 ± 1.18	6.31 ± 1.74	**6.33 ± 1.09**	**7.22 ± 1.62***
NEU# (10^9/L)	**2.94 ± 0.77**	**3.62 ± 1.35***	**3.26 ± 0.77**	**4.16 ± 1.31#**
LYM# (10^9/L)	2.23 ± 0.58	2.27 ± 0.56	2.53 ± 0.43	2.30 (0.42)
MON# (10^9/L)	0.25 (0.10)	0.28 (0.10)	0.51 ± 0.14	0.53 ± 0.13
EOS# (10^9/L)	0.10 (0.13)	0.14 ± 0.09	0.11 (0.09)	0.15 ± 0.09
NEU% (%)	52.13 ± 8.07	56.09 ± 8.00	**51.04 ± 6.75**	**56.70 ± 6.59#**
LYM% (%)	40.03 ± 7.95	36.75 ± 7.68	**37.70 ± 6.45**	**32.82 ± 6.13***
MON% (%)	4.67 ± 1.07	4.43 ± 1.01	8.10 ± 1.73	7.66 ± 1.14
EOS% (%)	2.70 (2.30)	2.70 (2.43)	1.90 (1.40)	2.07 ± 1.36
RBC (10^{12}/L)	4.94 (0.46)	5.07 ± 0.37	5.41 (0.46)	5.51 ± 0.42
HGB (g/L)	149.00 (11.00)	150.09 ± 10.04	161.74 ± 11.04	165.95 ± 11.03
HCT (%)	45.03 ± 3.24	45.05 ± 3.05	48.09 ± 2.91	48.92 ± 2.91
RET# (10^9/L)	**37.93 ± 12.25**	**45.41 ± 9.52***	No data	
RET% (%)	**0.76 ± 0.25**	**0.89 (0.22)***	No data	

*HAH+, participants with high-altitude headache (HAH); HAH−, participants without HAH; BMI, body mass index; SBP, systolic blood pressure; DBP, diastolic blood pressure; HR, heart rate; SpO_2, pulse oxygen saturation. *P-value is 0.05 or less; #P-value is 0.01 or less; The bold data represent significant.*

Predictors and Risk Factors for HAH

Among the pre-exposure parameters, the univariate logistic regression analyses revealed that only RET# was significantly associated with HAH ($P < 0.05$, **Table 3**, Supplementary Table 2C). Among the post-exposure parameters, the univariate analyses revealed that HAH was significantly associated with WBC, NEU#, NEU%, and LYM% (all $P < 0.05$, **Table 4**, Supplementary Table 2C). The adjusted logistic regression analyses revealed that HAH was independently predicted by pre-exposure low RET#, and that low post-exposure NEU% was an independent risk factor for HAH (all $P < 0.05$, **Table 5**).

DISCUSSION

The present study revealed that some hematological parameters may be novel independent risk factors/predictors for HAH. For example, HAH was associated with low pre-exposure values for RET#, RET%, and NEU#. In addition, the HAH group had low post-exposure values for NEU#, NEU%, and WBC, as well as high values for LYM%. Moreover, HAH was independently predicted by low pre-exposure RET#, while low post-exposure NEU% was an independent risk factor for HAH.

HAH Is Associated with Reticulocyte and Neutrophil Counts at Sea Level

The present study revealed that low pre-exposure RET# was associated with the development of HAH at an altitude of 3,700 m. Furthermore, the severity of HAH was negatively associated with RET#. In this context, reticulocytes are immature RBCs and circulate in the bloodstream for approximately 1–4 days before developing into young mature RBCs (Lombardi et al., 2013). Interestingly, hypoxia stress can stimulate the production of reticulocytes (MacNutt et al., 2013), and young mature RBCs have greater affinity for oxygen plus more efficient oxygen delivery to the tissues, compared to old RBCs (Samaja et al., 1991; Cohen and Matot, 2013). Moreover, a recent open-label randomized controlled trial revealed that erythropoietin (which stimulates hematopoiesis) is an effective prophylaxis for AMS (Heo et al., 2014). Therefore, our results may support the prevention of HAH using prophylactic induction of hematopoiesis in case with anticipated acute exposure to a hypoxic environment.

Our results also indicate that the HAH+ group had significantly lower pre-exposure NEU#, compared to the HAH−

TABLE 2 | Relationships between HAH severity score and all the variables.

	Variables at sea level		Variables at 3,700 m	
	With HAH score *r*	*P*-value	With HAH score *R*	*P*-value
DEMOGRAPHIC DATA				
Age (year)	0.276	0.066	The same as sea level	
BMI (kg/m^2)	−0.017	0.914	The same as sea level	
PHYSIOLOGICAL PARAMETERS				
SBP (mmHg)	0.088	0.565	0.046	0.764
DBP (mmHg)	0.000	0.999	0.125	0.414
HR (beat/min)	−0.218	0.150	−0.278	0.064
SpO_2 (%)	−0.151	0.323	0.145	0.341
HEMATOLOGICAL PARAMETERS				
WBC (10^9/L)	−0.266	0.078	**−0.319**	**<0.05**
NEU# (10^9/L)	−0.260	0.085	**−0.383**	**<0.01**
LYM# (10^9/L)	−0.026	0.866	0.285	0.058
MON# (10^9/L)	−0.190	0.210	−0.113	0.460
EOS# (10^9/L)	−0.007	0.966	−0.038	0.805
NEU% (%)	−0.238	0.115	**−0.437**	**<0.01**
LYM% (%)	0.237	0.117	**0.348**	**<0.05**
MON% (%)	0.123	0.421	0.168	0.270
EOS% (%)	−0.055	0.720	0.040	0.793
RBC (10^{12}/L)	−0.115	0.451	−0.252	0.096
HGB (g/L)	−0.066	0.665	−0.236	0.119
HCT (%)	0.036	0.813	−0.218	0.151
RET# (10^9/L)	**−0.315**	**<0.05**	No data	
RET% (%)	−0.283	0.059	No data	

HAH, High-altitude headache; BMI, body mass index; SBP, systolic blood pressure; DBP, diastolic blood pressure; HR, heart rate; SpO_2, pulse oxygen saturation. The bold data represent significant.

TABLE 3 | Univariate logistic regression for each variable at sea level.

			95% CI		
Risk factors	β-coefficient	Odds ratio	Lower	Upper	*P*-value
DEMOGRAPHIC DATA					
Age (year)	0.208	1.231	0.965	1.572	0.095
BMI (kg/m^2)	−0.506	0.603	0.091	4.008	0.601
Smoking	0.199	1.220	0.626	2.378	0.560
Drinking	−0.043	0.958	0.699	1.313	0.789
PHYSIOLOGICAL PARAMETERS					
SBP (mmHg)	0.008	1.008	0.931	1.092	0.845
DBP (mmHg)	−0.006	0.994	0.905	1.092	0.903
HR (beat/min)	−0.037	0.964	0.905	1.028	0.261
SpO_2 (%)	−0.527	0.590	0.249	1.401	0.232
HEMATOLOGICAL PARAMETERS					
WBC (10^9/L)	−0.376	0.687	0.415	1.136	0.143
NEU# (10^9/L)	−0.679	0.507	0.252	1.023	0.058
LYM# (10^9/L)	−0.126	0.882	0.310	2.505	0.813
MON# (10^9/L)	−3.168	0.042	0.000	19.531	0.312
EOS# (10^9/L)	1.173	3.233	0.044	237.534	0.593
NEU% (%)	−0.064	0.938	0.867	1.015	0.111
LYM% (%)	0.057	1.058	0.977	1.146	0.167
MON% (%)	−0.082	0.921	0.736	1.153	0.473
EOS% (%)	0.964	2.623	0.016	443.888	0.713
RBC (10^{12}/L)	−0.572	0.565	0.190	1.679	0.304
HGB (g/L)	−0.022	0.979	0.922	1.039	0.478
HCT (%)	−0.003	0.997	0.825	1.206	0.975
RET# (10^9/L)	**−0.065**	**0.937**	**0.882**	**0.996**	**<0.05**
RET% (%)	−2.701	0.067	0.004	1.125	0.060

CI, Confidence interval; BMI, body mass index; SBP, systolic blood pressure; DBP, diastolic blood pressure; HR, heart rate; SpO_2, pulse oxygen saturation. The bold data represent significant.

TABLE 4 | Univariate logistic regression for each variable at 3,700 m.

Risk factors	β-coefficient	Odds ratio	95% CI Lower	95% CI Upper	*P*-value
DEMOGRAPHIC DATA (THE SAME AS SEA LEVEL)					
Physiological parameters					
SBP (mmHg)	−0.005	0.995	0.948	1.044	0.845
DBP (mmHg)	0.021	1.021	0.959	1.086	0.518
HR (beat/min)	−0.042	0.959	0.906	1.014	0.143
SpO_2 (%)	0.167	1.182	0.952	1.468	0.130
Hematological parameters					
WBC (10^9/L)	**−0.579**	**0.561**	**0.315**	**0.996**	**<0.05**
NEU# (10^9/L)	**−0.961**	**0.382**	**0.177**	**0.825**	**<0.05**
LYM# (10^9/L)	1.038	2.823	0.642	12.417	0.170
MON# (10^9/L)	−1.445	0.236	0.002	22.793	0.536
EOS# (10^9/L)	0.737	2.089	0.017	252.777	0.763
NEU% (%)	**−0.128**	**0.880**	**0.796**	**0.973**	**<0.05**
LYM% (%)	**0.126**	**1.134**	**1.020**	**1.261**	**<0.05**
MON% (%)	0.213	1.238	0.815	1.880	0.317
EOS% (%)	0.102	1.107	0.798	1.536	0.543
RBC (10^{12}/L)	−0.907	0.404	0.096	1.697	0.216
HGB (g/L)	−0.036	0.964	0.912	1.020	0.206
HCT (%)	−0.103	0.902	0.730	1.114	0.338

CI, Confidence interval; BMI, body mass index; SBP, systolic blood pressure; DBP, diastolic blood pressure; HR, heart rate; SpO_2, pulse oxygen saturation. The bold data represent significant.

TABLE 5 | Adjusted logistic regression for HAH at sea level and 3,700 m.

Risk factors	β-coefficient	Odds ratio	95% CI Lower	95% CI Upper	*P*-value
VARIABLES AT SEA LEVEL					
RET# (10^9/L)	−0.065	0.937	0.882	0.996	<0.05
VARIABLES AT 3,700 M					
NEU% (%)	−0.128	0.880	0.796	0.973	<0.05

CI, Confidence interval.

group. Previous studies have demonstrated that neutrophils undergo cellular adhesion and trans-endothelial migration from the blood stream during inflammation (Hall, 2015). In addition, hypobaric hypoxia could readily amplify pre-existing inflammation, which might lead to cerebral edema and AMS (Eltzschig and Carmeliet, 2011; Song et al., 2016). Furthermore, a recent study demonstrated that inflammation at sea level could predict the development of AMS (Lu et al., 2016). Thus, our results may indicate that inflammation at sea level is a risk factor for HAH.

Neutrophil Recruitment during HAH

Our results indicate that the HAH+ had significantly lower values for NEU# and NEU%, and higher values for LYM%. Furthermore, HAH severity was negatively associated with NEU# and NEU%, while HAH severity was positively associated with LYM%. Although the relevance of these findings is unclear, there are several potential explanations.

The first potential explanation is that neutrophils undergo trans-endothelial migration from the blood stream during inflammation, which is related to the similar mechanisms underlying stroke and AMS (Jin et al., 2010; Julian et al., 2011; Hall, 2015). Moreover, neutrophils are among the first cells to infiltrate the ischemic brain (within 30 min to a few hours after developing focal cerebral ischemia), where they amplify the inflammatory response with the help of cytokines (e.g., interleukin-1β [IL-1β], IL-6, and tumor necrosis factor-α [TNF-α]) that are produced by activated microglial cells (Ziemka-Nalecz et al., 2017). Intriguingly, our previous study revealed that plasma levels of IL-1β, IL-6, and TNF-α were positively correlated with AMS severity at 3,700 m, and another recent study revealed that plasma IL-6 levels were positively associated with AMS severity at 4,450 m and 5,129 m (Boos et al., 2016; Song et al., 2016). Thus, we speculate that hypobaric hypoxia induces brain injury by recruiting circulating neutrophils that aggravate neurogenic inflammation and lead to the development of HAH.

The second potential explanation is that neutrophil recruitment may be due to dampened anti-inflammatory IL-10 and upregulated C-C Motif Chemokine Ligand 8 (CCL8). For example, our recent transcriptome analysis revealed that IL-10 is downregulated in AMS, whereas CCL8 is upregulated (Liu et al., 2017). In addition, IL-10 is a general suppressor of the inflammatory response, while CCL8 promotes neutrophil recruitment (O'Boyle et al., 2007; Ouyang et al., 2011). Thus, we speculate that the lower NEU# and NEU% in patients with HAH are associated with the reduction of IL-10 and upregulation of CCL8, and this topic warrants urgent investigation. The third potential explanation is that the relatively high LYM% in patients with HAH could be the result of lower NEU%, as patients with and without HAH had similar values for LYM#.

Independent Predictors and Risk Factors for HAH

The adjusted logistic regression analyses revealed that low post-exposure NEU% was a risk factor for HAH. This may be because of the inflammatory response that is induced during HAH development. In addition, HAH was independently predicted by low RET#. This may reflect an impaired ability to produce young mature RBCs, which would decrease oxygen delivery to the tissues at high altitudes.

Limitations

Ours is the first study to examine the hematological characteristics of HAH, and provides the first step toward linking the fields of hematology and HAH. However, the study also has several limitations. First, we only examined a small cohort of young Chinese men, which could have introduced age- or sex-related bias. Second, we did not have access to post-exposure reticulocyte data. Thus, our findings should be validated using larger and more heterogeneous cohorts, as well as more complete experimental data.

CONCLUSION

The present study is the first to examine the hematological characteristics of HAH, and revealed that HAH was closely associated with WBC, NEU#, NEU%, LYM%, RET#, and RET%. In addition, HAH was independently predicted by low pre-exposure RET#, and low post-exposure NEU% was an independent risk factor for HAH.

AUTHOR CONTRIBUTIONS

YG conceived and designed the study. BL and GW oversaw laboratory analyses and HH provided the overall supervision of the study. GX and BS did the statistical analysis or contributed the laboratory experiments. Both GW and BL contributed to sample and physiological data collections. HH drafted the report. All authors contributed to the interpretation of results, critical revision of the manuscript and approved the final manuscript. YG is the guarantor.

ACKNOWLEDGMENTS

This work was supported by the Key Projects in the Military Science & Technology Pillar Program during the 13 5-year Plan Period (AWS14C007), by the Key Research Project of PLA (BWS11J042, AWS16J023).

REFERENCES

Alizadeh, R., Ziaee, V., Aghsaeifard, Z., Mehrabi, F., and Ahmadinejad, T. (2012). Characteristics of headache at altitude among trekkers; a comparison between acute mountain sickness and non-acute mountain sickness headache. *Asian J. Sports Med.* 3, 126–130. doi: 10.5812/asjsm.34714

Ayhan, S., Ozturk, S., Erdem, A., Ozlu, M. F., Memioglu, T., Ozyasar, M., et al. (2013). Hematological parameters and coronary collateral circulation in patients with stable coronary artery disease. *Exp. Clin. Cardiol.* 18, e12–e15.

Bartsch, P., and Swenson, E. R. (2013). Acute high-altitude illnesses. *N. Engl. J. Med.* 369, 1666–1667. doi: 10.1056/NEJMcp1214870

Bian, S. Z., Jin, J., Li, Q. N., Yu, J., Tang, C. F., Rao, R. S., et al. (2015). Hemodynamic characteristics of high-altitude headache following acute high altitude exposure at 3700 m in young Chinese men. *J. Headache Pain* 16:527. doi: 10.1186/s10194-015-0527-3

Bian, S. Z., Zhang, J. H., Gao, X. B., Li, M., Yu, J., Liu, X., et al. (2013). Risk factors for high-altitude headache upon acute high-altitude exposure at 3700 m in young Chinese men: a cohort study. *J. Headache Pain* 14:35. doi: 10.1186/1129-2377-14-35

Boos, C. J., Woods, D. R., Varias, A., Biscocho, S., Heseltine, P., and Mellor, A. J. (2016). High altitude and acute mountain sickness and changes in circulating endothelin-1, interleukin-6, and interleukin-17a. *High Alt. Med. Biol.* 17, 25–31. doi: 10.1089/ham.2015.0098

Broessner, G., Rohregger, J., Wille, M., Lackner, P., Ndayisaba, J. P., and Burtscher, M. (2016). Hypoxia triggers high-altitude headache with migraine features: a prospective trial. *Cephalalgia* 36, 765–771. doi: 10.1177/0333102415610876

Burtscher, M., Mairer, K., Wille, M., and Broessner, G. (2011). Risk factors for high-altitude headache in mountaineers. *Cephalalgia* 31, 706–711. doi: 10.1177/0333102410394678

Carod-Artal, F. J. (2014). High-altitude headache and acute mountain sickness. *Neurologia* 29, 533–540. doi: 10.1016/j.nrl.2012.04.015

Celikbilek, A., Zararsiz, G., Atalay, T., and Tanik, N. (2013). Red cell distribution width in migraine. *Int. J. Lab. Hematol.* 35, 620–628. doi: 10.1111/ijlh.12100

Cohen, B., and Matot, I. (2013). Aged erythrocytes: a fine wine or sour grapes? *Br. J. Anaesth.* 111(Suppl. 1), i62–i70. doi: 10.1093/bja/aet405

Davis, C., and Hackett, P. (2017). Advances in the prevention and treatment of high altitude illness. *Emerg. Med. Clin. North Am.* 35, 241–260. doi: 10.1016/j.emc.2017.01.002

Devasena, T. (ed.). (2017). "Biomarkers," in *Therapeutic and Diagnostic Nanomaterials* (Singapore: Springer), 29–40.

Dong, T., Liu, Z., Xuan, Q., Wang, Z., Ma, W., and Zhang, Q. (2017). Tumor LDH-A expression and serum LDH status are two metabolic predictors for triple negative breast cancer brain metastasis. *Sci. Rep.* 7:6069. doi: 10.1038/s41598-017-06378-7

Eltzschig, H. K., and Carmeliet, P. (2011). Hypoxia and inflammation. *N. Engl. J. Med.* 364, 656–665. doi: 10.1056/NEJMra0910283

Guo, W. Y., Bian, S. Z., Zhang, J. H., Li, Q. N., Yu, J., Chen, J. F., et al. (2017). Physiological and psychological factors associated with onset of high-altitude headache in Chinese men upon acute high-altitude exposure at 3700 m. *Cephalalgia* 37, 336–347. doi: 10.1177/0333102416646761

Hackett, P. H., and Roach, R. C. (2004). High altitude cerebral edema. *High Alt. Med. Biol.* 5, 136–146. doi: 10.1089/1527029041352054

Hall, J. E. (2015). *Guyton and Hall Textbook of Medical Physiology E-Book.* Philadelphia, PA: Elsevier Health Sciences.

Heo, K., Kang, J. K., Choi, C. M., Lee, M. S., Noh, K. W., and Kim, S. B. (2014). Prophylactic effect of erythropoietin injection to prevent acute mountain sickness: an open-label randomized controlled trial. *J. Korean Med. Sci.* 29, 416–422. doi: 10.3346/jkms.2014.29.3.416

Hsueh, C., Tao, L., Zhang, M., Cao, W., Gong, H., Zhou, J., et al. (2017). The prognostic value of preoperative neutrophils, platelets, lymphocytes, monocytes and calculated ratios in patients with laryngeal squamous cell cancer. *Oncotarget.* 8, 60514–60527. doi: 10.18632/oncotarget.16234

Imray, C., Wright, A., Subudhi, A., and Roach, R. (2010). Acute mountain sickness: pathophysiology, prevention, and treatment. *Prog. Cardiovasc. Dis.* 52, 467–484. doi: 10.1016/j.pcad.2010.02.003

Jin, R., Yang, G., and Li, G. (2010). Inflammatory mechanisms in ischemic stroke: role of inflammatory cells. *J. Leukoc. Biol.* 87, 779–789. doi: 10.1189/jlb.1109766

Julian, C. G., Subudhi, A. W., Wilson, M. J., Dimmen, A. C., Pecha, T., and Roach, R. C. (2011). Acute mountain sickness, inflammation, and permeability: new insights from a blood biomarker study. *J. Appl. Physiol.* 111, 392–399. doi: 10.1152/japplphysiol.00391.2011

Kim, B. S., Moon, H. S., Sohn, J. H., Cha, M. J., Song, T. J., Kim, J. M., et al. (2016). Short-term diagnostic stability of probable headache disorders based on the International classification of headache disorders, 3rd edition beta version, in first-visit patients: a multicenter follow-up study. *J. Headache Pain* 17:13. doi: 10.1186/s10194-016-0605-1

Lawley, J. S. (2011). Identifying the possible risk factors for high-altitude headache in mountaineers. *Cephalalgia* 31, 1677–1678. doi: 10.1177/0333102411422385

Lippi, G., Cervellin, G., and Mattiuzzi, C. (2014). Migraine and erythrocyte biology: a review. *Int. J. Lab. Hematol.* 36, 591–597. doi: 10.1111/ijlh.12199

List, A. F., Baer, M. R., Steensma, D. P., Raza, A., Esposito, J., Martinez-Lopez, N., et al. (2012). Deferasirox reduces serum ferritin and labile plasma iron in RBC transfusion-dependent patients with myelodysplastic syndrome. *J. Clin. Oncol.* 30, 2134–2139. doi: 10.1200/JCO.2010.34.1222

Liu, B., Chen, J., Zhang, L., Gao, Y., Cui, J., Zhang, E., et al. (2017). IL-10 Dysregulation in acute mountain sickness revealed by transcriptome analysis. *Front. Immunol.* 8:628. doi: 10.3389/fimmu.2017.00628

Liu, B., Huang, H., Wang, S. X., Wu, G., Xu, G., Sun, B. D., et al. (2016). Physiological adjustments and circulating MicroRNA reprogramming are involved in early acclimatization to high altitude in Chinese Han Males. *Front. Physiol.* 7:601. doi: 10.3389/fphys.2016.00601

Lombardi, G., Colombini, A., Lanteri, P., and Banfi, G. (2013). Reticulocytes in sports medicine: an update. *Adv. Clin. Chem.* 59, 125–153. doi: 10.1016/B978-0-12-405211-6.00005-X

Lu, H., Wang, R., Li, W., Xie, H., Wang, C., Hao, Y., et al. (2016). Plasma cytokine profiling to predict susceptibility to acute mountain sickness. *Eur. Cytokine Netw.* 27, 90–96. doi: 10.1684/ecn.2016.0383

MacNutt, M. J., Rupert, J. L., and Sheel, A. W. (2013). Haematological acclimation and re-acclimation to hypoxia in the mouse. *Respir. Physiol. Neurobiol.* 189, 153–161. doi: 10.1016/j.resp.2013.07.018

Marmura, M. J., and Hernandez, P. B. (2015). High-altitude headache. *Curr. Pain Headache Rep.* 19:483. doi: 10.1007/s11916-015-0483-2

Nayak, A. R., Kashyap, R. S., Kabra, D., Deoras, P., Purohit, H. J., Taori, G. M., et al. (2011). Evaluation of routinely performed hematological and biochemical parameters for the prognosis of acute ischemic stroke patients. *Neurol. Sci.* 32, 855–860. doi: 10.1007/s10072-011-0718-x

O'Boyle, G., Brain, J. G., Kirby, J. A., and Ali, S. (2007). Chemokine-mediated inflammation: identification of a possible regulatory role for CCR2. *Mol. Immunol.* 44, 1944–1953. doi: 10.1016/j.molimm.2006.09.033

Ouyang, W., Rutz, S., Crellin, N. K., Valdez, P. A., and Hymowitz, S. G. (2011). Regulation and functions of the IL-10 family of cytokines in inflammation and disease. *Annu. Rev. Immunol.* 29, 71–109. doi: 10.1146/annurev-immunol-031210-101312

Pennardt, A. (2013). High-altitude pulmonary edema: diagnosis, prevention, and treatment. *Curr. Sports Med. Rep.* 12, 115–119. doi: 10.1249/JSR.0b013e318287713b

Sahin, I., Karabulut, A., Kaya, A., Gungor, B., Avci, I. I., Okuyan, E., et al. (2015). Increased level of red cell distribution width is associated with poor coronary collateral circulation in patients with stable coronary artery disease. *Turk Kardiyol. Dern. Ars.* 43, 123–130. doi: 10.5543/tkda.2015.24819

Samaja, M., Rovida, E., Motterlini, R., and Tarantola, M. (1991). The relationship between the blood oxygen transport and the human red cell aging process. *Adv. Exp. Med. Biol.* 307, 115–123. doi: 10.1007/978-1-4684-5985-2_11

Silber, E., Sonnenberg, P., Collier, D. J., Pollard, A. J., Murdoch, D. R., and Goadsby, P. J. (2003). Clinical features of headache at altitude: a prospective study. *Neurology* 60, 1167–1171. doi: 10.1212/01.WNL.0000055876.267 37.B9

Soderholm, M., Borne, Y., Hedblad, B., Persson, M., and Engstrom, G. (2015). Red cell distribution width in relation to incidence of stroke and carotid atherosclerosis: a population-based cohort study. *PLoS ONE* 10:e0124957. doi: 10.1371/journal.pone.0124957

Song, T. T., Bi, Y. H., Gao, Y. Q., Huang, R., Hao, K., Xu, G., et al. (2016). Systemic pro-inflammatory response facilitates the development of cerebral edema during short hypoxia. *J. Neuroinflamm.* 13:63. doi: 10.1186/s12974-016-0 528-4

Wilson, M. H., Newman, S., and Imray, C. H. (2009). The cerebral effects of ascent to high altitudes. *Lancet Neurol.* 8, 175–191. doi: 10.1016/S1474-4422(09)70014-6

Ziemka-Nalecz, M., Jaworska, J., and Zalewska, T. (2017). Insights into the neuroinflammatory responses after neonatal Hypoxia-Ischemia. *J. Neuropathol. Exp. Neurol.* 76, 644–654. doi: 10.1093/jnen/n lx046

Zorlu, A., Bektasoglu, G., Guven, F. M., Dogan, O. T., Gucuk, E., Ege, M. R., et al. (2012). Usefulness of admission red cell distribution width as a predictor of early mortality in patients with acute pulmonary embolism. *Am. J. Cardiol.* 109, 128–134. doi: 10.1016/j.amjcard.2011.08.015

2

The Influence of CO_2 and Exercise on Hypobaric Hypoxia Induced Pulmonary Edema in Rats

Ryan L. Sheppard[1,2], Joshua M. Swift[2], Aaron Hall[2] and Richard T. Mahon[2]*

[1] Department of Submarine Medicine and Survival Systems Groton, Naval Submarine Medical Research Laboratory, Groton, CT, United States, [2] Department of Undersea Medicine, Walter Reed Army Institute of Research and Naval Medical Research Center, Silver Spring, MD, United States

***Correspondence:**
Ryan L. Sheppard
ryan.l.sheppard.mil@mail.mil

Introduction: Individuals with a known susceptibility to high altitude pulmonary edema (HAPE) demonstrate a reduced ventilation response and increased pulmonary vasoconstriction when exposed to hypoxia. It is unknown whether reduced sensitivity to hypercapnia is correlated with increased incidence and/or severity of HAPE, and while acute exercise at altitude is known to exacerbate symptoms the effect of exercise training on HAPE susceptibility is unclear.

Purpose: To determine if chronic intermittent hypercapnia and exercise increases the incidence of HAPE in rats.

Methods: Male Wistar rats were randomized to sedentary (sed-air), CO_2 (sed-CO_2,) exercise (ex-air), or exercise + CO_2 (ex-CO_2) groups. CO_2 (3.5%) and treadmill exercise (15 m/min, 10% grade) were conducted on a metabolic treadmill, 1 h/day for 4 weeks. Vascular reactivity to CO_2 was assessed after the training period by rheoencephalography (REG). Following the training period, animals were exposed to hypobaric hypoxia (HH) equivalent to 25,000 ft for 24 h. Pulmonary injury was assessed by wet/dry weight ratio, lung vascular permeability, bronchoalveolar lavage (BAL), and histology.

Results: HH increased lung wet/dry ratio (HH 5.51 $\pm$ 0.29 vs. sham 4.80 $\pm$ 0.11, $P < 0.05$), lung permeability (556 $\pm$ 84 u/L vs. 192 $\pm$ 29 u/L, $P < 0.001$), and BAL protein (221 $\pm$ 33 μg/ml vs. 114 $\pm$ 13 μg/ml, $P < 0.001$), white blood cell (1.16 $\pm$ 0.26 vs. 0.66 $\pm$ 0.06, $P < 0.05$), and platelet (16.4 $\pm$ 2.3, vs. 6.0 $\pm$ 0.5, $P < 0.001$) counts in comparison to normobaric normoxia. Vascular reactivity was suppressed by exercise (−53% vs. sham, $P < 0.05$) and exercise+CO_2 (−71% vs. sham, $P < 0.05$). However, neither exercise nor intermittent hypercapnia altered HH-induced changes in lung wet/dry weight, BAL protein and cellular infiltration, or pulmonary histology.

Conclusion: Exercise training attenuates vascular reactivity to CO_2 in rats but neither exercise training nor chronic intermittent hypercapnia affect HH- induced pulmonary edema.

Keywords: vascular reactivity, HAPE, chemoreflex, hypercapnia, exercise

INTRODUCTION

Rapid ascent to altitudes greater than 2,500 m by non-acclimatized individuals can induce a form of altitude sickness known as high altitude pulmonary edema (HAPE). Clinical symptoms of HAPE include reduced exercise capacity, tachycardia, dyspnea, cough, frothy sputum, chest tightness (Houston, 1960), crackles on exam and the hallmark bilateral patchy infiltrates observable via chest radiography (Vock et al., 1989). Symptoms typically present and worsen within 2 days of significant altitude exposure in the unacclimatized, particularly when physical exertion is involved. Though HAPE is rare at altitudes below 3,000 m (Maggiorini et al., 1990; Gabry et al., 2003), subclinical HAPE has been estimated to occur in up to 75% of individuals at 4,500 m elevation (Cremona et al., 2002)

HAPE progression is driven by pulmonary vasoconstriction that occurs with prolonged exposure to hypoxia. Pulmonary vascular pressures subsequently increase and can stress the delicate alveolar capillary barrier and induce mechanical stress failure. This pulmonary vascular response likely has multiple driving mechanisms, including increased plasma norepinephrine and sympathetic tone (Duplain et al., 1999), elevated endothelin-1 (Ali et al., 2012; Barker et al., 2016), and decreased levels of exhaled nitric oxide (Duplain et al., 2000; Busch et al., 2001) and nitric oxide metabolite concentrations in both the systemic circulation and bronchoalveolar lavage (BAL) fluid (Swenson et al., 2002; Berger et al., 2005; Bailey et al., 2010). Numerous studies have indicated that HAPE susceptible individuals have a reduced hypoxic ventilation response (HVR) accompanied by lower pO_2 levels and greater hypoxic pulmonary vasoconstriction than non-HAPE sensitives (Hyers et al., 1979; Matsuzawa et al., 1989; Hohenhaus et al., 1995; Bartsch et al., 2002), though a reduced HVR does not appear necessary for HAPE to develop (Selland et al., 1993). The mechanism of reduced HVR is multifactorial, but blunted central and peripheral chemoreceptor sensitivity likely plays a central role (Albert and Swenson, 2014).

Although there is ample evidence of the impact of hypoxia on chemoreceptor reflex, HVR and HAPE, the impact of hypercapnia is less clear. While it has been reported that HAPE-susceptible individuals demonstrate reduced sensitivity to CO_2 (Mathew et al., 1983), the effect of chronic CO_2 exposure on HAPE susceptibility has not been investigated. It is also widely acknowledged that acute exercise exacerbates HAPE symptoms however the role of chronic exercise training in HAPE development is unclear. Exercise training increases cardiac output, which may enhance the heterogeneous pulmonary capillary pressures and leakage induced by hypoxia. Indeed, increased pulmonary fluid and BAL solute concentrations have been confirmed in conditioned endurance athletes after hypoxic exercise (Eldridge et al., 2006), but overall the data is very limited. This study examines the effect of chronic intermittent CO_2 exposure, with and without concomitant exercise training, on the development of hypobaric hypoxia (HH) induced pulmonary edema in a rat model. We hypothesized that chronic CO_2 exposure would result in an increased incidence and severity of HAPE, and that this effect would be exacerbated by exercise training.

MATERIALS AND METHODS

Animals

All experiments were reviewed and approved by the Walter Reed Army Institute of Research/Naval Medical Research Center Institutional Animal Care and Use Committee in compliance with DoDI 3216.01 and SECNAVINST 3900.38C and all applicable Federal regulations governing the protection of animals in research. The facility is AAALAC accredited, and all animals were maintained under the surveillance of licensed veterinarians. Eight to ten week old male Wistar rats (Charles River Laboratories) were pair-housed at the animal care facility and maintained on a 12 h light/dark cycle and provided standard rodent chow (Harlan Teklad 8604) and water *ad libitum*. Animals were quarantined for 1 week (as per institutional policy) before being randomly assigned to one of 5 groups, $N = 8$ per group (**Table 1**); (1) sham (no HH, no CO_2, no exercise), (2) sedentary animals exposed to room air only, (3) sedentary animals exposed to a custom 3.5% CO_2 gas mix, (4) exercised animals exposed to room air, (5) exercised animals exposed to a 3.5% CO_2 mix. A separate cohort of animals, $N = 8$/group, was utilized for all CO_2 reactivity experiments.

CO_2 Exposure and Exercise Training

A 3.5% CO_2 level was chosen as the target exposure level with consideration of the following; (1) the US Occupational Safety and Health Administration maximum short-term exposure limit for CO_2 in humans is 3%, (2) 3–4% CO_2 is noticeable by human subjects and induces moderate respiratory stimulation, (3) one treatment group would be receiving CO_2 simultaneously with exercise. For the exercise groups, 3–5 short familiarization runs were performed prior to beginning the 1 month training period in order to identify animals with poor treadmill running compliance. Approximately one in eight animals was removed from the study during the familiarization period due to failure to keep up a steady running pace, repeatedly falling back and touching the end plate (set to deliver a very mild electrical shock), or refusing to move off of the end plate altogether, on two or more occasions. Treadmill exercise training was conducted at 15 m/min, 10% grade, for 1 h/day, 5 days/week for 4 weeks on a metabolic modular treadmill (Columbus Instruments, Columbus

TABLE 1 | Treatment groups.

Group	HH	CO_2	Exercise
(1) Sham	–	–	–
(2) Sed-Air	+	–	–
(3) Sed-CO_2	+	+	–
(4) Ex-Air	+	–	+
(5) Ex-CO_2	+	+	+

HH, hypobaric hypoxia.

OH). The treadmill lanes were set up to an air-tight configuration and either room air or a custom mixture (3.5% CO_2, 20% O_2, balance N2) was supplied at a rate of 4 L/min. The 4 L/min flow rate was sufficient to maintain CO_2 and O_2 levels within each treadmill chamber at 3.5 and 20%, respectively, throughout the daily training period (9600-A1BTP O_2/CO_2 Analyzer, Alpha Omega Instruments, Lincoln, RI). In non-exercising groups the animals were placed on an inactive treadmill ventilated with either room air or the CO_2 mix for 1 h/day.

Hypobaric Hypoxia (HH)

Custom-built methylacrylic cylinders measuring 38 cm in length by 20 cm in diameter were constructed in house (**Figure 1**). Evacuation of the chambers was driven by a GAST 6066 vacuum pump (GAST Manufacturing, Benton Harbor MI) through a side port. Fresh air was supplied at a rate of 2–2.5 L/min from compressed air banks; this flow rate was sufficient to prevent any buildup of CO_2 (9600-A1BTP O_2/CO_2 Analyzer, Alpha Omega Instruments, Lincoln, RI). Chamber temperatures during operation did not differ significantly from the ambient room temperature (23–26°C). Chambers were furnished with rodent chow, water and a hide box for each animal to reduce overall stress. An atmospheric pressure equivalent to 25,000 ft of altitude (282.0 torr, CPA2501 digital air indicator, Mensor, TX) was chosen as the target for HH exposure. We arrived at this value after extensive model development testing revealed that this pressure reliably induced a significant increase in mean lung wet/dry weight ratios, whereas greater atmospheric pressures did not reliably increase wet/dry ratios after 24 h (data not shown). Longer duration exposures were not employed due to extreme dehydration (animals refused fluids during the exposures), and further reduced atmospheric pressures dramatically increased mortality. During all experiments the chambers were de-pressurized/re-pressurized at an equivalent rate of 1,000 ft/min. Intake/outtake valves were adjusted to maintain the targeted altitude equivalent of 25,000 ft ± 500 ft at all times. After 24 h, chambers were re-pressurized (1,000 ft/min) and animals were euthanized by overdose of a sodium pentobarbital solution (150 mg/kg, IP) upon return to sea level. Sham group animals were placed in the hypobaric chambers for 24 h with air flow of 2–2.5 L/min, but the chambers were not subjected to vacuum and remained at ambient room pressures.

Vascular CO_2 Reactivity

Cerebral blood flow (CBF) following acute exposure to CO_2 was assessed after completing the 4-week training program via rheoencephalography (REG) as described (Ainslie and Duffin, 2009). Animals were anesthetized via urethane (1,000 mg/kg, IP) and electrodes were prepared and placed as previously described (Bodo et al., 2005). After electrode positioning baseline REG readings were recorded. A 12% CO_2/20% O_2 gas mixture was then supplied for 30 s, followed by a 5 min recovery period on room air. The CO_2 pulse was repeated a second time, and changes in REG amplitude were averaged for each animal.

Lung Tissue Preparation and Bronchoalveolar Lavage (BAL)

Tracheal cannulas were placed and tied in and lungs were removed en bloc within 10 min of returning to ambient room pressure. A small portion of each right lobe was flash frozen in liquid N_2 for later gene expression analysis, while the majority was weighed, dried at 55°C for 72 h, and weighed again to determine the wet to dry weight ratio. BAL samples were obtained by gently infusing 1 ml of PBS into the left lung a total of 3 times, pooled, and stored on ice. Portions of each

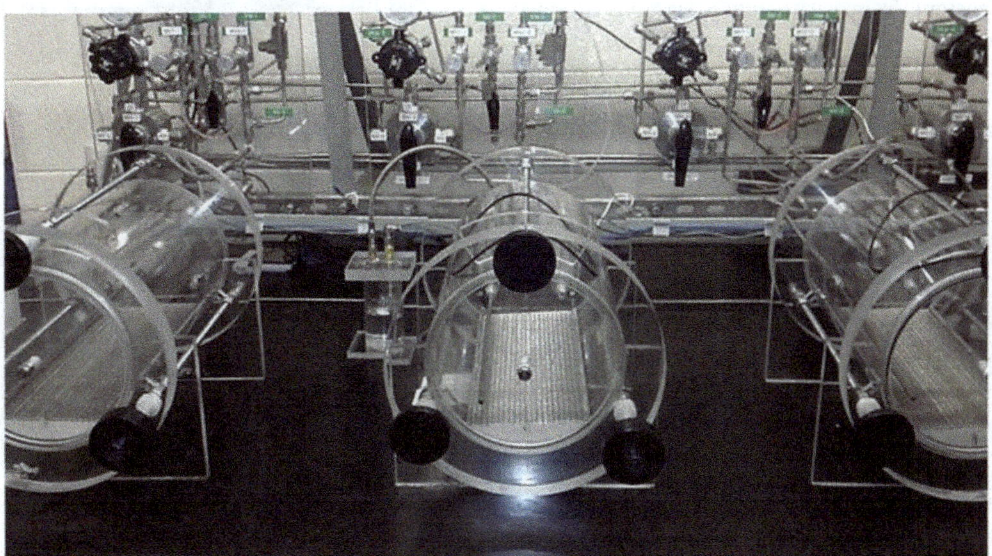

FIGURE 1 | Hypobaric chambers.

left lobe were preserved in a 10% formalin solution, sectioned 5 μm thick at equidistant points using a microtome and tissue block, hematoxylin/eosin stained, and examined by a board certified veterinary pathologist for evidence of fibrin thrombi, edema, endothelial damage, cellular infiltrates, thickening of the alveolar septum, hemorrhage or necrosis. Tissues were assigned quantitative values for each category on a 0–3 scoring system; 0 = no significant lesions, 1 = ≤ 20% of tissue affected, 2 = 20–50% of tissue affected, 3 = ≥ 50% of tissue affected. To ensure accuracy in scoring, 5 individual sections per animal were examined. Lavage fluid was spun at 1,500 g for 5 min, and the resulting pellets were then re-suspended in 1 ml of ice-cold PBS and immediately analyzed for cell type (Advia 120 Hematology System, Siemens Healthcare, Tarrytown, NJ). The supernatant was analyzed for lactate dehydrogenase activity and total protein content (Pierce BCA Protein Assay, Thermo Scientific, Rockford, IL).

Lung Vascular Permeability

Lung vascular permeability was examined *in vivo* after exposure to HH or normobaric conditions for 24 h. Sodium fluorescein dye (5 ml/kg, 2% solution; F6377-500G; Sigma-Aldrich, St. Louis, MO) was injected through the tail vein in a separate cohort of rats immediately after normobaric or hypobaric exposure. Thirty minutes after fluorescein injection rats were anesthetized with a ketamine/xylazine cocktail (80 and 10 mg/kg, respectively, IP) and transcardially perfused with PBS to remove the fluorescent tracer prior to harvesting the lungs. Lungs were rinsed with cold saline and homogenized with 2 ml of PBS. After homogenization, 2 ml of 50% TCA solution was added and the samples were vortexed to mix for 30 s to precipitate proteins in the lung samples. The resultant sample solution was cooled at 4°C for 30 min and covered to ensure no light exposure to the sample. Upon completion of cooling the samples were centrifuged for 10 min at 3,300 × g in 4°C. One mL of supernatant from each sample was placed into a 1.5 ml microcentrifuge tube and centrifuge at 16,000 × g at 4°C for 10 min. 200 ul of supernatant from each sample was added to a 96-well microplate along with 12 standards and read via spectrofluorometer according to manufacturer directions. Results are expressed as relative fluorescence units per liter.

Analysis

All data are expressed as means ± SEM and analyzed using GraphPad Prism (GraphPad Software, La Jolla, CA). Two-way ANOVA (sedentary/exercised X air/CO_2) was used to analyze for main effect and interactions between factors for each dependent variable. Tukey's *post-hoc* test with multiplicity adjusted *P*-value was used for pairwise comparisons. The sham group was not included in ANOVA as comparisons of sham vs. HH with CO_2/exercise trained groups were not of interest. Instead, unpaired *t*-tests were used to determine the effects of HH (sham vs. sed-air only) on each dependent variable. Statistical significance was accepted at $P \leq 0.05$.

RESULTS

Rat HH Induces Pulmonary Edema

HH exposed animals exhibited signs of pulmonary injury consistent with HAPE. Lung wet-to-dry weight ratios in sed-air animals increased 15% over sham animals ($P = 0.014$; **Figure 2**). Pulmonary vascular permeability in the sed-air group, assessed by sodium fluorescein dye leakage, was increased 190% over sham ($P < 0.001$). Total protein content, white blood cell concentration, and platelet concentration in BAL fluid were significantly increased by HH (**Table 2**), while there was no change in lactate dehydrogenase activity in the BAL fluid, and no red blood cells were detected in either group. Histological examination revealed no evidence of gross pulmonary pathology.

Exercise Training Attenuates CO_2-Induced Increases in CBF

Exposure to a 30 s, 12% CO_2 pulse increased REG amplitude by 343% ± 63.9, 185% ± 33, 161% ± 45, and 100% ± 28, in sed-air, sed-CO_2, ex-air, and ex-CO_2 groups, respectively (**Figure 3**). Daily CO_2 exposure (sed-CO_2) resulted in an apparent reduction

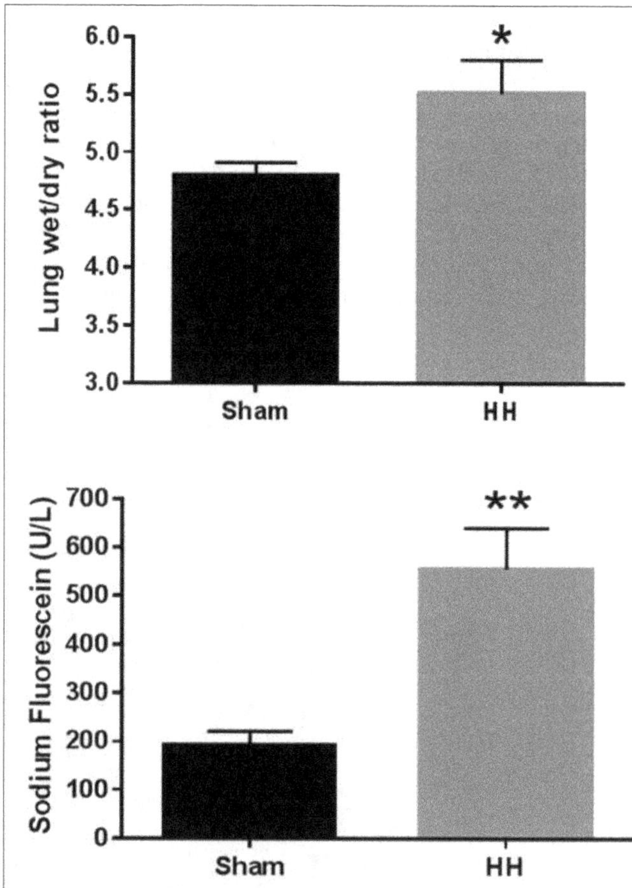

FIGURE 2 | Effects of HH on pulmonary fluid accumulation (**A**, top) and pulmonary vascular permeability (**B**, bottom). Animals were exposed to atmospheric pressure equivalent to 25,000 ft elevation or ambient pressure for 24 h. *$P < 0.05$, **$P < 0.001$. $N = 8$ per group.

TABLE 2 | Hypobaric hypoxia exposure vs. sham control.

	Sham	Sed-air	Sed-CO_2	Ex-air	Ex-CO_2
MASS					
Pre	391 ± 8 g	464 ± 17 g	458 ± 15 g	464 ± 17 g	464 ± 17 g
Post	375 ± 7 g	423 ± 16 g	420 ± 14 g	423 ± 16 g	423 ± 16 g
Δ	16	41	37	37	36
% change	(−4.3%)	(−8.9%)^{**a}	(−8.0%)	(−9.2%)	(−9.2%)
BAL					
Protein (μg/ml)	114 ± 14	$222 \pm 33^{**a}$	171 ± 22	151 ± 14	186 ± 21
LDH (U/L)	261 ± 13	305 ± 31	269 ± 29	274 ± 29	274 ± 26
Platelet (1 × 106^3/uL)	6.0 ± 0.6	$16.4 \pm 2.3^{**a}$	11.8 ± 1.3	$8.8 \pm 1.1^{*b}$	11.8 ± 1.2
WBC (1 × 10^3/uL)	0.68 ± 0.07	$1.16 \pm 0.26^{*a}$	0.79 ± 0.09	$0.47 \pm 0.07^{*b}$	0.69 ± 0.10
RBC	ND	ND	ND	ND	ND

*ND, not detected, *$P \leq 0.05$, **$P \leq 0.001$, in compares on to [a]sham, [b]sed-air. Hypobaric hypoxia groups are compared to each other; Sham is compared to sed-air group only.*

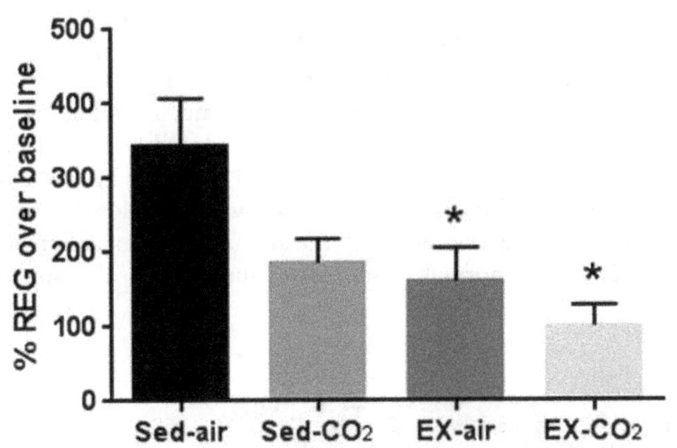

FIGURE 3 | Changes in cerebral blood flow after acute exposure to 12% CO_2. Rheoencephalogram amplitude after acute CO_2 exposure was compared to baseline recordings on room air. *Indicates significant difference ($P < 0.05$) from sedentary-air group. Sed-air ($N = 6$), sed-CO_2 ($N = 8$), ex-air ($N = 6$), ex-CO_2 ($N = 7$).

in the CO_2 pulse-induced REG increase but this effect did not reach statistical significance ($P = 0.062$), while exercise alone (ex-air) and exercise w/CO_2 (ex-CO_2) attenuated the CO_2-pulse induced REG increase by 53% ($P = 0.038$) and 71% ($P = 0.003$) vs. sed-air, respectively. REG values in the sed-CO_2, ex-air, and ex-CO_2 groups were not significantly different from each other and there was no interactive effect. One animal in the ex-air group was removed from the study due to a foot injury that precluded treadmill running, and two animals in the sed-air and one animal from the ex-CO_2 group died due to complications from anesthesia and/or REG electrode placement.

CO_2 and Exercise Training Do Not Affect the Incidence or Severity of HH-Induced Pulmonary Edema

To assess the effects of chronic exercise and CO_2 exposure on the development of HAPE in rodents, we exposed each of the four groups to HH equivalent to 25,000 ft of altitude for 24 h. Though the lung tissues were edematous in comparison to non-altitude exposed tissues, exercise and CO_2 exposure had no effect on between group wet-to-dry weight ratios (**Figure 4**). BAL analysis revealed no difference in total protein content or LDH activity between any of the groups however the ex-air group did have decreased platelet and total white blood cell concentrations in the BAL fluid (**Table 2**). Upon histological examination the tissues from each group were indistinguishable and relatively unremarkable, showing minimal signs of cellular infiltrates, septal thickening, hemorrhage, or necrosis (**Figure 5**).

DISCUSSION

The primary aim of this study was to determine how chronic intermittent CO_2 exposure may affect HAPE susceptibility in rats. HAPE development is largely dependent upon an inappropriately high level of pulmonary vascular constriction concurrent with exposure to hypoxia. Repeated hypoxic exposures appear to alter the chemoreceptor reflex (Berkenbosch et al., 1992; Mahamed and Duffin, 2001), and we hypothesized that chronic intermittent CO_2 exposure would also affect chemoreceptor sensitivity, exacerbate the pulmonary vasoconstriction effect of hypoxia, and worsen the symptoms and severity of HAPE. We also hypothesized that chronic CO_2 would reduce HVR, further exacerbating HAPE development. As most individuals acutely exposed to altitude are also performing relatively strenuous exercise (mountaineers, extreme sport athletes, military personnel, etc.) an exercise component was included to assess the interaction of chronic intermittent CO_2 and cardiovascular conditioning on HAPE susceptibility. The results presented here do not support our hypotheses, but do include some interesting findings.

Our HAPE model successfully induced pulmonary edema where previously published efforts to develop rat models of HAPE have met with mixed success. The methodology and exposure protocols have varied considerably, and while some studies have reported significant changes in wet-to-dry weight ratios after various altitude exposure profiles (Shukla et al., 2011; Lee et al., 2013), others did not demonstrate any differences in wet/dry ratio (Omura et al., 2000; Berg et al., 2004), used other methods to identify and quantify pulmonary edema (Li et al., 2011; Lin et al., 2011), or used very severe exposure protocols to induce pulmonary edema (Bai et al., 2010). Though our model was generally well tolerated the animals were lethargic, did not consume food or water during the exposure, and lost a significant amount of bodyweight (see **Table 2**). Despite a robust HAPE model however, exercise training and chronic intermittent hypercapnia did not affect HH-induced pulmonary edema. It is possible that simulated altitude of 25,000 ft for 24 h (greater than what most humans are likely to experience) was sufficient to elicit a maximal level of pulmonary vascular stress and that any effects of hypercapnia and exercise were masked or comparatively minor. Lower pressures and/or longer exposure times dramatically increased mortality and morbidity, which lends some support to this hypothesis. A more modest simulated altitude exposure may allow for more differentiation between the treatment groups, but our preliminary tests at higher atmospheric pressures were insufficient to reliably induce an appreciable level of pulmonary edema.

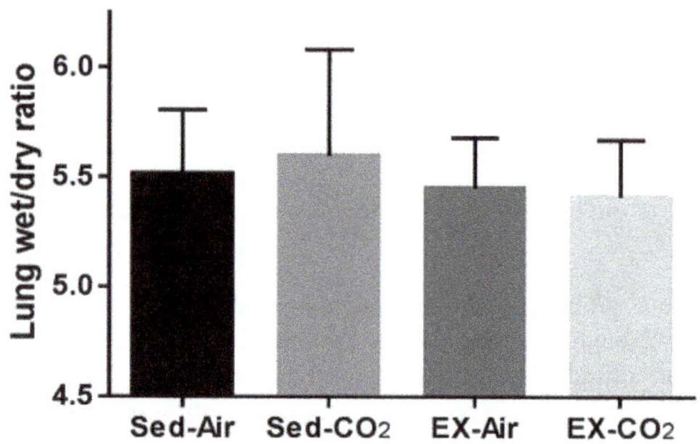

FIGURE 4 | Effects of HH on pulmonary fluid accumulation after 1 month of exercise and CO_2 exposure. Results are following exposure to atmospheric pressure equivalent to 25,000 ft elevation for 24 h. Sed-air (*N* = 8), sed-CO_2 (*N* = 8), ex-air (*N* = 6), ex-CO_2 (N = 8).

The level of bodyweight loss in HH-exposed animals was quite striking with most animals losing ~9% of total bodyweight in 24 h. Similar bodyweight losses have been reported in mice after exposure to ~14,000 ft of altitude for 3 days, however most of this was due to adipose lipolysis (Hannon and Rogers, 1975) which is unlikely to account for much of the losses here, and previous studies have reported reduced fluid intake in rodents exposed to altitude (Jones et al., 1981). The bodyweight reductions seen here were likely mostly due to loss of total body water, however preloading the animals with subcutaneous fluid (25–30 ml normal saline) and humidifying the supply

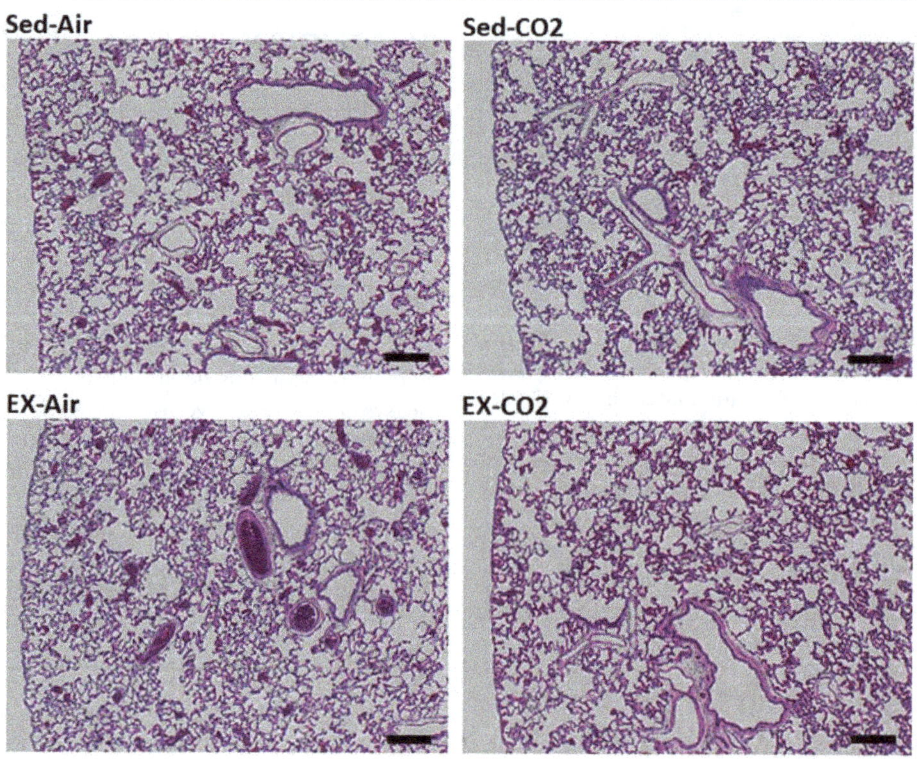

FIGURE 5 | Histology of HH exposed left lung lobe. Representative sections for each treatment group. Tissues were assigned quantitative pathology scores by a veterinary pathologist. Black bar = 200 μm.

air to ~60% during HH also had no discernible effect on bodyweight loss or lung wet/dry weight ratios in a separate cohort of animals. Sham animals that were not exposed to HH averaged 4.3% loss of total bodyweight over the same time period, indicating roughly half of the bodyweight reduction can be attributed to non-HH factors. Nevertheless the additional bodyweight reductions seen in HH-exposed animals may still have been sufficient to appreciably reduce plasma and interstitial fluid volume. As HAPE is driven by heterogeneously high pulmonary vascular pressures, such a reduction in total blood volume may have been sufficient to attenuate HH-induced increases in pulmonary vascular pressures. We did not perform direct measurements of pulmonary artery pressure or compare pre-post-total body water levels, so this possibility cannot be ruled out.

We hypothesized that chronic CO_2 exposure would suppress respiratory drive with HH and the study was designed with the intent to periodically measure respiration throughout the HH exposure period. Despite successful preliminary optimization runs, complications during the collection period made the respiratory data unreliable and it was not feasible to repeat the experiments. This is a significant limitation of the study and without this data we can only speculate, however the central and peripheral chemoreceptors responsible for respiratory regulation are highly sensitive to pCO_2 /H^+ (Nattie, 1999) and a stimulus that was sufficient to alter the CBF response to hypercapnia could be expected to also affect respiratory drive.

While direct measurement of pulmonary artery pressure via catheterization or echocardiogram would have been preferable, we used CBF as a general indicator of a systemic vascular response to CO_2, and not as a surrogate of pulmonary vascular reactivity. Exercise markedly suppressed CO_2-mediated increases in CBF, indicating that the vasculature was not responding to the increased pCO_2 levels with the degree of dilation seen in control animals. There are several potential mechanisms for this. An increase in circulating H^+ resulting from CO_2 metabolism would normally have a direct effect on peripheral vascular smooth muscle leading to vessel dilation (Kontos et al., 1977), but chronic exercise and CO_2 exposure may have desensitized the vasculature to elevated H^+ and disrupted normal cerebrovascular autoregulation. Alternatively, CO_2 and H^+ can induce formation of reactive oxygen and reactive nitrogen species and may influence brainstem mediated adaptations to hypercapnia and hypoxia (Dean, 2010). Though both cerebral and pulmonary tissues demonstrate a high degree of blood flow autoregulation, local responses to hypoxia are quite different and it is possible this extends to hypercapnia as well. Further investigations comparing vascular autoregulation in the brain vs. lung would be informative. Our findings may also be of interest in the context of High Altitude Cerebral Edema, which was not studied here.

CONCLUSION

Chronic intermittent CO_2 exposure and exercise training do not affect the incidence of HAPE in rats, but exercise training does attenuate CO_2 induced increases in CBF.

AUTHOR CONTRIBUTIONS

RS, AH, and RM were responsible for study design and conceptualization. RS and JS collected and analyzed the data. RS compiled the initial manuscript. RS, JS, AH, and RM revised the manuscript and approved the submitted version.

FUNDING

This work was supported by the Office of Naval Research work unit# 0602236N.0000.000.A1509.

ACKNOWLEDGMENTS

The authors are grateful to Amber Zhou, Eve Laurent, William Porter, William Hickman, Austin Headley, and Michael Bodo for their technical assistance.

REFERENCES

Ainslie, P. N., and Duffin, J. (2009). Integration of cerebrovascular CO_2 reactivity and chemoreflex control of breathing: mechanisms of regulation, measurement, and interpretation. *Am. J. Physiol. Regul. Integr. Comp. Physiol.* 296, R1473–R1495. doi: 10.1152/ajpregu.91008.2008

Albert, T. J., and Swenson, E. R. (2014). Peripheral chemoreceptor responsiveness and hypoxic pulmonary vasoconstriction in humans. *High Alt. Med. Biol.* 15, 15–20. doi: 10.1089/ham.2013.1072

Ali, Z., Mishra, A., Kumar, R., Alam, P., Pandey, P., Ram, R., et al. (2012). Interactions among vascular-tone modulators contribute to high altitude pulmonary edema and augmented vasoreactivity in highlanders. *PLoS ONE* 7:e44049. doi: 10.1371/journal.pone.0044049

Bai, C., She, J., Goolaerts, A., Song, Y., Shen, C., Shen, J., et al. (2010). Stress failure plays a major role in the development of high-altitude pulmonary oedema in rats. *Eur. Respir. J.* 35, 584–591. doi: 10.1183/09031936.00001709

Bailey, D. M., Dehnert, C., Luks, A. M., Menold, E., Castell, C., Schendler, G., et al. (2010). High-altitude pulmonary hypertension is associated with a free radical-mediated reduction in pulmonary nitric oxide bioavailability. *J. Physiol.* 588(Pt 23), 4837–4847. doi: 10.1113/jphysiol.2010.194704

Barker, K. R., Conroy, A. L., Hawkes, M., Murphy, H., Pandey, P., Kain, K. C., et al. (2016). Biomarkers of hypoxia, endothelial and circulatory dysfunction among climbers in Nepal with AMS and HAPE: a prospective case-control study. *J. Travel Med.* 23:taw005. doi: 10.1093/jtm/taw005

Bartsch, P., Swenson, E. R., Paul, A., Julg, B., and Hohenhaus, E. (2002). Hypoxic ventilatory response, ventilation, gas exchange, and fluid balance in acute mountain sickness. *High Alt. Med. Biol.* 3, 361–376. doi: 10.1089/15270290260512846

Berg, J. T., Ramanathan, S., and Swenson, E. R. (2004). Inhibitors of hypoxic pulmonary vasoconstriction prevent high-altitude pulmonary edema in rats. *Wilderness Environ. Med.* 15, 32–37. doi: 10.1580/1080-6032(2004)015[0032:IOHPVP]2.0.CO;2

Berger, M. M., Hesse, C., Dehnert, C., Siedler, H., Kleinbongard, P., Bardenheuer, H. J., et al. (2005). Hypoxia impairs systemic endothelial function in individuals prone to high-altitude pulmonary edema. *Am. J. Respir. Crit. Care Med.* 172, 763–767. doi: 10.1164/rccm.200504-654OC

Berkenbosch, A., Dahan, A., DeGoede, J., and Olievier, I. C. (1992). The ventilatory response to CO2 of the peripheral and central chemoreflex loop before and after sustained hypoxia in man. *J. Physiol. (Lond).* 456, 71–83. doi: 10.1113/jphysiol.1992.sp019327

Bodo, M., Pearce, F. J. Baranyi, L., and Armonda, R. A. (2005). Changes in the intracranial rheoencephalogram at lower limit of cerebral blood flow autoregulation. *Physiol. Meas.* 26, S1–S17. doi: 10.1088/0967-3334/26/2/001

Busch, T., Bärtsch, P., Pappert, D., Grünig, E., Hildebrandt, W., Elser, H., et al. (2001). Hypoxia decreases exhaled nitric oxide in mountaineers susceptible to high-altitude pulmonary edema. *Am. J. Respir. Crit. Care Med.* 163, 368–373. doi: 10.1164/ajrccm.163.2.2001134

Cremona, G., Asnaghi, R., Baderna, P., Brunetto, A., Brutsaert, T., Cavallaro, C., et al. (2002). Pulmonary extravascular fluid accumulation in recreational climbers: a prospective study. *Lancet* 359, 303–309. doi: 10.1016/S0140-6736(02)07496-2

Dean, J. B. (2010). Hypercapnia causes cellular oxidation and nitrosation in addition to acidosis: implications for CO2 chemoreceptor function and dysfunction. *J. Appl. Physiol. (1985).* 108, 1786–1795. doi: 10.1152/japplphysiol.01337.2009

Duplain, H., Sartori, C., Lepori, M., Egli, M., Allemann, Y., Nicod, P., et al. (2000). Exhaled nitric oxide in high-altitude pulmonary edema: role in the regulation of pulmonary vascular tone and evidence for a role against inflammation. *Am. J. Respir. Crit. Care Med.* 162, 221–224. doi: 10.1164/ajrccm.162.1.9908039

Duplain, H., Vollenweider, L., Delabays, A., Nicod, P., Bärtsch, P., Scherrer, U., et al. (1999). Augmented sympathetic activation during short-term hypoxia and high-altitude exposure in subjects susceptible to high-altitude pulmonary edema. *Circulation* 99, 1713–1718. doi: 10.1161/01.CIR.99.13.1713

Eldridge, M. W., Braun, R. K., Yoneda, K. Y., and Walby, W. F. (2006). Effects of altitude and exercise on pulmonary capillary integrity: evidence for subclinical high-altitude pulmonary edema. *J. Appl. Physiol. (1985).* 100, 972–980. doi: 10.1152/japplphysiol.01048.2005

Gabry, A. L., Ledoux, X., Mozziconacci, M., and Martin, C. (2003). High-altitude pulmonary edema at moderate altitude (< 2,400 m; 7,870 feet): a series of 52 patients. *Chest* 123, 49–53. doi: 10.1378/chest.123.1.49

Hannon, J. P., and Rogers, B. G. (1975). Body composition of mice following exposure to 4300 and 6100 meters. *Aviat. Space Environ. Med.* 46, 1232–1235.

Hohenhaus, E., Paul, A., McCullough, R. E., Kucherer, H., and Bartsch, P. (1995). Ventilatory and pulmonary vascular response to hypoxia and susceptibility to high altitude pulmonary oedema. *Eur. Respir. J.* 8, 1825–1833. doi: 10.1183/09031936.95.08111825

Houston, C. S. (1960). Acute pulmonary edema of high altitude. *N. Engl. J. Med.* 263, 478–480. doi: 10.1056/NEJM196009082631003

Hyers, T. M., Scoggin, C. H., Will, D. H., Grover, R. F., and Reeves, J. T. (1979). Accentuated hypoxemia at high altitude in subjects susceptible to high-altitude pulmonary edema. *J. Appl. Physiol. Respir. Environ. Exerc. Physiol.* 46, 41–46. doi: 10.1152/jappl.1979.46.1.41

Jones, R. M., Terhaard, C., Zullo, J., and Tenney, S. M. (1981). Mechanism of reduced water intake in rats at high altitude. *Am. J. Physiol.* 240, R187–R191. doi: 10.1152/ajpregu.1981.240.3.R187

Kontos, H. A., Raper, A. J., and, Patterson, J. L. (1977). Analysis of vasoactivity of local pH, PCO2 and bicarbonate on pial vessels. *Stroke* 8, 358–360. doi: 10.1161/01.STR.8.3.358

Lee, S. Y., Li, M. H., Shi, L. S., Chu, H., Ho, C. W., Chang, T. C., et al. (2013). Rhodiola crenulata extract alleviates hypoxic pulmonary edema in rats. *Evid. Based Complement. Alternat. Med.* 2013:718739. doi: 10.1155/2013/718739

Li, Z., Gao, C., Wang, Y., Liu, F., Ma, L., Deng, C., et al. (2011). Reducing pulmonary injury by hyperbaric oxygen preconditioning during simulated high altitude exposure in rats. *J. Trauma* 71, 673–679. doi: 10.1097/TA.0b013e3181f5b073

Lin, H. J., Wang, C. T., Niu, K. C., Gao, C., Li, Z., Lin, M. T., et al. (2011). Hypobaric hypoxia preconditioning attenuates acute lung injury during high-altitude exposure in rats via up-regulating heat-shock protein 70. *Clin. Sci.* 121, 223–231. doi: 10.1042/CS20100596

Maggiorini, M., Buhler, B., Walter, M., and Oelz, O. (1990). Prevalence of acute mountain sickness in the Swiss Alps. *BMJ* 301, 853–855. doi: 10.1136/bmj.301.6756.853

Mahamed, S., and Duffin, J. (2001). Repeated hypoxic exposures change respiratory chemoreflex control in humans. *J. Physiol.* 534(Pt 2), 595–603. doi: 10.1111/j.1469-7793.2001.00595.x

Mathew, L., Gopinathan, P. M., Purkayastha, S. S., Sen Gupta, J., and Nayar, H. S. (1983). Chemoreceptor sensitivity and maladaptation to high altitude in man. *Eur. J. Appl. Physiol. Occup. Physiol.* 51, 137–144. doi: 10.1007/BF00952546

Matsuzawa, Y., Fujimoto, K., Kobayashi, T., Namushi, N. R., Harada, K., Kohno, H., et al. (1989). Blunted hypoxic ventilatory drive in subjects susceptible to high-altitude pulmonary edema. *J. Appl. Physiol. (1985).* 66, 1152–1157.

Nattie, E. (1999). CO_2, brainstem chemoreceptors and breathing. *Prog. Neurobiol.* 59, 299–331. doi: 10.1016/S0301-0082(99)00008-8

Omura, A., Roy, R., and Jennings, T. (2000). Inhaled nitric oxide improves survival in the rat model of high-altitude pulmonary edema. *Wilderness Environ. Med.* 11, 251–256. doi: 10.1580/1080-6032(2000)011[0251:INOISI]2.3.CO;2

Selland, M. A., Stelzner, T. J., Stevens, T., Mazzeo, R. S., McCullough, R. E., Reeves, J. T., et al. (1993). Pulmonary function and hypoxic ventilatory response in subjects susceptible to high-altitude pulmonary edema. *Chest* 103, 111–116. doi: 10.1378/chest.103.1.111

Shukla, D., Saxena, S., Purushothaman, J., Shrivastava, K., Singh, M., Shukla, S., et al. (2011). Hypoxic preconditioning with cobalt ameliorates hypobaric hypoxia induced pulmonary edema in rat. *Eur. J. Pharmacol.* 656, 101–109. doi: 10.1016/j.ejphar.2011.01.038

Swenson, E. R., Maggiorini, M., Mongovin, S., Gibbs, J. S., Greve, I., Mairbäurl, H., et al. (2002). Pathogenesis of high-altitude pulmonary edema: inflammation is not an etiologic factor. *JAMA* 287, 2228–2235. doi: 10.1001/jama.287.17.2228

Vock, P., Fretz, C., Franciolli, M., and Bartsch, P. (1989). High-altitude pulmonary edema: findings at high-altitude chest radiography and physical examination. *Radiology* 170(3 Pt 1), 661–666. doi: 10.1148/radiology.170.3.2916019

3

Sensory Processing and Integration at the Carotid Body Tripartite Synapse: Neurotransmitter Functions and Effects of Chronic Hypoxia

*Erin M. Leonard, Shaima Salman and Colin A. Nurse**

Department of Biology, McMaster University, Hamilton, ON, Canada

***Correspondence:**
Colin A. Nurse
nursec@mcmaster.ca

Maintenance of homeostasis in the respiratory and cardiovascular systems depends on reflexes that are initiated at specialized peripheral chemoreceptors that sense changes in the chemical composition of arterial blood. In mammals, the bilaterally-paired carotid bodies (CBs) are the main peripheral chemoreceptor organs that are richly vascularized and are strategically located at the carotid bifurcation. The CBs contribute to the maintenance of O_2, CO_2/H^+, and glucose homeostasis and have attracted much clinical interest because hyperactivity in these organs is associated with several pathophysiological conditions including sleep apnea, obstructive lung disease, heart failure, hypertension, and diabetes. In response to a decrease in O_2 availability (hypoxia) and elevated CO_2/H^+ (acid hypercapnia), CB receptor type I (glomus) cells depolarize and release neurotransmitters that stimulate apposed chemoafferent nerve fibers. The central projections of those fibers in turn activate cardiorespiratory centers in the brainstem, leading to an increase in ventilation and sympathetic drive that helps restore blood PO_2 and protect vital organs, e.g., the brain. Significant progress has been made in understanding how neurochemicals released from type I cells such as ATP, adenosine, dopamine, 5-HT, ACh, and angiotensin II help shape the CB afferent discharge during both normal and pathophysiological conditions. However, type I cells typically occur in clusters and in addition to their sensory innervation are ensheathed by the processes of neighboring glial-like, sustentacular type II cells. This morphological arrangement is reminiscent of a “tripartite synapse” and emerging evidence suggests that paracrine stimulation of type II cells by a variety of CB neurochemicals may trigger the release of “gliotransmitters” such as ATP via pannexin-1 channels. Further, recent data suggest novel mechanisms by which dopamine, acting via D2 receptors (D2R), may inhibit action potential firing at petrosal nerve endings. This review will update current ideas concerning the presynaptic and postsynaptic mechanisms that underlie chemosensory processing in the CB. Paracrine signaling pathways will be highlighted, and particularly those that allow the glial-like type II cells to participate in the integrated sensory response during exposures to chemostimuli, including acute and chronic hypoxia.

Keywords: carotid body, chemoreceptor type I cells, glial-like type II cells, purinergic signaling, neurotransmitters, sensory transmission, petrosal neurons

INTRODUCTION

Oxygen (O_2) is essential to the survival of aerobic organisms that rely on oxidative phosphorylation for the production of ATP as a major energy source. Consequently, both water- and air-breathing vertebrates have evolved mechanisms for monitoring O_2 levels in the environmental water, pulmonary airways, and/or arterial blood. In conditions of O_2 deficiency (hypoxia), strategically-located sensors in the gills of water-breathers and peripheral chemoreceptor organs of air-breathers initiate compensatory respiratory and cardiovascular reflex responses so as to maintain homeostasis (Gonzalez et al., 1994; Cutz and Jackson, 1999; Milsom and Burleson, 2007; Kumar and Prabhakar, 2012). In mammals, the main peripheral chemoreceptor organs are the carotid bodies (CBs), which contain O_2- and CO_2/H^+-sensitive detectors known as glomus or type I cells (Gonzalez et al., 1994; Peers and Buckler, 1995; López-Barneo et al., 2016). While the chemoreceptive properties of the CB have been well established over much of the last century (Gonzalez et al., 2014), current views consider the CBs as general metabolic sensors capable of detecting not only the respiratory gases and blood acidity, but also blood glucose and circulating insulin levels (López-Barneo, 2003; Conde et al., 2014; Thompson et al., 2016).

The CBs are located bilaterally at the carotid bifurcation where they monitor blood O_2 just before it reaches the brain, an organ that is a critically sensitive to O_2 deprivation. In keeping with their role as circulatory chemical sensors, they are reputed to be the most richly vascularized organs in the body (Gonzalez et al., 1994). The gross morphology of the CB reveals a network of fenestrated capillaries that penetrate clusters of chemoreceptor type I cells which receive sensory innervation from the carotid sinus nerve (CSN) (McDonald, 1981). The type I cells share an intimate association with neighboring glial-like, sustentacular type II cells in a ratio of ~4:1 (McDonald, 1981; Kondo, 2002), and there is evidence of synapse-like specializations between these two cell types (Platero-Luengo et al., 2014). Thus, the CB chemoreceptor complex, consisting of clusters of receptor type I cells, type II glial cells, and the abutting sensory nerve terminals, displays the features of a "tripartite synapse" that provides the substrate for synaptic integration at many sites in the central nervous system (CNS) (Eroglu and Barres, 2010). During chemoexcitation, the CB output is relayed as an increase in action potential frequency in chemosensory fibers of the CSN whose cell bodies are located in the petrosal ganglia. These fibers terminate centrally in the nucleus tractus solitarius where they help control lung ventilation and sympathetic outflow to the cardiovascular system (Claps and Torrealba, 1988; Gonzalez et al., 1994; Kumar and Prabhakar, 2012).

Over the last ~30 years there have been numerous studies on the transduction mechanisms by which CB receptor type I cells sense a reduction in PO_2 (hypoxia) and an elevation in PCO_2/H^+ and how these signals are relayed to the brain via the CSN. On the presynaptic side, there is a consensus that acute hypoxia causes inhibition of background K^+ channels in type I cells, and this is a key step in chemotransduction leading to voltage-gated Ca^{2+} entry and neurotransmitter release (Buckler, 2015; López-Barneo et al., 2016). However, despite significant recent progress, the identity of the PO_2 sensor is still debatable though there is strong support for a role of the mitochondrial electron transport chain (Buckler, 2015; López-Barneo et al., 2016; Chang, 2017; Prabhakar and Peng, 2017; Rakoczy and Wyatt, 2017). On the postsynaptic side, there has been significant progress in elucidating the roles of several neurochemicals, especially the purines ATP and its metabolite adenosine, in shaping the afferent CSN discharge (Iturriaga and Alcayaga, 2004; Nurse, 2005, 2010; Conde et al., 2012a; Nurse and Piskuric, 2013). However, this task has become more challenging given the increasing number of neuroactive agents present in the CB, and the growing evidence that the glial-like type II cells may not be silent partners during sensory transmission (Tse et al., 2012; Nurse and Piskuric, 2013; Nurse, 2014). An understanding of the roles of these neurochemicals and the mechanisms underlying synapse integration in the CB is important given that alterations in CB sensitivity and CSN discharge are now linked to several cardiorespiratory abnormalities in humans (Kumar and Prabhakar, 2012; Iturriaga, 2017). For example during obstructive sleep apnea, a condition where patients are exposed to bouts of chronic intermittent hypoxia (CIH), CB chemosensitivity becomes exaggerated leading to long-term facilitation (LTF) of the sensory discharge and increased risk of hypertension (Prabhakar et al., 2015). Also, CB chemosensitivity is enhanced in chronic heart failure (CHF), leading to sympathetic hyperactivity and exacerbation of the disease progression (Schultz et al., 2015). In this article, we review the role of several neurotransmitters and neuromodulators in the integrative sensory response at the CB tripartite synapse. In particular, we consider the major transmitters involved in the interactions between type I cells and the sensory nerve ending during chemotransduction, as well as the contribution of paracrine signaling mechanisms to synaptic integration and crosstalk among type I cells, type II cells, and the sensory nerve endings. Finally, we consider how synaptic plasticity mechanisms during exposures to chronic sustained hypoxia might contribute to alterations in neurochemical signaling at the tripartite synapse.

SYNAPTIC TRANSMISSION BETWEEN CHEMORECEPTOR TYPE I CELLS AND SENSORY NERVE TERMINALS

During chemotransduction type I cells release neurotransmitters resulting in an increase in CSN action potential frequency. As discussed below, the main transmitters responsible for this postsynaptic excitatory response are likely ATP and adenosine; however, contributions from other CB transmitters including ACh, histamine, and 5-HT cannot be ignored and may well depend on developmental age, species under investigation, or the presence or absence of pathophysiological conditions (Zhong et al., 1999; Iturriaga and Alcayaga, 2004; Nurse, 2005, 2010; Lazarov et al., 2006; Del Rio et al., 2008; Conde et al., 2012a; Kumar and Prabhakar, 2012). Further, the magnitude of the CSN excitatory response appears to be blunted by the concurrent action of inhibitory neurotransmitters such as GABA and dopamine (Alcayaga et al., 1999; Iturriaga et al., 2009; Nurse, 2010). In the case of dopamine, it is possible that its release from activated afferent C fibers during chemoexcitation may lead to autocrine-paracrine stimulation of inhibitory D2 receptors (D2R) on nearby type I cells and/or afferent nerve terminals (Benot and Lopez-Barneo, 1990; Almaraz et al., 1993; Iturriaga et al., 2003).

Role of ATP and Postsynaptic P2X2/3 Receptors

The stimulatory effects of intracarotid administration of ATP on ventilation and CSN discharge have been known for some time (reviewed by Zapata, 2007). However, use of a co-culture model of rat type I cell clusters and juxtaposed petrosal neurons demonstrated that blockers of purinergic P2X2/3 receptors, i.e., suramin and PPADS, inhibited the postsynaptic response elicited by hypoxia and/or hypercapnia (Zhang et al., 2000; Prasad et al., 2001; Zhang and Nurse, 2004; Nurse and Piskuric, 2013). A central role of ATP acting via postsynaptic P2X2/3 receptors during chemoexcitation was confirmed by the following observations: (i) Chemosensitive petrosal neurons in co-culture expressed functional P2X2/3 receptors (Zhang et al., 2000); (ii) Immunoreactive P2X2 and P2X3 subunits were localized to petrosal terminals opposed to type I cells in CB tissue sections *in situ* (Zhang et al., 2000; Prasad et al., 2001); (iii) P2X2 knockout mice showed a markedly attenuated hypoxic ventilatory response (Rong et al., 2003); (iv) Acute hypoxia induced Ca^{2+}-dependent, vesicular ATP release from isolated whole CB, CB slices, and cultured CB cells (Buttigieg and Nurse, 2004; Conde et al., 2012a); (v) In intact CB-sinus nerve preparations *in vitro*, P2X2/3 and selective P2X3 receptor antagonists inhibited the CSN discharge evoked by hypoxia (He et al., 2006; Reyes et al., 2007; Niane et al., 2011); and (vi) In the co-culture model, the selective P2X receptor blocker PPADS inhibited the hypoxia-induced postsynaptic response in the petrosal neuron, but not the presynaptic receptor potential in type I cells (**Figures 1A1,A2**). Though most of the preceding data were obtained in rodent preparations, an excitatory postsynaptic role of ATP acting via ligand-gated receptor channels has also been observed in the cat CB (Iturriaga and Alcayaga, 2004; Reyes et al., 2007; Zapata, 2007).

Role of Adenosine and Postsynaptic A2a Receptors

The excitatory effects of exogenous adenosine on both ventilation and CSN discharge were first confirmed in the 1980's and appear to be species independent (McQueen and Ribeiro, 1983; Monteiro and Ribeiro, 1987; Conde et al., 2006, 2009). While presynaptic adenosine A2a and A2b receptors on type I cells are well described (see later), the excitatory effects of exogenous adenosine appear to be mainly postsynaptic, involving high affinity A2a receptors (A2aR) that are expressed in petrosal chemoafferent neurons (Gauda, 2002; Conde et al., 2006, 2009). During acute hypoxia and hypercapnia a significant fraction of the CSN sensory discharge is dependent on the stimulation of postsynaptic A2aR (Conde et al., 2006; Zhang et al., 2017). The extracellular adenosine level at the CB chemosensory synapse is generated via equilibrative nucleoside transporters (ENTs) in type I cells and/or breakdown of extracellular ATP by ectonucleotidases (Conde and Monteiro, 2004). More recently, molecular characterization and immunolocalization of surface-located nucleotidases in the rat CB have revealed the presence of

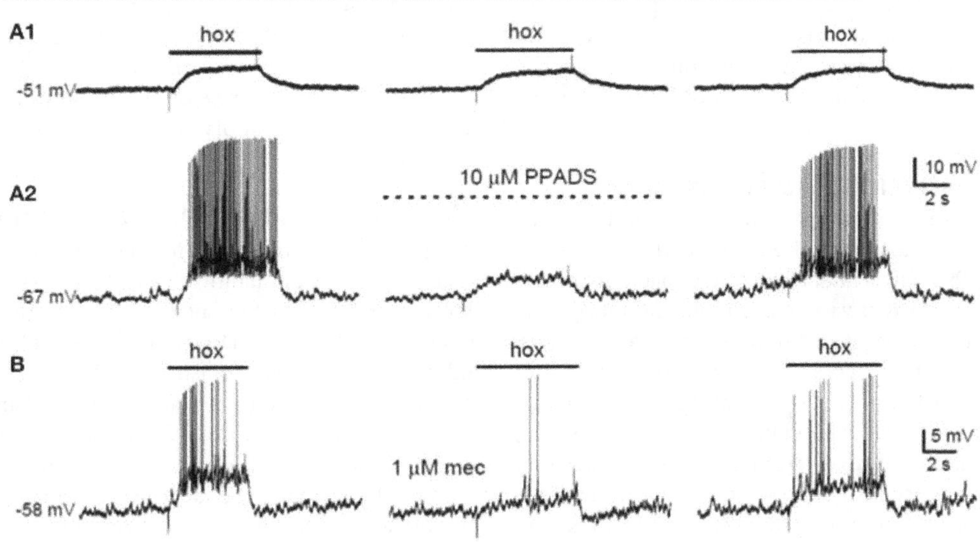

FIGURE 1 | Effects of purinergic and nicotinic receptor blockers on hypoxic chemotransmission in co-cultures. **(A)** Simultaneous recordings of membrane potential from a type I cell **(A1)** and a petrosal neuron **(A2)** in co-culture. The P2X2/3 receptor blocker PPADS (10 μM) reversibly suppressed the "postsynaptic" neuronal response **(A2)**, but had negligible effect on the "presynaptic" type I cell response **(A1)**. **(B)** The hypoxia (hox)-induced sensory discharge in a co-cultured petrosal neuron (left trace) was reversibly inhibited by the nicotinic cholinergic blocker mecamylamine (mec; 1 μM; middle trace). Data adapted from Nurse (2010).

nucleotidase triphosphate diphospho-hydrolase (NTPDase)2,3 and ecto-5′nucleotidase(ecto-5′Nt/CD73) in association with type I cell clusters (Salman et al., 2017). The NTPDase 2,3 pair efficiently hydrolyses ATP to AMP and ADP, while ecto-5′Nt hydrolyses AMP to adenosine (Zimmermann, 2000). Interestingly, in a recent study pharmacological inhibition of ecto-5′NT, but not ENTs, caused a reduction in basal and hypoxia-evoked CB sensory discharge, as well as in the hypoxic ventilatory response in adult rats (Holmes et al., 2017). These data suggest that the principal source of adenosine that contributes to the increase in CSN discharge during acute hypoxia is from the catabolism of extracellular ATP. However, in a previous study, pharmacological inhibition of ENT was found to increase adenosine release from rat CBs especially at high-intensity hypoxia, at least when adenosine deaminase was simultaneously inhibited (Conde et al., 2012a). Thus, the relative contributions of ecto-5′Nt and ENT to extracellular adenosine during acute hypoxia may well depend on the PO_2 level. A plausible mechanism by which adenosine, acting via postsynaptic A2aR, increases excitability in petrosal afferent neurons was recently proposed (Zhang et al., 2017). In that study on rat CB co-cultures, adenosine caused a depolarizing shift in the voltage dependence of activation of a hyperpolarization-activated cyclic nucleotide gated cation current *I*h in chemosensory neurons. Consistent with the involvement of high affinity A2aR, the effect was mediated by nanomolar concentrations of adenosine and was reversibly inhibited by the selective A2aR blocker, SCH58261. In concert with the known effects of the *I*h current in regulating firing frequency in a variety of cell types (Biel et al., 2009), adenosine was also shown to increase membrane excitability and action potential frequency in identified chemosensory petrosal neurons in co-culture (Zhang et al., 2017). Moreover, HCN4 immunoreactive subunits were localized to chemosensory, tyrosine hydroxylase (TH)-positive petrosal neurons in tissue sections of rat petrosal ganglia *in situ* (Zhang et al., 2017); HCN4 subunits are known to contribute to *I*h channel currents and to increases in action potential frequency through elevations in intracellular cAMP in different cell types (Biel et al., 2009).

Role of ACh and Nicotinic Receptors

The role of ACh as a major excitatory neurotransmitter in the CB has had a controversial history (Eyzaguirre and Zapata, 1984; Nurse and Zhang, 1999; Fitzgerald, 2000; Iturriaga and Alcayaga, 2004). There is no doubt that various nicotinic and muscarinic ACh receptors (AChR) are expressed in the CB of several species, though whether or not type I cells synthesize and store ACh in all cases is controversial (Gauda, 2002; Iturriaga and Alcayaga, 2004; Zhang and Nurse, 2004; Shirahata et al., 2007). However, hypoxia-induced release of ACh from intact CBs has been detected in several species including cats, rabbits, and humans (Fitzgerald, 2000; Shirahata et al., 2007; Zapata, 2007; Kåhlin et al., 2014). Moreover, in the co-culture model of the rat CB a combination of nicotinic and purinergic blockers were required to inhibit most of the hypoxia-induced postsynaptic response (Zhang et al., 2000); often, only partial inhibition was seen when either blocker was present alone (**Figures 1A2,B**). In concert with these results, systemic blockade of both nicotinic and purinergic P2X receptors inhibited ventilation in newborn rats (Niane et al., 2012). Additional evidence supporting ACh as an important CB excitatory neurotransmitter was obtained in the following studies: (i) functional nicotinic AChR were present on >65% of isolated rat petrosal neurons (Zhong and Nurse, 1997) and in the majority of petrosal neurons that were functionally connected to the cat CB (Varas et al., 2003; Iturriaga and Alcayaga, 2004); (ii) in the isolated rat and cat CB-sinus nerve preparations *in vitro* nicotinic AChR blockers inhibited the hypoxia-induced chemosensory discharge (Iturriaga and Alcayaga, 2004; He et al., 2005; Zapata, 2007; Niane et al., 2009); and (iii) consistent with a postsynaptic role for ACh, α7 nAChR immunoreactivity has been localized to nerve endings surrounding type I clusters in rat and cat CB *in situ* (Shirahata et al., 2007; Niane et al., 2009), and there is electrophysiological evidence consistent with the presence of functional α7 nAChR in cat petrosal neurons (Alcayaga et al., 2007).

Role of Histamine and H1-3 Receptors

Histamine is synthesized, stored (in considerably higher amounts than dopamine), and released from the CB during acute hypoxia (Koerner et al., 2004; Del Rio et al., 2008). In addition, histamine receptors (H1, H2, H3) have been localized to both the CB and petrosal ganglion (Lazarov et al., 2006). Application of H1R and H3R agonists to the rat CB had a mild stimulatory effect on ventilatory output (Lazarov et al., 2006). In the cat, H1R antagonists reduced, whereas H3R antagonists enhanced, the excitatory effect of histamine on the sinus nerve discharge (Del Rio et al., 2008). In the latter study, though histamine increased sinus nerve discharge when applied to both the isolated superfused and perfused CB *in vitro*, it had no effect on the isolated petrosal ganglion discharge. This suggests a direct effect of histamine on the CB parenchymal cells and/or a selective effect on petrosal terminals that is not replicated at the soma. In isolated rat type I cells, H3R agonists inhibited the rise in Ca^{2+} elicited by muscarinic agonists (Thompson et al., 2010). Further work is required to clarify the role of histamine and its receptors in the CB though both excitatory and inhibitory pathways appear to be present.

Role of Inhibitory Neurotransmitters

The preceding sections have focused on postsynaptic interactions that are predominantly excitatory. However, inhibitory mechanisms appear to play an important role in regulating the CB sensory discharge. Dopamine is probably the best-described inhibitory CB neurotransmitter (Benot and Lopez-Barneo, 1990), yet it was only recently that a plausible postsynaptic mechanism was proposed (Zhang et al., 2017). In the latter study on rat CB co-cultures, dopamine caused a hyperpolarizing shift in the voltage dependence of I_h activation and a decrease in membrane excitability in chemosensory petrosal neurons. This effect was opposite to that discussed above for adenosine, where the voltage dependence of I_h activation was shifted in the depolarizing direction and resulted in increased membrane excitability. The effect of dopamine on I_h was prevented during co-incubation with the selective D2 receptor (D2R) antagonist, sulpiride (Zhang et al., 2017). These data suggest that stimulation of D2R on chemosensory petrosal neurons and their terminals causes a decrease in intracellular cAMP leading to inhibition of the cAMP-gated I_h channels containing HCN4 subunits (Zhang et al., 2017). In this scenario, the source of dopamine is predominantly from nearby type I cells though it may include terminals of excited catecholaminergic C fibers of petrosal CB chemoafferents (Almaraz et al., 1993; Iturriaga et al., 2003).

There is also evidence that GABA, acting via ionotropic GABA(A) receptors on petrosal afferent terminals, can inhibit the chemosensory discharge by a shunting mechanism which diminishes the depolarizing action of excitatory inputs (Zhang et al., 2009). GABA is synthesized and stored in type I cells and its release during chemoexcitation has been inferred since pharmacological blockade of GABA(A) receptors using bicuculline facilitates the hypoxia-induced sensory discharge in cat and rat carotid body (Igarashi et al., 2009; Zhang et al., 2009). Moreover benzodiazepines, which enhance GABA(A) receptor activity, suppress ventilation in cats and inhibit the CB chemosensory discharge evoked by acute hypoxia (Igarashi et al., 2009).

AUTOCRINE-PARACRINE INTERACTIONS INVOLVING CHEMORECEPTOR TYPE I CELLS AND GLIAL-LIKE TYPE II CELLS

As discussed above, purinergic transmission from CB type I cells to the sensory nerve endings involves fast-acting ionotropic P2X receptors and slow-acting metabotropic adenosine P1 receptors. However, both autocrine and paracrine signaling mechanisms mediated mainly via metabotropic receptors on type I and glial-like type II cells can further fine-tune the synaptic neurotransmitter pool near the sensory nerve endings. In addition to direct synaptic interactions between type I cells and sensory nerve terminal the following cell- cell interactions are possible: (i) type I cell to type I cell; (ii) type I cell to type II cell; (iii) type II cell to type I cell; and (iv) direct communication between type II cells and the sensory nerve ending. Electrical coupling between adjacent type I cells, and between type I cells and the sensory nerve ending, is also possible as reviewed elsewhere (Eyzaguirre, 2007).

Autocrine-Paracrine Signaling Among Neighboring Type I Cells

These pathways may involve either negative or positive feedback mechanisms. Perhaps the best-studied pathway involves the negative feedback role of dopamine acting on inhibitory D2R on the same or neighboring type I cells. For example, selective blockade of D2R using domperidone or haloperidol caused a concentration dependent enhancement of basal, high K^+-, and hypoxia-evoked catecholamine release from intact rat CB (Conde et al., 2008). The effect is likely due to a negative feedback inhibition of intracellular Ca^{2+} signaling because dopamine was found to inhibit L-type Ca^{2+} currents in isolated type I cells (Benot and Lopez-Barneo, 1990), whereas selective D2R agonists inhibited the hypoxia-evoked rise in intracellular Ca^{2+} (Carroll et al., 2005). In addition to DA, there is evidence that ATP and GABA may also inhibit type I cell function via negative feedback mechanisms. For example, ATP was found to inhibit the hypoxia-induced rise in intracellular Ca^{2+} in type I cells via metabotropic P2Y1R (Xu et al., 2005) or P2Y12R (Carroll et al., 2012). Because ADP is also an effective ligand for both these receptors, and P2Y12Rs are highly expressed in type I cells (Zhou et al., 2016), it is possible that degradation of ATP by the surface-located nucleotidases NTPDase2,3 (Salman et al., 2017), generates sufficient ADP to further inhibit type I cells. Under normoxic conditions, NTPDase2 mRNA expression in the CB is much higher than NTPDase3 mRNA (Salman et al., 2017). Assuming parallel changes in the corresponding proteins, this expression pattern favors elevated ADP levels since NTPDase2 is relatively ineffective at hydrolyzing ADP to AMP (Zimmermann, 2000). GABA acting on autocrine-paracrine GABA(B) receptors was reported to inhibit the hypoxia-evoked receptor potential in type I cells (Fearon et al., 2003). In the latter study, the signaling mechanism involved activation of a resting TASK-like K^+ conductance via a pertussis toxin- sensitive and PKA-dependent pathway.

The type I cell response to chemostimuli such as acute hypoxia may also be modified by positive feedback mechanisms. For example, the ATP metabolite adenosine has been shown to enhance intracellular Ca^{2+} signaling in type I cells by triggering membrane depolarization and voltage-gated Ca^{2+} entry via adenylate cyclase-PKA dependent inhibition of background TASK channels (Xu et al., 2006). Also, there is evidence that 5-HT acting via 5-HT2a receptors (5-HT2aR) can enhance the hypoxia-evoked receptor potential in type I cells via an autocrine-paracrine positive feedback mechanism involving PKC-mediated inhibition of resting and Ca^{2+}-dependent K^+ conductances (Zhang et al., 2003).

ATP Release From Type 1 Cells During Chemostimulation Can Lead to Intracellular Ca^{2+} Elevations in Nearby Type II Cells

The idea that glial-like type II cells may participate in the integrative CB sensory response was first suggested by the observation that the excitatory transmitter ATP can elicit a rise in intracellular Ca^{2+} in isolated type II cells (Xu et al., 2003). Though these cells display small voltage-dependent outward currents, they lack significant inward Na^+ or Ca^{2+} currents (Duchen et al., 1988; Xu et al., 2003; Zhang et al., 2012), consistent with an intracellular source for the ATP-mediated Ca^{2+} rise (Xu et al., 2003). This effect of ATP was mimicked by selective P2Y2 receptor (P2Y2R) agonists such as UTP, and P2Y2R immunoreactivity was detectable in spindle-shaped type II cells in tissue sections of the rat CB *in situ* (Xu et al., 2003). As exemplified in **Figure 2C**, subsequent studies using the agonist UTP confirmed the P2Y2R-mediated increase in intracellular Ca^{2+} in rat type II cells (Piskuric and Nurse, 2012; Zhang et al., 2012). P2Y2Rs typically couple via G_q-proteins to activate the phospholipase C-IP3-PKC signaling pathway

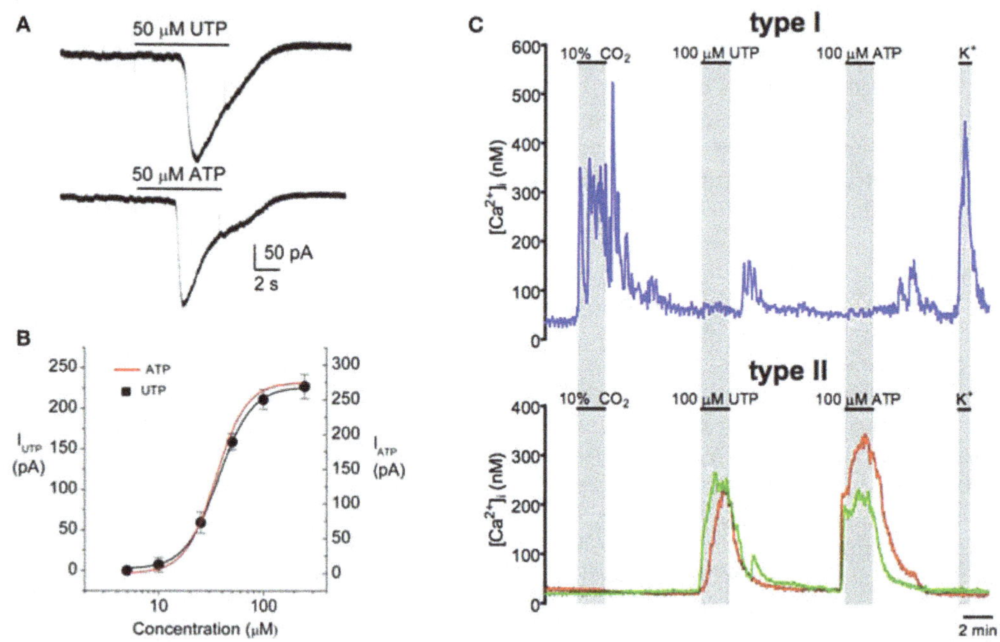

FIGURE 2 | Purinergic activation of the inward current in type II cells is mediated by P2Y2 receptors in association with a rise in intracellular Ca^{2+}. Both **(A)** ATP (50 μM) and **(B)** UTP (50 μM) induced similar inward currents (at −60 mV) in the same type II cell as expected for P2Y2 receptors. **(B)** Dose–response relation (black curve) for the UTP-evoked currents in a group of type II cells; data are represented as means ± SEM ($n = 4$) and fitted with the Hill equation with an $EC_{50} = 37$ μM. The dose–response curve for ATP (red) is superimposed and is indistinguishable from that for UTP. **(C)** Intracellular Ca^{2+} $[Ca^{2+}]_i$ responses monitored simultaneously in type I and type II cells. Both hypercapnia (10% CO_2) and high K^+ (30 mM) induced $[Ca^{2+}]_i$ responses in the type I cell (upper trace), but not in the two type II cells (lower red and green traces). Conversely, ATP and UTP induced similar $[Ca^{2+}]_i$ responses in the type II cells, but the type I cell was unresponsive. Data taken from Zhang et al. (2012).

and mobilize Ca^{2+} from internal stores (von Kügelgen, 2006), suggesting this mechanism is likely responsible for the Ca^{2+} elevation in type II cells. Because ATP is a key excitatory CB neurotransmitter the question arose whether paracrine stimulation of type II cells by ATP occurs during normal CB chemoexcitation. To address this, isolated rat type I cell clusters containing contiguous type II cells where challenged with chemosensory stimuli such as acute hypoxia and hypercapnia, as well as the depolarizing stimulus, high (30 mM) K^+ (Murali and Nurse, 2016). As expected, all three stimuli evoked rapid intracellular Ca^{2+} elevations in receptor type I cells but, interestingly, nearby type II cells frequently responded with a delayed, secondary increase in intracellular Ca^{2+} (Murali and Nurse, 2016), as illustrated in **Figures 3A,B**. The paracrine action of ATP released from type I cells appeared to be responsible for the secondary type II cell Ca^{2+} responses because the latter were reversibly inhibited by the P2Y2R antagonist, suramin (**Figure 3A**), as well as by the nucleoside hydrolase, apyrase (**Figure 3B**).

Several Other CB Neurochemicals Stimulate a Rise in Intracellular Ca^{2+} in Type II Cells

In addition to ATP (see above), several other neuroactive chemicals in the CB cause a rise in intracellular Ca^{2+} when applied to a significant proportion of isolated type II cells. For example, the small molecule neurotransmitters ACh and 5-HT, acting via metabotropic muscarinic and 5-HT2 receptors respectively, stimulated intracellular Ca^{2+} transients in ~53 and 67% of UTP-sensitive type II cells respectively (Tse et al., 2012; Murali et al., 2015, 2017). In addition, nanomolar concentrations of the neuropeptide angiotensin II stimulated a rise in intracellular Ca^{2+} in a significant proportion (~75%) of type II cells via losartan-sensitive AT_1 receptors (Tse et al., 2012; Murali et al., 2014). The biosynthetic pathway for producing angiotensin II, including angiotensin converting enzyme (ACE) and the precursor angiotensinogen, is expressed in type I cells (Leung et al., 2000; Lam and Leung, 2003), suggesting it could play a paracrine role in the CB. In all cases, the intracellular Ca^{2+} response in type II cells persisted in Ca^{2+}-free extracellular solutions and/or following store depletion with thapsigargin or cyclopiazonic acid, suggesting Ca^{2+} release from internal stores (Tse et al., 2012; Murali et al., 2014, 2017). Although less well-studied, another neuropeptide, i.e., endothelin-1 (ET-1), that is synthesized and released by type I cells during hypoxia (Chen et al., 2002; Platero-Luengo et al., 2014), is also capable of evoking intracellular Ca^{2+} responses in type II cells at nanomolar concentrations (Murali et al., 2015). Whether or not all of these neuroactive agents combine to enhance Ca^{2+} signaling in type II cells during chemoexcitation, as described above for ATP, remains to be determined. It is also possible that

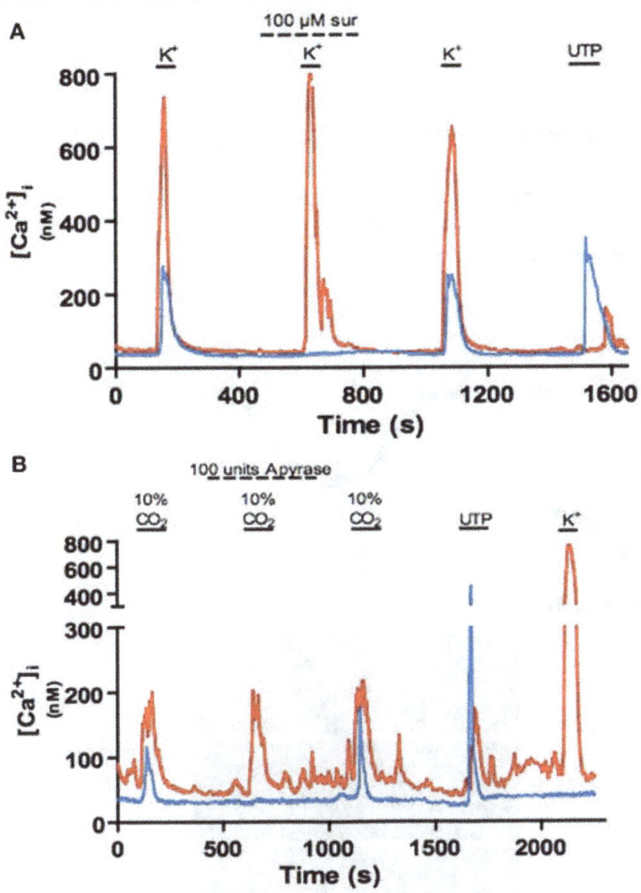

FIGURE 3 | Blockade of P2Y2 receptors with suramin or degradation of extracellular ATP with apyrase inhibits crosstalk from type I to type II cells. **(A)** Example intracellular Ca^{2+} traces showing the reversible inhibition of the delayed or indirect Ca^{2+} response in a type II cell (blue) by the P2Y2R blocker suramin (100 μM) during stimulation of nearby type I cells (red) with high K^+ (30 mM). **(B)** Application of apyrase (a nucleoside hydrolase) reversibly inhibits the delayed Ca^{2+} response in a type II cell during stimulation of nearby type I cells with high (10%) CO_2. Data adapted from Murali and Nurse (2016).

their actions may become more relevant in pathophysiological conditions associated with chronic or intermittent hypoxia, when their expression level and/or that of their cognate receptors are elevated (Chen et al., 2002; Lam et al., 2004).

DOWNSTREAM EFFECTS OF NEUROTRANSMITTER-MEDIATED INTRACELLULAR Ca^{2+} SIGNALING IN TYPE II CELLS

There is abundant evidence that glial cells in the CNS contribute to synapse integration by generating intracellular Ca^{2+} signals and releasing gliotransmitters such as ATP, GABA, and glutamate (Eroglu and Barres, 2010; Bazargani and Attwell, 2016). As discussed above, several CB neurotransmitters elicited intracellular Ca^{2+} elevations in type II cells raising questions about the downstream consequence, and particularly whether this led to the release of gliotransmitters.

Carotid Body Neurotransmitters Activate Pannexin-1 (Panx-1) Channels in Type II Cells

In electrophysiological studies on isolated type II cells, the P2Y2R agonists ATP or UTP activated an inward current at the resting membrane potential (Zhang et al., 2012), as illustrated in **Figures 2A,B**. This current reversed direction near 0 mV and, as illustrated in **Figure 4A**, was reversibly inhibited by low concentrations of carbenoxolone (5 μM), a putative blocker of pannexin-1 (Panx-1) channels. Panx-1 immunoreactivity also co-localized with isolated GFAP-positive type II cells in dissociated CB cultures (see **Figure 4D**), and stained processes of type II cells in CB tissue sections (Zhang et al., 2012). Panx-1 channels assemble as hexamers in the plasma membrane and though structurally similar to gap junction hemichannels, Panx-1 sequences show closer homology to the invertebrate innexins (Dahl, 2015; Penuela et al., 2015). In addition to ATP, other CB neurotransmitters that evoked a rise in intracellular Ca^{2+} in type II cells such as angiotensin II, ACh, and 5-HT also activated an inward Panx-1-like current based on its sensitivity to carbenoxolone (Murali et al., 2014, 2015, 2017). However, carbenoxolone is also a well-known blocker of gap junctional connexins, albeit at typically higher (>10x) concentrations (Lohman and Isakson, 2014), raising questions about the true identity of the channels. In recent studies, the UTP-evoked inward current in type II cells was reversibly inhibited by a more specific Panx-1 mimetic peptide channel blocker ^{10}Panx (100 μM) (see **Figures 4B,C**), but not by similar concentrations of scrambled control peptide ^{sc}Panx (Murali et al., 2017). Taken together, the combined pharmacological and immunocytochemical data, summarized in **Figure 4**, support the notion that Panx-1 channels mediate the neurotransmitter-activated inward currents in type II cells.

Activation of Pannexin-1 Channels in Type II Cells Is Dependent on Intracellular Ca^{2+}

The observation that several neurotransmitters that elicited a rise in intracellular Ca^{2+} also activated Panx-1 currents in type II cells led to an investigation of a possible link between the two events (Murali et al., 2014). Indeed, as illustrated in **Figures 5A–D**, the Panx-1 inward current activated by either angiotensin II or ATP was reversibly inhibited when the membrane-permeable Ca^{2+} chelator BAPTA-AM was present in the extracellular solution (Murali et al., 2014). These results are in concert with previous demonstrations that: (i) ATP activated an inward current at negative potentials in oocytes co-expressing Panx-1 channels and P2Y2R (Locovei et al., 2006); (ii) in inside-out patches from these oocytes Panx-1 channels were strongly activated at negative potentials when the cytoplasmic face was exposed to micromolar (but not 0) Ca^{2+}; and (iii) in other glial cell types, e.g., microglia and astrocytes, Panx-1 channel opening is regulated by intracellular Ca^{2+} (Dahl, 2015). However, it should be noted that the activation of Panx-1 channels by cytoplasmic Ca^{2+}

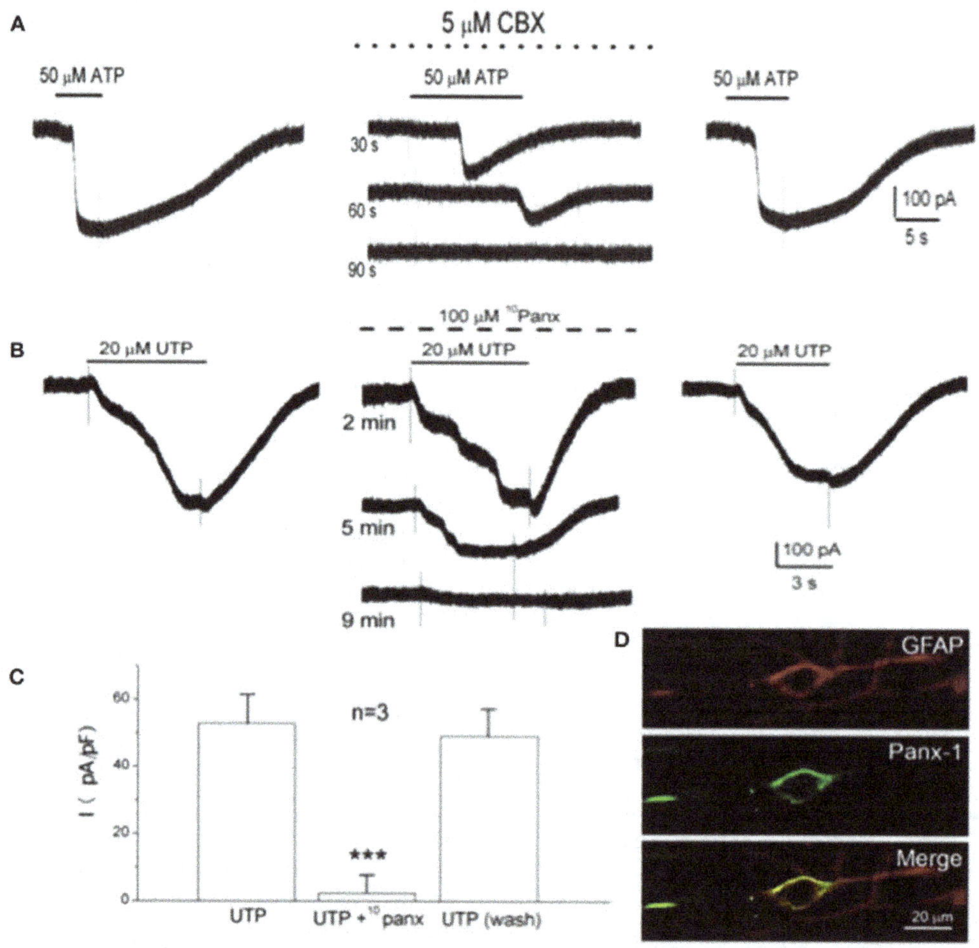

FIGURE 4 | Inhibition of the P2Y2R-activated inward current by selective Panx-1 channel blockers and localization of Panx-1 immunoreactivity in type II cells. The selective Panx-1 blockers, carbenoxolone (CBX; 5 μM) and ^{10}Panx peptide (100 μM), reversibly inhibited the inward current in type II cells elicited by 50 μM ATP **(A)** and 20 μM UTP **(B)**, respectively. **(C)** UTP-activated inward current (plotted as current density pA/pF) for three cells before, during and after (wash) treatment with 100 μM ^{10}Panx peptide; ***$P < 0.001$. **(D)** Confocal images of pannexin-1 (Panx-1) immunostaining of a solitary, GFAP-positive, spindle-shaped type II cell in a 6-day-old culture of dissociated rat carotid body; note co-localization of GFAP-ir with Panx-1-ir in the type II cell. Adapted from Zhang et al. (2012) and Murali et al. (2017).

may be dependent on cell type, since in hippocampal neurons Panx-1 channel activation is Ca^{2+}-independent (Thompson, 2015).

Pannexin-1 Channels as Conduits for Release of the "Gliotransmitter" ATP From Type II Cells

Panx-1 channels have pores large enough to allow passage of molecules <1.5 kDa in various cell types including astrocytes and central neurons (Dahl, 2015; Penuela et al., 2015; Thompson, 2015). These molecules include "gliotransmitters" such as ATP, GABA, and glutamate. Given the central role of ATP in CB neurotransmission (Nurse, 2014), it was of interest to determine whether the Panx-1 channels in type II cells acted as ATP release channels. To test this, P2XR-expressing petrosal neurons served as ATP biosensors in the CB co-cultures containing type I/type II cell clusters (Zhang et al., 2012). In that study, selective stimulation of P2Y2R on type II cells with UTP led to depolarization and/or increased firing in several nearby petrosal neurons. These petrosal responses were reversibly inhibited by blockers of P2X2/3 receptors (PPADS) or Panx-1 channels (carbenoxolone) suggesting they arose from ATP released through Panx-1 channels (Zhang et al., 2012). Though petrosal neurons functioned as ATP biosensors in the latter study, the results led to the intriguing possibility that simply stimulating type II glial cells alone was sufficient to excite petrosal afferent terminals at the CB tripartite synapse, apparently without type I cell involvement. This occurred in spite of the unfavorably geometry present in this monolayer co-culture model, increasing the likelihood that it may also occur *in vivo*. If so, the proposed interaction could be facilitated by the close relation between type II cell processes and the afferent terminal (Platero-Luengo et al., 2014), as well as the possibility of physical coupling

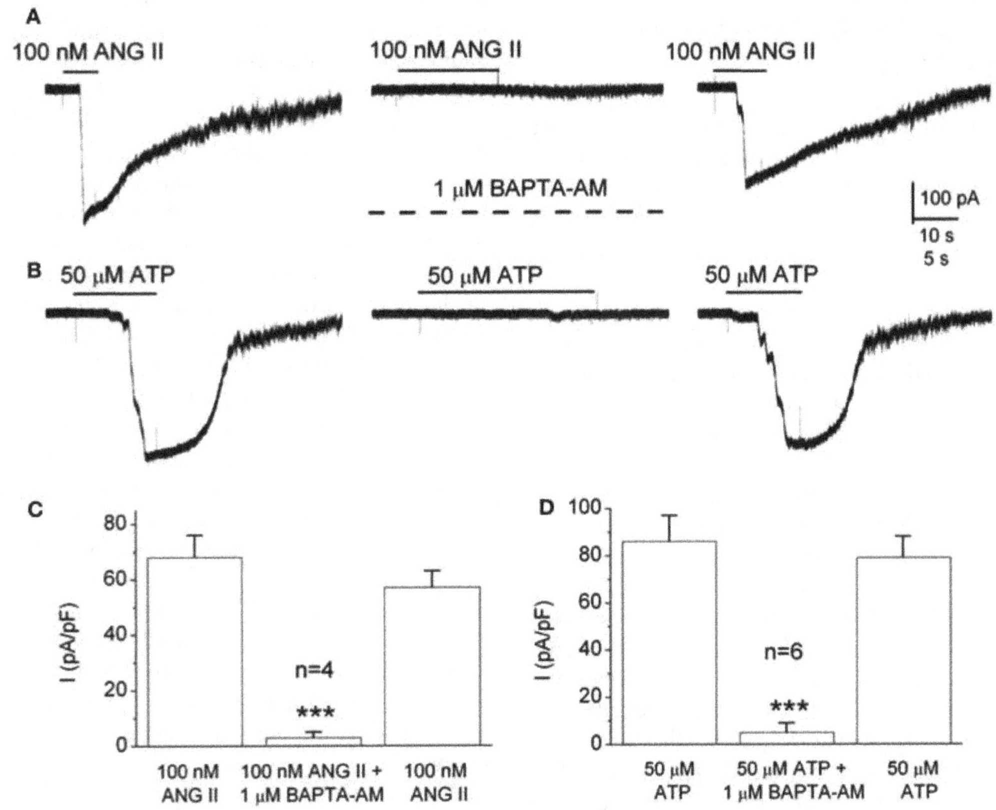

FIGURE 5 | Chelating intracellular Ca^{2+} in type II cells with BAPTA prevents Panx-1 current activation by angiotensin II and ATP. **(A)** The ANG II-induced Panx-1 current was almost completely and reversibly inhibited during incubation with the membrane permeable Ca^{2+} chelator, BAPTA-AM (1 μM; middle trace). **(B)** Similarly, the same result was obtained when ATP was used as the agonist. **(C,D)** Summary data show the reversible inhibition of the Panx-1 current evoked by ANG II and ATP respectively, when BAPTA-AM was present (**C**, $n = 4$, and **D**, $n = 6$); $^{***}p < 0.001$. Data taken from Murali et al., 2014.

between P2X2/3R and Panx-1 channels as recently shown in co-immunoprecipitation studies (Li et al., 2017). This potential for type II cells alone to directly excite petrosal nerve endings via ATP release has further implications. For example, conditions associated with an increase in circulating levels of compounds such as angiotensin II, e.g., CIH-induced hypertension and CHF (Schultz et al., 2015), could lead to enhanced CB excitation solely via stimulation of AT_1 receptors on type II cells. Additional independent support for the posit that type II cells can release ATP through Panx-1 channels was obtained in experiments using fura-2 Ca^{2+} imaging to test for possible crosstalk from type II to type I cells (Murali and Nurse, 2016). In that study carbenoxolone reversibly inhibited ATP-dependent crosstalk from type II to type I cells, as discussed further below. The ability of the spindle-shaped type II cells to release ATP, coupled with their expression of P2Y2R, also raise the possibility that intercellular Ca^{2+} waves may propagate within the network of interconnected type II cells and thereby facilitate delivery of ATP to the synaptic region.

ATP-Dependent Crosstalk From Type II to Type I Cells

The P2Y2R-$[Ca^{2+}]_i$-Panx-1 pathway discussed in the preceding sections implied a potential role for type II cells as ATP amplifiers due to the mechanism of "ATP-induced ATP release." In addition to causing excitation at the sensory nerve terminal via P2X2/3R, ATP released through Panx-1 channels could in turn inhibit type I cells by negative feedback mechanisms involving P2Y1R or P2Y12R as discussed earlier. However, extracellular ATP at the CB chemosensory synapse can be metabolized by ectonucleotidases to adenosine (Conde and Monteiro, 2004; Holmes et al., 2017; Salman et al., 2017), which is excitatory at both the sensory nerve ending and type I cells (see above). This raised the question whether P2Y2R-mediated activation of Panx-1 channels in type II cells could lead to positive feedback stimulation of neighboring type I cells. Indeed, stimulation of type II cells with UTP often led to a delayed secondary rise in intracellular Ca^{2+} in nearby type I cells (Murali and Nurse, 2016). Consistent with a role for adenosine, generated from ATP catabolism after release through Panx-1 channels, the delayed type II cell Ca^{2+} response was strongly inhibited by the Panx-1 blocker carbenoxolone, the adenosine A2aR blocker SCH58261, and the ecto-5′-nucleotidase blocker AOPCP (Murali and Nurse, 2016). Thus, type II cells may participate in the integrated sensory response of CB by contributing to both ATP and adenosine synaptic pools.

PLASTICITY IN CB NEUROTRANSMITTER FUNCTIONS DURING EXPOSURE TO CHRONIC HYPOXIA

A prominent feature of the CB is its remarkable plasticity following exposure of animals to different patterns of hypoxia including chronic sustained and chronic intermittent hypoxia or CIH (Kumar and Prabhakar, 2012). The reader is referred to other excellent reviews for a discussion of CB plasticity following CIH (Prabhakar et al., 2015; Iturriaga, 2017). Changes in ion channel expression leading to increased membrane excitability of type I cells, as well as alterations in a variety of neurotransmitter systems, are well-described CB plasticity mechanisms that occur during exposures to chronic sustained hypoxia (Prabhakar and Jacono, 2005; Powell, 2007). We focus here mainly on purinergic neurotransmitter mechanisms underlying CB plasticity during chronic hypoxia, as may occur during ascent to altitude. In the latter condition, an adaptive process known as ventilatory acclimatization to hypoxia (VAH) ensures an increase in sensitivity of the CB chemoreflex such that for a given PO_2 there is an augmented CSN discharge frequency over and above that present before acclimatization (Prabhakar and Jacono, 2005; Powell, 2007; Kumar and Prabhakar, 2012). Given the central role of ATP and adenosine in CB chemoexcitation as previously discussed, perhaps it is not surprising that alterations in purinergic signaling pathways have been implicated in VAH. For example, when adult rats were reared under chronic hypoxia (12% O_2) for 7 days, infusion of the non-specific adenosine receptor antagonist 8-sulpho-phenyltheophylline (8-SPT) attenuated the increase in respiratory frequency evoked by acute hypoxia (Walsh and Marshall, 2006). Similarly when caffeine, a non-specific adenosine receptor antagonist, was included in the drinking water of chronically-hypoxic rats the CB sensory output was markedly inhibited (Conde et al., 2012b). These data point to a major contribution of adenosine signaling to the mechanisms underlying VAH.

Because surface-located ectonucleotidases control adenosine levels at the CB tripartite synapse (see above), it was of interest to determine whether expression of these enzymes was regulated by chronic hypoxia as occurs in other cell types, e.g., smooth muscle cells (Koszalka et al., 2004; Robson et al., 2005). In a recent study, exposure of rats to chronic hypobaric hypoxia (~60 kPa, simulating an altitude of ~4,300 m) for 5–7 days led to an ~2x increase in expression of NTPDase3 and ecto-5′-nucleotidase/CD73 mRNAs, concomitant with a significant decrease in expression of NTPDasel and NTPDase2 mRNAs (Salman et al., 2017). Assuming changes in mRNA expression correlate with parallel changes in protein expression, the modifications seen in chronic hypoxia favor a shift toward adenosine signaling in the CB because NTPDase3 efficiently hydrolyses ATP to AMP, whereas ecto-5′-nucleotidase catalyzes the conversion of AMP to adenosine in the rate-limiting step (Zimmermann, 2000). This shift could be further aided by the rapid depletion of the ATP and ADP pools because both purines are natural physiological inhibitors of ecto-5′-nucleotidase (Lecka et al., 2010). Further, the tendency of ecto-5′nucleotidase and adenosine A2aR to co-localize, as previously demonstrated in the striatum (Augusto et al., 2013), could enable the efficiency of adenosine-A2aR interactions at the membranes of both type I cells and sensory nerve terminals. The proposed depletion of extracellular ATP and ADP pools during chronic hypoxia could facilitate type I cell depolarization and increased sensitivity by diminishing their negative feedback influences mediated by interactions with P2Y1R and/or P2Y12R on type I cells (Xu et al., 2006; Carroll et al., 2012). Evidence for an increased role for adenosine signaling during VAH is further supported by the observation that acute hypoxia-evoked adenosine release is markedly potentiated in isolated whole CBs from chronically hypoxic rats (Conde et al., 2012b). It is also possible that autoregulatory "push-pull" mechanisms could prevent adenosine-mediated overexcitation. For example, high levels of adenosine in the micromolar range could activate low affinity A2bR on type I cells and facilitate secretion of dopamine (Conde et al., 2008; Livermore and Nurse, 2013), which inhibits CB function via pre- and postsynaptic D2R on type I cells and petrosal nerve endings (see earlier discussion). Indeed, an increase in both basal and hypoxia-evoked dopamine release has been reported for chronically hypoxic CB chemoreceptor cells (Jackson and Nurse, 1997; Conde et al., 2012b). Taken together, these studies support a major shift toward adenosine-A2R signaling in the CB after exposure to chronic hypoxia *in vivo*.

CONCLUSIONS AND FUTURE DIRECTIONS

In this review we considered the evidence that the integrated CB output is determined largely by neurochemical interactions at the tripartite synapse formed by type I chemoreceptor cells, type II glial cells, and sensory nerve endings. Several of these interactions involving fast-acting ionotropic receptors and slower-acting G-protein coupled receptors are summarized in **Figure 6**. There is a growing consensus that the purines ATP and adenosine are key players in mediating CB chemoexcitation and their actions involve P2 and P1 receptors located at pre- and postsynaptic sites. While the evidence in most species has long favored an inhibitory role for dopamine acting via D2R on type I cells, we considered novel data showing that dopamine-D2R signaling might also inhibit the sensory afferent discharge via modulation of the I_h current that controls action potential frequency. Moreover, recent evidence suggests that the excitatory effects of P2Y2R-mediated Ca^{2+} signaling in varying subpopulations of type II cells might be inhibited by dopamine (Leonard and Nurse, 2017), or histamine (Nurse et al., 2018). The possibility that other CB neurochemicals including small molecules (e.g., histamine and 5-HT) and neuropeptides (e.g., angiotensin II) might act postsynaptically on I_h so as to regulate firing frequency requires future investigation. We also considered several G-protein coupled pathways by which type II glial cells might contribute to synapse integration; all of these converge on the Ca^{2+}-dependent activation of Panx-1 channels which act as conduits for ATP release. These channels

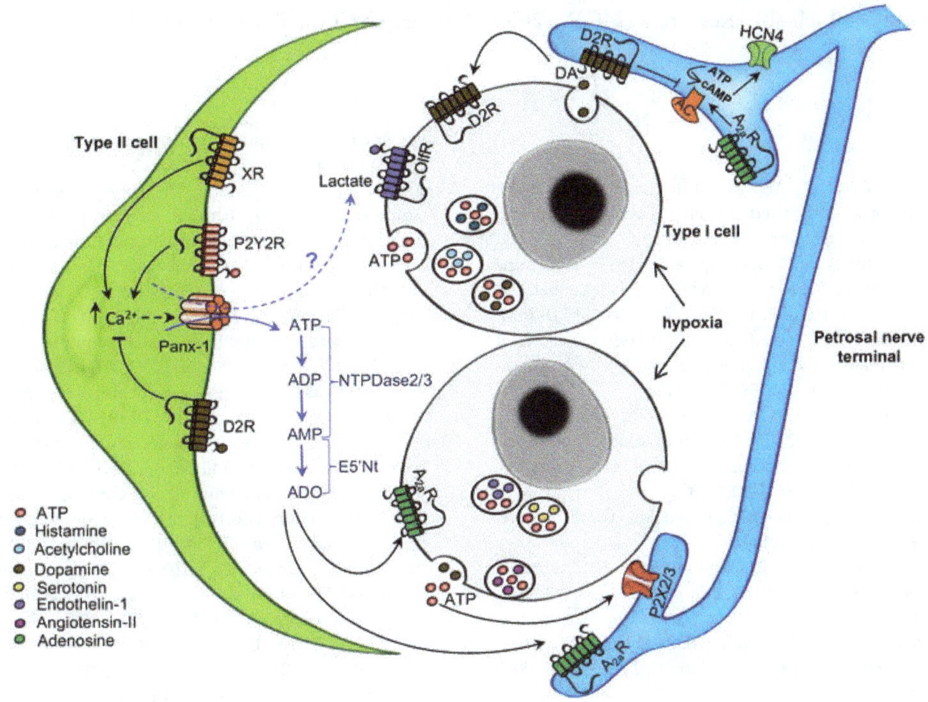

FIGURE 6 | Schematic representation of neurotransmitter functions at the tripartite synapse of the rat carotid body. The diagram shows some of the neurotransmitter mechanisms that are likely to operate at the carotid body sensory synapse during acute hypoxia. Chemoreceptor type I cells depolarize and release ATP, dopamine (DA), and other neurochemicals (X) during hypoxia. ATP acts postsynaptically on ionotropic P2X2/3R on petrosal nerve terminals causing excitation. ATP also activates P2Y2R on adjacent glial-like type II cells, leading to a rise in intracellular Ca^{2+} and activation of pannexin-1 (Panx-1) channels which act as conduits for the further release of ATP; Panx-1 channels may also release other "gliotransmitters" such as lactate, a potential ligand for Olf78 receptors present on type I cells. Extracellular ATP is degraded by a series of surface-located nucleotidases, including NTPDase2,3 and ecto-5-nucleotidase, to adenosine (ADO). ADO could then act in a paracrine manner to activate A2aR on nearby type I cells (causing inhibition of TASK channels) and sensory nerve terminals (causing modulation HCN4-containing I_h channels), leading to increased excitation. DA released during hypoxia may act on inhibitory D2R present on adjacent type I cells, and possibly type II cells, so as to inhibit intracellular Ca^{2+} signaling. Also, DA may act postsynaptically on the sensory nerve terminal to inhibit the HCN channels and action potential frequency. Other released neurochemicals (X), including angiotensin II, 5-HT, ACh, and ET-1, may act on corresponding G-protein coupled receptors (XR) on type II (and likely type I) cells to increase intracellular Ca^{2+} signaling and activate Panx-1 channels. The action of some of these neurochemicals may become more relevant in pathophysiological conditions (e.g., after chronic or intermittent hypoxia) when carotid body sensitivity is augmented. Omitted for clarity are: (i) negative feedback inhibition of type I cell function by ATP and ADP acting via P2Y1 or P2Y12 receptors; (ii) stimulatory effect of low affinity A2b receptors on DA secretion from type II cells; and (iii) inhibitory effects of GABA on presynaptic GABA(B) receptors on type I cells and on postsynaptic GABA(A) receptors on the sensory nerve terminal. Figure adapted from Murali et al. (2017).

are known to release other "gliotransmitters" in the CNS, raising the possibility that type II cells may also release other neuroactive chemicals to further shape or fine-tune the CB sensory output. For example, open Panx-1 channels in CNS astrocytes may stimulate release of lactate which serves as an extracellular energy substrate as well as a signaling molecule for glia-neuron communication (Karagiannis et al., 2016). In this regard, the lactate receptor Olfr78 that is highly expressed in type I cells has been proposed as a potential "hypoxia sensor" (Chang, 2017), raising the possibility that this pathway could be activated during acute hypoxia by lactate release from type II cells via Panx-1 channels (see **Figure 6**). Finally, this review considered some of the purinergic mechanisms that are likely to contribute to the increased sensitivity of the CB during exposure to chronic hypoxia. Whether similar or overlapping changes occur during pathophysiological conditions that lead to increased CB chemosensitivity, e.g., exposure to intermittent hypoxia (Kumar and Prabhakar, 2012), requires future investigation.

AUTHOR CONTRIBUTIONS

EL performed experiments, analyzed data, helped prepare figures, reviewed literature and contributed to first draft. SS performed experiments, analyzed data, helped prepare figures, reviewed literature and contributed to first draft. CN organized review subheadings, helped interpret data, helped prepare figures, reviewed literature and contributed to first draft.

ACKNOWLEDGMENTS

We thank several colleagues especially Min Zhang, Nikol Piskuric, Sindy Murali, and Cathy Vollmer for their contributions to some of the ideas and to several of the figures presented in this review. Grant support to CAN was provided by the Canadian Institutes of Health Research (MOP 12037 and MOP 142469) and the Natural Sciences and Engineering Research Council of Canada.

REFERENCES

Alcayaga, C., Varas, R., Valdés, V., Cerpa, V., Arroyo, J., Iturriaga, R., et al. (2007). ATP- and ACh-induced responses in isolated cat petrosal ganglion neurons. *Brain Res.* 1131, 60–67. doi: 10.1016/j.brainres.2006.11.012

Alcayaga, J., Varas, R., Arroyo, J., Iturriaga, R., and Zapata, P. (1999). Dopamine modulates carotid nerve responses induced by acetylcholine on the cat petrosal ganglion *in vitro*. *Brain Res.* 831, 97–103. doi: 10.1016/S0006-8993(99)01402-X

Almaraz, L., Wang, Z. Z., Stensaas, L. J., and Fidone, S. J. (1993). Release of dopamine from carotid sinus nerve fibers innervating type I cells in the cat carotid body. *Biol. Signals* 2, 16–26. doi: 10.1159/000109474

Augusto, E., Matos, M., Sévigny, J., El-Tayeb, A., Bynoe, M. S., Müller, C. E., et al. (2013). Ecto-5′-nucleotidase (CD73)-mediated formation of adenosine is critical for the striatal adenosine A2A receptor functions. *J. Neurosci.* 33, 11390–11399. doi: 10.1523/JNEUROSCI.5817-12.2013

Bazargani, N., and Attwell, D. (2016). Astrocyte calcium signaling: the third wave. *Nat. Neurosci.* 19, 182–189. doi: 10.1038/nn.4201

Benot, A. R., and Lopez-Barneo, J. (1990). Feedback inhibition of Ca^{2+} currents by dopamine in glomus cells of the carotid body. *Eur. J. Neurosci.* 2, 809–812. doi: 10.1111/j.1460-9568.1990.tb00473.x

Biel, M., Wahl-Schott, C., Michalakis, S., and Zong, X. (2009). Hyperpolarization-activated cation channels: from genes to function. *Physiol. Rev.* 89, 847–885. doi: 10.1152/physrev.00029.2008

Buckler, K. J. (2015). TASK channels in arterial chemoreceptors and their role in oxygen and acid sensing. *Pflugers Arch.* 467, 1013–1025. doi: 10.1007/s00424-015-1689-1

Buttigieg, J., and Nurse, C. A. (2004). Detection of hypoxia-evoked ATP release from chemoreceptor cells of the rat carotid body. *Biochem. Biophys. Res. Commun.* 322, 82–87. doi: 10.1016/j.bbrc.2004.07.081

Carroll, J. L., Agarwal, A., Donnelly, D. F., and Kim, I. (2012). Purinergic modulation of carotid body glomus cell hypoxia response during postnatal maturation in rats. *Adv. Exp. Med. Biol.* 758, 249–253. doi: 10.1007/978-94-007-4584-1_34

Carroll, J. L., Boyle, K. M., Wasicko, M. J., and Sterni, L. M. (2005). Dopamine D2 receptor modulation of carotid body type 1 cell intracellular calcium in developing rats. *Am. J. Physiol. Lung Cell. Mol. Physiol.* 288, L910–L916. doi: 10.1152/ajplung.00414.2003

Chang, A. J. (2017). Acute oxygen sensing by the carotid body: from mitochondria to plasma membrane. *J. Appl. Physiol.* 123, 1335–1343. doi: 10.1152/japplphysiol.00398.2017

Chen, J., He, L., Dinger, B., Stensaas, L., and Fidone, S. (2002). Role of endothelin and endothelin A-type receptor in adaptation of the carotid body to chronic hypoxia. *Am. J. Physiol. Lung Cell. Mol. Physiol.* 282, L1314–L1323. doi: 10.1152/ajplung.00454.2001

Claps, A., and Torrealba, F. (1988). The carotid body connections: a WGA-HRP study in the cat. *Brain Res.* 455, 123–133. doi: 10.1016/0006-8993(88)90121-7

Conde, S. V., Gonzalez, C., Batuca, J. R., Monteiro, E. C., and Obeso, A. (2008). An antagonistic interaction between A2B adenosine and D2 dopamine receptors modulates the function of rat carotid body chemoreceptor cells. *J. Neurochem.* 107, 1369–1381. doi: 10.1111/j.1471-4159.2008.05704.x

Conde, S. V., and Monteiro, E. C. (2004). Hypoxia induces adenosine release from the rat carotid body. *J. Neurochem.* 89, 1148–1156. doi: 10.1111/j.1471-4159.2004.02380.x

Conde, S. V., Monteiro, E. C., Obeso, A., and Gonzalez, C. (2009). Adenosine in peripheral chemoreception: new insights into a historically overlooked molecule–invited article. *Adv. Exp. Med. Biol.* 648, 145–159. doi: 10.1007/978-90-481-2259-2_17

Conde, S. V., Monteiro, E. C., Rigual, R., Obeso, A., and Gonzalez, C. (2012a). Hypoxic intensity: a determinant for the contribution of ATP and adenosine to the genesis of carotid body chemosensory activity. *J. Appl. Physiol.* 112, 2002–2010. doi: 10.1152/japplphysiol.01617.2011

Conde, S. V., Obeso, A., Vicario, I., Rigual, R., Rocher, A., and Gonzalez, C. (2006). Caffeine inhibition of rat carotid body chemoreceptors is mediated by A2A and A2B adenosine receptors. *J. Neurochem.* 98, 616–628. doi: 10.1111/j.1471-4159.2006.03912.x

Conde, S. V., Ribeiro, M. J., Obeso, A., Rigual, R., Monteiro, E. C., and Gonzalez, C. (2012b). Chronic caffeine intake in adult rat inhibits carotid body sensitization produced by chronic sustained hypoxia but maintains intact chemoreflex output. *Mol. Pharmacol.* 82, 1056–1065. doi: 10.1124/mol.112.081216

Conde, S. V., Sacramento, J. F., Guarino, M. P., Gonzalez, C., Obeso, A., Diogo, L. N., et al. (2014). Carotid body, insulin, and metabolic diseases: unraveling the links. *Front. Physiol.* 5:418. doi: 10.3389/fphys.2014.00418

Cutz, E., and Jackson, A. (1999). Neuroepithelial bodies as airway oxygen sensors. *Respir. Physiol.* 115, 201–214. doi: 10.1016/S0034-5687(99)00018-3

Dahl, G. (2015). ATP release through pannexon channels. *Philos. Trans. R. Soc. Lond. B. Biol. Sci.* 370:20140191. doi: 10.1098/rstb.2014.0191

Del Rio, R., Moya, E. A., Koenig, C. S., Fujiwara, K., Alcayaga, J., and Iturriaga, R. (2008). Modulatory effects of histamine on cat carotid body chemoreception. *Respir. Physiol. Neurobiol.* 164, 401–410. doi: 10.1016/j.resp.2008.09.005

Duchen, M. R., Caddy, K. W., Kirby, G. C., Patterson, D. L., Ponte, J., and Biscoe, T. J. (1988). Biophysical studies of the cellular elements of the rabbit carotid body. *Neuroscience* 26, 291–311. doi: 10.1016/0306-4522(88)90146-7

Eroglu, C., and Barres, B. A. (2010). Regulation of synaptic connectivity by glia. *Nature* 468, 223–231. doi: 10.1038/nature09612

Eyzaguirre, C. (2007). Electric synapses in the carotid body-nerve complex. *Respir. Physiol. Neurobiol.* 157, 116–122. doi: 10.1016/j.resp.2007.01.013

Eyzaguirre, C., and Zapata, P. (1984). Perspectives in carotid body research. *J. Appl. Physiol.* 57, 931–957. doi: 10.1152/jappl.1984.57.4.931

Fearon, I. M., Zhang, M., Vollmer, C., and Nurse, C. A. (2003). GABA mediates autoreceptor feedback inhibition in the rat carotid body via presynaptic GABAB receptors and TASK-1. *J. Physiol.* 553, 83–94. doi: 10.1113/jphysiol.2003.048298

Fitzgerald, R. S. (2000). Oxygen and carotid body chemotransduction: the cholinergic hypothesis - a brief history and new evaluation. *Respir. Physiol.* 120, 89–104. doi: 10.1016/S0034-5687(00)00091-8

Gauda, E. B. (2002). Gene expression in peripheral arterial chemoreceptors. *Microsc. Res. Tech.* 59, 153–167. doi: 10.1002/jemt.10190

Gonzalez, C., Almaraz, L., Obeso, A., and Rigual, R. (1994). Carotid body chemoreceptors: from natural stimuli to sensory discharges. *Physiol. Rev.* 74, 829–898. doi: 10.1152/physrev.1994.74.4.829

Gonzalez, C., Conde, S. V., Gallego-Martín, T., Olea, E., Gonzalez-Obeso, E., Ramirez, M., et al. (2014). Fernando de Castro and the discovery of the arterial chemoreceptors. *Front. Neuroanat.* 8:25. doi: 10.3389/fnana.2014.00025

He, L., Chen, J., Dinger, B., Stensaas, L., and Fidone, S. (2006). Effect of chronic hypoxia on purinergic synaptic transmission in rat carotid body. *J. Appl. Physiol.* 100, 157–162. doi: 10.1152/japplphysiol.00859.2005

He, L., Dinger, B., and Fidone, S. (2005). Effect of chronic hypoxia on cholinergic chemotransmission in rat carotid body. *J. Appl. Physiol.* 98, 614–619. doi: 10.1152/japplphysiol.00714.2004

Holmes, A. P., Ray, C. J., Pearson, S. A., Coney, A. M., and Kumar, P. (2017). Ecto-5′-nucleotidase (CD73) regulates peripheral chemoreceptor activity and cardiorespiratory responses to hypoxia. *J. Physiol.* doi: 10.1113/JP274498. [Epub ahead of print].

Igarashi, A., Zadzilka, N., and Shirahata, M. (2009). Benzodiazepines and GABA-GABAA receptor system in the cat carotid body. *Adv. Exp. Med. Biol.* 648, 169–175. doi: 10.1007/978-90-481-2259-2_19

Iturriaga, R. (2017). Translating carotid body function into clinical medicine. *J. Physiol.* doi: 10.1113/JP275335. [Epub ahead of print].

Iturriaga, R., and Alcayaga, J. (2004). Neurotransmission in the carotid body: transmitters and modulators between glomus cells and petrosal ganglion nerve terminals. *Brain Res. Brain Res. Rev.* 47, 46–53. doi: 10.1016/j.brainresrev.2004.05.007

Iturriaga, R., Alcayaga, J., and Gonzalez, C. (2009). Neurotransmitters in carotid body function: the case of dopamine–invited article. *Adv. Exp. Med. Biol.* 648, 137–143. doi: 10.1007/978-90-481-2259-2_16

Iturriaga, R., Cerpa, V., Zapata, P., and Alcayaga, J. (2003). Catecholamine release from isolated sensory neurons of cat petrosal ganglia in tissue culture. *Brain Res.* 984, 104–110. doi: 10.1016/S0006-8993(03)03118-4

Jackson, A., and Nurse, C. (1997). Dopaminergic properties of cultured rat carotid body chemoreceptors grown in normoxic and hypoxic environments. *J. Neurochem.* 69, 645–654. doi: 10.1046/j.1471-4159.1997.69020645.x

Kåhlin, J., Mkrtchian, S., Ebberyd, A., Hammarstedt-Nordenvall, L., Nordlander, B., Yoshitake, T., et al. (2014). The human carotid body releases acetylcholine, ATP and cytokines during hypoxia. *Exp. Physiol.* 99, 1089–1098. doi: 10.1113/expphysiol.2014.078873

Karagiannis, A., Sylantyev, S., Hadjihambi, A., Hosford, P. S., Kasparov, S., and Gourine, A. V. (2016). Hemichannel-mediated release of lactate. *J. Cereb. Blood Flow Metab.* 36, 1202–1211. doi: 10.1177/0271678X15611912

Koerner, P., Hesslinger, C., Schaefermeyer, A., Prinz, C., and Gratzl, M. (2004). Evidence for histamine as a transmitter in rat carotid body sensor cells. *J. Neurochem.* 91, 493–500. doi: 10.1111/j.1471-4159.2004.02740.x

Kondo, H. (2002). Are there gap junctions between chief (glomus, type I) cells in the carotid body chemoreceptor? A review. *Microsc. Res. Tech.* 59, 227–233. doi: 10.1002/jemt.10196

Koszalka, P., Ozüyaman, B., Huo, Y., Zernecke, A., Flögel, U., Braun, N., et al. (2004). Targeted disruption of cd73/ecto-5′-nucleotidase alters thromboregulation and augments vascular inflammatory response. *Circ. Res.* 95, 814–821. doi: 10.1161/01.RES.0000144796.82787.6f

Kumar, P., and Prabhakar, N. R. (2012). Peripheral chemoreceptors: function and plasticity of the carotid body. *Compr. Physiol.* 2, 141–219. doi: 10.1002/cphy.c100069

Lam, S. Y., Fung, M. L., and Leung, P. S. (2004). Regulation of the angiotensin-converting enzyme activity by a time-course hypoxia in the carotid body. *J. Appl. Physiol.* 96, 809–813. doi: 10.1152/japplphysiol.00684.2003

Lam, S. Y., and Leung, P. S. (2003). Chronic hypoxia activates a local angiotensin-generating system in rat carotid body. *Mol. Cell. Endocrinol.* 203, 147–153. doi: 10.1016/S0303-7207(03)00087-X

Lazarov, N., Rozloznik, M., Reindl, S., Rey-Ares, V., Dutschmann, M., and Gratzl, M. (2006). Expression of histamine receptors and effect of histamine in the rat carotid body chemoafferent pathway. *Eur. J. Neurosci.* 24, 3431–3444. doi: 10.1111/j.1460-9568.2006.05241.x

Lecka, J., Rana, M. S., and Sévigny, J. (2010). Inhibition of vascular ectonucleotidase activities by the pro-drugs ticlopidine and clopidogrel favours platelet aggregation. *Br. J. Pharmacol.* 161, 1150–3460. doi: 10.1111/j.1476-5381.2010.00951.x

Leonard, E. M., and Nurse, C. A. (2017). "Evidence for dopaminergic inhibitory cell-cell interactions in the rat carotid body," in *XXth Meeting of the International Society of Arterial Chemoreception (ISAC)* (Baltimore, MD), database (A1).

Leung, P. S., Lam, S. Y., and Fung, M. L. (2000). Chronic hypoxia upregulates the expression and function of AT(1) receptor in rat carotid body. *J. Endocrinol.* 167, 517–524. doi: 10.1677/joe.0.1670517

Li, S., Bjelobaba, I., and Stojilkovic, S. S. (2017). Interactions of Pannexin1 channels with purinergic and NMDA receptor channels. *Biochim. Biophys. Acta.* 1860, 166–173. doi: 10.1016/j.bbamem.2017.03.025

Livermore, S., and Nurse, C. A. (2013). Enhanced adenosine A2b receptor signaling facilitates stimulus-induced catecholamine secretion in chronically hypoxic carotid body type I cells. *Am. J. Physiol. Cell Physiol.* 305, C739–C750. doi: 10.1152/ajpcell.00137.2013

Locovei, S., Wang, J., and Dahl, G. (2006). Activation of pannexin 1 channels by ATP through P2Y receptors and by cytoplasmic calcium. *FEBS Lett.* 580, 239–244. doi: 10.1016/j.febslet.2005.12.004

Lohman, A. W., and Isakson, B. E. (2014). Differentiating connexin hemichannels and pannexin channels in cellular ATP release. *FEBS Lett.* 588, 1379–1388. doi: 10.1016/j.febslet.2014.02.004

López-Barneo, J. (2003). Oxygen and glucose sensing by carotid body glomus cells. *Curr. Opin. Neurobiol.* 13, 493–499. doi: 10.1016/S0959-4388(03)00093-X

López-Barneo, J., González-Rodríguez, P., Gao, L., Fernández-Agüera, M. C., Pardal, R., and Ortega-Sáenz, P. (2016). Oxygen sensing by the carotid body: mechanisms and role in adaptation to hypoxia. *Am. J. Physiol. Cell Physiol.* 310, C629–C642. doi: 10.1152/ajpcell.00265.2015

McDonald, D. M. (1981). "Peripheral chemoreceptors: structure-function relationships of the carotid body," in *Regulation of Breathing, Lung Biology in Health and Disease,* Vol. 17, ed T. F. Horbein (New York, NY: Marcel Dekker), 105–320.

McQueen, D. S., and Ribeiro, J. A. (1983). On the specificity and type of receptor involved in carotid body chemoreceptor activation by adenosine in the cat. *Br. J. Pharmacol.* 80, 347–354. doi: 10.1111/j.1476-5381.1983.tb10040.x

Milsom, W. K., and Burleson, M. L. (2007). Peripheral arterial chemoreceptors and the evolution of the carotid body. *Respir. Physiol. Neurobiol.* 157, 4–11. doi: 10.1016/j.resp.2007.02.007

Monteiro, E. C., and Ribeiro, J. A. (1987). Ventilatory effects of adenosine mediated by carotid body chemoreceptors in the rat. *Naunyn Schmiedebergs. Arch. Pharmacol.* 335, 143–148. doi: 10.1007/BF00177715

Murali, S., and Nurse, C. A. (2016). Purinergic signalling mediates bidirectional crosstalk between chemoreceptor type I and glial-like type II cells of the rat carotid body. *J. Physiol.* 594, 391–406. doi: 10.1113/JP271494

Murali, S., Zhang, M., and Nurse, C. A. (2014). Angiotensin II mobilizes intracellular calcium and activates pannexin-1 channels in rat carotid body type II cells via AT1 receptors. *J. Physiol.* 592, 4747–4762. doi: 10.1113/jphysiol.2014.279299

Murali, S., Zhang, M., and Nurse, C. A. (2015). Paracrine signaling in glial-like type II cells of the rat carotid body. *Adv. Exp. Med. Biol.* 860, 41–47. doi: 10.1007/978-3-319-18440-1_5

Murali, S., Zhang, M., and Nurse, C. A. (2017). Evidence that 5-HT stimulates intracellular Ca^{2+} signalling and activates pannexin-1 currents in type II cells of the rat carotid body. *J. Physiol.* 595, 4261–4277. doi: 10.1113/JP273473

Niane, L., Joseph, V., and Bairam, A. (2009). Role of cholinergic-nicotinic receptors on hypoxic chemoreflex during postnatal development in rats. *Respir. Physiol. Neurobiol.* 169, 323–332. doi: 10.1016/j.resp.2009.09.014

Niane, L. M., Donnelly, D. F., Joseph, V., and Bairam, A. (2011). Ventilatory and carotid body chemoreceptor responses to purinergic P2X receptor antagonists in newborn rats. *J. Appl. Physiol.* 110, 83–94. doi: 10.1152/japplphysiol.00871.2010

Niane, L. M., Joseph, V., and Bairam, A. (2012). Systemic blockade of nicotinic and purinergic receptors inhibits ventilation and increases apnoea frequency in newborn rats. *Exp. Physiol.* 97, 981–993. doi: 10.1113/expphysiol.2012.065011

Nurse, C. A. (2005). Neurotransmission and neuromodulation in the chemosensory carotid body. *Auton. Neurosci.* 120, 1–9. doi: 10.1016/j.autneu.2005.04.008

Nurse, C. A. (2010). Neurotransmitter and neuromodulatory mechanisms at peripheral arterial chemoreceptors. *Exp. Physiol.* 95, 657–667. doi: 10.1113/expphysiol.2009.049312

Nurse, C. A. (2014). Synaptic and paracrine mechanisms at carotid body arterial chemoreceptors. *J. Physiol.* 592, 3419–3426. doi: 10.1113/jphysiol.2013.269829

Nurse, C. A., Leonard, E. M., and Salman, S. (2018). The role of glial-like type II cells as paracrine modulators of carotid body chemoreception. *Physiol. Gemomics.* doi: 10.1152/physiolgenomics.00142.2017. [Epub ahead of print].

Nurse, C. A., and Piskuric, N. A. (2013). Signal processing at mammalian carotid body chemoreceptors. *Semin. Cell Dev. Biol.* 24, 22–30. doi: 10.1016/j.semcdb.2012.09.006

Nurse, C. A., and Zhang, M. (1999). Acetylcholine contributes to hypoxic chemotransmission in co-cultures of rat type 1 cells and petrosal neurons. *Respir. Physiol.* 115, 189–199. doi: 10.1016/S0034-5687(99)00017-1

Peers, C., and Buckler, K. J. (1995). Transduction of chemostimuli by the type I carotid body cell. *J. Membr. Biol.* 144, 1–9. doi: 10.1007/BF00238411

Penuela, S., Gehi, R., and Laird, D. W. (2015). The biochemistry and function of pannexin channels. *Biochim. Biophys. Acta* 1828, 15–22. doi: 10.1016/j.bbamem.2012.01.017

Piskuric, N. A., and Nurse, C. A. (2012). Effects of chemostimuli on $[Ca^{2+}]$i responses of rat aortic body type I cells and endogenous local neurons: comparison with carotid body cells. *J. Physiol.* 590, 2121–2135. doi: 10.1113/jphysiol.2012.229468

Platero-Luengo, A., Gonzalez-Granero, S., Duran, R., Diaz-Castro, B., Piruat, J. I., Garcia-Verdugo, J. M., et al. (2014). An O_2-sensitive glomus cell-stem cell synapse induces carotid body growth in chronic hypoxia. *Cell* 156, 291–303. doi: 10.1016/j.cell.2013.12.013

Powell, F. L. (2007). The influence of chronic hypoxia upon chemoreception. *Respir. Physiol. Neurobiol.* 157, 154–161. doi: 10.1016/j.resp.2007.01.009

Prabhakar, N. R., and Jacono, F. J. (2005). Cellular and molecular mechanisms associated with carotid body adaptations to chronic hypoxia. *High Alt. Med. Biol.* 6, 112–120. doi: 10.1089/ham.2005.6.112

Prabhakar, N. R., and Peng, Y. J. (2017). oxygen sensing by the carotid body: past and present. *Adv. Exp. Med. Biol.* 977, 3–8. doi: 10.1007/978-3-319-55231-6_1

Prabhakar, N. R., Peng, Y. J., Kumar, G. K., and Nanduri, J. (2015). Peripheral chemoreception and arterial pressure responses to intermittent hypoxia. *Compr. Physiol.* 5, 561–577. doi: 10.1002/cphy.c140039

Prasad, M., Fearon, I. M., Zhang, M., Laing, M., Vollmer, C., and Nurse, C. A. (2001). Expression of P2X2 and P2X3 receptor subunits in rat carotid body afferent neurones: role in chemosensory signalling. *J. Physiol.* 537, 667–677. doi: 10.1113/jphysiol.2001.012836

Rakoczy, R. J., and Wyatt, C. N. (2017). Acute oxygen-sensing by the carotid body: a rattlebag of molecular mechanisms. *J. Physiol.* doi: 10.1113/JP274351. [Epub ahead of print].

Reyes, E. P., Fernández, R., Larraín, C., and Zapata, P. (2007). Effects of combined cholinergic-purinergic block upon cat carotid body chemoreceptors *in vitro*. *Respir. Physiol. Neurobiol.* 156, 17–22. doi: 10.1016/j.resp.2006.07.007

Robson, S. C., Wu, Y., Sun, X., Knosalla, C., Dwyer, K., and Enjyoji, K. (2005). Ectonucleotidases of CD39 family modulate vascular inflammation and thrombosis in transplantation. *Semin. Thromb. Hemost.* 31, 217–233. doi: 10.1055/s-2005-869527

Rong, W., Gourine, A. V., Cockayne, D. A., Xiang, Z., Ford, A. P., Spyer, K. M., et al. (2003). Pivotal role of nucleotide P2X2 receptor subunit of the ATP-gated ion channel mediating ventilatory responses to hypoxia. *J. Neurosci.* 23, 11315–11321.

Salman, S., Vollmer, C., McClelland, G. B., and Nurse, C. A. (2017). Characterization of ectonucleotidase expression in the rat carotid body: regulation by chronic hypoxia. *Am. J. Physiol. Cell Physiol.* 313, C274–C284. doi: 10.1152/ajpcell.00328.2016

Schultz, H. D., Marcus, N. J., and Del Rio, R. (2015). Mechanisms of carotid body chemoreflex dysfunction during heart failure. *Exp. Physiol.* 100, 124–129. doi: 10.1113/expphysiol.2014.079517

Shirahata, M., Balbir, A., Otsubo, T., and Fitzgerald, R. S. (2007). Role of acetylcholine in neurotransmission of the carotid body. *Respir. Physiol. Neurobiol.* 157, 93–105. doi: 10.1016/j.resp.2006.12.010

Thompson, C. M., Troche, K., Jordan, H. L., Barr, B. L., and Wyatt, C. N. (2010). Evidence for functional, inhibitory, histamine H3 receptors in rat carotid body Type I cells. *Neurosci. Lett.* 471, 15–19. doi: 10.1016/j.neulet.2009.12.077

Thompson, E. L., Ray, C. J., Holmes, A. P., Pye, R. L., Wyatt, C. N., Coney, A. M., et al. (2016). Adrenaline release evokes hyperpnoea and an increase in ventilatory CO_2 sensitivity during hypoglycaemia: a role for the carotid body. *J. Physiol.* 594, 4439–4452. doi: 10.1113/JP272191

Thompson, R. J. (2015). Pannexin channels and ischaemia. *J. Physiol.* 593, 3463–3470. doi: 10.1113/jphysiol.2014.282426

Tse, A., Yan, L., Lee, A. K., and Tse, F. W. (2012). Autocrine and paracrine actions of ATP in rat carotid body. *Can. J. Physiol. Pharmacol.* 90, 705–711. doi: 10.1139/y2012-054

Varas, R., Alcayaga, J., and Iturriaga, R. (2003). ACh and ATP mediate excitatory transmission in cat carotid identified chemoreceptor units *in vitro*. *Brain Res.* 988, 154–163. doi: 10.1016/S0006-8993(03)03366-3

von Kügelgen, I. (2006). Pharmacological profiles of cloned mammalian P2Y-receptor subtypes. *Pharmacol. Ther.* 110, 415–432. doi: 10.1016/j.pharmthera.2005.08.014

Walsh, M. P., and Marshall, J. M. (2006). The role of adenosine in the early respiratory and cardiovascular changes evoked by chronic hypoxia in the rat. *J. Physiol.* 575, 277–289. doi: 10.1113/jphysiol.2006.108779

Xu, F., Xu, J., Tse, F. W., and Tse, A. (2006). Adenosine stimulates depolarization and rise in cytoplasmic $[Ca^{2+}]$ in type I cells of rat carotid bodies. *Am. J. Physiol. Cell Physiol.* 290, C1592–C1598. doi: 10.1152/ajpcell.00546.2005

Xu, J., Tse, F. W., and Tse, A. (2003). ATP triggers intracellular Ca^{2+} release in type II cells of the rat carotid body. *J. Physiol.* 549, 739–747. doi: 10.1113/jphysiol.2003.039735

Xu, J., Xu, F., Tse, F. W., and Tse, A. (2005). ATP inhibits the hypoxia response in type I cells of rat carotid bodies. *J. Neurochem.* 92, 1419–1430. doi: 10.1111/j.1471-4159.2004.02978.x

Zapata, P. (2007). Is ATP a suitable co-transmitter in carotid body arterial chemoreceptors? *Respir. Physiol. Neurobiol.* 157, 106–115. doi: 10.1016/j.resp.2007.01.002

Zhang, M., Clarke, K., Zhong, H., Vollmer, C., and Nurse, C. A. (2009). Postsynaptic action of GABA in modulating sensory transmission in co-cultures of rat carotid body via GABA(A) receptors. *J. Physiol.* 587, 329–344. doi: 10.1113/jphysiol.2008.165035

Zhang, M., Fearon, I. M., Zhong, H., and Nurse, C. A. (2003). Presynaptic modulation of rat arterial chemoreceptor function by 5-HT: role of K^+ channel inhibition via protein kinase C. *J. Physiol.* 551, 825–842. doi: 10.1113/jphysiol.2002.038489

Zhang, M., and Nurse, C. A. (2004). CO2/pH chemosensory signaling in co-cultures of rat carotid body receptors and petrosal neurons: role of ATP and ACh. *J. Neurophysiol.* 92, 3433–3445. doi: 10.1152/jn.01099.2003

Zhang, M., Piskuric, N. A., Vollmer, C., and Nurse, C. A. (2012). P2Y2 receptor activation opens pannexin-1 channels in rat carotid body type II cells: potential role in amplifying the neurotransmitter ATP. *J. Physiol.* 590, 4335–4350. doi: 10.1113/jphysiol.2012.236265

Zhang, M., Vollmer, C., and Nurse, C. A. (2017). Adenosine and dopamine oppositely modulate a hyperpolarization-activated current I_h in chemosensory neurons of the rat carotid body in co-culture. *J. Physiol.* doi: 10.1113/JP274743. [Epub ahead of print].

Zhang, M., Zhong, H., Vollmer, C., and Nurse, C. A. (2000). Co-release of ATP and ACh mediates hypoxic signalling at rat carotid body chemoreceptors. *J. Physiol.* 525(Pt 1), 143–158. doi: 10.1111/j.1469-7793.2000.t01-1-00143.x

Zhong, H., and Nurse, C. A. (1997). Nicotinic acetylcholine sensitivity of rat petrosal sensory neurons in dissociated cell culture. *Brain Res.* 766, 153–161. doi: 10.1016/S0006-8993(97)00526-X

Zhong, H., Zhang, M., and Nurse, C. A. (1999). Electrophysiological characterization of 5-HT receptors on rat petrosal neurons in dissociated cell culture. *Brain Res.* 816, 544–553.

Zhou, T., Chien, M. S., Kaleem, S., and Matsunami, H. (2016). Single cell transcriptome analysis of mouse carotid body glomus cells. *J. Physiol.* 594, 4225–4251. doi: 10.1113/JP271936

Zimmermann, H. (2000). Extracellular metabolism of ATP and other nucleotides. *Naunyn Schmiedebergs. Arch. Pharmacol.* 362, 299–309. doi: 10.1007/s002100000309

4

Long-Term Intermittent Work at High Altitude: Right Heart Functional and Morphological Status and Associated Cardiometabolic Factors

Julio Brito[1], Patricia Siques[1], Rosario López[2], Raul Romero[1], Fabiola León-Velarde[3], Karen Flores[1], Nicole Lüneburg[4], Juliane Hannemann[4] and Rainer H. Böger[4]*

[1] Institute of Health Studies, University Arturo Prat, Iquique, Chile, [2] Department of Preventive Medicine and Public Health, University Autonoma of Madrid, Madrid, Spain, [3] Department of Biological and Physiological Sciences, Facultad de Ciencias y Filosofía/IIA, University Peruana Cayetano Heredia, Lima, Peru, [4] Institute of Clinical Pharmacology and Toxicology, University Medical Center Hamburg-Eppendorf, Hamburg, Germany

***Correspondence:**
Julio Brito
jbritor@tie.cl

Background: Living at high altitude or with chronic hypoxia implies functional and morphological changes in the right ventricle and pulmonary vasculature with a 10% prevalence of high-altitude pulmonary hypertension (HAPH). The implications of working intermittently (day shifts) at high altitude (hypobaric hypoxia) over the long term are still not well-defined. The aim of this study was to evaluate the right cardiac circuit status along with potentially contributory metabolic variables and distinctive responses after long exposure to the latter condition.

Methods: A cross-sectional study of 120 healthy miners working at an altitude of 4,400–4,800 m for over 5 years in 7-day commuting shifts was designed. Echocardiography was performed on day 2 at sea level. Additionally, biomedical and biochemical variables, Lake Louise scores (LLSs), sleep disturbances and physiological variables were measured at altitude and at sea level.

Results: The population was 41.8 ± 0.7 years old, with an average of 14 ± 0.5 (range 5–29) years spent at altitude. Most subjects still suffered from mild to moderate symptoms of acute mountain sickness (mild was an LLS of 3–5 points, including cephalea; moderate was LLS of 6–10 points) (38.3%) at the end of day 1 of the shift. Echocardiography showed a 23% mean pulmonary artery pressure (mPAP) >25 mmHg, 9% HAPH (≥30 mmHg), 85% mild increase in right ventricle wall thickness (≥5 mm), 64% mild right ventricle dilation, low pulmonary vascular resistance (PVR) and fairly good ventricle performance. Asymmetric dimethylarginine (ADMA) (OR 8.84 (1.18–66.39); $p < 0.05$) and insulin (OR: 1.11 (1.02–1.20); $p < 0.05$) were associated with elevated mPAP and were defined as a cut-off. Interestingly, the correspondence analysis identified association patterns of several other variables (metabolic, labor, and biomedical) with higher mPAP.

Conclusions: Working intermittently at high altitude involves a distinctive pattern. The most relevant and novel characteristics are a greater prevalence of elevated mPAP and HAPH than previously reported at chronic intermittent hypobaric hypoxia (CIHH), which is accompanied by subsequent morphological characteristics. These findings are associated with cardiometabolic factors (insulin and ADMA). However, the functional repercussions seem to be minor or negligible. This research contributes to our understanding and surveillance of this unique model of chronic intermittent high-altitude exposure.

Keywords: high-altitude pulmonary hypertension, chronic intermittent hypobaric hypoxia, altitude, right heart, insulin and ADMA

INTRODUCTION

The right cardiac circuit (rather than the left) of high-altitude populations living in chronic hypobaric hypoxia (CH) undergoes major changes. These changes are characterized by elevated pulmonary artery pressure (PAP), right ventricle hypertrophy, and heart and pulmonary vessel remodeling. Some individuals develop high-altitude pulmonary hypertension (HAPH). Individuals who relocate to live permanently at altitude display the same phenomena (Penaloza and Arias-Stella, 2007). A complex series of pathophysiological and physiological mechanisms are responsible for the responses to hypoxia. The first described mechanism is hypoxic pulmonary vasoconstriction (HPV) (von Euler and Liljestrand, 1946), which is followed by several metabolic and molecular alterations, such as an imbalance between endothelial vasoconstrictors and vasodilators, reactive oxygen species (ROS) (Chen et al., 2012), and some associated factors, including insulin and asymmetric dimethylarginine (ADMA) (Richalet and Pichon, 2014; Lüneburg et al., 2016).

Recently, a new type of exposure to altitude has been of interest: long-term chronic intermittent hypobaric hypoxia (CIHH), which has been acknowledged as a distinct pathophysiological condition, including higher blood pressure at altitude and acute mountain sickness persistence on day 1 (Richalet et al., 2002; Brito et al., 2007). This exposure implies long-term exposure to shifts of 4 to 15 days at an altitude above 3,500 m, which are followed by a resting period of the same number of days at sea level (Richalet et al., 2002; West, 2002). Mining, observatory, army, and frontier control personnel are frequently exposed to these conditions, and their numbers are dramatically increasing. In Chile alone, it has been estimated that there are over 65,000 workers exposed to this condition (Brito et al., 2007). Therefore, many aspects of the underlying molecular mechanisms and clinical consequences are not well-known. Some studies in humans have demonstrated changes in the right heart circulation that are similar to those occurring in CH, such as a rise in PAP and right ventricular enlargement and/or hypertrophy (Richalet et al., 2002; Sarybaev et al., 2003; Brito et al., 2007). Remodeling of pulmonary vessels has also been demonstrated in animal models (Brito et al., 2015). Notwithstanding, there is scarce research assessing these changes over long durations in larger groups of individuals or looking for new potential associations with other physiological and biochemical variables as associated factors.

The endothelium has been known to play an important role in the regulation of systemic and pulmonary vascular tone, which mainly occurs by secreting the potent vasodilator nitric oxide (NO). NO is synthesized by endothelial NO synthase (NOS), which is competitively inhibited by the endogenous compound asymmetric dimethylarginine ADMA (Böger, 2006). In contrast to ADMA, symmetric dimethylarginine (SDMA) does not directly interfere with NOS activity. Elevated levels of ADMA are a cause of vasoconstriction and high blood pressure and have been associated with a high risk of cardiovascular events and mortality (Zoccali et al., 2001; Böger et al., 2009a,b).

Animal research has already provided some information about molecular or functional interactions in CIHH. Interestingly, NO bioavailability and ROS production have been demonstrated to play a major role in vascular adaptation to altitude hypoxia (Siques et al., 2014b; Lüneburg et al., 2016; Waypa et al., 2016). The morphological, physiological and molecular changes appear to be similar to those occurring in CH, but they may be less pronounced in CIHH (Brito et al., 2008; Siques et al., 2014b; Lüneburg et al., 2016).

Thus, it was expected that altered right heart circuit status and possible associated factors (metabolic, labor, and physiological) would be found in people undergoing long intermittent work at high altitude. Therefore, a cross-sectional study was performed with the aim of determining the morphological and functional status of the right cardiac circuit in miners working intermittently at an altitude between 4,400 and 4,800 m for a period of more than 5 years. Moreover, the study assessed several physiological and metabolic factors to determine whether they were associated with cardiac parameters and whether some of these featured a distinctive response in the evaluated condition.

MATERIALS AND METHODS

Subjects and Study Design

A cross-sectional study was performed in a random sample of 120 healthy native Chilean male miners working in a mine settlement in the northern part of Chile at an altitude of 4,400 or 4,800 m (53

Abbreviations: BP, Blood pressure; SBP, Systolic blood pressure; DBP, Diastolic blood pressure; SPAP, Systolic pulmonary artery pressure; mPAP, Mean pulmonary artery pressure; RVWT, Right ventricle wall thickness; FCRV, Four-chamber right ventricle; RVOT, Right ventricle outflow track; RAA, Right atrium area; PVR, Pulmonary vascular resistance; LVEF, Left ejection fraction; AD, Aortic diameter; TAPSE, Tricuspid annular plane systolic excursion; RV, Right ventricle; RVH, Right ventricle hypertrophy; ADMA, Asymmetric dimethylarginine; SDMA, Symmetric dimethylarginine; HP, Pulmonary hypertension; HAPH, High-altitude pulmonary hypertension; CIHH, Chronic intermittent hypobaric hypoxia; HPV, Hypoxic pulmonary vasoconstriction; WP, Waist perimeter; SL, Sea level.

and 47% of the study population, respectively) in a shift regimen (7 days at altitude followed by a resting period of 7 days at sea level). The miners slept at 3,800 m and worked a 12-h day shift at highest altitude, with the trip from the dormitories to the pit lasting 30 min. All subjects had undergone a medical examination and laboratory tests to determine altitude fitness. The inclusion criteria were working in shifts (7X7) at high altitude (above 4,000 m) for more than 5 years and a healthy status without serious comorbidities. The exclusion criteria were diabetes, hypertension, diagnosed obstructive sleep apnea, supplementary oxygen in the dormitories and any cardiopulmonary disease.

Written informed consent was obtained from all participants in accordance with the Declaration of Helsinki. The study was approved by the Research Ethics Committee of Universidad Arturo Prat, Iquique, Chile.

Measured Variables

Measures were taken (1) at altitude (at the mine's health facility) early in the morning 18 h after arrival (after one night's sleep) and (2) at sea level (SL) at an ambulatory medical facility in Iquique, Chile during day 2 of the resting period. An exact definition of the measurement time of each variable is provided below.

General Data

Age, weight, height, body mass index (BMI), calculated as weight (kg) divided by height squared (m^2), waist perimeter (WP), smoking habit, years at altitude, physical activity and medical status were assessed during the basal screening at SL.

Physiological Parameters

Systolic blood pressure (SBP), diastolic blood pressure (DBP), heart rate (HR), and hemoglobin oxygen saturation (SaO2) were determined at each study time point (at altitude and SL) in the morning. SBP and DBP were measured in the right arm of each participant while seated and after 5 min of rest using appropriately sized cuffs and calibrated standard mercury sphygmomanometers according to international guidelines (Chobanian et al., 2003; European Society of Hypertension-European Society of Cardiology Guidelines Committee, 2003). Heart rate was measured with an HR-100C Omron device (Omron, Health Care Inc.®, Bethesda, Maryland; USA), and SaO2 was determined using a finger pulse oximeter (POX050, Mediaid®, Cerritos, CA; USA). The mean of two measurements separated by a 5-min interval was taken as a valid determination of BP, HR, and SaO2. Same measures were obtained at SL for comparison.

Acute Mountain Sickness (AMS) and Sleep Measurements

The Lake Louise Score-AMS self-assessment test (LLS; Roach et al., 1993), validated in similar Chilean populations (Richalet et al., 2002; Brito et al., 2007), was performed at altitude 18 h after arrival, including the first night's sleep. AMS was diagnosed when headache and at least one other symptom occurred and a LLSs of ≥ 3 was reached. Severity was assessed according to the following categories: mild (3–4), moderate (5–10), and severe (11–15) (Hackett, 2003). The modified Spiegel questionnaire, validated in similar populations (Richalet et al., 2002; Brito et al., 2007), was recorded to assess sleep status at the same time. Both scores were obtained at SL for comparison.

Hematological and Biochemical Measurements

Blood samples were taken at SL in the morning after 8 h of fasting through venous puncture without stasis: hematocrit (Htc), hemoglobin (Hb), lipid profile, glycemia, and insulin. Additionally, insulin sensitivity or resistance [homeostatic model assessment (HOMA-IR) index] was calculated by HOMA program V.2.2 (Diabetes trial unit, University of Oxford). The biomarkers asymmetric dimethylarginine (ADMA) and symmetric dimethylarginine (SDMA) were measured using a validated liquid chromatographic–tandem mass spectrometric assay as described previously (Schwedhelm, 2005). The ADMA reference range is ≤ 0.732 μmol/L, which was derived from a large population-based cohort (Schwedhelm et al., 2009). An SDMA reference range of ≤ 0.53 μmol/L was later established by the same author (Schwedhelm et al., 2011).

Echocardiographic Assessment

An echocardiographic assessment was performed by two experienced cardiologists at SL facilities, in the morning after a 1 h rest, using an echocardiograph (GE Vivid-I®, GE Healthcare Systems, Tirat Carmel, Israel) with a 1.5–3.6 MHz phased array probe. Left ventricular end diastolic and end systolic measurements and left ventricular septal and posterior wall thicknesses were obtained from parasternal long axis view in M-mode with the ultrasound beam aligned to tips of mitral leaflets. Left ventricular ejection fraction (LVEF) was calculated from the M-mode recordings using Teichholtz formula (Teichholz et al., 1976). Right heart measurements were obtained after aligning the tip of ultrasound beam at true left ventricular apex. Pulmonary ejection time and pulmonary acceleration times were obtained with pulse Doppler recordings of the pulmonary valve from a parasternal short axis view at aortic valve level. Mean pulmonary artery pressure (mPAP) was calculated from pulmonary acceleration time according to Mahan formulas (Dabestani et al., 1987). Tricuspid annular systolic excursion was measured in M-mode from an apical four-chamber view with the ultrasound beam aligned to the lateral aspect of the tricuspid annulus. Right ventricular free wall thickness (RVWT) was obtained from a subcostal four-chamber view. Tricuspid annular plane systolic excursion (TAPSE index) was used for right ventricle (RV) performance (Kaul et al., 1984; López et al., 2012). Pulmonary vascular resistance (PVR) was calculated according to the formula described by Abbas et al. (2003). Similarly, other authors have noted that echocardiography for right heart assessment, including pulmonary hypertension, has shown a high correlation (r^2) with invasive right heart catheterization (Kojonazarov et al., 2007; Taleb et al., 2013). All measurements and reference values were acquired according to American Society of Echocardiography Guidelines (Rudski et al., 2010). Two separate cut-off criteria were studied to define pulmonary hypertension (PH): (a) HAPH's consensus (León-Velarde et al., 2005), which is defined at mPAP ≥ 30 mmHg, and (b) SL PH's criteria (Rubin and American College of Chest Physicians, 2004), which is defined at mPAP ≥25 mmHg. The reason for including the SL cut-off was two-fold: (1) because the echocardiogram was performed at SL and (2) to have a comparative panorama since the current condition under examination entailed a substantial period of both high-altitude and SL exposure.

Data Analysis

All data were entered into a database and analyzed using IBM SPSS, V21.0® statistical package (Armonk, NY, USA). For qualitative variables, absolute and relative frequencies were calculated. For quantitative variables, proportions, means, standard deviations, and standard errors were calculated. Normality of the distribution was checked using Kolmogorov–Smirnov test. All variables, except for LLS, were normally distributed. Therefore, a non-parametric Wilcoxon Test was used for LLS. Student's t-test for related or independent samples was used as appropriate. Pearson's chi-square test was used for proportional differences for independent variables. Additionally, Pearson's correlation was performed between quantitative variables. Binary logistic regression models were used to assess the association of all variables measured with the mPAP using two different cut-offs (<30 vs. ≥30 mmHg and <25 vs. ≥25 mmHg). After univariate analyses of all variables, the statistically significant variables were introduced into a multivariable logistic regression model using the forward stepwise method. The results were presented as crude (mutually adjusted) odds ratios (OR) and 95% confidence intervals (CI). The significance level was established at $p < 0.05$.

To look for association patterns, a multiple correspondence analysis was performed between categorical variables, which might display a more comprehensive panorama. Biomedical, occupational and metabolic variables were chosen and dichotomized at their normal values. The graph and variances of each dimension are provided. Angles <60° are considered as association and the longer distance of the variable from its origin the better represented. A Cronbach's alpha of >0.50 was considered appropriate.

RESULTS

General Characteristics

The study group was 120 miners with a mean age of 41.8 ± 0.7 years and a mean exposure to CIHH of 14 ± 0.5 years. Most study participants were overweight (BMI: 26.3 ± 0.3 kg/m^2) and sedentary (<3 weekly <30 min moderate exercise sessions, according to Chilean criteria) (MINSAL Ministerio de Salud, 2006), and a third of them were current smokers. **Table 1** gives a complete overview of the demographic and anthropometric characteristics of the study group.

TABLE 1 | General characteristics of chronic intermittent hypoxia group.

Variables	$\bar{X}$ ± SE; (range)	%
Age (years old)	41.8 ± 0.7 (20–58)	
<40		40.8
≥40		59.2
Years at altitude	13.9 ± 0.5 (05–29)	
5–<10		20.8
≥10		79.2
Altitude of work (m)	4.600 ± 0.2 (4.400–4.800)	
4,400		53.3
4,800		46.7
BMI (kg/m^2)	26.3 ± 0.3 (16.6–34.9)	
<25		36.7
≥25–<29.9		52.5
≥30		10.8
Waist Perimeter (cm)	97.1 ± 09 (61–121)	
≤100		67.5
>100		32.5
Smoking Status		
Yes		34.2
No		65.8
Sedentary		
Yes		80.2
No		19.2

Values for quantitative variables are means ($\bar{X}$) ± standard error (SE) and ranges; values for qualitative variables are proportions (%).

TABLE 2 | Physiological parameters.

Variables	$\bar{X}$ +SE SL	$\bar{X}$ +SE Altitude	p
SBP	109.4 ± 1.0	126.2 ± 1.0	<0.001
DBP	69.9 ± 0.9	81.0 ± 0.7	<0.001
HR	71.5 ± 1.1	82.0 ± 1.0	<0.001
SaO2	97.7 ± 0.1	89.6 ± 0.3	<0.001
LL	0.61 ± 0.1	2.7 ± 0.2	<0.001
Spiegel test	10.6 ± 0.3	14.5 ± 0.4	<0.001

Systolic blood pressure (SBP; mmHg), diastolic blood pressure (DBP; mmHg), heart rate (HR; b/m), hemoglobin oxygen saturation (SaO2; %), Lake Louise (score) and Spiegel test (score), at sea level (SL) and at altitude. Values are means ($\bar{X}$)±SE (standard error), and p was obtained from t-test of related samples.

Physiological Parameters

As expected, both SBP and DBP were higher at altitude than at SL, along with a slight increase in HR. Approximately 40% of the subjects had elevated SBP at altitude (≥130 mmHg, $p < 0.01$), and 18% had elevated DBP (≥90 mmHg, $p < 0.05$). SaO2 differed between SL and altitude in proportion to the level of altitude. However, 30% of the study population had SaO2 levels ≤88% at altitude (**Table 2**).

AMS and Sleep Disturbances

Despite long exposure to high altitude, a rather high proportion of individuals showed AMS (38.4%) on the first day, which was mainly moderate, and remarkably many study participants had cephalea (47.5%). Most individuals declared that they had mainly regular non-satisfactory sleep (75%), whereas the sleep disturbances and AMS measured at SL were minimal (20% and

TABLE 3 | Hematological and biochemical measurements at sea level.

Variables	$\overline{X}$± SE	Reference range
Hematocrit (%)	47.6 ± 0.3	41–49
Hemoglobin (mg/dL)	16.2 ± 0.1	13.0–17.5
Total cholesterol (mg/dL)	193.1 ± 3.3	50–200
HDL-cholesterol (mg/dL)	43.3 ± 0.8	40–60
LDL-cholesterol (mg/dL)	114.5 ± 2.8	80–125
VLDL-cholesterol (mg/dL)	35.3 ± 1.8	10–35
Triglycerides (mg/dL)	175.9 ± 8.9	30–150
Total cholesterol/ HDL-cholesterol	4.5 ± 0.1	3
LDL-cholesterol/HDL-cholesterol	2.8 ± 0.9	3
Glycemia (mg/dL)	89.4 ± 1.3	90–110
Insulinemia (IU)	11.4 ± 0.6	10–20
Homeostatic model assessment (HOMA-IR)	1.4 ± 0.8	2.6
Asymmetric dimethylarginine (ADMA; μmol/L)	0.83 ± 0.2	0.73
Symmetric dimethylarginine (SDMA; μmol/L)	0.54 ± 0.2	0.53

Values are means ($\overline{X}$) ±standard error (SE) and reference range.

12.5%, respectively). The presence of AMS was significantly associated with mPAP ≥25 and mPAP ≥30 mmHg ($p < 0.05$).

Hematocrit and Hemoglobin

Mean Htc and Hb were almost within the normal range (70% below 17 mg/dL). Only two individuals had Hb values of 19 mg/dL, and none had Hb above 21 mg/dL (**Table 3**).

Lipid Profile

In 48% of the individuals, triglycerides were elevated above 150 mg/dL, and mean triglycerides and VLDL-cholesterol was also elevated. Although mean total cholesterol was within the normal range, 42% of the study participants had values over 200 mg/dL. Mean HDL-cholesterol and LDL-cholesterol were within the respective normal ranges. The Castelli index (total cholesterol and HDL-cholesterol) was within its upper limit, and HDL/LDL index was normal (**Table 3**), although 20% of subjects had low HDL, and 30% had elevated LDL.

Glycemia, Insulin, and HOMA-IR

Mean glycemia and insulin values were within normal ranges. The mean HOMA-IR index was also normal (**Table 3**). However, for subjects with insulin above 20 IU (11%), the HOMA-IR index was 3.3 ± 0.2. Insulin was found to significantly correlate ($p < 0.01$) with BMI ($r = 0.34$); WP ($r = 0.39$), SBP at altitude ($r = 0.25$), VLDL and triglycerides (TG) (both $r = 0.25$) and mPAP ($r = 0.22$; $p < 0.05$).

Upon further analysis of the association of mean insulin levels with mPAP values, a distinctive difference in insulin concentrations at each cut-off point of mPAP was found. At mPAP ≥30 mmHg, mean insulin was 16.9 ± 2.14 IU, whereas at mPAP <30 mmHg, a lower mean insulin value was observed (10.6 ± 0.32 IU; p <0.01, **Figure 1A**). Those with high insulin levels had a higher HOMA-IR (**Figure 1B**). Moreover, this association was further corroborated by the correlation of HOMA-IR with higher mPAP ($r = 0.24$, p <0.001).

ADMA

Mean ADMA concentration was slightly elevated (0.83 ± 0.2 μmol/L) compared to the reference range (**Table 3**). Half of the subjects had ADMA concentrations ≥0.80 μmol/L. ADMA was positively correlated ($p < 0.05$) with WP ($r = 0.21$), Hb ($r = 0.20$), and SDMA ($r = 0.82$; $p < 0.001$). Most importantly, ADMA was correlated with mPAP ($r = 0.21$; $p < 0.05$) and RVWT ($r = 0.30$; p <0.001). Distinctly, mean ADMA concentration was 1.01 ± 0.15 μmol/L in subjects with mPAP ≥30 mmHg, as opposed to 0.81 ± 0.18 μmol/L in subjects with mPAP <30 mmHg ($p < 0.001$; **Figure 2**).

Echocardiographic Findings (mPAP and Morphological Status)

Most individuals had mPAP within normal ranges (73.9%) with wide variability. Nevertheless, 26.1% of the subjects had elevated values at a cut-off point of 25 mmHg, but only 9.2% could be categorized as truly HAPH (≥30 mmHg), and none exceeded an mPAP of 36 mmHg (**Table 4**).

Regarding morphological status, it was noted that 85% of the individuals had mild right ventricle hypertrophy (RVH), and over half showed a grade of right ventricular (RV) dilation supported by an increase in FCVR and right ventricle outflow track (RVOT) values. However, a minimal percentage (15%) of right atrium enlargement is seen (**Table 4**). A representative figure of RVH is shown in **Figure 3A**, and pulmonary acceleration curve at outflow tract in **Figure 3B**.

Most subjects display PVR within the normal range, except for 4.8% of the individuals, who have slightly increased PVR. Despite the latter finding, the subjects with mPAP ≥30 mmHg had a value of 1.33 Wood units vs. 1.04 Wood units with mPAP <30 mmHg (p <0.001). The RV performance index (TAPSE) shows no impairment and good performance in this group. For the left ventricle, the left ventricle ejection fraction is within the normal range and the aortic diameter is only mildly enlarged in 22.6% of the individuals (**Table 4**).

Some significantly positive correlations ($p < 0.01$) were found in all correlations performed between echocardiographic variables: (a) mPAP vs. RVWT $r = 0.39$, RVOT $r = 0.35$, and PVR $r = 0.40$; (b) RVWT vs. RVOT $r = 0.30$ and PVR $r = 0.22$; and (c) right atrium area (RAA) vs. four-chamber right ventricle (FCRV) $r = 0.44$ and PVR $r = 0.21$.

However, only two associations were shown when both cut-off values for mPAP (25 and 30 mmHg) were used in the univariate logistic regression and in the forward stepwise logistic multivariate regression final model. At the cut-off value of 25 mmHg, ADMA (OR 8.84; CI 1.18–66.39, $p < 0.05$) and insulin (OR: 1.07, CI 1.01–1.13, $p < 0.05$) showed an association. At the cut-off value of 30 mmHg, the same associations were observed: ADMA (OR: 10.74, CI 1.16–99.9, $p < 0.05$) and insulin (OR: 1.11, CI 1.02–1.20, $p < 0.05$). All OR were adjusted by smoking status, age, and BMI.

Multiple Correspondence Analysis

Because only two associations were found, a multiple correspondence analysis was performed. This statistical tool allows visualize association patterns or profiles between

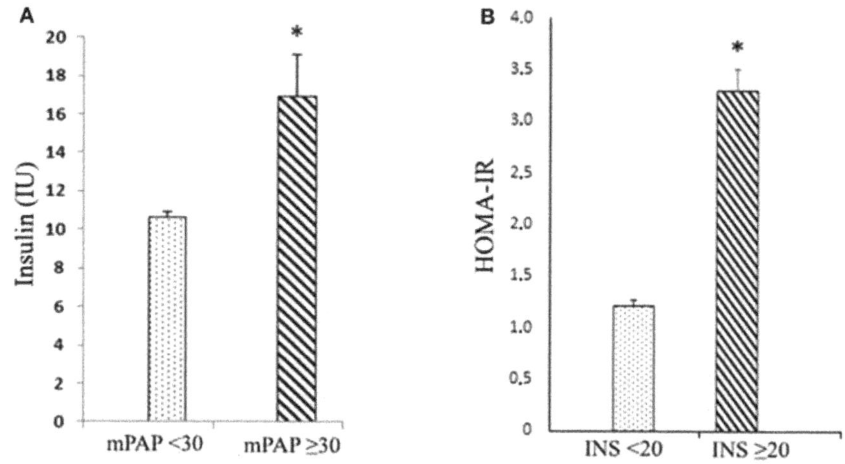

FIGURE 1 | Comparison between insulin, mPAP, and HOMA-IR **(A)** insulin (INS; IU) according to mean pulmonary artery pressure values (mPAP; mmHg); cut-off point $< \geq 30$ mmHg; and **(B)** homeostatic model assessment (HOMA-IR; Index) according to insulin values: cut-off point $< \geq 20$ IU. Values are means $(\bar{X}) \pm$SE (standard error); $^*p < 0.01$.

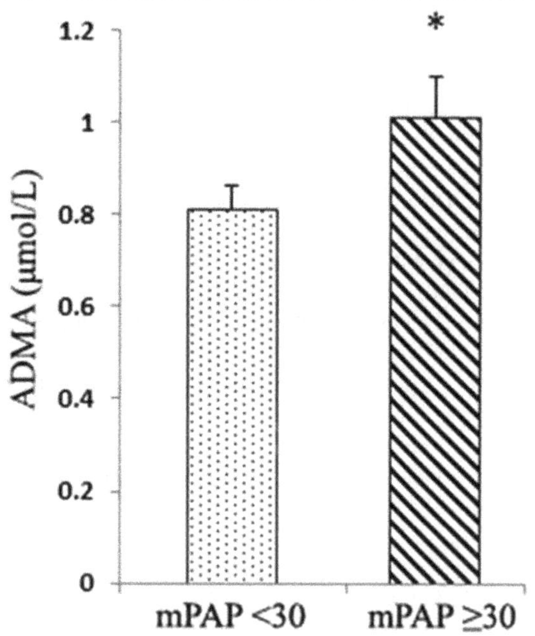

FIGURE 2 | Comparison of ADMA and mPAP (cut-off point $< \geq 30$ mmHg). Asymmetric dimethylarginine (ADMA; μmol/L); mean pulmonary artery pressures (mPAP; mmHg). Values are means $(\bar{X}) \pm$SE (standard error); $^*p <$ 0.01.

different dichotomized variables to be determined: occupational and biomedical (years old and years at altitude), metabolic (ADMA, insulin, triglycerides, BMI, and waist perimeter) and echocardiographic (right ventricle wall thickness and mPAP) were introduced. To interpret the graphical representation, category associations can be detected by their proximity whose reference is the angle formed with the coordinates origin (small angles between two categories indicates greater association) and the relative distance to the origin.

Therefore, on one hand, two different profiles are shown. In one profile, metabolic variables were within normal values, and age < 40 and years at altitude <15 were associated with mPAP $<$ 25. In the other profile, altered metabolic values, higher age, and over 15 years at altitude were found to be associated with mPAP $\geq$ 25. On the other hand, that mPAP $>$ 25 and $>$ 15HAyears are strongly associated (small angle), mPAP $>$25 and insulin $>$ 20 are moderately associated (medium angle) and mPAP $>$ 25 and age $<$ 40 (180 degree angle) suggest opposite directions (no association) are depicted (**Figure 4**). Interestingly, when the same procedure was performed with mPAP $\geq$ 30, the results were similar.

DISCUSSION

This cross-sectional study, in long-term CIHH working shifts at high altitude, has the following main findings: (1) a distinctive and unique pattern of physiological responses was determined, wherein a third of subjects showed moderate AMS persistence; (2) high proportions of elevated mPAP (26.1%) and HAPH (9.2%) were found by echocardiography; and (3) specific cardiometabolic variables (high triglycerides, insulin resistance, high ADMA, increased waist perimeter and BMI) appeared to be associated factors, with insulin and ADMA clearly associated with elevated mPAP.

General Aspects

This cross-sectional study with a large number of subjects working intermittently in a long-term CIHH at high altitude contributes three important concepts (mentioned above), which will be individually discussed for methodological reasons; however, these concepts appear to be related and intertwined as a whole.

TABLE 4 | Echocardiographic findings at sea level.

Variables	$\bar{X}$+ SE	Range	SL reference value	Out of reference value (%)
SPAP (mmHg)	27.6 ± 0.5	13.0–38.0	30	36
mPAP (mmHg) Mahan	20.2 ± 0.6	10.2–35.8	<25	73.9
≥25 overall	–		–	26.1
≥25–<30	–		–	16.9
≥30	–		–	9.2
RVWT (mm)	6.3 ± 0.1	4.0–10.0	<5	85
<5 mm				15
≥5 mm				85
FCRV (mm)	30.8 ± 0.4	23.0–43.0	<28	64
RVOT short axis (mm)	29.6 ± 0.4	23.0–39.0	27-30	45
<30 mm				55
≥30 mm				45
RAA (cm^2)	15.1 ± 0.2	10.0–24.0	<18	15
PVR (Wood units; 240 din/cm*s^2)	1.08 ± 0.02	0.59–1.76	<1.5	4.8
LVEF (%)	70.1 ± 0.7	50.0–87.0	≥56	4.2
AD (mm)	30.5 ± 0.3	21.0–41.0	<34	22.6
TAPSE index (cm)	2.3 ± 0.3	1.25–2.90	≥1.6	0.9

Systolic pulmonary artery pressure (SPAP), mean pulmonary artery pressure by Mahan (mPAP, right ventricle wall thickness (RVWT, four-chamber right ventricle (FCRV), right ventricle outflow track (RVOT), right atrium area (RAA), pulmonary vascular resistance (PVR), left ventricle ejection fraction (LVEF), aortic diameter (AD) and tricuspid annular plane systolic excursion (TAPSE). Values are means ($\bar{X}$) ± standard error (SE), range, sea level (SL) cut-off values (reference: American Society of Echocardiography; Rudski et al., 2010) and proportions out of reference value (%).

The first concept is that this population seems to share distinctive and unique features. In fact, there is a remarkable proportion of overweight and sedentarism, as has been previously reported (Esenamanova et al., 2014). Smoking habit proportion is similar to Chilean prevalence. Physiological responses are also coincident with previous reports in that BP rises at altitude but reaches normal values at SL. Moreover, it has been described that BP decreases after day 2 during the shift at high altitude, but it does not reach SL values (Richalet et al., 2002; Brito et al., 2007); nonetheless, a certain proportion of individuals maintain an SBP and DBP within a rather elevated range at altitude according to previous reports (Siques et al., 2009). Conversely, SaO2 drops at altitude and is fully recovered at SL, and the mean SaO2 reached at altitude is similar to acclimatized subjects; however, almost one-third of the subjects have lower SaO2 values, which could be explained by individual variability or a poor response to altitude (day 1's impact) (Brito et al., 2007). Additionally, coincident with previous reports in humans, Htc and Hb do not show pathological values or excessive erythrocytosis (Richalet et al., 2002; Brito et al., 2007; Siques et al., 2007). The latter adds support to the suggestion that under this regimen, high or excessive erythrocytosis is rare. Likewise, consistently high AMS presence (mostly moderate), cephalea and sleep disturbances despite the extensive elapsed time are additional distinctive features. These findings are also coincident with previous studies in which AMS was present during the first 1 or 2 days of a shift at high altitude (Richalet et al., 2002; Brito et al., 2007). However, some cohort studies have described a decline during following exposures (Richalet et al., 2002; Wu et al., 2009). The reasons are beyond the scope of this study, but may be due to an inability to acclimatize properly, the loss of acclimatization during the shift at SL or rapid ascent.

Metabolic Responses

Lipid Profile: TG and Total Cholesterol (T-Chol)

Another relevant result of this study are the changes in lipid profiles. It has been assumed by several authors that under CH or CIHH, individuals are prone to good metabolic features (Anderson and Honigman, 2011; Ezzati et al., 2012). However, recent evidence has shown that there is an increasing proportion of individuals with marked metabolic alteration (Mohanna et al., 2006), which would be related to chronic mountain sickness (Miele et al., 2016) and other altitude diseases (San Martin et al., 2017). In fact, our results support this observation; in this model of exposure, a rather high proportion (almost half of the subjects) displayed an altered lipid profile. Previous studies have consistently reported an increase in TG and contradictory results for T-Chol (Li et al., 2007; Siques et al., 2007). The most remarkable changes seen in this study are an increase in TG, VLDL and T-Chol, but the mean Castelli index remains at its upper limit.

Hypoxemia may disturb lipid metabolism by upregulating hepatic SCD-1, leading to *de novo* TG synthesis, an increase of adipose tissue lipolysis, lipoprotein secretion and decrease of lipoprotein clearance (Li et al., 2007; Drager et al., 2012; Siques et al., 2014a). Thus, it could be surmised that TG alteration could be another distinctive feature of exposure to CIHH and may be a matter of concern. Recognition of TG alteration as a cardiovascular risk factor is a growing issue (Assmann et al., 1996).

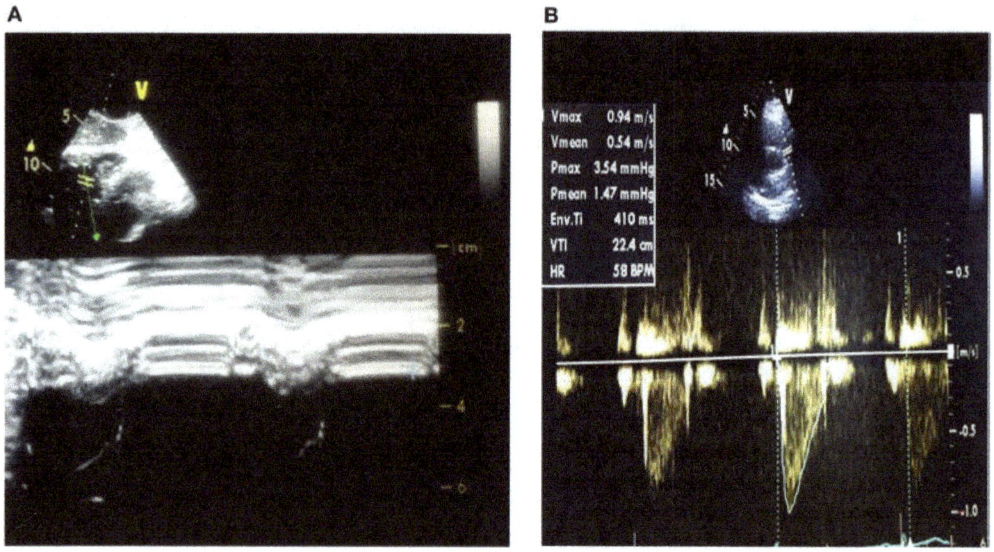

FIGURE 3 | Representative echocardiographic images **(A)** right ventricular hypertrophy and **(B)** Acceleration curve of pulmonary flow at pulmonary artery outflow tract.

Insulin, Insulin Resistance (IR)

Complementary to the above metabolic findings, insulin and IR have been noted as tightly related to the development of PH and could be considered associated factors (Zamanian et al., 2009). Their relation to HAPH is still to be demonstrated. However, the finding that the insulin level correlated to anthropometric variables (BMI and WP) and to mPAP—and this population is mostly overweight—might suggest a similar role in HAPH as has been reported either for IR (McLaughlin and Rich, 2004) and/or PH (Tarasevicìute and Voelkel, 2006) at SL. The findings of a cut-off point of different insulin values according to mPAP and that higher insulin values are also associated with higher mPAP further support insulin's role. IR may also share other pathophysiological conditions that are present under hypoxia, such as elevation of cytokines (interleukin-6, monocyte chemotactic protein) and ADMA (Zamanian et al., 2009). Recently, an inverse relationship between oxygen hemoglobin saturation and IR has been described in chronic hypoxia. There are many physiopathological explanations (Miele et al., 2016), including the disruption of leptin pathways (Polotsky et al., 2003).

ADMA as a Marker of Cardiometabolic Risk

ADMA is a competitive NOS inhibitor that has been identified as a regulator of NO production (Böger, 2006). ADMA is endogenously present in the human body and inhibits NO-dependent vasodilation *in vitro* (Vallance et al., 1992) and *in vivo* (Böger et al., 1998). ADMA is degraded by dimethylarginine dimethylaminohydrolase (DDAH). Disruption of the ADMA/DDAH pathway causes endothelial dysfunction and elevated blood pressure in the systemic and pulmonary circulation (Leiper et al., 2007). Therefore, the possible role of ADMA in HAPH is a focus of current research. The current results show a significant elevation of ADMA at altitude, and for the first time, they show a correlation of ADMA with both mPAP and right ventricle wall thickness, suggesting a pivotal pathophysiological role of this pathway in the development of pulmonary vascular dysfunction at high altitude. Moreover, a clear cut-off value of ADMA was observed according to mPAP.

Recently published data support the current findings. In rats subjected to long-term CIHH, an impaired NO pathway secondary to elevated ADMA and increased ROS were found (Siques et al., 2014b; Lüneburg et al., 2016). Furthermore, young healthy adults first exposed to CIHH develop elevated ADMA concentrations over the time (Lüneburg et al., 2017). Therefore, ADMA may be a useful biomarker for subjects with HAPH.

PAP and Right Heart Status

An increase in PAP is a well-known physiological response to hypoxia (von Euler and Liljestrand, 1946). Additionally, permanent residents have changes in their pulmonary vascular circuit that might account for a prevalence up to 10% of HAPH (León-Velarde et al., 2005; Penaloza and Arias-Stella, 2007). Unfortunately, most information comes from acute or chronic exposure and rarely from long-term CIHH; therefore, the described changes might not be entirely applicable to CIHH. Research conducted under different commuting exposure regimes in humans (2-year cohort, 30 × 30 shift; 2-year cohort, 7 × 7 shift) and in a 12-year cross-sectional study (5 × 2 shift) at altitudes between 3,550 and 4,400 m) also described an increase in mPAP, right ventricle enlargement or ventricle hypertrophy, although a small number of subjects was included (Richalet et al., 2002; Sarybaev et al., 2003; Brito et al., 2007). The latter author determined a 4% prevalence of HAPH in CIHH at 3,550 m. Interestingly, experimental studies in rats led to the suggestion that RV changes were achieved to a lesser extent in CIHH than in CH (Corno et al., 2004; Brito et al., 2008).

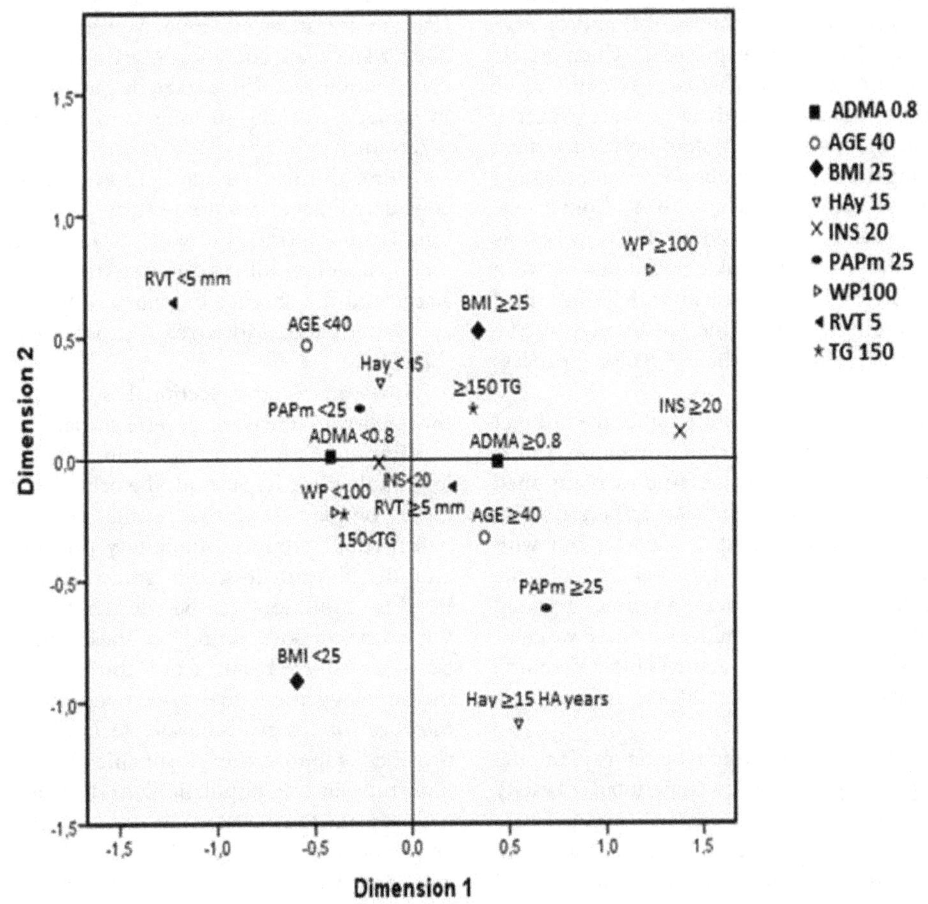

FIGURE 4 | Association patterns between variables by multiple correspondence analysis. Variables and cut-off points: asymmetric dimethylarginine (ADMA; μmol/L; $< \geq 0.8$), age (years old; $< \geq 40$), body mass index (BMI; kg/ m^2; $< \geq 25$), high-altitude years (HAy; $< \geq 15$ years), insulin (INS; IU; $< \geq 20$), mean pulmonary artery pressure (PAPm, mmHg; $< \geq 25$), waist perimeter (WP; cm; $< \geq 100$), right ventricle wall thickness (RVT; mm; $< \geq 5$) and triglycerides (TG; mg/dL; $< \geq 150$). Explained proportion of total variance of dimension 1 = 57.3% and dimension 2 = 42%. Cronbach's alpha: 0.594.

Despite several limitations (cross-sectional study, echocardiogram performed at SL, only clinical functional capacity assessment and previously selected subjects for high-altitude work) of the current study, the results showed a strikingly high proportion of mPAP over 25 mmHg with a proportion of HAPH greater than previously reported that is similar to the prevalence in CH. Likewise, it could well be inferred that subsequent pulmonary vasculature remodeling triggered by HPV was present, as reported in CH (Penaloza and Arias-Stella, 2007; Sylvester et al., 2012) and reproduced in rats under long-term CIHH (Brito et al., 2015). Similarly, in light of the results and despite the concept of "turn on-turn off" biological responses in this condition (Powell and Garcia, 2000), it seems reasonable to infer that in the current model, individuals undertake a more prolonged pulmonary hypertensive state than expected in this condition at high altitude.

Moreover, the HAPH levels found in this study could be considered mild, which is supported by the fact that no subjects had mPAP values over 36 mmHg and that the subjects had a current healthy status without claims of functional capacity impairment. The lack of functional repercussions (Penaloza et al., 1963) and a mild or moderate HAPH have been described for CH and acute hypoxia (Naeije and Dedobbeleer, 2013); this phenomenon has been noted as the paradox of HAPH (Grover, 2014). Nevertheless, some disputes still exist regarding exercise capacity at high altitude and HAPH. In fact, a recent study of Kyrgyz highlanders with HAPH found a mild reduction in exercise performance and reduced quality of life (Latshang et al., 2017). Accordingly, these rather contradictory findings have led to introduction of the concept of "pulmonary vascular reserve" as a complex mechanism that determines good or poor exercise capacity (Groepenhoff et al., 2012; Naeije and Dedobbeleer, 2013; Pavelescu et al., 2013).

Likewise, this study also shows a striking proportion of RVWT enlargement, suggesting that in the long term, almost all subjects experience RV remodeling and that an mPAP value of 25 mmHg would be sufficient to generate significant changes in the right heart. Whether this is merely an acclimatization response in this model of exposure that causes the RV to increase its performance as a consequence of its homeometric adaptation to afterload increase (Kolár and Ostádal, 1991; Naeije and Dedobbeleer, 2013; Richalet and Pichon, 2014) and/or ROS activation by hypoxia of AMP kinase proteins (Chen et al., 2012; Waypa et al., 2016) or other mechanisms remains to be elucidated. Additionally, a vascular hyperdynamic state triggered by adrenergic activation and autonomic system imbalance must be considered for exerting its influence on the above variables and possibly in RV dilation (Richalet and Pichon, 2014). Conversely, right atrium morphological changes account for a very low proportion. Complementary, several weak correlations between RV morphological parameters showed linearity with RV afterload (mPAP value). These findings support the consistency of the measurements, and they are in line with the PH evolving process (ACCF/AHA, 2009).

Further analysis of the PVR results is limited since the indirect method of measurement could bias their interpretation and is also controversial. In fact, although some studies mentioned above support a high correlation with right heart catheterization, some others have described this method as accurate but with only moderate precision (Naeije, 2003; Rudski et al., 2010; Naeije and Dedobbeleer, 2013). If these results were accurate, it would support a more hyperdynamic state and milder surmised vascular remodeling, most likely as the result of greater NO bioavailability, as shown in CIHH rats (Siques et al., 2014b; Brito et al., 2015).

Hence, the above considerations would better explain the mild HAPH with apparently almost no functional capacity repercussion. In fact, the TAPSE index of ventricle performance is good. The left ventricle does not seem to be affected, except for a low proportion of aortic dilation, which could also be explained by the hyperdynamic state of this model. The latter findings agree with a previous report regarding left ventricle changes under hypoxia (Richalet and Pichon, 2014).

Moreover, as mentioned, the correspondence analysis using both mPAP values depicted two distinctive patterns of associations with metabolic, biomedical and occupational factors. This tool, albeit is a descriptive method, has allowed to demonstrate the association of elevated mPAP with others variables not found in the regression model. In fact, >15 years of working in this model is strongly associated to elevated mPAP, and additionally, the association of insulin >20 with elevated mPAP further and consistently support what was previously found. The findings obtained with this correspondence analysis are of utmost interest, plausible and depict a sort of signature of this exposure model; however, its role in understanding the pathophysiological process of HAPH remains to be determined. Because this analysis only allows association patterns to be determined, its potential usefulness for screening or prediction will require further studies.

Therefore, the current study highlights a rather novel finding, as discussed previously, in which an association of insulin and ADMA with high mPAP and HAPH was found. Also, the years spent at altitude in this CIHH model might be considered. It is worth noting that some of the above-mentioned associated variables to elevated mPAP, have been previously found to individually contribute to PH and HAPH (Parameswaran et al., 2006; Wu et al., 2009; Zamanian et al., 2009; Kane et al., 2016; San Martin et al., 2017). Until now, their contribution as a whole to right cardiac circuit parameter values in subjects working in long-term CIHH had not been clearly determined.

Although this study design has some limitations, its use was considered necessary to evaluate right cardiac status during long-term intermittent work at high altitude. First, a cross-sectional design allows the determination of only association, status and the absence of changes, but no predictive factors or cause and effect. Moreover, a prospective study might be very difficult.

However, a cross-sectional study has the advantages of the ability to measure several variables, lower cost, and the identification of important points to be studied in a future longitudinal study. Second, the echocardiogram was performed at SL on day 2 of the resting period for logistic reasons, which could produce pulmonary pressures lower than at high altitude. Nevertheless, this study allowed important findings in this condition to be determined. As a whole, while the characteristics found in these subjects could eventually be assumed to result from the study design, the rigorous methodology used, the strict selection and exclusion criteria, the use of more accurate technology and the literature provided support the reasonable validity of the findings of this study in this population. Additionally, altitude differences may explain the elevated proportions of altered morphological and functional right cardiac parameters found in this study compared with those in a previous cross-sectional study (Brito et al., 2007). In fact, the latter study was conducted at 3,550 m, while the subjects in the current study worked at over 4,400 m.

CONCLUSIONS

In summary, this study contributes to the knowledge of long-term CIHH working conditions at altitude, a rather unique biological situation of hypoxia exposure. Thus, it corroborates the persistence of AMS and lack of excessive erythrocytosis. However, this study highlights some novel findings: a high prevalence of HAPH, which is similar to that reported in CH, and with higher numbers of subjects with elevated mPAP and RVWT. In addition to determining the right circuit morphological and functional status, this study is the first, to our knowledge, to identify an association between increased cardiometabolic variables and others with elevated mPAP in CIHH. Therefore, these findings are likely to have important implications for defining the epidemiological and biological features of this model or prompting actions for public health.

AUTHOR CONTRIBUTIONS

JB, PS, and RL: conceived of and designed the study, analyzed and interpreted the data, drafted the manuscript, critically revised important intellectual content in the manuscript, and provided overall supervision; RR, KF, NL, JH, and RB: performed data acquisition, analysis, or interpretation and critically revised important intellectual content in the manuscript; FL-V: assisted with critical decisions and revisions; JB, PS, RL, RR, FL-V, KF, NL, JH, and RB: contributed to the interpretation of results and critical revision of the manuscript, approved the final manuscript and agreed to be accountable for all aspects of the work.

FUNDING

This work was supported by grants from AECID # A/030027/10 and FIC-TARAPACA BIP 30477541-0 and from the German Federal Ministry of Research 01DN17046 DECIPHER.

ACKNOWLEDGMENTS

We would like to thank Jacobo Alarcon (RN) and Gabriela Lamas for their technical assistance.

REFERENCES

Abbas, A. E., Fortuin, F. D., Schiller, N. B., Appleton, C. P., Moreno, C. A., and Lester, S. J. (2003). A simple method for noninvasive estimation of pulmonary vascular resistance. *J. Am. Coll. Cardiol.* 41, 1021–1027. doi: 10.1016/S.0735-1097(02)02973-X

ACCF/AHA (2009). Expert consensus document on pulmonary hypertension: McLaughlin, V.V., Archer, S.L., Badesch, D.B., Barst, R.J., Farber, H.W., Lindner, J.R., et al. (2009). ACCF/AHA 2009 expert consensus document on pulmonary hypertension a report of the American College of Cardiology Foundation Task Force on Expert Consensus Documents and the American Heart Association developed in collaboration with the American College of Chest Physicians; American Thoracic Society, Inc.; and the Pulmonary Hypertension Association. *J. Am. Coll. Cardiol.* 53, 1573–1619. doi: 10.1016/j.jacc.2009.01.004

Anderson, J. D., and Honigman, B. (2011). The effect of altitude-induced hypoxia on heart disease: do acute, intermittent, and chronic exposures provide cardioprotection? *High Alt. Med. Biol.* 12, 45–55. doi: 10.1089/ham.2010.1021

Assmann, G., Schulte, H., and von Eckardstein, A. (1996). Hypertriglyceridemia and elevated lipoprotein (a) are risk factors for major coronary events in middle-aged men. *Am. J. Cardiol.* 77, 1179–1184.

Böger, R. H. (2006). Asymmetric dimethylarginine (ADMA): a novel risk marker in cardiovascular medicine and beyond. *Ann. Med.* 38, 126–136. doi: 10.1080/07853890500472151

Böger, R. H., Bode-Böger, S. M., Szuba, A., Tsao, P. S., Chan, J. R., Tangphao, O., et al. (1998). Asymmetric dimethylarginine (ADMA): a novel risk factor for endothelial dysfunction: its role in hypercholesterolemia. *Circulation* 98, 1842–1847. doi: 10.1161/01.CIR.98.18.1842

Böger, R. H., Maas, R., Schulze, F., and Schwedhelm, E. (2009a). Asymmetric dimethylarginine (ADMA) as a prospective marker of cardiovascular disease and mortality-an update on patient populations with a wide range of cardiovascular risk. *Pharmacol. Res.* 60, 481–487. doi: 10.1016/j.phrs.2009.07.001

Böger, R. H., Sullivan, L. M., Schwedhelm, E., Wang, T. J., Maas, R., Benjamin, E. J., et al. (2009b). Plasma asymmetric dimethylarginine and incidence of cardiovascular disease and death in the community. *Circulation* 119, 1592–1600. doi: 10.1161/CIRCULATIONAHA.108.838268

Brito, J., Siques, P., Arribas, S. M., López de Pablo, A. L., González, M. C., Naveas, N., et al. (2015). Adventitial alterations are the main features in pulmonary artery remodeling due to long-term chronic intermittent hypobaric hypoxia in rats. *BioMed. Res. Int.* 2015:169841. doi: 10.1155/2015/169841

Brito, J., Siques, P., León-Velarde, F., De La Cruz, J. J. D. L., Barlaro, T., López, V., et al. (2008). Varying exposure regimes to long term chronic intermittent hypoxia exert different outcomes and morphological effects on Wistar rats at 4600 m. *Toxicol. Environ. Chem.* 90, 169–179. doi: 10.1080/02772240701382206

Brito, J., Siques, P., León-Velarde, F., De La Cruz, J. J., López, V., and Herruzo, R. (2007). Chronic intermittent hypoxia at high altitude exposure for over 12 years: assessment of hematological, cardiovascular, and renal effects. *High Alt. Med. Biol.* 8, 236–244. doi: 10.1089/ham.2007.8310

Chen, F., Haigh, S., Barman, S., and Fulton, D. J. (2012). From form to function: the role of Nox4 in the cardiovascular system. *Front. Physiol.* 3:412. doi: 10.3389/fphys.2012.00412

Chobanian, A. V., Bakris, G. L., Black, H. R., Cushman, W. C., Green, L. A., Izzo, J. L. Jr., et al. (2003). Seventh report of the Joint National Committee on Prevention, Detection, Evaluation, and Treatment of High blood pressure. *Hypertension* 42, 1206–1252. doi: 10.1161/01.HYP.0000107251.49515.c2

Corno, A. F., Milano, G., Morel, S., Tozzi, P., Genton, C. Y., Samaja, M., et al. (2004). Hypoxia: unique myocardial morphology? *J. Thorac. Cardiovasc. Surg.* 127, 1301–1308. doi: 10.1016/j.jtcvs.2003.06.012

Dabestani, A., Mahan, G., Gardin, J. M., Takenaka, K., Burn, C., Allfie, A., et al. (1987). Evaluation of pulmonary artery pressure and resistance by pulsed Doppler echocardiography. *Am. J. Cardiol.* 59, 662–668. doi: 10.1016/0002-9149(87)91189-1

Drager, L. F., Li, J., Shin, M. K., Reinke, C., Aggarwal, N. R., Jun, J. C., et al. (2012).Intermittent hypoxia inhibits clearance of triglyceride-rich lipoproteins and inactivates adipose lipoprotein lipase in a mouse model of sleep apnoea. *Eur. Heart J.* 33, 783–790. doi: 10.1093/eurheartj/ehr097

Esenamanova, M. K., Kochkorova, F. A., Tsivinskaya, T. A., Vinnikov, D., and Aikimbaev, K. (2014). Chronic intermittent high altitude exposure, occupation, and body mass index in workers of mining industry. *High Alt. Med. Biol.* 15, 412–417. doi: 10.1089/ham.2013.1150

European Society of Hypertension-European Society of Cardiology Guidelines Committee (2003). 2003 European Society of Hypertension-European Society of Cardiology guidelines for the management of arterial hypertension. *J. Hypertens.* 21, 1011–1053. doi: 10.1097/00004872-200306000-00001

Ezzati, M., Horwitz, M. E., Thomas, D. S., Friedman, A. B., Roach, R., Clark, T., et al. (2012). Altitude, life expectancy and mortality from ischaemic heart disease, stroke, COPD and cancers: national population-based analysis of US counties. *J. Epidemiol. Commun. Health* 66:e17. doi: 10.1136/jech.2010.112938

Groepenhoff, H., Overbeek, M. J., Mulè, M., van der Plas, M., Argiento, P., Villafuerte, F. C., et al. (2012). Exercise pathophysiology in patients with chronic mountain sickness exercise in chronic mountain sickness. *Chest* 142, 877–884. doi: 10.1378/chest.11-2845

Grover, R. F. (2014). The paradox of hypoxic pulmonary hypertension (2013 Grover Conference series). *Pulm. Circ.* 4, 151–157. doi: 10.1086/676837

Hackett, P. H. (2003). "Acute mountain sickness and high altitude cerebral edema: a review for the practitioner," in *Health and Heigh: Proceedings of the 5th World Congress on Mountain Medicine and High Altitude Physiology,* eds G. Viscor and A. Ricart (Spain: Universitat de Barcelona), 9–22.

Kane, G. C., Sachdev, A., Villarraga, H. R., et al. (2016). Impact of age on pulmonary artery systolic pressures at rest and with exercise. *Echo Res. Pract.* 3, 53–61. doi: 10.1530/ERP-16-0006

Kaul, S., Tei, C., Hopkins, J. M., and Shah, P. M. (1984). Assessment of right ventricular function using two-dimensional echocardiography. *Am. Heart J.* 107, 526–531. doi: 10.1016/0002-8703(84)90095-4

Kojonazarov, B. K., Imanov, B. Z., Amatov, T. A., Mirrakhimov, M. M., Naeije, R., Wilkins, M. R., et al. (2007). Noninvasive and invasive evaluation of pulmonary arterial pressure in highlanders. *Eur. Respir. J.* 29, 352–356. doi: 10.1183/09031936.00137605

Kolár, F., and Ostádal, B. (1991). Right ventricular function in rats with hypoxic pulmonary hypertension. *Pflugers Arch.* 419, 121–126. doi: 10.1007/BF00372996

Latshang, T. D., Furian, M., Aeschbacher, S. S., Ulrich, S., Osmonov, B., Mirrakhimov, E. M., et al. (2017). Association between sleep apnoea and pulmonary hypertension in Kyrgyz highlanders. *Eur. Respir. J.* 49, 1601530. doi: 10.1183/13993003.01530-2016

Leiper, J., Nandi, M., Torondel, B., Murray-Rust, J., Malaki, M., O'Hara, B., et al. (2007). Disruption of methylarginine metabolism impairs vascular homeostasis. *Nat. Med.* 13, 198–203. doi: 10.1038/nm1543

León-Velarde, F., Maggiorini, M., Reeves, J. T., Aldashev, A., Asmus, I., Bernardi, L., et al. (2005). Consensus statement on chronic and subacute high altitude diseases. *High Alt. Med. Biol.* 6, 147–157. doi: 10.1089/ham.2005.6.147

Li, J., Nanayakkara, A., Jun, J., Savransky, V., and Polotsky, V. Y. (2007). Effect of deficiency in SREBP cleavage-activating protein on lipid metabolism during intermittent hypoxia. *Physiol. Genomics* 31, 273–280. doi: 10.1152/physiolgenomics.00082.2007

López, N., Escobar, C. I., López, F., Durango, L., Fernández, R., and Franco, G. (2012). Función longitudinal del ventrículo derecho estimada por el desplazamiento sistólico del anillo tricúspide (TAPSE) en 557 pacientes sano. *Rev. Colomb. Cardiol.* 19, 281–286. doi: 10.1016/S0120-5633(12)70147-X

Lüneburg, N., Siques, P., Brito, J., Arriaza, K., Pena, E., Klose, H., et al. (2016). Long-term chronic intermittent hypobaric hypoxia in rats causes an imbalance in the asymmetric dimethylarginine/nitric oxide pathway and ROS Activity: a possible synergistic mechanism for altitude pulmonary hypertension? *Pulm. Med.* 2016:6578578. doi: 10.1155/2016/6578578

Lüneburg, N., Siques, P., Brito, J., De La Cruz, J. J., León-Velarde, F., Hannemann, J., et al. (2017). Long-term intermittent exposure to high altitude elevates asymmetric dimethylarginine in first exposed young adults. *High Alt. Med. Biol.* 18, 226–233. doi: 10.1089/ham.2016.0123

McLaughlin, V. V., and Rich, S. (2004). Pulmonary hypertension. *Curr. Probl. Cardiol.* 29, 575–634. doi: 10.1016/S0146-2806(04)00149-5

Miele, C. H., Schwartz, A. R., Gilman, R. H., Pham, L., Wise, R. A., Davila-Roman, V. G., et al. (2016). Increased cardiometabolic risk and worsening hypoxemia at high altitude. *High Alt. Med. Biol.* 17, 93–100. doi: 10.1089/ham.2015.0084

MINSAL Ministerio de Salud (2006). *II Encuesta de Calidad de Vida y Salud Chile 2006*. Available online at: http://www.crececontigo.gob.cl/wp-content/uploads/2015/11/ENCAVI-2006.pdf

Mohanna, S., Baracco, R., and Seclén, S. (2006). Lipid profile, waist circumference, and body mass index in a high altitude population. *High Alt. Med. Biol.* 7, 245–255. doi: 10.1089/ham.2006.7.245

Naeije, R. (2003). Pulmonary vascular resistance. A meaningless variable? *Intensive Care Med.* 29, 526–529. doi: 10.1007/s00134-003-1693-3

Naeije, R., and Dedobbeleer, C. (2013). Pulmonary hypertension and the right ventricle in hypoxia. *Exp. Physiol.* 98, 1247–1256. doi: 10.1113/expphysiol.2012.069112

Parameswaran, K., Todd, D. C., and Soth, M. (2006). Altered respiratory physiology in obesity. *Can. Respir. J.* 13, 203–210. doi: 10.1155/2006/834786

Pavelescu, A., Faoro, V., Guenard, H., de Bisschop, C., Martinot, J. B., Mélot, C., et al. (2013). Pulmonary vascular reserve and exercise capacity at sea level and at high altitude. *High Alt. Med. Biol.* 14, 19–26. doi: 10.1089/ham.2012.1073

Penaloza, D., and Arias-Stella, J. (2007). The heart and pulmonary circulation at high altitudes: healthy highlanders and chronic mountain sickness. *Circulation* 115, 1132–1146. doi: 10.1161/CIRCULATIONAHA.106.624544

Penaloza, D., Banchero, N., Sime, F., and Gamboa, R. (1963). The heart in chronic hypoxia. *Biochem. Clin.* 2, 283–298.

Polotsky, V. Y., Li, J., Punjabi, N. M., Rubin, A. E., Smith, P. L., Schwartz, A. R., et al. (2003). Intermittent hipoxia increases insulin resistance in genetically obese mice. *J. Physiol.* 552, 253–264. doi: 10.1113/jphysiol.2003.048173

Powell, F. L., and Garcia, N. (2000). Physiological effects of intermittent hypoxia. *High Alt. Med. Biol.* 1, 125–136. doi: 10.1089/15270290050074279

Richalet, J. P., and Pichon, A. (2014). "Right ventricle and high altitude," in *The Right Heart*, eds S. P. Gaine, R. Naeije, and A. J. Peacock (London: Springer-Verlag Press), 117–129.

Richalet, J. P., Donoso, M. V., Jiménez, D., Antezana, A. M., Hudson, C., Cortès, G., et al. (2002). Chilean miners commuting from sea level to 4500 m: a prospective study. *High Alt. Med. Biol.* 3, 159–166. doi: 10.1089/15270290260131894

Roach, R. C., Bartsch, P., Hackett, P. H., and Oelz, O. (1993). "The Lake Louise acute mountain sickness scoring system," in *Hypoxia and Molecular Medicine: Proceedings of the Eighth International Hypoxia Symposium, Lake Louise, Alberta, Canada,* eds J. R. Sutton, C. S. Houston, and G. Coates (Burlington, VT: Queen City Printers), 272–274.

Rubin, L. J., and American College of Chest Physicians (2004). Diagnosis and management of pulmonary arterial hypertension: ACCP evidence-based clinical practice guidelines. *Chest* 126(1 Suppl.), 7S–10S. doi: 10.1378/chest.126.1_suppl.4S

Rudski, L. G., Lai, W. W., Afilalo, J., Hua, L., Handschumacher, M. D., Chandrasekaran, K., et al. (2010). Guidelines for the echocardiographic assessment of the right heart in adults: a report from the American Society of Echocardiography endorsed by the European Association of Echocardiography, a registered branch of the European Society of Cardiology, and the Canadian Society of Echocardiography. *J. Am. Soc. Echocardiogr.* 23, 685–713; quiz: 786. doi: 10.1016/j.echo.2010.05.010

San Martin, R., Brito, J., Siques, P., and León-Velarde, F. (2017). Obesity as a conditioning factor for high-altitude diseases. *Obes. Facts* 10, 363–372. doi: 10.1159/000477461

Sarybaev, A. S., Palasiewicz, G., Usupbaeva, D. A., Plywaczewski, R., Maripov, A. M., Sydykov, A. S., et al. (2003). Effects of intermittent exposure to high altitude on pulmonary hemodynamics: a prospective study. *High Alt. Med. Biol.* 4, 455–463. doi: 10.1089/1527029033226 16209

Schwedhelm, E. (2005). Quantification of ADMA: analytical approaches. *Vasc. Med.* 10(Suppl. 1):S89–S95. doi: 10.1177/1358836X0501000113

Schwedhelm, E., Xanthakis, V., Maas, R., Sullivan, L. M., Atzler, D., Lüneburg, N., et al. (2011). Plasma symmetric dimethylarginine reference limits from the Framingham offspring cohort. *Clin. Chem. Lab. Med.* 49, 1907–1910. doi: 10.1515/cclm.2011.679

Schwedhelm, E., Xanthakis, V., Maas, R., Sullivan, L. M., Schulze, F., Riederer, U., et al. (2009). Asymmetric dimethylarginine reference intervals determined with liquid chromatography-tandem mass spectrometry: results from the Framingham offspring cohort. *Clin. Chem.* 55, 1539–1545. doi: 10.1373/clinchem.2009.124263

Siques, P., Brito, J., Banegas, J. R., León-Velarde, F., de la Cruz-Troca, J. J., López, V., et al. (2009). Blood pressure responses in young adults first exposed to high altitude for 12 months at 3550 m. *High Alt. Med. Biol.* 10, 329–335. doi: 10.1089/ham.2008.1103

Siques, P., Brito, J., León-Velarde, F., Barrios, L., De La Cruz, J. J., López, V., et al. (2007). Hematological and lipid profile changes in sea-level natives after exposure to 3550-m altitude for 8 months. *High Alt. Med. Biol.* 8, 286–295. doi: 10.1089/ham.2007.8405

Siques, P., Brito, J., Naveas, N., Pulido, R., De la Cruz, J. J., Mamani, M., et al. (2014a). Plasma and liver lipid profiles in rats exposed to chronic hypobaric hypoxia: changes in metabolic pathways. *High Alt. Med. Biol.* 15, 388–395. doi: 10.1089/ham.2013.1134

Siques, P., López de Pablo, A. L., Brito, J., Arribas, S. M., Flores, K., Arriaza, K., et al. (2014b). Nitric oxide and superoxide anion balance in rats exposed to chronic and long term intermittent hypoxia. *Biomed. Res. Int.* 2014:610474. doi: 10.1155/2014/610474

Sylvester, J. T., Shimoda, L. A., Aaronson, P. I., and Ward, J. P. (2012). Hypoxic pulmonary vasoconstriction. *Physiol. Rev.* 92, 367–520. doi: 10.1152/physrev.00041.2010

Taleb, M., Khuder, S., Tinkel, J., and Khouri, S. J. (2013). The diagnostic accuracy of Doppler echocardiography in assessment of pulmonary artery systolic pressure: a meta-analysis. *Echocardiography* 30, 258–265. doi: 10.1111/echo.12061

Taraseviciute, A., and Voelkel, N. F. (2006). Severe pulmonary hypertension in postmenopausal obese women. *Eur. J Med Res* 11, 198–202.

Teichholz, L. E., Kreulen, T., Herman, M. V., and Gorlin, R. (1976). Problems in echocardiographic volume determinations: echocardiographic-angiographic correlations in the presence of absence of asynergy. *Am. J. Cardiol.* 37, 7–11. doi: 10.1016/0002-9149(76)90491-4

Vallance, P., Leone, A., Calver, A., Collier, J., and Moncada, S. (1992). Endogenous dimethylarginine as an inhibitor of nitric oxide synthesis. *J. Cardiovasc. Pharmacol.* 20(Suppl. 12), S60–S62. doi: 10.1097/00005344-199204002-00018

von Euler, U. S., and Liljestrand, G. (1946). Observations on the pulmonary arterial blood pressure in the cat. *Acta Physiol. Scand.* 12, 301–320. doi: 10.1111/j.1748-1716.1946.tb00389.x

Waypa, G. B., Dudley, V., and Schumacker, P. T. (2016). Role of pulmonary arterial smooth muscle and endothelial mitochondrial complex III in chronic hypoxia-induced pulmonary hypertension. *Am. J. Respir. Crit. Care Med.* 193:A3884.

West, J. B. (2002). Intermittent exposure to high altitude. *High Alt. Med. Biol.* 3, 141–143. doi: 10.1089/15270290260131858

Wu, T. Y., Ding, S. Q., Liu, J. L., Yu, M. T., Jia, J. H., Duan, J. Q., et al. (2009). Reduced incidence and severity of acute mountain sickness in Qinghai–Tibet railroad construction workers after repeated 7-month exposures despite 5-month low altitude periods. *High Alt. Med. Biol.* 10, 221–232. doi: 10.1089/ham.2009.1012

Zamanian, R. T., Hansmann, G., Snook, S., Lilienfeld, D., Rappaport, K. M., Reaven, G. M., et al. (2009). Insulin resistance in pulmonary arterial hypertension. *Eur. Respir. J.* 33, 318–324. doi: 10.1183/09031936.00000508

Zoccali, C., Bode-Böger, S., Mallamaci, F., Benedetto, F., Tripepi, G., Malatino, L., et al. (2001). Plasma concentration of asymmetrical dimethylarginine and mortality in patients with end-stage renal disease: a prospective study. *Lancet* 358, 2113–2117. doi: 10.1016/S0140-6736(01)07217-8

5

Leptin Signaling in the Carotid Body Regulates a Hypoxic Ventilatory Response Through Altering TASK Channel Expression

Fang Yuan[1,2], Hanqiao Wang[3], Jiaqi Feng[1], Ziqian Wei[1], Hongxiao Yu[1], Xiangjian Zhang[2,4], Yi Zhang[1,2] and Sheng Wang[1,2]**

[1] Department of Physiology, Hebei Medical University, Shijiazhuang, China, [2] Hebei Key Laboratory of Vascular Homeostasis and Hebei Collaborative Innovation Center for Cardio-Cerebrovascular Disease, Shijiazhuang, China, [3] Department of Sleep, Third Hospital of Hebei Medical University, Shijiazhuang, China, [4] Department of Neurology, Second Hospital of Hebei Medical University, Shijiazhuang, China

***Correspondence:**
Yi Zhang
yizhanghebmu@163.com
Sheng Wang
wangsheng@hebmu.edu.cn

Leptin is an adipose-derived hormone that plays an important role in the regulation of breathing. It has been demonstrated that obesity-related hypoventilation or apnea is closely associated with leptin signaling pathways. Perturbations of leptin signaling probably contribute to the reduced sensitivity of respiratory chemoreceptors to hypoxia/hypercapnia. However, the underlying mechanism remains incompletely understood. The present study is to test the hypothesis that leptin signaling contributes to modulating a hypoxic ventilatory response. The respiratory function was assessed in conscious obese Zucker rats or lean littermates treated with an injection of leptin. During exposure to hypoxia, the change in minute ventilation was lower in obese Zucker rats than chow-fed lean littermates or high fat diet-fed littermates. Such a change was abolished in all groups after carotid body denervation. In addition, the expression of phosphorylated signal transducers and activators of transcription 3 (pSTAT3), as well as putative O_2-sensitive K^+ channels including TASK-1, TASK-3 and TASK-2 in the carotid body, was significantly reduced in obese Zucker rats compared with the other two phenotype littermates. Chronic administration of leptin in chow-fed lean Zucker rats failed to alter basal ventilation but vigorously increased tidal volume, respiratory frequency, and therefore minute volume during exposure to hypoxia. Likewise, carotid body denervation abolished such an effect. In addition, systemic leptin elicited enhanced expression of pSTAT3 and TASK channels. In conclusion, these data demonstrate that leptin signaling facilitates hypoxic ventilatory responses probably through upregulation of pSTAT3 and TASK channels in the carotid body. These findings may help to better understand the pathogenic mechanism of obesity-related hypoventilation or apnea.

Keywords: leptin, hypoventilation, hypoxic ventilatory response, carotid body, TASK channels, STAT3

INTRODUCTION

Leptin, a peptide hormone secreted mainly by adipocytes, regulates multiple physiological functions including metabolism, cardiovascular activity, and breathing (Grill et al., 2002; Bassi et al., 2015). Leptin's role in controlling breathing has been implicated in recent studies, with its participation in sleep-related breathing disorders including obesity hypoventilation syndrome

(OHS) and obstructive sleep apnea (Malhotra and White, 2002). In animal models, leptin deficient mice exhibit impaired ventilatory responses to CO_2 which can be rescued by leptin replacement therapy, in favor of facilitation of breathing by leptin (O'Donnell et al., 2000). Leptin receptors (ob-Rs) are composed of six isoforms termed from ob-Ra to -Rf, with the long form of ob-Rb mediating the majority of leptin's intracellular signal transduction (Tartaglia, 1997). Although the role of leptin signaling pathways in mediating various physiological actions has been investigated intensively, the molecular mechanism underlying its action on breathing remains incompletely understood.

The peripheral respiratory chemoreflex serves as a homeostatic regulatory mechanism by which enough oxygen must be supplied to the organism when challenged by hypoxia through altering respiratory amplitude and frequency. The carotid body (CB) chemoreceptors, located near the fork of the carotid artery, are activated shortly after exposure to hypoxia and then send information to the nucleus tractus solitarius and high integrative centers, with the outcome of adaptive ventilatory responses (Gonzalez-Martin et al., 2011; Ciriello and Caverson, 2014). Accumulated evidence indicates the presence of ob-Rb in the CB cells (Porzionato et al., 2011; Messenger et al., 2013), and that leptin signaling contributes to CB-mediated ventilatory responses (Olea et al., 2015; Ribeiro et al., 2017). However, it remains controversial whether the CB mediates the acute effect of leptin on hypoxic ventilatory response (HVR) because leptin's role may involve the change in gene expression and protein synthesis, requiring hours even days for full effects (Hall et al., 2010). We thereby predicted that the stimulatory effect of leptin on HVR may require chronic activation of CBs, but such a confirmation is yet to be put forward.

In the CBs, leptin signaling pathways involve the downstream signaling proteins of ob-R signal transducers and activators of transcription 3 (STAT3), suppressor of cytokine signaling 3 (SOCS3), and extracellular-signal-regulated kinase 1/2 (ERK1/2) (Messenger et al., 2013; Moreau et al., 2015), reminiscent of modulatory effects of these molecules on carotid chemoreceptor sensitivity. Emerging evidence has shown that the chemosensitivity of glomus cells in CBs requires two-pore K^+ channels including TWIK-related acid-sensitive K (TASK)-1 channels and acid-sensitive ion channels (Trapp et al., 2008; Tan et al., 2010). However, very little is known concerning whether the activation of the ob-R and downstream signaling molecules modulates the sensitization of CB chemoreceptors via affecting these ion channels.

We sought to address herein whether the leptin signaling pathway in the CB contributes to regulating HVR and the possible mechanism involved. We utilized whole body plethysmography (WBP) to assess HVR in obese Zucker rats (ob-R deficiency) or in lean littermate controls treated with injections of leptin. The main findings suggest that chronic application of leptin contributes to facilitation of HVRs probably through upregulation of phosphorylated STAT3 (pSTAT3) and TASK channel expression.

MATERIALS AND METHODS

Animals

The experiments were carried out in 12~20-week-old male obese Zucker rats (OZR) and lean littermates (LZR) obtained from the Charles River Laboratories (USA). Animals, synchronized for a 12:12 h light-dark cycle (lights on at 8 am, lights off at 8 pm), were housed individually and allowed to move freely in standard plastic cages in a climate-controlled room (22 ± 1°C). Food and water were provided *ad libitum* for LZRs and OZRs. In some cases, a group of LZRs were placed on a high-fat diet (HFD, 45% kcal/g fat, Research Diets D12451) for 8 weeks and used as a simple obesity control (LHZR). The LHZR and OZR groups were weight-matched to determine the effect of simple obesity-induced mechanical resistance on ventilation. Body weight was measured once a week ($n = 20$ for each phenotype). All experiments were performed in accordance to ethical guidelines of the Animal Protection Association and were approved by Animal Care and Ethical Committee of Hebei Medical University. When the animal experiments were completed, an overdose of intraperitoneal injection of sodium pentobarbital (> 200 mg/kg) was carried out for euthanasia.

Breathing Measurement

Breathing was studied by WBP in conscious, freely moving rats (EMKA Technologies, France) as described previously (Kumar et al., 2015; Fu et al., 2017). In brief, rats were placed in the WBP chamber on the day before the testing protocol (2 h acclimation period). For acute hypoxia, rats were exposed to 10% O_2 (balance N_2) for up to ~7 min by a gas mixture devices (1,500 ml/min, GSM-3, CWE, USA). Ventilatory flow signals were recorded, amplified, digitized and analyzed using IOX 2.7 (EMKA Technologies) to determine breathing parameters over sequential 20 s epochs (~50 breaths) during periods of behavioral quiescence and regular breathing. Minute volume (V_E; ml/min/g) was calculated as the product of the respiratory frequency (f_R, breaths/min) and tidal volume (V_T; ml/kg), normalized to rat body weight (g). To further confirm the CB-mediated effect of leptin, breathing parameters were also measured in rats with carotid body denervation (CBD). The carotid sinus nerves were sectioned as depicted before (Kumar et al., 2015). Shortly, anesthesia was induced with 4% halothane in 100% O_2 and maintained by reducing the inspired halothane concentration to 1.5~1.8%. The depth of anesthesia was assessed by an absence of the corneal and hindpaw withdrawal reflex. Body temperature of all mice was maintained at 37°C using a temperature-controlled heating pad. To prevent any functional regeneration of chemosensory fibers, the carotid sinus nerves were removed completely from the cranial pole of the CB until reaching the branch to the glossopharyngeal nerve. The wound was carefully sutured and disinfected with 10% of polividone iodine. Conscious chemodenervated rats were exposed to ventilatory challenge 5–7 days after recovery. No significant weight loss was observed. All the three groups of rats (LZR, LHZR and OZR) were submitted to surgery.

To examine whether hypoventilation resulted in retention of CO_2 in obese rats, arterial blood gas was measured using an

OPTI-CCA blood gas analyzer (OPTI Medical Systems, USA) at a steady state in halothane-anesthetized, paralyzed rats. General anesthesia was induced with 4% halothane in room air as depicted above. Arterial blood (200 μl per sample) was drawn from the femoral artery in the three animal groups. Arterial blood measurements of interest included partial pressure of arterial O_2 (P_aO_2), partial pressure of CO_2 (P_aCO_2) and pH.

Plasma Leptin Levels and Hypodermic Leptin Injections

Measurements of plasma levels of leptin were performed at room air (21% O_2) in anesthetized rats. After general anesthesia as described above, whole blood samples were taken through a cardiac puncture. Blood samples were drawn into collection tubes containing the anticoagulant EDTA (Sigma-Aldrich, USA) and kept on ice. After centrifugation, the plasma was stored at−80°C for leptin analysis by ELISA kit (#ab100773, Abcam, USA), an *in vitro* enzyme-linked immunosorbent assay for the quantitative measurement as previously described (Panetta et al., 2017). The assay was read using a power wave XS2 plate reader (Biotek Instruments, USA).

To confirm whether the chronic activation of leptin signaling pathways played a part in the HVR, subcutaneous injections of leptin (60 μg/kg) or equal volume of vehicle (saline) were carried out once daily for 7 days in CBI LZRs ($n = 8$ for each group), and breathing parameters were measured after 7 day injections during exposure to room air or hypoxia. To further confirm the CB's role, subcutaneous injections of leptin or saline were performed 7 days after the carotid sinus nerves were sectioned in each group ($n = 8$ for both).

Carotid Body Protein Extracts and Western Blot Analysis

Rats were deeply anesthetized by isoflurane (2–3%) inhalation and then decapitated. The carotid bifurcation was exposed and both CBs were removed and cleaned. The CB ($n = 8$) were pooled from 4 rats in each group and homogenized in 100 μl of RIPA buffer solution (150 mM NaCl, 1 mM EDTA, 1% Triton-X 100, 50 mM Tris–HCl at pH of 7.5) with a protease inhibitor cocktail (Roche Diagnostics, Canada). The homogenate was centrifuged at 4°C for 20 min at 13200 rpm. The resultant supernatant was retained as the protein preparation. Equal concentrations of extracted proteins normalized by colorimetric BCA Protein Assay (Pierce Corp., USA). After denaturation, the protein (~30 μg) in each lane was fractionated in 10% polyacrylamide gel and then transferred onto apolyvinylidene fluoride membrane. The membranes were blocked with bovine serum albumin and incubated at 4°C overnight with primary antibodies anti-ob-R (1:2000, #ab5593, Abcam, USA), anti-TASK-1 (1:200, #APC024, Alomone labs, Israel), anti-TASK-2 (1:200, #APC037, Alomone labs, Israel), anti-TASK-3 (1:200, #APC044, Alomone labs, Israel), anti-pSTAT3 (1:2000, #9145, Cell Signaling Technology, USA), anti-STAT3 (1:1000, #9139, Cell Signaling Technology, USA), and anti-β-actin (1:3,000, #T0022, Affinity Biosciences, USA). The membranes were then incubated with corresponding secondary antibodies for 1 h at room temperature. The reaction was visualized using the enhanced chemiluminescence (ECL) method, and the bands were analyzed by ImageJ software (NIH, USA). The protein contents were normalized to β-actin. See Supplementary Material for original gel images.

Data Acquisition and Processing

Data are expressed as mean ± SEM. Unless indicated otherwise, two-tailed unpaired *t*-test, one-way ANOVA with Dunnett's or Tukey's *post-hoc* test and two-way ANOVA with Bonferroni *post-hoc* test were used to compare significant difference between different groups. Differences within or between groups with *P*-values of <0.05 were considered significant.

RESULTS

Reduced Basal Ventilation in OZRs

Adult OZRs exhibit many abnormal physiological attributes due to the deficiency of the ob-R, representing a good animal model to study the obesity-related hypoventilation as observed in humans. We thus addressed leptin's role using this phenotype and the littermate control rat. First, we measured the body weight of three groups of rats ($n = 20$ for each group). The averaged body weight was larger in LHZRs (492 ± 30 g) and OZRs (512 ± 49 g) than LZRs (382 ± 14 g, $P < 0.01$ vs. LHZR or OZR). In addition, weight gain was accompanied by higher levels of blood plasma leptin level in OZRs (15.28 ± 0.55 μg/L) in relative to LHZRs (7.45 ± 0.50 μg/L, $P < 0.01$ vs. OZR) or LZRs (7.34 ± 0.38 μg/L, $P < 0.01$ vs. OZR; $P > 0.05$, vs. LHZR).

Baseline breathing parameters were measured in the three groups of animals while breathing room air (21% O_2). Compared with the LZRs, V_E and V_T were considerably lower in OZRs and LHZRs ($P < 0.01$ for both, vs. LZRs, **Figures 1A,C**), whereas the OZR has a faster f_R than the other two groups ($P < 0.01$ for both). Of interest, although no remarkable difference in basal V_E was observed between OZRs and LHZRs, V_T and f_R were comparable ($P < 0.01$ for both, **Figure 1B**), indicative of a different breathing pattern. To evaluate whether hypoventilation resulted in hypercapnia or respiratory acidosis in obese animals, the arterial blood gas was measured at a steady-state. Apparently, hypercapnia, acidosis and normal P_aO_2 were observed in LHZRs and OZRs (**Table 1**). Therefore, both OZRs and LHZRs exhibit basal hypoventilation, overweight and hypercapnia, with the exception of hyperleptinemia in OZRs but not LHZRs.

Impairment of HVR in OZRs

To address whether the ob-R deficiency yielded a diminished HVR, hypoxia was achieved while inhaling 10% O_2 to activate peripheral respiratory chemoreflex. When acutely challenged with hypoxia, all three phenotypes displayed robust increases in f_R and V_E except for V_T, with the smallest change in the HVR in OZRs (**Figures 1A–C**). In addition, the hypoxia-stimulated increment of V_E was far less in OZRs compared to the other two groups ($P < 0.01$, **Figure 1E**). Interestingly, LZRs and LHZRs displayed a similar change in V_E during hypoxia

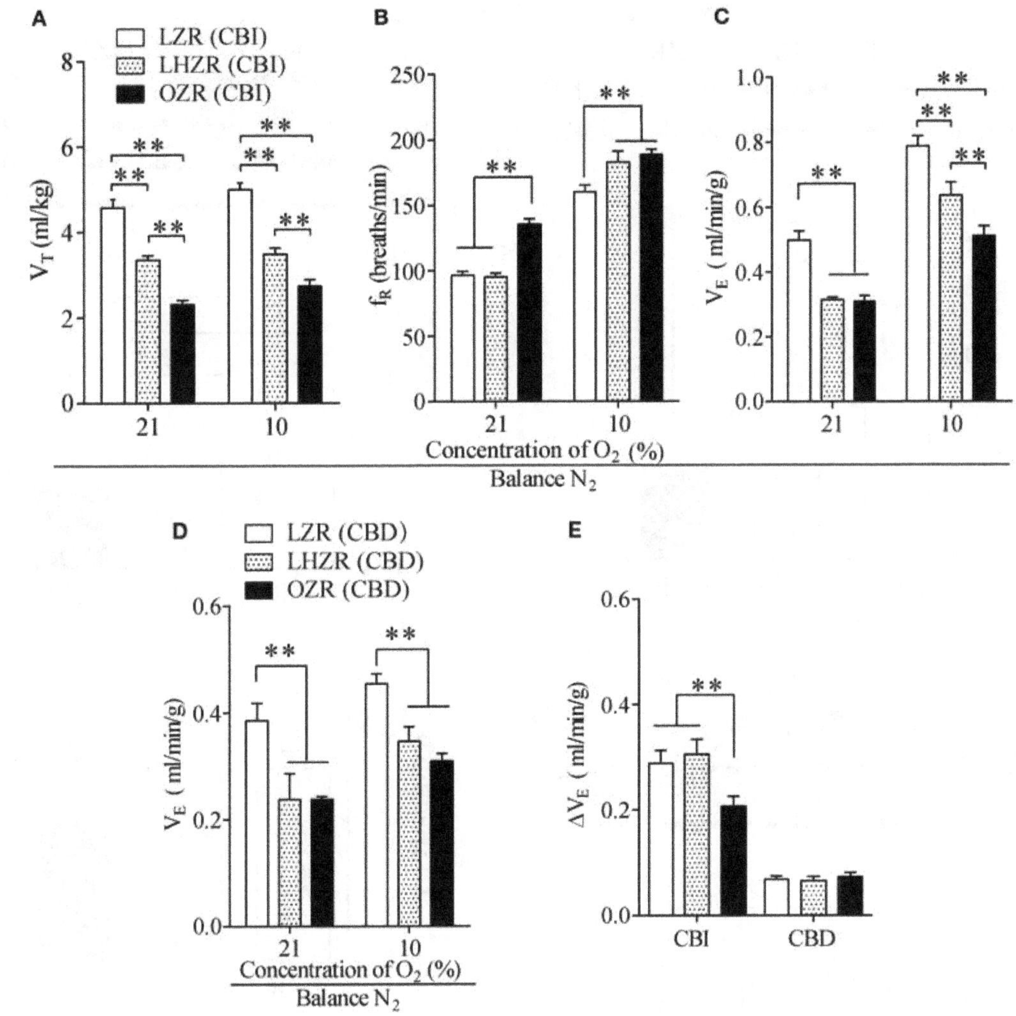

FIGURE 1 | The OZR exhibits impaired HVR. **(A–C)** Effect of hypoxia on V_T, f_R, and V_E in the three groups of rats. **(D)** The stimulatory effect of hypoxia on V_E in three groups of CBD rats. **(E)** Changes in V_E during exposure to 10% O_2 between CBI and CBD rats. $n = 20$ for each group, $^{**}P < 0.01$ as drawn by two-way ANOVA with Bonferroni *post-hoc* test. V_T, tidal volume; f_R, respiratory frequency; V_E, minute ventilation; CBI, carotid body innervation; CBD, carotid body denervation.

TABLE 1 | Blood gas analysis during exposure to room air.

Group	P_aCO_2(mmHg)	P_aO_2(mmHg)	pH
LZR	37.9 ± 1.8	102.5 ± 5.9	7.32 ± 0.02
LHZR	51.6 ± 1.0**	93.8 ± 2.7	7.24 ± 0.01*
OZR	50.9 ± 0.6**	87.6 ± 2.8*	7.22 ± 0.01*

LZR, lean Zucker rats; LHZR, HFD-fed LZR; OZR, obese Zucker rats; $n = 12$ for each group; $^{*}P < 0.05$, $^{**}P < 0.01$ by one-way ANOVA with Tukey's post-hoc test, vs. LZRs.

($P > 0.05$, **Figure 1E**). In spite of similar degree of body weight, OZRs exhibited far more severe hypoventilation in response to hypoxia compared to LHZRs ($P < 0.01$, **Figures 1A–C**). However, exposure to hypoxia caused no significant difference in increments of V_E in all three groups of rats after sectioning carotid sinus nerves ($P > 0.05$, **Figures 1D,E**), in favor of the involvement of CBs in such an effect. Collectively, the ob-R deficiency (OZR), instead of simple obesity (LHZR), plays a predominant role in the impaired HVR.

Downregulation of pSTAT3 and TASK Channels in OZR CBs

The pSTAT3/STAT3 signaling has been implicated in mediating major effects of the ob-R. To determine the expression level of ob-R and STAT3, the quantitative analysis was made using Western blot in the three groups ($n = 4$ for each group). Compared with LZRs and LHZRs, pSTAT3/STAT3 (**Figures 2C,D**) were remarkably downregulated in the CBs of OZRs ($P < 0.01$), reliably correlating pSTAT3/STAT3 expression with the ob-R deficiency (**Figures 2A,B**). Several lines of evidence demonstrated that the chemosensitivity is associated with TASK-1 and TASK-3 in CB glomus cells and TASK-2 in retrotrapezoid nucleus neurons (Trapp et al., 2008; Gestreau et al., 2010; Wang et al., 2013). The reduced sensitivity of CBs to hypoxia in OZRs

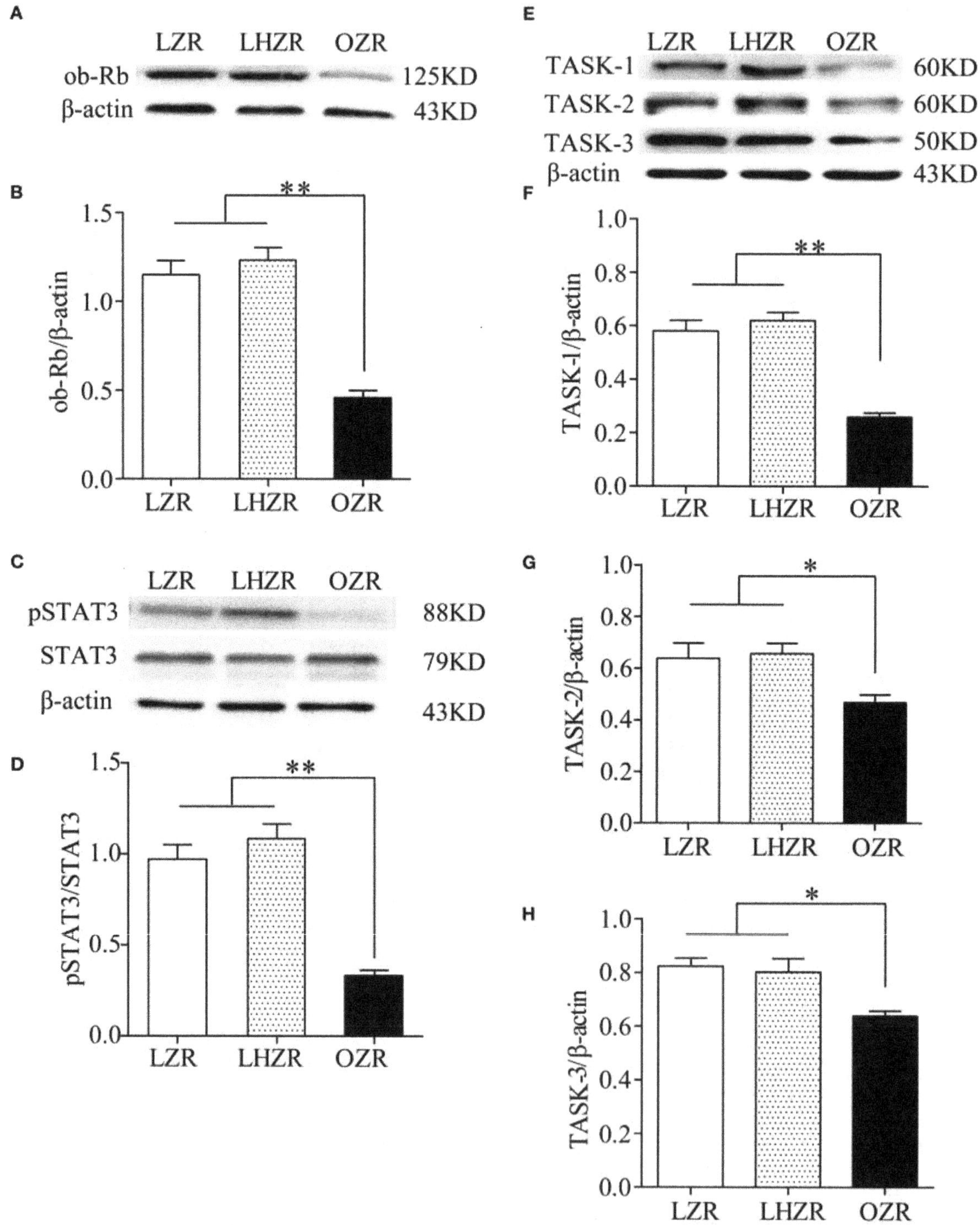

FIGURE 2 | Downregulation of pSTAT3/STAT3 and TASK-1,-2,-3 channels in CBs. Gel images and bar charts showing quantitative analysis of expression of ob-Rb **(A,B)**, pSTAT3/STAT3 **(C,D)**, and TASK-1,-2,-3 **(E–H)** in the CB ($n = 8$) from each group ($n = 4$). $^{*}P < 0.05$, $^{**}P < 0.01$ by one-way ANOVA with Dunnett's *post-hoc* test. ob-Rb, leptin receptor type b; STAT3, signal transducers and activators of transcription 3; pSTAT3, phosphorylated STAT3.

was probably associated with these ion channels. Evidently, the expression level of TASK-1, TASK-2, TASK-3 in OZR CBs was lower in relative to the other two groups ($P < 0.05 \sim 0.01$, **Figures 2E–H**). However, no statistical significance in these channel expression was found between LZRs and LHZRs ($P > 0.05$ for all, **Figures 2E–H**). Hence, the ob-R deficiency contributes to reduced expression of pSTAT3 and TASK channels.

Facilitation of HVR by Chronic Application of Leptin

To examine the effect of activation of ob-Rs on the HVR, subcutaneous injections of leptin (60 μg/kg) or equal volume of normal saline were carried out once daily for 7 days in LZRs ($n = 8$ for each group), and breathing parameters were measured at different time points separated by 7 days. As shown in **Table 2**, compared with the vehicle control (8.2 ± 0.4 μg/L), the plasma levels of leptin was raised to 13.1 ± 0.6 μg/L ($P < 0.01$) over 7-day treatment and restored to control level after 1 week. Chronic administration of leptin for 7 days produced no significant change in body weight ($P > 0.05$, data not shown) and basal breathing parameters (V_T, f_R and V_E) in relative to the vehicle control (**Figures 3A–C**). Neither P_aCO_2 nor blood pH changed significantly in leptin-injected rats (data not shown). During exposure to 10% O_2, V_T, f_R, and V_E were all increased in either leptin- or saline-injected LZRs ($P < 0.05\sim0.01$) but the change in V_E was greater in leptin-injected rats in relative to the vehicle controls (**Figure 3E**). The stimulatory effect of leptin on HVR persisted for at least 2 weeks (**Table 3**). After bilaterally sectioning carotid sinus nerves, leptin-induced increase in V_E was abolished (**Figures 3D,E**). Collectively, chronic administration of leptin potentiated the HVR.

Effect of Leptin on Expression of pSTAT3 and TASK Channels

To investigate the possible mechanism underlying exogenous application of leptin action on the HVR, we tested the expression of ob-R and the downstream pSTAT3 and TASK-1, TASK-2, TASK-3 channels in CBs after injection of leptin for 7 days. The findings indicated that leptin administration caused greater upregulation of ob-R and of pSTAT3 ($P < 0.01$, $n = 4$ for each group, **Figures 4A,B**). Furthermore, leptin also enhanced expression of TASK-1, TASK-2, TASK-3 ($P < 0.01$, $n = 4$ for each group, **Figures 4C–E**). The results suggest that the stimulatory effect of leptin on HVR are closely associated with enhanced expression of pSTAT3 and TASK channels, which may contribute to the regulation of CB's chemosensitivity.

DISCUSSION

We demonstrate herein that the ob-R deficiency, rather than simple obesity, not only reduces baseline ventilation but also inhibits the HVR, with decreased pSTAT3 expression in CBs. Chronic administration of leptin has no marked effects on basal ventilation but considerably enhances the HVR, accompanied by increased expression of pSTAT3. Additionally, either ob-R deficiency or leptin administration is reliably associated with changes in expression of TASK-1, TASK-2, and TASK-3 channels. These findings suggest that leptin signaling in the CB contributes to potentiation of HVR probably through enhancement of pSTAT3 and TASK channels expressions.

The obese Zucker rat represents a good model of ob-R deficiency and manifests relatively early onset obesity (Bray and York, 1971). One line of early evidence shows that respiratory system compliance was significantly lower in the OZR compared with the lean phenotype, and that resting ventilatory parameters (uncorrected for body weight) were similar between obese and lean animals, with similar ventilatory response to hypoxia between two phenotypes (Farkas and Schlenker, 1994). In the present study, we compared the difference between obese and lean phenotypes using the previously described method (Kumar et al., 2015; Fu et al., 2017) to normalize breathing parameters to body weight. Interestingly, with this analysis method, the OZRs exhibited fast f_R, reduced V_T and thus lower V_E during exposure to room air. This outcome interprets occurrence of hypercapnia and respiratory acidosis observed in OZRs. Based on these attributes, the OZR resembles an animal model of leptin resistance. The LHZR, a simple obesity control carrying genotype of the LZR, displayed hypercapnia, respiratory acidosis, relatively normal serum leptin, basal hypoventilation and moderate response to hypoxia, probably representing a model of simple obesity rather than leptin resistance. In obese patients, a higher level of leptin is found to cause an increase in basal ventilation associated with excess body mass, with OHS patients exhibiting an even higher serum leptin level than eucapnic individuals matched for body mass index (Phipps et al., 2002). In animal models, HFD rats exhibit an unchanged (Olea et al., 2014) or enhanced basal V_E (Ribeiro et al., 2017). Importantly, Ribeiro et al. found 3 weeks of HFD blunted leptin responses to hypoxia in the CB, probably due to development of CB leptin resistance, suggesting at least 3 weeks required for the establishment of leptin resistance. However, in the present study, hyperleptinaemia and leptin resistance did not occur in the LHZR most likely because of the genetic manipulation which makes the difference and the hypoventilation thus appears to be a restrictive ventilatory pattern. Another explanation may be supported by previous findings suggesting that elevation of leptin levels is a consequence of hypoxia and not of fat accumulation (Tatsumi et al., 2005). Taken together, our findings support that the impaired basal ventilation and HVR in OZRs is ascribed mainly to ob-R deficiency rather than mere obesity. We did not measure chest wall mechanics and compare the difference in chest wall impedance between two obese rats, whereas it would be expected that obesity-induced increase in chest wall impedance must play a relatively small part in such effects. This also helps better understanding of the results that ΔV_E induced by hypoxia is insignificant between LZRs and LHZRs.

Leptin's actions involve fast or slow onset, thus requiring minutes, several hours, even days before major changes occur. Its acute effects on breathing has been implicated in prior studies

TABLE 2 | Blood plasma levels of leptin in response to chronic application of saline and leptin.

Day	Saline group (Leptin, μg/L)	Leptin group (Leptin, μg/L)
0 day	7.8 ± 0.5	7.6 ± 0.5
7th day	8.2 ± 0.4	13.1 ± 0.6**
14th day	7.6 ± 0.5	9.3 ± 0.6
21st day	8.0 ± 0.6	8.6 ± 1.0

*n = 8 for each group; **P < 0.01 by two-tailed unpaired t-test, vs. saline.*

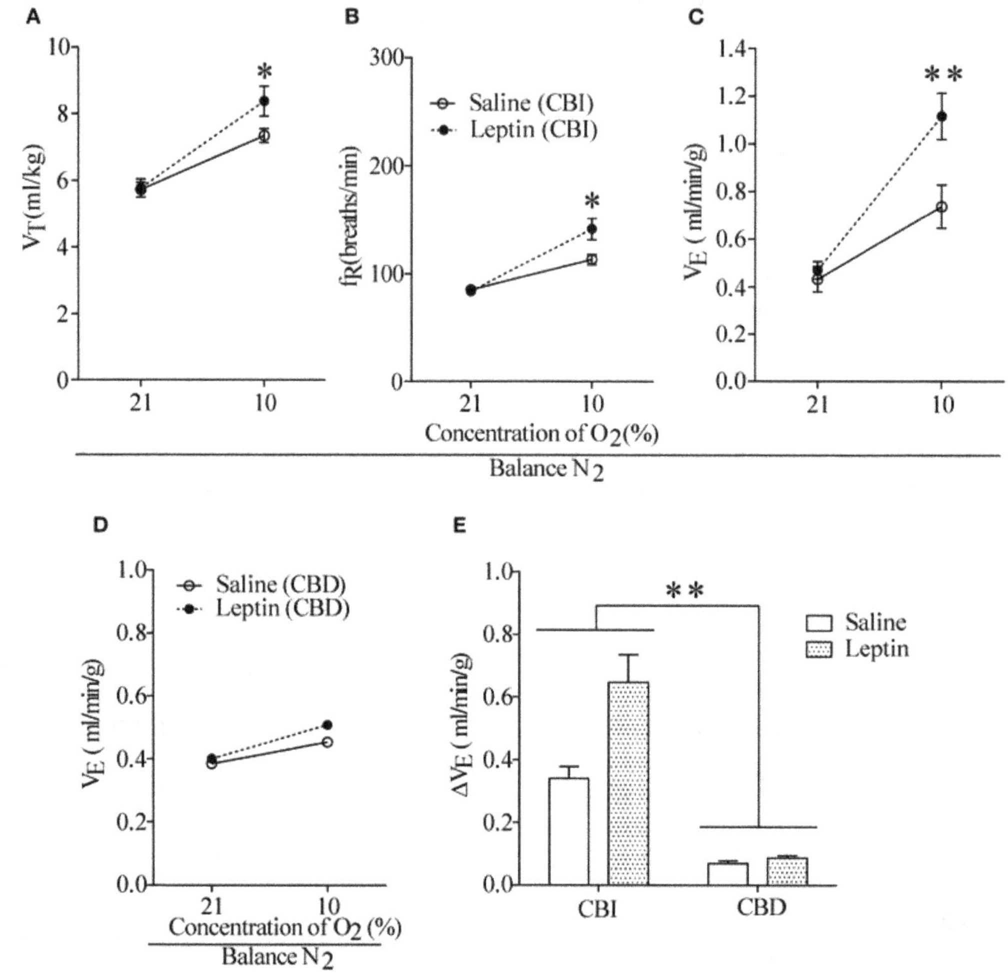

FIGURE 3 | Effect of hypodermic injection of Leptin on breathing parameters. **(A–C)** Injection of leptin raised V_T, f_R, and V_E measured on 7th day in the LZR with CBI. **(D)** The stimulatory effect of hypoxia was reduced in two groups of rats with CBD. **(E)** Changes in V_E during exposure to 10% O_2 in CBI and CBD groups. $n = 8$ for each group, $^*P < 0.05$, $^{**}P < 0.01$ by two-way ANOVA with Bonferroni *post-hoc* test, Leptin vs. Saline group.

TABLE 3 | V_E measured during exposure to room air and hypoxia.

Day	O_2 level	Saline group (V_E ml/min/g)	Leptin group (V_E ml/min/g)
0 day	Air	469 ± 41	451 ± 21
	10%O_2	810 ± 24	819 ± 26
7th day	Air	479 ± 26	470 ± 36
	10%O_2	819 ± 44	1117 ± 97**
14th day	Air	463 ± 17	481 ± 32
	10%O_2	819 ± 32	1036 ± 88**
21st day	Air	468 ± 36	438 ± 24
	10%O_2	771 ± 75	914 ± 48

V_E, minute ventilation, $n = 8$ for each group, $^{**}P < 0.01$ by two-way ANOVA with Bonferroni post-hoc test, vs. Saline.

(Chang et al., 2013; Olea et al., 2015; Pye et al., 2015; Ribeiro et al., 2017). For example, Olea et al. have found that acute application of leptin in anaesthetized animals augmented basal V_E and potentiated the ischemic hypoxia-induced V_E in a dose-dependent manner (Olea et al., 2015). More recently, Ribeiro et al. reported that leptin increases V_E both in basal and hypoxic conditions in control rats but such effects were blunted in high fat diet fed rats (Ribeiro et al., 2017). In contrast, acute application of leptin in isolated CB type I cells failed significantly to alter the resting membrane potential and acidification-induced depolarization was unaffected by leptin, thereby suggesting that acute leptin stimulation did not alter CB's chemosensitivity (Pye et al., 2015). In addition to acute effects, chronic treatment with leptin *in vivo* also has been shown to potentiate respiratory chemoreflex (Bassi et al., 2014). Acute or chronic actions may be mediated by different leptin signaling pathways. Chronic administration of leptin in the present study did not augment basal ventilation but potentiated HVR in conscious rats, an effect persisting for ≥7 days. This appears to play an essential role in reinforcing ventilation to supply more oxygen when challenged by hypoxia. The plasma levels of leptin after 7 days treatment are quite similar to those quantified in plasma for the

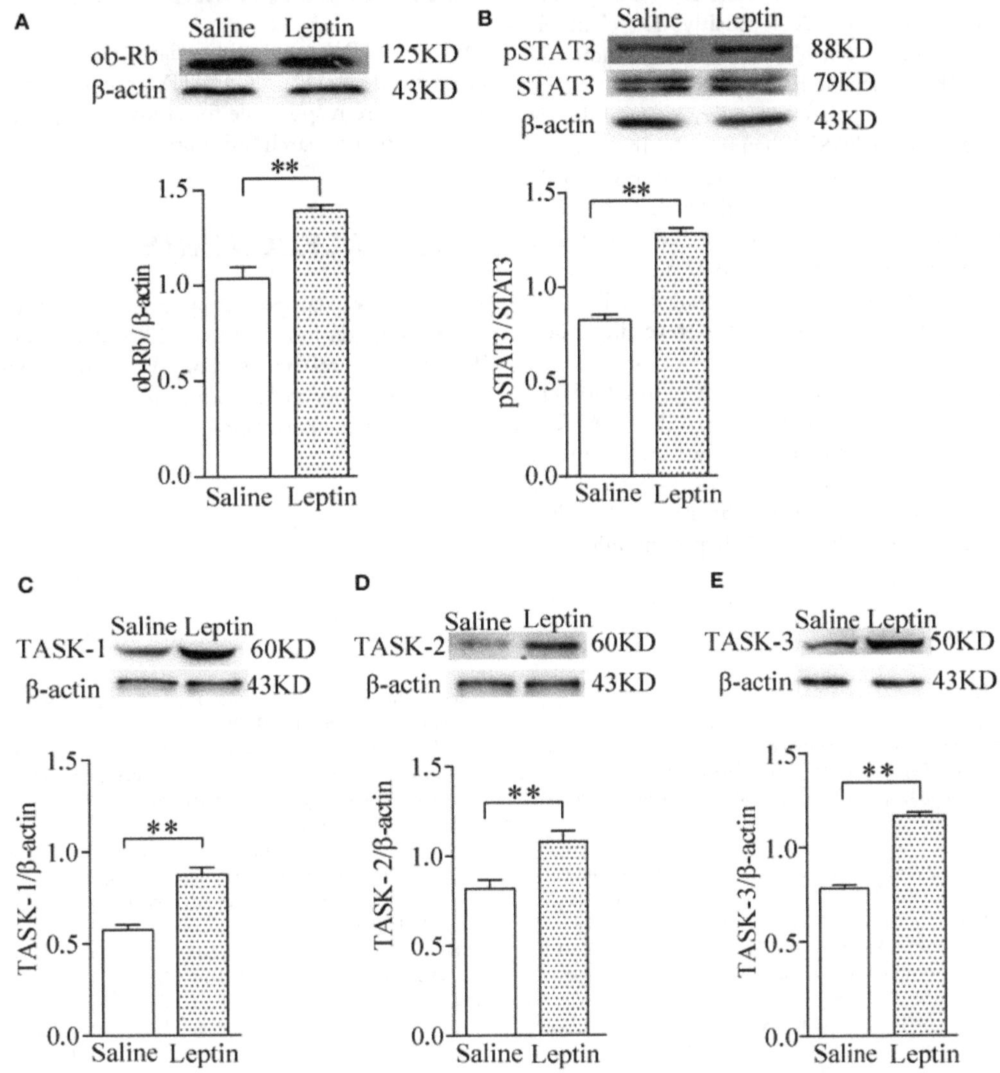

FIGURE 4 | Stimulatory effect of leptin on pSTAT3/STAT3 and TASK-1,-2,-3 channel protein expression in CBs. Gel images and bar charts showing quantitative analysis of leptin-stimulated expression of ob-Rb **(A)** pSTAT3/STAT3 **(B)** and TASK-1,-2,-3 **(C–E)** in the CB ($n = 8$) of each group ($n = 4$). $^{**}P < 0.01$ by two-tailed unpaired t-test.

OZRs, taken together with the enhancement of HVR with 7 day leptin administration and the impairment of HVR in OZRs rats, indicates that 7 day stimulatory effects of leptin did not result in leptin resistance.

The reason why the basal ventilation was herein not enhanced by the chronic application of leptin would be attributable to animal's state (anesthetized vs. conscious) and the dose of leptin administered. The dose of leptin applied to our animals was chosen based on what was chronically applied previously (Wjidan et al., 2015), and lower than that used in prior reports examining the acute effects of leptin on cardiovascular (Rahmouni et al., 2002; Rahmouni and Morgan, 2007) and respiratory functions (O'Donnell et al., 2000; Bassi et al., 2012). Moreover, in the case of potentially therapeutic utilizations, this dose would be expected to specifically exert a respiratory but not excessive cardiovascular effects. Higher concentrations of leptin would be expected to saturate plasma carrier molecules and some of unbound leptin would be degradated. Furthermore, since the amount of leptin to cross blood-brain barrier is relied on receptor-mediated transport mechanism (Morris and Rui, 2009), access to the brain should be limited somehow.

Leptin's intracellular signal transduction has been extensively investigated, with exception of molecular mechanisms underlying its effect on respiratory chemosensitivity. It remains poor understood how the activation of leptin signaling affects O_2-sensitive channels which may determine CB's chemosensitivity. Along with recent studies indicating that the chemosensitivity of CBs is closely associated with TASK-1 and TASK-3 channels (Trapp et al., 2008; Tan et al., 2010), TASK-2 channels has also been evidenced to set central respiratory CO_2 and O_2 sensitivity

(Gestreau et al., 2010). In addition, activation of ob-Rs appears to regulate ion channels including ATP-sensitive K^+ channels and voltage-gated K^+ channels (Gavello et al., 2016). Although STAT3, SOCS3, and ERK1/2 may mediate leptin's role in the CBs, the critical information is lacking to data concerning modulatory effects of these molecules on TASK channels. In the present study, we did not directly address how the activation of ob-Rs and downstream signaling proteins regulated TASK-1, TASK-3, and TASK-2 channels, but notably, the altered expression levels of these channels would be expected to be attributable to leptin signaling and contribute to leptin-stimulated facilitation of the HVR. Future work is required for revealing such mechanisms.

In summary, leptin signaling participates in setting CB's O_2 sensitivity probably through the modulation of TASK-1, TASK-3, and TASK-2 channels and thus contributes to the potentiation of HVR. This line of cellular evidence extends our understanding of molecular mechanism of leptin action on breathing, shedding light on the etiology of obesity-related hypoventilation or apnea.

AUTHOR CONTRIBUTIONS

FY, JF, and HW acquired the data; FY, JF, and ZW analyzed and interpreted data; FY, XZ, and HY drafted the manuscript; FY, SW, and YZ were responsible for study concept and design; YZ and SW obtained research funding.

ACKNOWLEDGMENTS

This study was supported by grants from the National Natural Science Foundation of China (31271223, 31671184) and from the Province Natural Science Foundation of Hebei (H2016206477). The experiments comply with the current laws of the country in which they were performed.

REFERENCES

Bassi, M., Furuya, W. I., Menani, J. V., Colombari, D. S., do Carmo, J. M., da Silva, A. A., et al. (2014). Leptin into the ventrolateral medulla facilitates chemorespiratory response in leptin-deficient (ob/ob) mice. *Acta Physiol.* 211, 240–248. doi: 10.1111/apha.12257

Bassi, M., Giusti, H., Leite, C. M., Anselmo-Franci, J. A., do Carmo, J. M., da Silva, A. A., et al. (2012). Central leptin replacement enhances chemorespiratory responses in leptin-deficient mice independent of changes in body weight. *Pflugers Arch.* 464, 145–153. doi: 10.1007/s00424-012-1111-1

Bassi, M., Werner, I. F., Zoccal, D. B., Menani, J. V., Colombari, E., Hall, J. E., et al. (2015). Control of respiratory and cardiovascular functions by leptin. *Life Sci.* 125, 25–31. doi: 10.1016/j.lfs.2015.01.019

Bray, G. A., and York, D. A. (1971). Genetically transmitted obesity in rodents. *Physiol. Rev.* 51, 598–646. doi: 10.1152/physrev.1971.51.3.598

Chang, Z., Ballou, E., Jiao, W., McKenna, K. E., Morrison, S. F., and McCrimmon, D. R. (2013). Systemic leptin produces a long-lasting increase in respiratory motor output in rats. *Front. Physiol.* 4:16. doi: 10.3389/fphys.2013.00016

Ciriello, J., and Caverson, M. M. (2014). Carotid chemoreceptor afferent projections to leptin receptor containing neurons in nucleus of the solitary tract. *Peptides* 58, 30–35. doi: 10.1016/j.peptides.2014.05.014

Farkas, G. A., and Schlenker, E. H. (1994). Pulmonary ventilation and mechanics in morbidly obese Zucker rats. *Am. J. Respir. Crit. Care Med.* 150, 356–362. doi: 10.1164/ajrccm.150.2.8049815

Fu, C., Xue, J., Wang, R., Chen, J., Ma, L., Liu, Y., et al. (2017). Chemosensitive Phox2b-expressing neurons are crucial for hypercapnic ventilatory response in the nucleus tractus solitarius. *J. Physiol.* 595, 4973–4989. doi: 10.1113/JP274437

Gavello, D., Carbone, E., and Carabelli, V. (2016). Leptin-mediated ion channel regulation: PI3K pathways, physiological role, and therapeutic potential. *Channels* 10, 282–296. doi: 10.1080/19336950.2016.1164373

Gestreau, C., Heitzmann, D., Thomas, J., Dubreuil, V., Bandulik, S., Reichold, M., et al. (2010). Task2 potassium channels set central respiratory CO_2 and O_2 sensitivity. *Proc. Natl. Acad. Sci. U.S.A.* 107, 2325–2330. doi: 10.1073/pnas.0910059107

Gonzalez-Martin, M. C., Vega-Agapito, M. V., Conde, S. V., Castaneda, J., Bustamante, R., Olea, E., et al. (2011). Carotid body function and ventilatory responses in intermittent hypoxia. Evidence for anomalous brainstem integration of arterial chemoreceptor input. *J. Cell Physiol.* 226, 1961–1969. doi: 10.1002/jcp.22528

Grill, H. J., Schwartz, M. W., Kaplan, J. M., Foxhall, J. S., Breininger, J., and Baskin, D. G. (2002). Evidence that the caudal brainstem is a target for the inhibitory effect of leptin on food intake. *Endocrinology* 143, 239–246. doi: 10.1210/endo.143.1.8589

Hall, J. E., da Silva, A. A., do Carmo, J. M., Dubinion, J., Hamza, S., Munusamy, S., et al. (2010). Obesity-induced hypertension: role of sympathetic nervous system, leptin, and melanocortins. *J. Biol. Chem.* 285, 17271–17276. doi: 10.1074/jbc.R110.113175

Kumar, N. N., Velic, A., Soliz, J., Shi, Y., Li, K., Wang, S., et al. (2015). Regulation of breathing by CO_2 requires the proton-activated receptor GPR4 in retrotrapezoid nucleus neurons. *Science* 348, 1255–1260. doi: 10.1126/science.aaa0922

Malhotra, A., and White, D. P. (2002). Obstructive sleep apnoea. *Lancet* 360, 237–245. doi: 10.1016/S0140-6736(02)09464-3

Messenger, S. A., Moreau, J. M., and Ciriello, J. (2013). Effect of chronic intermittent hypoxia on leptin and leptin receptor protein expression in the carotid body. *Brain Res.* 1513, 51–60. doi: 10.1016/j.brainres.2013.03.022

Moreau, J. M., Messenger, S. A., and Ciriello, J. (2015). Effects of angiotensin II on leptin and downstream leptin signaling in the carotid body during acute intermittent hypoxia. *Neuroscience* 310, 430–441. doi: 10.1016/j.neuroscience.2015.09.066

Morris, D. L., and Rui, L. (2009). Recent advances in understanding leptin signaling and leptin resistance. *Am. J. Physiol. Endocrinol. Metab.* 297, E1247–E1259. doi: 10.1152/ajpendo.00274.2009

O'Donnell, C. P., Tankersley, C. G., Polotsky, V. P., Schwartz, A. R., and Smith, P. L. (2000). Leptin, obesity, and respiratory function. *Respir. Physiol.* 119, 163–170. doi: 10.1016/S0034-5687(99)00111-5

Olea, E., Agapito, M. T., Gallego-Martin, T., Rocher, A., Gomez-Niño, A., Obeso, A., et al. (2014). Intermittent hypoxia and diet-induced obesity: effects on oxidative status, sympathetic tone, plasma glucose and insulin levels, and arterial pressure. *J. Appl. Physiol. (1985)* 117, 706–719. doi: 10.1152/japplphysiol.00454.2014

Olea, E., Ribeiro, M. J., Gallego-Martin, T., Yubero, S., Rigual, R., Masa, J. F., et al. (2015). The carotid body does not mediate the acute ventilatory effects of leptin. *Adv. Exp. Med. Biol.* 860, 379–385. doi: 10.1007/978-3-319-18440-1_43

Panetta, P., Berry, A., Bellisario, V., Capoccia, S., Raggi, C., Luoni, A., et al. (2017). Long-term sex-dependent vulnerability to metabolic challenges in prenatally stressed rats. *Front. Behav. Neurosci.* 11:113. doi: 10.3389/fnbeh.2017.00113

Phipps, P. R., Starritt, E., Caterson, I., and Grunstein, R. R. (2002). Association of serum leptin with hypoventilation in human obesity. *Thorax* 57, 75–76. doi: 10.1136/thorax.57.1.75

Porzionato, A., Rucinski, M., Macchi, V., Stecco, C., Castagliuolo, I., Malendowicz, L. K., et al. (2011). Expression of leptin and leptin receptor isoforms in the rat and human carotid body. *Brain Res.* 1385, 56–67. doi: 10.1016/j.brainres.2011.02.028

Pye, R. L., Dunn, E. J., Ricker, E. M., Jurcsisn, J. G., Barr, B. L., and Wyatt, C. N. (2015). Acutely administered leptin increases $[Ca^{2+}]_i$ and BK Ca currents but does not alter chemosensory behavior in rat carotid body type I cells. *Adv. Exp. Med. Biol.* 860, 61–67. doi: 10.1007/978-3-319-18440-1_8

Rahmouni, K., Haynes, W. G., Morgan, D. A., and Mark, A. L. (2002). Selective resistance to central neural administration of leptin in agouti obese mice. *Hypertension* 39, 486–490. doi: 10.1161/hy0202.102836

Rahmouni, K., and Morgan, D. A. (2007). Hypothalamic arcuate nucleus mediates the sympathetic and arterial pressure responses to leptin. *Hypertension* 49, 647–652. doi: 10.1161/01.HYP.0000254827.59792.b2

Ribeiro, M. J., Sacramento, J. F., Gallego-Martin, T., Olea, E., Melo, B. F., Guarino, M. P., et al. (2017). High fat diet blunts the effects of leptin on ventilation and on carotid body activity. *J. Physiol.* doi: 10.1113/JP275362. [Epub ahead of print].

Tan, Z. Y., Lu, Y., Whiteis, C. A., Simms, A. E., Paton, J. F., Chapleau, M. W., et al. (2010). Chemoreceptor hypersensitivity, sympathetic excitation, and overexpression of ASIC and TASK channels before the onset of hypertension in SHR. *Circ. Res.* 106, 536–545. doi: 10.1161/CIRCRESAHA.109.206946

Tartaglia, L. A. (1997). The leptin receptor. *J. Biol. Chem.* 272, 6093–6096. doi: 10.1074/jbc.272.10.6093

Tatsumi, K., Kasahara, Y., Kurosu, K., Tanabe, N., Takiguchi, Y., and Kuriyama, T. (2005). Sleep oxygen desaturation and circulating leptin in obstructive sleep apnea-hypopnea syndrome. *Chest* 127, 716–721. doi: 10.1378/chest.127.3.716

Trapp, S., Aller, M. I., Wisden, W., and Gourine, A. V. (2008). A role for TASK-1 (KCNK3) channels in the chemosensory control of breathing. *J. Neurosci.* 28, 8844–8850. doi: 10.1523/JNEUROSCI.1810-08.2008

Wang, S., Benamer, N., Zanella, S., Kumar, N. N., Shi, Y., Bévengut, M., et al. (2013). TASK-2 channels contribute to pH sensitivity of retrotrapezoid nucleus chemoreceptor neurons. *J. Neurosci.* 33, 16033–16044. doi: 10.1523/JNEUROSCI.2451-13.2013

Wjidan, K., Ibrahim, E., Caszo, B., Gnanou, J., and Singh, H. (2015). Dysregulation of glucose homeostasis following chronic exogenous administration of leptin in healthy sprague-dawley rats. *J. Clin. Diagn. Res.* 9, OF06–OF09. doi: 10.7860/JCDR/2015/15594.7003

6

Revisiting the Role of TRP, Orai, and ASIC Channels in the Pulmonary Arterial Response to Hypoxia

Roberto V. Reyes[1,2], Sebastián Castillo-Galán[1], Ismael Hernandez[1], Emilio A. Herrera[1,2], Germán Ebensperger[1,2] and Aníbal J. Llanos[1,2]*

[1] *Unidad de Fisiología y Fisiopatología Perinatal, Programa de Fisiopatología, Instituto de Ciencias Biomédicas, Facultad de Medicina, Universidad de Chile, Santiago, Chile,* [2] *International Center for Andean Studies, Universidad de Chile, Santiago, Chile*

***Correspondence:**
Roberto V. Reyes
vicreyes@med.uchile.cl;
virreyc@gmail.com

The pulmonary arteries are exquisitely responsive to oxygen changes. They rapidly and proportionally contract as arterial PO_2 decrease, and they relax as arterial PO_2 is re-established. The hypoxic pulmonary vasoconstriction (HPV) is intrinsic since it does not require neural or endocrine factors, as evidenced in isolated vessels. On the other hand, pulmonary arteries also respond to sustained hypoxia with structural and functional remodeling, involving growth of smooth muscle medial layer and later recruitment of adventitial fibroblasts, secreted mitogens from endothelium and changes in the response to vasoconstrictor and vasodilator stimuli. Hypoxic pulmonary arterial vasoconstriction and remodeling are relevant biological responses both under physiological and pathological conditions, to explain matching between ventilation and perfusion, fetal to neonatal transition of pulmonary circulation and pulmonary artery over-constriction and thickening in pulmonary hypertension. Store operated channels (SOC) and receptor operated channels (ROC) are plasma membrane cationic channels that mediate calcium influx in response to depletion of internal calcium stores or receptor activation, respectively. They are involved in both HPV and pathological remodeling since their pharmacological blockade or genetic suppression of several of the Stim, Orai, TRP, or ASIC proteins in SOC or ROC complexes attenuate the calcium increase, the tension development, the pulmonary artery smooth muscle proliferation, and pulmonary arterial hypertension. In this Mini Review, we discussed the evidence obtained in *in vivo* animal models, at the level of isolated organ or cells of pulmonary arteries, and we identified and discussed the questions for future research needed to validate these signaling complexes as targets against pulmonary hypertension.

Keywords: store operated channels, receptor operated channels, hypoxia, hypoxic pulmonary vasoconstriction, pulmonary arterial remodeling, pulmonary hypertension

INTRODUCTION

The pulmonary arteries have distinctive properties all along the individual's life, compared to systemic arteries. During gestation, the gas exchange is carried out by the placenta, the pulmonary vascular resistance (PVR) is high and the pulmonary blood flow is low, receiving less than 10–20% of the combined fetal cardiac output (CO). In fact, fetal pulmonary arteries have a narrow lumen and a thick medial layer with immature smooth muscle cells, increased synthesis and signaling of vasoconstrictors as well as low oxygen tension (PaO_2) in the fetal arterial blood, among other factors, which contribute to the pulmonary high resistance, low flow state. At birth, PVR quickly decreases and the pulmonary blood flow increases ~10 times to accommodate the totality of the CO, allowing the lungs to replace the placenta as gas exchanger at the first minutes of postnatal life (Rudolph, 1979; Suresh and Shimoda, 2016). Increases of PaO_2 and signaling mechanisms favoring the vasodilation contribute to this fetal to neonatal physiological transition. The pulmonary arteries also undergo a quick and dramatic structural transition at birth: the pulmonary artery smooth muscle cells (PASMC) of the medial layer flattens and their cytoskeleton reorganizes deriving in wall thinning and luminal enlargement. These changes finally allow the establishment of postnatal pulmonary circulation with thin pulmonary arterial wall and low mean pulmonary arterial pressure (mPAP ~8–20 mmHg at rest for humans) compared to systemic circulation (Peñaloza and Arias-Stella, 2007; Gao and Raj, 2010; Gao and Raj, 2011; Nayr and Lakshminrusimha, 2014). A unique feature of the pulmonary arteries is their intrinsic sensitivity to hypoxia, possessing a vasoconstrictor response to acute hypoxia called "hypoxic pulmonary vasoconstriction" (HPV), which is already present in fetal pulmonary arteries and continues to exist in every life stages. HPV is a rapid and reversible contraction of pulmonary arteries, whose intensity is proportional to the degree of hypoxia and it occurs independently of neural or humoral factors (Sylvester et al., 2012). HPV contributes to the physiologically high PVR state during fetal life, while it allows to optimize the ratio between ventilation and perfusion during the postnatal life (Dunham-Snary et al., 2017; Hussain et al., 2017). Pulmonary arteries also mount a maladaptive response to chronic hypoxia, known as pathological pulmonary arterial remodeling, characterized by the hyperplasic and hypertrophic thickening of medial layer and later thickening of adventitia and intima, with increased extracellular matrix deposition. An example of the later is the exposure to chronic hypoxia during pregnancy, early birth or adult life, resulting in pulmonary hypertension, a condition characterized by elevated pulmonary arterial mPAP and PVR, pathological pulmonary artery remodeling, often complicated with right ventricular hypertrophy and cardiac failure (Herrera et al., 2015; Suresh and Shimoda, 2016).

STORE OPERATED CHANNELS, RECEPTOR OPERATED CHANNELS, STRUCTURE, FUNCTION, AND PHARMACOLOGY

Cytosolic free Ca^{2+} [(Ca^{2+})i] is pivotal for PASMC contraction, differentiation and proliferation, as well as for synthesis of vasoactive compounds from the pulmonary artery endothelial cells (PAEC). The $[Ca^{2+}]$i may increases through its release from sarcoplasmic reticulum (SR) stores mediated by ryanodine receptors (RyR) or Inositol triphosphate receptors (IP3R), or through calcium influx mediated by voltage operated calcium channels (VOC), receptor operated calcium channels (ROC), or store operated calcium channels (SOC) from plasma membrane (Kuhr et al., 2012).

The SOC is a functional definition for plasma membrane cationic channels that are physiologically activated as calcium stores of SR are gradually depleted by agonists coupled to IP3R or RyR, ensuring a mechanism to refill intracellular Ca^{2+} stores and enabling to maintain long term $[Ca^{2+}]$i signals. The most useful strategy to evaluate SOC function is to measure $[Ca^{2+}]$i in isolated cells pre-loaded with a fluorescent Ca^{2+}-sensitive dye like FURA-2AM. The cells are superfused in a Ca^{2+}-free medium with nifedipine to block VOC, intracellular calcium stores are passively depleted by inhibition of SR Ca^{2+} pump (SERCA) with thapsigargin or cyclopiazonic acid, and $[Ca^{2+}]$i changes are evaluated after restoration of extracellular Ca^{2+}. This Ca^{2+} influx is referred as store operated calcium entry (SOCE). Alternatively, SOCE is also evaluated as the rate of fluorescence quenching by Mn^{2+} which enters the cell after store depletion as Ca^{2+} surrogate and reduces fluorescence through binding the dye (Bird et al., 2008). Concerning their structure, early studies suggested that SOC were formed by pore-forming subunits of the canonical transient receptor potential (TRPC) proteins. However, posterior discoveries showed a complex formed by Orai1 protein and stromal interacting molecule-1 (Stim1) as basic components able to generate store operated calcium influx, raising a controversy about the real molecular identity of SOCs (Earley and Brayden, 2015). This model suggests that SOC are hexamers of Orai proteins (Orai1, 2 or 3) and/or tetramers of TRPC proteins (TRPC1, 3, 4, 5, 6, or 7) that form the pore, and need the interaction mainly with Stim1 protein as calcium sensor of the SR to be activated. Store depletion of SR calcium results in redistribution of Stim1 from a homogeneous pattern in the bulk SR in resting cells, to a localized pattern into regions of SR called *punctae*, close to plasma membrane, allowing its interaction with Orai1 or TRPC proteins and their gating. Stim1-Orai complexes generate the Ca^{2+}-release-activated Ca^{2+} currents (I_{crac}) associated with oscillations of Ca^{2+} and characterized as a small inwardly rectifying and selective Ca^{2+} currents in electrophysiological studies. These oscillations are necessary to further recruit TRPC subunits, mainly TRPC1, to form Stim-TRPC complexes that generate additional but sometimes less selective Ca^{2+} currents. The selectivity probably depends on the type of TRPC subunits that tetramerize to form the active complex. The recruitment of both currents results in a sustained Ca^{2+} elevation termed the store operated calcium current (I_{soc}) (Ambudkar et al., 2017; Putney, 2017). This model is consistent with the ability of different sub-types of Stim, TRPC, and Orai proteins to generate SOCE in pulmonary arteries (Fernandez et al., 2012; Earley and Brayden, 2015; Wang et al., 2017). Moreover, other TRP channels such as transient receptor potential vanilloid-4 (TRPV4) and structurally unrelated Na^{+}- and Ca^{2+}-permeable cation channels such as acid-sensing ion channels-1 (ASIC1) may also contribute to SOC signaling in PASMC (Goldenberg et al., 2015; Jernigan, 2015). Whether the mechanism linking store depletion and ASIC1 activation to generate SOCE is related with association of ASIC1 with Stim, Orai, TRPC proteins, or other unknown signal has not been elucidated. Next to SOC complexes, TRP proteins also work as ROC. After receptor activation by agonist binding, phospholipase C (PLC) isozymes convert phosphatidylinositol-4,5-bisphosphate (PIP2) into inositoltriphosphate (IP3) and diacylglycerol (DAG), and DAG or its synthetic analog OAG, used to identify receptor operated Ca2+ entry (ROCE) are common activators of all TRPC channels (Dietrich et al., 2005; Fernandez et al., 2012; Storch et al., 2017) except TRPC1 whose role as an ion channel or channel regulator is still a matter of debate (Dietrich et al., 2014).

Inhibitors targeting Stim, Orai, and TRP proteins are increasing in number and potency. Nevertheless, for many of these molecules, their mechanism of action, specificity, and toxicity needs further investigation to allow *in vivo* assays or clinical trials. For instance, two old useful inhibitors are SKF-96365 and 2-APB, are reported to block TRPC3/5, and the Stim/Orai interaction, respectively, at micromolar concentrations, but they also block VOC and IP3R at a similar concentration range (Putney, 2010; Bon and Beech, 2013). Lanthanides, such as La^{3+} or Gd^{3+} strongly inhibit Orai but their use is limited because their water solubility is poor in the presence of proteins and multivalent anions (Bird et al., 2008). Other blockers such as ML-9, BTP2, some GSK-compounds and RO2959 target other molecules in addition to Stim, Orai, or TRP subunits and/or are poorly soluble in physiological solutions (Prakriya and Lewis, 2015; Tian et al., 2016). Some recently characterized inhibitors show improved potency and selectivity: compound 8009-5364 and larixyl acetate block TRPC6 OAG-induced currents (Urban et al., 2012, 2016), AncoA4 blocks Orai channels and prevents its binding with Stim1 (Sadaghiani et al., 2014) while GSK2193874, GSK2220691, and HC067047 block TRPV4 currents (Everaerts et al., 2010; Thorneloe et al., 2012; Balakrishna et al., 2014). These inhibitors are promising tools to study the role of these channels on pulmonary vascular function (**Table 1**). The development of new agents specific for other TRP or Orai isoforms, combining potency and water-solubility should be helpful to study the composition and stoichiometry of native SOC/ROC complexes in pulmonary arteries and to validate them as potential pharmacological targets for pulmonary hypertension treatment.

THE ROLE OF TRP, STIM, ORAI, AND ASIC PROTEINS IN THE PULMONARY ARTERIAL RESPONSE TO ACUTE HYPOXIA

The SOCE and different TRP, Orai, Stim, and ASIC proteins are robustly expressed in rodent pulmonary arteries and PASMC (Lin et al., 2004; Wang et al., 2006, 2017; Jernigan et al., 2009; Fernandez et al., 2015). Indeed, in PASMC from distal pulmonary arteries the increase of $[Ca^{2+}]i$ in response to acute hypoxia, SOCE and the expression of Stim1, TRPC1, 4, and 6 are greater than in proximal pulmonary arteries (Lu et al., 2008). Moreover, evidence from knockdown, knockout, or overexpression experiments show that in rodent PASMC, Stim1 and 2, Orai 1, 2 and 3, TRPC1 and 6, and ASIC1 contribute to SOCE (Lin et al., 2004; Jernigan et al., 2009; Nitta et al., 2014; Fernandez et al., 2015; Wang et al., 2017). Both, hypoxia-induced $[Ca^{2+}]i$ increase and HPV responses, are biphasic with a rapid and transient first phase of 5–20 min, followed by a slower and more sustained second phase of more than 180 min (Sommer et al., 2016). The first phase is abolished in TRPC6−/− mice, while knockdown of Stim1 suppresses the second phase (Weissmann et al., 2006; Lu et al., 2009). HPV, SOCE, and ROCE are also attenuated in ASIC1−/− mice compared to ASIC+/+ controls (Nitta et al., 2014). In lung of adult rat, SOC blockade with SKF-96365 inhibits HPV in a concentration-dependent manner (Weigand et al., 2005). The first phase of HPV is also suppressed by TRPC6 blockade with compound 800-5364 and larixyl acetate in mouse isolated lung (Urban et al., 2012, 2016). A significant decrease of HPV is also observed in knockout mice for transient receptor potential vanilloid-4 channel (TRPV4), and there is evidence of "promiscuous" TRPC6/TRPV4 heteromers assembly to generate SOC (Goldenberg et al., 2015). Transcripts of TRPC1, 3, 5, and 6 are detected in PASMC from late gestation ovine fetuses (Resnik et al., 2007) while TRPC1, 3, 4, 5, 6, Orai1, and Stim1 messengers are expressed in lungs from newborn lambs. Moreover the HPV recorded *in vivo* is significantly suppressed through SOC blockade with 2-APB in lambs (Parrau et al., 2013). Taken together, these data clearly show that at least in neonatal sheep and in adult rodents, SOC/ROC are key for contractile response to acute hypoxia, and that at least Stim1, TRPC6, and TRPV4 form part of the molecular complex involved in HPV. Nevertheless, as active Orai and TRPC complexes are hexamers and tetramers, respectively, the possibility of heteromeric association incorporating other Orai or TRPC subtypes to generate Ca^{2+} influx associated to HPV cannot be excluded.

Currently, the mechanism linking hypoxia and SOC/ROC activation is a matter of research. For instance, increase of reactive oxygen species (ROS) during hypoxia is proposed to directly and indirectly activate RyR to deplete SR calcium stores, activate SOC, and increase $[Ca^{2+}]i$ and contraction (Sommer et al., 2016; Suresh and Shimoda, 2016). Hypoxia and ischemia/reperfusion provokes DAG accumulation and TRPC6 activation in PASMC and PAEC, respectively, where H_2O_2 directly and indirectly mediates this effect (Weissmann et al., 2006, 2012). Interestingly H_2O_2 resulting from increased ROS, also promotes the interaction of Stim1, with Orai1 and TRPC1, and upregulates these proteins to mediate SOCE in PASMC (Chen et al., 2017). H_2O_2 also promotes Src family kinase-mediated stimulation of TPRV4 in lung microvascular endothelial cells (Suresh et al., 2015), but it is not elucidated if this mechanism also occurs in PASMC. It also remains to be demonstrated if the rate and the potency of the responses evoked by H_2O_2 is consistent with tension development observed in HPV. Indeed, in PASMC, $[Ca^{2+}]i$ evokes contraction through its binding to calmodulin (CaM) and activation of myosin light chain kinase (MLCK), to phosphorylate the 20 kDa myosin light chain (MLC_{20}), and increase the $pMLC_{20}/MLC_{20}$ ratio (Ogut and Brozovich, 2008; Kuhr et al., 2012). Despite this obvious link between $[Ca^{2+}]i$ and contraction, the relation between $pMLC_{20}/MLC_{20}$ ratio and SOC has been demonstrated only for

TABLE 1 | Current inhibitors of store operated channels and receptor operated channels.

Inhibitor/type	Observed target or action	Potency	Selectivity	Solubility	Reference
La^{3+}, Ga^{3+}/ Lanthanides	Block pore of Orai1 and Orai3 channels	IC_{50} = 0.2–0.5 μM	Selective at effective concentrations to block Orai	Water soluble, precipitates in the presence of soluble proteins and polyvalent anions	Bird et al., 2008; Prakriya and Lewis, 2015
SKF-96365/ phenyle-thyl-imidazole	Block recombinant TRPC3 and TRPC6 currents and Icrac currents	IC_{50} = 0.6–14 μM	Block voltage-gated calcium channels (T-type) and cAMP-gated-chloride channels	Water soluble	Putney, 2010; Bon and Beech, 2013; Tian et al., 2016
2-APB/ organoborated	Inteference of Stim1-Orai1 interaction	IC_{50} = 10 μM	Inhibits IP3R, TRPM7 channels, connexins gap junction	Dimethyl sulfoxide (DMSO)	Putney, 2010; Prakriya and Lewis, 2015
ML-9/pyrazol derivative	Inhibits Stim1 translocation	IC_{50} = 10 μM	Inhibits MLCK, PKA and PKC	DMSO	Prakriya and Lewis, 2015; Tian et al., 2016
BTP2/pyrazol derivative	Blocks recombinant TRPC3 and TRPC5 currents and Icrac currents	IC_{50} = 0.1 μM	Activates TRPM4 channels	DMSO, Ethanol	Prakriya and Lewis, 2015; Tian et al., 2016
RO2959	Blocks recombinant Stim1/Orai1, Stim1/Orai2 and Stim1/Orai3 currents	IC_{50} = 25 nM for Orai1 currents and 530 nM for Orai3 currents	Other targets not described	DMSO	Prakriya and Lewis, 2015
GSK5498A, GSK5503A, GSK7975A/ pyrazol derivatives	Block recombinant Stim1/Orai1 and Stim1/Orai3 currents	IC_{50} = 1–4 μM	Block TRPV6 channels	DMSO	Prakriya and Lewis, 2015; Tian et al., 2016
GSK2193874/ piperidin derivative	Blocks TRPV4 currents and Ca^{2+} entry	IC_{50} = 2–40 nM depending on species	Block hERG and CaV1.2 channels with low potency	DMSO	Thorneloe et al., 2012
GSK2220691	Blocks TRPV4 currents	IC_{50} = 2.5–10 nM	Selective	0.5% methylcellulose	Balakrishna et al., 2014
HC067047	Blocks TRPV4 currents	IC_{50} = 17–133 nM depending on species	Blocks hERG K^+ channels and TRPM8	DMSO, ethanol	Everaerts et al., 2010
8009-5364/ β-carboline derivative	Blocks TRPC6/TRPC3 OAG-induced and agonist-induced Ca^{2+} entry	IC_{50} = 5 μM and 13 μm for OAG-stimulated TRPC6 and TRPC3, respectively.	Blocks TRPA1 channel	DMSO	Urban et al., 2012
Larixyl acetate/larch-derived diterpene	Blocks TRPC6/TRPC3 OAG-induced and agonist-induced Ca^{2+} entry	IC_{50} = 0.58 μM and 6.38 μm for OAG-stimulated TRPC6 and TRPC3, respectively.	Block TRPC7, TRPC4, and TRPC5 with IC_{50} at 2.9–19.3 μM range	Chloroform, ethyl acetate	Urban et al., 2016
AncoA4/tricyclic chromone-fused analog	Blocks Orai1 Ca^{2+} entry and prevents Stim1/Orai1 binding	IC_{50} = 0.88 μM	No other targets described	DMSO	Sadaghiani et al., 2014

The IC_{50} values reported correspond to endogenous Icrac currents or to heterologous expressed TRPC/V, Orai, or Stim currents.

TRPV4 (Goldenberg et al., 2015), while it has not still been demonstrated for other SOC forming subunits. Further, the relation of SOC/ROC with other mechanisms regulating PASMC contraction such as calcium sensitization remains unexplored.

TRP, STIM, ORAI, AND ASIC PROTEINS: TENSION DEVELOPMENT AND PULMONARY ARTERIAL REMODELING IN RESPONSE TO CHRONIC HYPOXIA

The pathological pulmonary arterial remodeling induced by chronic hypoxia is the result of an imbalance between proliferation and apoptosis of PASMC, changes in the differentiation state of PASMC and fibroblasts, and secretion of vasoactive compounds from PAEC (Suresh and Shimoda, 2016).

The PASMC and pulmonary arterial rings from rats exposed to chronic hypoxia have increased basal $[Ca^{2+}]$I and arterial tension, which are reduced by SOC blockade. In contrast, SOC blockade have minimal effects on normoxic controls. Interestingly, protein levels of Orail and 2, TRPC1 and 6, Stim1 and 2, ASIC1, and SOCE are greater in pulmonary vasculature of hypoxic animals than control rats (Lin et al., 2004; Wang et al., 2006, 2009, 2017; Jernigan et al., 2012; Hou et al., 2013; He et al., 2018). ASIC1−/− mice show decreased SOCE and attenuated hypoxic pulmonary hypertension compared to ASIC+/+ controls (Nitta et al., 2014). Moreover, chronically hypoxic newborn lambs gestated and born at 3,600 m altitude, have pulmonary hypertension, increased HPV, and upregulated TRPC4 and Stim1 pulmonary transcripts. In these animals, SOC blockade with a single dose of 2-APB evokes a greater attenuation of HPV compared to normoxic controls (Parrau et al., 2013). In another ovine model with partial gestation under chronic hypoxia, the newborn lambs show pulmonary hypertension that persists at sea level and increased TRPC4 and Orai1 expression. Further, an experimental therapy with 2-APB reduces mPAP, PVR, and pathological pulmonary arterial remodeling, both at the level of the medial and adventitial layer in these lambs (Castillo-Galán et al., 2016).

For TRPC1 and 6, as for Orai2, the hypoxic upregulation depends on hypoxia inducible factor-1α (HIF-1α), a cardinal transcription factor involved in the control of oxygen-regulated genes (Wang et al., 2006, 2017). An additional increase of TRPC1 transcription is mediated by nuclear factor of activated T-cells c3 (NFATc3), a calcium-sensitive transcription factor, allowing an amplification of the initial hypoxic induction (Wang et al., 2009). Induction of ASIC1-dependent SOCE by chronic hypoxia is due to increased membrane localization mediated by RhoA activation rather than increased transcription (Herbert et al., 2017). In addition, hypoxia may induce the synthesis and secretion of mitogens from PAEC. These mitogens function as paracrine regulators of PASMC proliferation, and SOC may contribute to both syntheses of these mitogens as to their proliferative signaling. For instance, hypoxia upregulates SOCE and TRPC4 in PAEC. This Ca^{2+} influx increases DNA binding activity of AP-1, a calcium-sensitive transcription factor, to activate transcription of AP-1 responsive genes like ET-1, PDGF, and VEGF among others. This is a mechanism that may contribute to pulmonary artery obliteration observed in pulmonary hypertension (Fantozzi et al., 2003). In turn, mitogens like platelet-derived growth factor (PDGF) and bone morphogenetic protein-4 (BMP4), a secreted ligand of the TGF-β superfamily, bind to receptors on PASMC. In doing so, PDGF and BMP4 further upregulate TRPC1, 4, 6, Orai1, and Stim1 expression, SOCE, and proliferation. PDGF-mediated upregulation of Orai1/Stim1 depends on Akt/mTOR proliferative pathway in both PASMC and pulmonary artery fibroblasts, while BMP4-mediated induction of TRPC1/4/6 depends on p38MAPK-ERK1/2 signaling (Ogawa et al., 2012; Zhang et al., 2014).

Other signaling mechanisms such as extracellular calcium sensing receptor (CaSR) and peroxisome-proliferator activated receptor-γ (PPAR-γ) are also involved in the pathogenesis of pulmonary hypertension and remodeling through SOCE. CaSR are G-coupled protein receptors activated by extracellular Ca^{2+} binding, and they are functionally coupled to TRPC6 activation to promote SOCE and ROCE, among other signaling mechanisms. CaSR are overexpressed in proliferating PASMC from hypoxic rodents or from patients with idiopathic pulmonary hypertension (IPAH), while their pharmacological or genetic suppression reduce proliferation and pulmonary hypertension (Yamamura et al., 2012, 2015; Smith et al., 2016; Tang et al., 2016). PPAR-γ is a member of the nuclear receptor hormone super family, and it is downregulated through TGF-β1 signaling in PASMC, whereas TRPC1 and 6 are upregulated in neonatal and adult rodents with hypoxic pulmonary hypertension. Conversely, stimulation of PPAR-γ reverses pulmonary hypertension and remodeling, and down regulates SOC expression (Gong et al., 2011; Yang et al., 2015; Jiang et al., 2016; Du et al., 2017).

To proliferate, PASMC undergo a de-differentiation, from a contractile and quiescent phenotype present in functional and healthy pulmonary vessels, to a synthetic and proliferative type, present in later stages of pathological remodeling. TRPC6, Orai2, and Stim2 contribute to the transition from the contractile to the synthetic phenotype (Fernandez et al., 2015). Theoretically, proliferative increase in response to SOCE may be mediated by direct stimulation of calmodulin kinase (CaMK) and p38-MAPK pathway, and activation of Ca^{2+}-sensitive transcription factors, such as NFATc3, CREB, and NF-Kβ (Kuhr et al., 2012). NFATc3 has been better studied in relation to PASMC proliferation and remodeling. Dephosphorylation of NFATc3 through Ca^{2+} and calcineurin promotes its nuclear translocation, to activate responsive genes related to PASMC proliferation, apoptosis resistance, and synthesis of contractile proteins, such as α-actin smooth muscle. Chronic hypoxia stimulates NFATc3 nuclear import. Parallel increase of ET-1 synthesis and activation of the RhoA-Rho kinase (RhoA/ROCK) pathway potentiates calcineurin-NFATc3 import (de Frutos et al., 2007, 2011; Ran et al., 2014). Moreover, the anti-proliferative effect of phosphodiesterase-5 (PDE5) inhibition with sildenafil on PASMC occurs with simultaneous inhibition of NFATc3 translocation, decreased SOCE, and TRPC1 downregulation. Additional SOCE decrease evoked by sildenafil may also be explained by PKG-dependent phosphorylation and inhibition of TRPC6 (Wang et al., 2009; Koitabashi et al., 2010). Conversely, the silencing of Stim1 reduces the proliferation of PASMC together with a decrease of NFATc3 translocation (Hou et al., 2013). Decreased NFATc3 nuclear import is also detected after genetic or pharmacological suppression of ASIC1-mediated SOCE (Gonzalez Bosc et al., 2016). Collectively, these data show that Ca^{2+} handling mediated by SOC/ROC stimulate PASMC proliferation through multiple signaling pathways. Several of these transduction pathways need further characterization related to the type of SOC/ROC complexes involved as well as for possible cross talk between them. **Figure 1** depicts the principal links of SOC/ROC with the pulmonary artery response to both acute and chronic hypoxia.

CONCLUSION AND PERSPECTIVES

Identification of Stim, Orai, and TRP proteins as part of the molecular components of SOCE/ROCE, and description of their direct or indirect regulation by oxygen allowed to gain understanding on their contribution to both hypoxic pulmonary vasoconstriction and remodeling. Nevertheless, some challenging developments are still needed in this field to

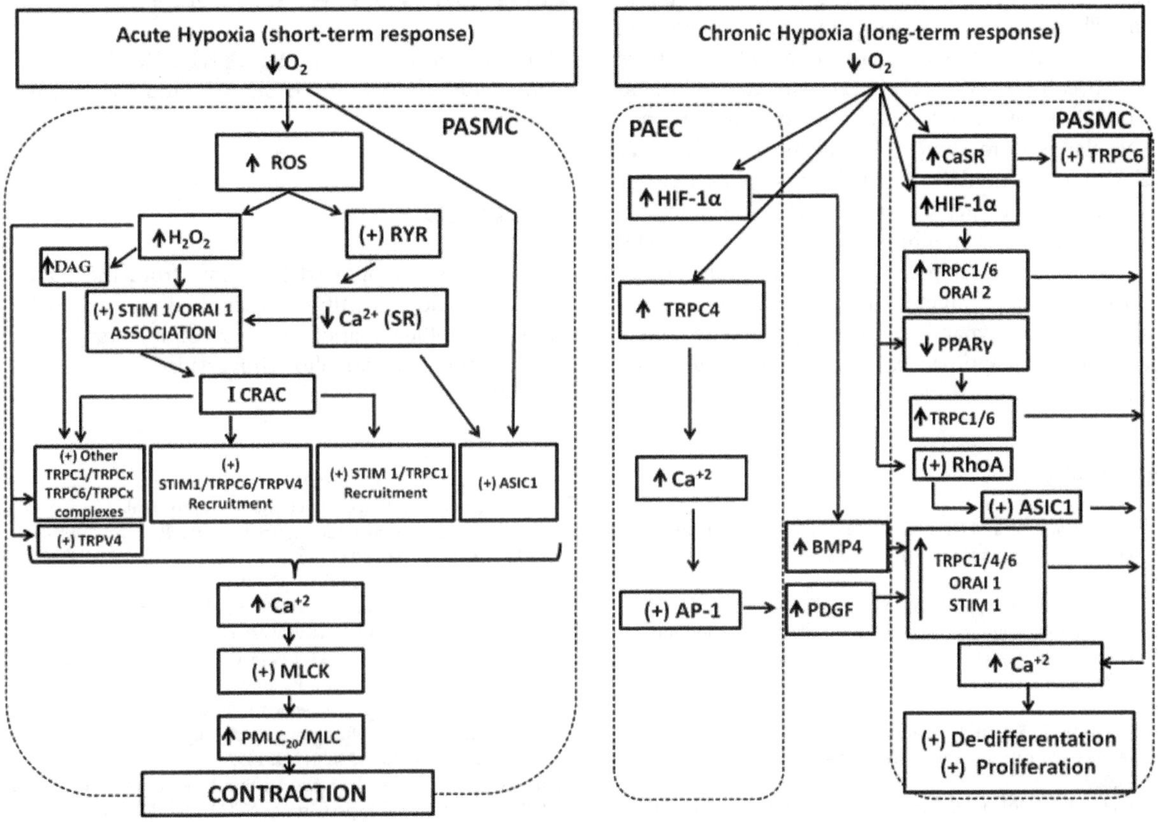

FIGURE 1 | SOC and ROC involvement in the pulmonary response to acute and chronic hypoxia. Acute hypoxia generates increase of ROS and H_2O_2. ROS stimulates RyR opening and depletion of SR-Ca^{2+} stores. Both H_2O_2 and depletion of SR-Ca^{2+} stores stimulates Stim1/Orai1 association to generate the calcium-release activated calcium current (Icrac), which in turn promotes further interaction of Stim1 with TRPC1, TRPC6, and TRPV4 proteins and recruitment to generate the store operated calcium (Isoc) current. The participation of other TRPC proteins in association with TRPC1 or 6 to generate Isoc cannot be discarded. Increase of DAG cell content promoted by H_2O_2 activates TRPC6/TRPCx channels. H_2O_2 can also directly activate TRPC6 and TRPV4 channels. Finally, ASIC1 also mediates hypoxic increase of SOC through an unknown mechanism. Increase of SOC and ROC results in the final increase of Ca^{2+}, stimulation of the myosin light chain kinase (MLCK), phosphorylation of myosin light chain, and contraction. Chronic hypoxia upregulates hypoxia inducible factor (HIF1) resulting in increased expression the secreted ligand bone morphogenetic protein-4 (BMP-4) from pulmonary artery endothelial cells (PAEC). Hypoxia also upregulates TRPC4 and Ca^{2+} increase, stimulates activator protein1 (AP-1) that in turn upregulates platelet-derived growth factor (PDGF). Secreted PDGF upregulates TRPC1, 4, 6, Orai1, and stim1 in pulmonary artery smooth muscle cells (PASMC). Hypoxia also upregulates the calcium sensing receptor (CaSR) coupled to TRPC6 stimulation and downregulates PPAR-γ in PASMC. Chronic hypoxia also stimulates RhoA protein, which stimulates ASIC1 incorporation to de membrane. The net result is an increase of expression and activity of TRPC1, 4, 6, Orai 1, 2, and ASIC1. The contribution of all these proteins to store and receptor operated calcium entry results in sustained Ca^{2+} increase to promote PASMC proliferation and remodeling.

fully understand SOC and ROC function in pulmonary arteries.

Despite Stim1, TRPC1, TRPC6, and TRPV4 are identified part of the SOC and ROC signaling complexes involved in HPV in pulmonary arteries, association of these subunits with other TRPC subtypes to form functional tetramers cannot be excluded. The same observation is valid for Orai complexes. The exact stoichiometry of native SOC and ROC complexes, if different homo/hetero multimer variants Orai, TRP, or ASIC are expressed along the development, and if they are associated to different SOCE and ROCE kinetics, is not elucidated.

Another question relates to the mechanism linking SR store depletion to ASIC1-mediated Ca^{2+} entry in PASMC. It is not known whether this mechanism is related to Stim as Ca^{2+} sensor of the SR, to association of ASIC1 with TRP proteins or to a totally different signal. The possibility to activate ion channels in response to store depletion by mechanisms different to those already discussed here cannot be ruled out.

There is no doubt that continuous chronic hypoxia upregulates Stim, Orai and TRPC proteins, SOCE/ROCE and evokes PASMC proliferation. Nevertheless, if different Stim, Orai, and TRPC proteins are responsive to hypoxia depending on development and duration of the stimulus is an unsolved question. Another form of hypoxia exposure is chronic intermittent hypoxia (CIH), for instance in obstructive sleep apnea (Iturriaga et al., 2014) or intermittent exposition to hypobaria (Herrera et al., 2015). Moreover, rats and mice exposed to CIH develop pulmonary hypertension and pathological remodeling, but the role of Ca2+ influx mediated by Stim, Orai, and ASIC channels on this condition is unexplored (Nisbet et al., 2009; Nara et al., 2015).

SOC and ROC are promising targets against pulmonary hypertension. There is an increasing number of inhibitors targeting Orai, TRP, and ASIC1, but many of them have not been tested in *in vivo* conditions to revert experimental pulmonary hypertension. SOC/ROC have a widespread distribution in the cardiovascular system, and side effects are likely. For instance, a 2-APB treatment decreases mPAP in hypoxic newborn lambs, but CO also diminishes transiently (Castillo-Galán et al., 2016). Therefore, novel SOC inhibitors targeting the pulmonary circulation need to be develop and tested in whole animals with the possibility to simultaneously record the systemic cardiovascular and hemodynamic responses possible to validate them as pharmacological approaches against hypoxic pulmonary hypertension.

AUTHOR CONTRIBUTIONS

RR drafted the manuscript. SC-G, IH, EH, GE, and AL edited the manuscript. RR, SC-G, IH, EH, GE, and AL approved the final submission.

FUNDING

This work was supported by grants from the Fondo Nacional de Investigación Científica y Tecnológica FONDECYT 1120605, 1130424, 1140647, and 1151119, and from Vicerrectoría de Investigación y Desarrollo, Universidad de Chile (VID-Enlace, ENL023f16).

REFERENCES

Ambudkar, I. S., de Souza, L. B., and Ong, H. L. (2017). TRPC1, Orai1, and STIM1 in SOCE: friends in tight spaces. *Cell Calcium* 63, 33–39. doi: 10.1016/j.ceca.2016.12.009

Balakrishna, S., Song, W., Achanta, S., Doran, S. F., Liu, B., Kaelberer, M. M., et al. (2014). TRPV4 inhibition counteracts edema and inflammation and improves pulmonary function and oxygen saturation in chemically induced acute lung injury. *Am. J. Physiol. Lung Cell. Mol. Physiol.* 307, L518–L172. doi: 10.1152/ajplung.00065.2014

Bird, G. S., DeHaven, W. I., Smyth, J. T., and Putney, J. W. (2008). Methods for studying store-operated calcium entry. *Methods* 46, 204–212. doi: 10.1016/j.ymeth.2008.09.009

Bon, R., and Beech, D. J. (2013). In pursuit of small molecule chemistry for calcium-permeable non-selective TRPC channels. Mirage or pot of gold? *Br. J. Pharmacol.* 170, 459–474. doi: 10.1111/bph.12274

Castillo-Galán, S., Quezada, S., Moraga, F. A., Ebensperger, G., Herrera, E. A., Beñaldo, F., et al. (2016). 2-aminoethyldiphenylborinate modifies the pulmonary circulation in pulmonary hypertensive newborn lambs partially gestated at high altitude. *Am. J. Physiol. Lung Cell. Mol. Physiol.* 311, L788–L799. doi: 10.1152/ajplung.00230.2016

Chen, T.-X., Xu, X.-Y., Zhao, Z., Zhao, F.-Y., Gao, Y.-M., Yan, X.-H., et al. (2017). Hydrogen peroxide is a critical regulator of the hypoxia-induced alterations of store-operated Ca^{2+} entry into rat pulmonary arterial smooth muscle cells. *Am. J. Physiol. Lung Cell. Mol. Physiol.* 312, L477–L487. doi: 10.1152/ajplung.00138.2016

de Frutos, S., Diaz, J. M., Nitta, C. H., Sherpa, M. L., and Bosc, L. V. (2011). Endothelin-1 contributes to increased NFATc3 activation by chronic hypoxia in pulmonary arteries. *Am. J. Physiol. Cell Physiol.* 301, C441–C450. doi: 10.1152/ajpcell.00029.2011

de Frutos, S., Spangler, R., Alò, D., and Bosc, L. V. (2007). NFATc3 mediates chronic hypoxia-induced pulmonary arterial remodeling with α-actin up-regulation. *J. Biol. Chem.* 282, 15081–15089. doi: 10.1074/jbc.M702679200

Dietrich, A., Falbusch, M., and Gudermann, T. (2014). Classic transient receptor potential 1 (TRPC1): channel or channel regulator? *Cells* 3, 939–962. doi: 10.3390/cells3040939

Dietrich, A., Mederos, Y., Schnitzler, M., Kalwa, H., Storch, U., and Gudermann, T. (2005). Functional characterization and physiological relevance of the TRPC3/6/7 subfamily of cation channels. *Naunyn Scmiedebergs Arch. Pharmacol.* 371, 257–265. doi: 10.1007/s00210-1052-8

Du, Y., Fu, J., Yao, L., Qiao, L., Liu, N., Xing, Y., et al. (2017). Altered expression of PPAR-γ and TRPC in neonatal rats with persistent pulmonary hypertension. *Mol. Med. Rep.* 16, 1117–1124. doi: 10.3892/mmr.2017.6744

Dunham-Snary, K. J., Wu, D., Sykes, E. A., Thakrar, A., Parlow, L. R., Mewburn, J. D., et al. (2017). Hypoxic pulmonary vasoconstriction. From molecular mechanisms to medicine. *Chest* 151, 181–192. doi: 10.1016/j.chest.2016.09.001

Earley, S., and Brayden, J. E. (2015). Transient receptor potential channels in the vasculature. *Physiol. Rev.* 95, 645–690. doi: 10.1152/physrev.00026.2014

Everaerts, W., Zhen, X., Ghosh, D., Vriens, J., Gevaert, T., Gilbert, J. P., et al. (2010). Inhibition of the cation channel TRPV4 improves bladder function in mice and rats with cyclophosphamide-induced cystitis. *Proc. Natl. Acad. Sci. U.S.A.* 107, 19084–19089. doi: 10.1073/pnas.1005.333.107

Fantozzi, I., Zhang, S., Platoshyn, O., Remillard, V., Cowling, R. T., and Yuan, J. X. (2003). Hypoxia increases AP-1 binding activity by enhancing capacitative Ca^{2+} entry in human pulmonary artery endothelial cells. *Am. J. Physiol. Lung Cell. Mol. Physiol.* 285, L1233–L1245. doi: 10.1152/ajplung.00445.2002

Fernandez, R. A., Sundivakkam, P., Smith, K. A., Zeifman, A. S., Drennan, A. R., and Yuan, J. X. (2012). Pathogenic role of store-operated and receptor-operated Ca^{2+} channels in pulmonary arterial hypertension. *J. Signal Transduct.* 2012:951497. doi: 10.1155/2012/951497

Fernandez, R. A., Wan, J., Song, S., Smith, K. A., Gu, Y., Tauseef, M., et al. (2015). Upregulated expression of STIM2, TRPC6, and Orai2 contributes to the transition of pulmonary arterial smooth muscle cells from a contractile to proliferative phenotype. *Am. J. Physiol. Cell Physiol.* 308, C581–C593. doi: 10.1152/ajpcell.00202.2014

Gao, Y., and Raj, J. U. (2010). Regulation of the pulmonary circulation in the fetus and the newborn. *Physiol. Rev.* 90, 1291–1335. doi: 10.1152/physrev.00032.2009

Gao, Y., and Raj, U. (2011). Hypoxic pulmonary hypertension of the newborn. *Compr. Physiol.* 1, 61–79. doi: 10.1002/cphy.c090015

Goldenberg, N. M., Wang, L., Ranke, H., Liedtke, W., Tabuchi, A., and Kuebler, W. M. (2015). TRPV4 is required for hypoxic pulmonary vasoconstriction. *Anesthesiology* 122, 1338–1348. doi: 10.1097/ALN.0000000000000647

Gong, K., Xing, D., Li, P., Aksut, B., Ambalavanan, N., Yang, Q., et al. (2011). Hypoxia induces downregulation of PPAR-γ in isolated pulmonary arterial smooth muscle cells and in rat lung via transforming growth factor-β signaling. *Am. J. Physiol. Lung Cell. Mol. Physiol.* 301, L899–L907. doi: 10.1152/ajplung.00062.2011

Gonzalez Bosc, L. V., Plomaritas, D. R., Herbert, L. M., Giermakowska, W., Browning, C., and Jernigan, N. L. (2016). ASIC1-mediated calcium entry stimulates NFATc3 nuclear translocation via PICK1 coupling in pulmonary arterial smooth muscle cells. *Am. J. Physiol. Lung Cell. Mol. Physiol.* 311, L48–L58. doi: 10.1152/ajplung.00040.2016

He, X., Song, S., Ayon, R. J., Balisterieri, A., Black, S. M., Makino, A., et al. (2018). Hypoxia selectively up-regulates cation channels and increases cytosolic $[Ca^{2+}]$ in pulmonary, but not coronary, arterial smooth muscle cells. 314, C504–C517. doi: 10.1152/ajpcell.00272.2017

Herbert, L. M., Resta, T. C., and Jernigan, N. L. (2017). RhoA increases ASIC1a plasma membrane localization and calcium influx in pulmonary arterial smooth muscle cells following chronic hypoxia. *Am. J. Cell Physiol.* 314, C166–C176. doi: 10.1152/ajpcell.00159.2017

Herrera, E. A., Farías, J. G., Ebensperger, G., Reyes, R. V., Llanos, A. J., and Castillo, R. L. (2015). Pharmacological approaches in either intermittent or permanent hypoxia: a tale of two exposures. *Pharmacol. Res.* 101, 94–101. doi: 10.1016/j.phrs.2015.07.011

Hou, X., Chen, J., Luo, Y., Liu, F., Xu, G., and Gao, Y. (2013). Silencing of STIM1 attenuates hypoxia-induced PASMCs proliferation via inhibition of the $SOC/Ca^{2+}/NFAT$ pathway. *Respir. Res.* 14:2. doi: 10.1186/1465-9921-14-12.

Hussain, A., Suleiman, M. S., George, S. J., Loubani, M., and Morice, A. (2017). Hypoxic pulmonary vasoconstriction in humans: tale or myth. *Open Cardiovasc. Med. J.* 11, 1–13. doi: 10.2174/1874192401711010001

Iturriaga, R., Andrade, D. C., and Del Rio, R. (2014). Enhanced carotid chemosensory activity and the cardiovascular alterations induced by intermittent hypoxia. *Front. Physiol.* 5:468. doi: 10.3389/fphys.2014.000468

Jernigan, N. L. (2015). Smooth muscle acid-sensing ion channel-1: pathophysiological implication in hypoxic pulmonary hypertension. *Exp. Physiol.* 100, 111–120. doi: 10.113/expphysiol.2014.081612

Jernigan, N. L., Herbert, L. M., Walker, B. R., and Resta, T. C. (2012). Chronic hypoxia upregulates pulmonary arterial ASIC1: a novel mechanism of enhanced store-operated Ca^{2+} entry and receptor-dependent vasoconstriction. *Am. J. Cell Physiol.* 302, C931–C940. doi: 10.1152/ajpcell00332.2011

Jernigan, N. L., Paffett, M. L., Walker, B. R., and Resta, T. C. (2009). ASIC1 contributes to pulmonary vascular smooth muscle store-operated Ca^{2+} entry. *Am. J. Physiol. Lung Cell. Mol. Physiol.* 297, L271–285. doi: 10.1152/ajplung.00020.2009

Jiang, Q., Lu, W., Yang, K., Hadadi, C., Fu, X., Chen, Y., et al. (2016). Sodium tanshinone IIA sulfonate inhibits hypoxia-induced enhancement of SOCE in pulmonary arterial smooth muscle cells via the PKG-PPAR-γ signaling axis. *Am. J. Physiol. Cell Physiol.* 311, C136–C149. doi: 10.1152/ajpcell.00252.201

Koitabashi, N., Aiba, T., Hesketh, G. G., Rowell, J., Zhang, M., Takimoto, E., et al. (2010). Cyclic GMP/PKG-dependent inhibition of TRPC6 channel activity and expression negatively regulates cardiomyocyte NFAT activation Novel mechanism of cardiac stress modulation by PDE5 inhibition. *J. Mol. Cell. Cardiol.* 48, 713–724. doi: 10.1016/j.yjmcc.2009.11.015

Kuhr, F. K., Smith, K. A., Song, M. Y., Levitan, I., and Yuan, J. X. (2012). New mechanisms of pulmonary arterial hypertension: role of Ca^{2+} signaling. *Am. J. Physiol. Heart Circ. Physiol.* 302, H1546–H1562. doi: 10.1152/ajpheart.00944.2011

Lin, M. J., Leung, G. P., Zhang, W. M., Yang. X. R., Yip, K. P., Tse, C. M., et al. (2004). Chronic hypoxia-induced upregulation of store-operated and receptor-operated Ca2+ channels in pulmonary arterial smooth muscle cells: a novel mechanism of hypoxic pulmonary hypertension. *Circ. Res.* 95, 496–505. doi: 10.1161/01.RES.0000138952.16382.ad

Lu, W., Wang, J., Peng, G., Shimoda, L. A., and Sylvester, J. T. (2009). Knockdown of stromal intaracting molecule 1 attenuates store-operated Ca^{2+} entry and Ca^{2+} responses to acute hypoxia in pulmonary arterial smooth muscle. *Am. J. Physiol. Lung Cell. Mol. Physiol.* 297, L17–L25. doi: 10.1152/ajplung.00063.2009

Lu, W., Wang, J., Shimoda, L. A., and Sylvester, J. T. (2008). Differences in STIM1 and TRPC expression in proximal and distal pulmonary arterial smooth muscle are associated with differences in Ca^{2+} responses to hypoxia. *Am. J. Physiol. Lung Cell. Mol. Physiol.* 295, L104–L113. doi: 10.1152/ajplung.00058.2008

Nara, A., Nagai, H., Shintani-Ishida, K., Ogura, S., Shimosawa, T., Kuwahira. I., et al. (2015). Pulmonary arterial hypertension in rats due to age-related arginase activation in intermittent hypoxia. *Am. J. Respir. Cell Mol. Biol.* 53, 184–192. doi: 10.1165/rcmb.2014-0163OC

Nayr, J., and Lakshminrusimha, S. (2014). Update on PPHN: mechanism and treatment. *Semin. Perinatol.* 38, 78–91. doi: 10.1053/j.semperi.2013.11.004

Nisbet, R. E., Graves, A. S., Kleinhenz, D. J., Rupnow, H. L., Reed, A. L., Fan, T. H., et al. (2009). The role of NADPH oxidase in chronic intermittent hypoxia-induced pulmonary hypertension in mice. *Am. J. Respir. Cell Mol. Biol.* 40, 601–609. doi: 10.1165/rcmb.2008-0145OC

Nitta, C. H., Osmond, D. A., Herbert, L. M., Beasley, B. F., Resta, T. C., Walker, B. R., et al. (2014). Role of ASIC1 in the development of chronic hypoxia-induced pulmonary hypertension. *Am. J. Physiol. Heart Circ. Physiol.* 306, H41–H52. doi: 10.1152/ajpheart.00269.2013

Ogawa, A., Firth, A. L., Smith, K. A., Maliakal, M. V., and Yuan, J. X. (2012). PDGF enhances store-operated Ca^{2+} entry by upregulating STIM1/Orai1 via activation of Akt/mTOR in human pulmonary arterial smooth muscle cells. *Am. J. Physiol. Cell Physiol.* 302, C405–C411. doi: 10.1152/ajpcell.00337.2011

Ogut, O., and Brozovich, F. (2008). The potential role of MLC phosphatase and MAPK signaling in the pathogenesis of vascular dysfunction in heart failure. *J. Cell Mol. Med.* 12, 2158–2164. doi: 10.1111/j.1582-4934.2008.00536.x

Parrau, D., Ebensperger, G., Herrera, E. A., Moraga, F., Riquelme, R. A., Ulloa, C. E., et al. (2013). Store operated channels in the pulmonary circulation of high- and low-altitude neonatal lambs. *Am. J. Physiol. Lung Cell. Mol. Physiol.* 304, L540–L548. doi: 10.1152/ajplung.00024.2012

Peñaloza, D., and Arias-Stella, J. (2007). The heart and pulmonary circulation at high altitudes: healthy highlanders and chronic Mountain sickness. *Circulation* 115, 1132–1146. doi: 10.1161/CIRCULATIONAHA.106.624544

Prakriya, M., and Lewis, R. S. (2015). Store-operated calcium channels. *Physiol. Rev.* 95, 1383–1436. doi: 10.1152/physrev.00020.2014

Putney, J. W. (2010). Pharmacology of store-operated calcium channels. *Mol. Interv.* 10, 209–218. doi: 10.1124/mi.10.4.4

Putney, J. W. (2017). Forms and function of store-operated calcium entry mediators, Stim and Orai. *Adv. Biol. Regul.* doi: 10.1016/j.jbior.2017.11.006 [Epub ahead of print].

Ran, Y., Wu, H., Wei, L., Yu, X., Chen, J., Li, S., Zhang, L., et al. (2014). NFATc3 pathway participates in the process that 15-LO/15-HETE protects pulmonary artery smooth muscle cells against apoptosis during hypoxia. *J. Recept. Signal Transduct. Res.* 34, 270–282. doi: 10.3109/10799893.2014.917322

Resnik, E. R., Keck, M., Sukovich, D. J., Herron, J. M., and Cornfield, D. M. (2007). Chronic intrauterine pulmonary hypertension increases capacitive calcium entry in fetal pulmonary artery smooth muscle cells. *Am. J. Physiol. Lung Cell. Mol. Physiol.* 292, L953–L959. doi: 10.1152/ajplung.00327.2006

Rudolph, A. M. (1979). Fetal and neonatal pulmonary circulation. *Annu. Rev. Physiol.* 41, 383–395. doi: 10.1146/annurev.ph.41.030179.002123

Sadaghiani, A. M., Lee, S. M., Odegaard, J. I., Leveson-Gower, D. B., McPherson, O. M., Novick, P., et al. (2014). Identification of Orai1 channel inhibitors by using minimal functional domains to screen small molecule microarrays. *Chem. Biol.* 21, 1278–1292. doi: 10.1016/j.chembiol.2014.08.016

Smith, K. A., Ayon, R. J., Tang, H., Makino, A., and Yuan, J. X. (2016). Calcium-sensing receptor regulates cytosolic $[Ca^{2+}]$ and plays a major role in the development of pulmonary hypertension. *Front. Physiol.* 7:517. doi: 10.3389/fphys.2016.00517

Sommer, N., Strielkov, L., Pak, O., and Weissman, N. (2016). Oxygen sensing and signal transduction in hypoxic pulmonary vasoconstriction. *Eur. Respir. J.* 47, 288–303. doi: 10.1183/13993003.00945-2015

Storch, U., Forst, A.-L., Pardatscher, F., Erdogmus, S., Philipp, M., Gregoritza, M., et al. (2017). Dynamic NHERF interaction with TRPC4/5 proteins is required for channel gating by diacylglycerol. *Proc. Natl. Acad. Sci. U.S.A.* 114, E37–E46. doi: 10.1073/pnas.1612263114

Suresh, K., Servinsky, L., Reyes, J., Baksh, S., Undem, C., Caterina, M., et al. (2015). Hydrogen peroxide-induced calcium influx in lung microvascular endotelial cells involves TRPV4. *Am. J. Physiol. Lung Cell. Mol. Physiol.* 309, L1467–L1477. doi: 10.1152/ajplung.00275.2015

Suresh, K., and Shimoda, L. A. (2016). Lung circulation. *Compr. Physiol.* 6, 897–943. doi: 10.1002/cphy.c140049

Sylvester, J. T., Shimoda, L. A., Aaronson, P. I., and Ward, J. P. (2012). Hypoxic pulmonary vasoconstriction. *Physiol. Rev.* 92, 367–520. doi: 10.1152/physrev.00041.2010

Tang, H., Yamamura, A., Yamamura, H., Song, S., Fraidenburg, D. R., Chen, J., et al. (2016). Pathogenic role of calcium-sensing receptors in the development and progression of pulmonary hypertension. *Am. J. Physiol. Lung Cell. Mol. Physiol.* 310, L849–L859. doi: 10.1152/ajplung.00050.2016

Thorneloe, K. S., Cheung, M., Bao, W., Alsaid, H., Lenhard, S., Jian, M.-Y., et al. (2012). An orally active TRPV4 channel blocker prevents and resolves pulmonary edema induced by heart failure. *Sci. Transl. Med.* 4:159ra148. doi: 10.1126/scitranslmed.3004276

Tian, C., Du, L., Zhou, Y., and Li, M. (2016). Store-operated CRAC channel inhibitors: opportunities and challenges. *Future Med. Chem.* 8, 817–832. doi: 10.4155/fmc-2016-0024

Urban, N., Hill, K., Wang, L., Kuebler, W. M., and Schaefer, M. (2012). Novel pharmacological TRPC inhibitors block hypoxia-induced vasoconstriction. *Cell Calcium* 51, 194–206. doi: 10.1016/j.ceca.2012.01.001

Urban, N., Wang, L., Kwiek, S., Rademann, J., Kuebler, W. M., and Schaefer, M. (2016). Identification and validation of larixyl acetate as a potent TRPC6 inhibitor. *Mol. Pharmacol.* 89, 197–213. doi: 10.1124/mol.115.100792

Wang, C., Li, J.-F., Zhao, L., Liu, J., Wang, J., Wang, Y. X., et al. (2009). Inhibition of SOC/Ca^{2+}/NFAT pathway is involved in the anti-proliferative effect of sildenafil on pulmonary artery smooth muscle cells. *Respir. Res.* 10, 123–136. doi: 10.1186/1465-9921-10-123

Wang, J., Weigand, L., Lu, W., Sylvester, J. T., Semenza, G. L., and Shimoda, L. A. (2006). Hypoxia inducible factor 1 mediates hypoxia-induced TRPC expression and elevated intracellular Ca^{2+} in pulmonary arterial smooth muscle cells. *Circ. Res.* 98, 1528–1537. doi: 10.1161/01.RES.0000227551.68124.98

Wang, J., Xu, C., Zheng, K., Yang, K., Lai, N., Wang, T., et al. (2017). Orai 1, 2, 3 and STIM1 promote store-operated calcium entry in pulmonary arterial smooth muscle cells. *Cell Death Discov.* 3:17074. doi: 10.1038/cddiscovery.2017.74

Weigand, L., Foxson, J., Wang, J., Shimoda, L. A., and Sylvester, J. T. (2005). Inhibition of hypoxic pulmonary vasoconstriction by antagonists of store-operated Ca^{2+} and nonselective cation channels. *Am. J. Physiol. Lung Cell. Mol. Physiol.* 289, L5–L13. doi: 10.1152/ajplung.00044.2005

Weissmann, N., Dietrich, A., Fuchs, B., Kalwa, H., Ay, M., Dimitrascu, R., et al. (2006). Classical transient receptor potential channel 6 (TRPC6) is essential for hypoxic pulmonary vasoconstriction and alveolar gas exchange. *Proc. Natl. Acad. Sci. U.S.A.* 103, 19093–19098. doi: 10.1073/pnas.0606728103

Weissmann, N., Sydykov, A., Kalwa, H., Storch, U., Fuchs, B., Mederos, Y., et al. (2012). Activation of TRPC6 channels is essential for lung ischaemia-reperfusion induced oedema in mice. *Nat. Commun.* 3:649. doi: 10.1038/ncomms1660

Yamamura, A., Guo, Q., Yamamura, H., Zimnicka, A., Pohl, N. M., Smith, K. A., et al. (2012). Enhanced Ca^{2+}-sensing receptor function in idiopathic pulmonary arterial hypertension. *Circ. Res.* 111, 469–48. doi: 10.1161/CIRCRESAHA.112.266361

Yamamura, A., Ohara, N., and Tsukamoto, K. (2015). Inhibition of excessive cell proliferation by calcilytics in idiopathic pulmonary arterial hypertension. *PLoS One* 10:e0138384. doi: 10.1371/journal.pone.0138384

Yang, K., Lu, W., Jiang, Q., Yun, X., Zhao, M., Jiang, H., et al. (2015). Peroxisome proliferator-activated receptor γ-mediated inhibition on hypoxia-triggered store-operated calcium entry. A caveolin-1-dependent mechanism. *Am. J. Respir. Cell Mol. Biol.* 53, 882–892. doi: 10.1165/rcmb.2015-0002OC

Zhang, Y., Wang, Y., Yang, K., Tian, L., Fu, X., Wang, Y., et al. (2014). BMP4 increases the expression of TRPC and basal $[Ca^{2+}]i$ via the p38MAPK and ERK1/2 pathways independent of BMPRII in PASMCs. *PLoS One* 9:e112695. doi: 10.1371/journal.pone.0112695

7

Plasmatic Concentrations of ADMA and Homocysteine in Llama (*Lama glama*) and Regulation of Arginase Type II: An Animal Resistent to the Development of Pulmonary Hypertension Induced by Hypoxia

Vasthi López[1], Fernando A. Moraga[2], Anibal J. Llanos[3], German Ebensperger[3], María I. Taborda[1] and Elena Uribe[4]*

[1] Laboratorio de Metabolismo de Aminoácidos e Hipoxia, Departamento de Ciencias Biomédicas, Universidad Católica del Norte, Coquimbo, Chile, [2] Laboratorio de Fisiología, Hipoxia y Función Vascular, Departamento de Ciencias Biomedicas, Facultad de Medicina, Universidad Católica del Norte, Coquimbo, Chile, [3] Laboratorio de Fisiología y Fisiopatología del Desarrollo, Departamento de Ciencias Biomédicas, Universidad de Chile, Santiago, Chile, [4] Laboratorio de Enzimología, Departamento de Bioquímica y Biología Molecular, Universidad of Concepción, Concepción, Chile

***Correspondence:**
Fernando A. Moraga
fmoraga@ucn.cl

There are animal species that have adapted to life at high altitude and hypobaric hypoxia conditions in the Andean highlands. One such species is the llama (*Lama glama*), which seem to have developed efficient protective mechanisms to avoid maladaptation resulting from chronic hypoxia, such as a resistance to the development of hypoxia -induced pulmonary hypertension. On the other hand, it is widely known that different models of hypertension can arise as a result of changes in endothelial function. The respect, one of the common causes of deregulation in endothelial vasodilator function have been associated with down-regulation of the NO synthesis and an increase in plasma levels of asymmetric dimethylarginine (ADMA) and homocysteine. Additionally, it is also known that NO production can be regulated by plasma levels of L-arginine as a result of the competition between nitric oxide synthase (NOS) and arginase. The objective of this study, was to determine the baseline concentrations of ADMA and homocysteine in llama, and to evaluate their effect on the arginase pathway and their involvement in the resistance to the development of altitude-induced pulmonary hypertension. METHOD: Lowland and highland newborn sheep and llama were investigated near sea level and at high altitude. Blood determinations of arterial blood gases, ADMA and homocysteíne are made and the effect of these on the arginase activity was evaluated. RESULTS: The basal concentrations of ADMA and homocysteine were determined in llama, and they were found to be significantly lower than those found in other species and in addition, the exposure to hypoxia is unable to increase its concentration. On the other hand, it was observed that the llama exhibited 10 times less arginase II activity as compared to sheep, and the expression was not induced by hypoxia.

Finally, ADMA y Hcy, has no effect on the type II arginase pathway. CONCLUSION: Based on our results, we propose that low concentrations of ADMA and homocysteine found in llamas, the low expression of arginase type II, DDAH-2 and CBS, as well as its insensitivity to activation by homocysteine could constitute an adaptation mechanism of these animals to the hypoxia.

Keywords: llama, ADMA, pulmonary hypertension, homocysteine, arginase

INTRODUCTION

Hypoxic pulmonary vasoconstriction (HPV) in distal pulmonary arteries is an intrinsic vasoconstrictor response to low oxygen levels. Once the normoxic condition returns, the vasoconstrictor response returns to normal levels. If the hypoxic stimulus becomes chronic it leads to structural and functional maladaptation of the pulmonary arterial bed, characterized by pulmonary artery remodeling and vasoconstriction. This results in sustained pulmonary arterial hypertension (PAH) that is often accompanied by right ventricular hypertrophy, heart failure and eventually death (Giordano, 2005; Pe-aloza, 2012). Species that have adapted to life at high altitude and hypobaric hypoxia conditions in the Andean *altiplano* have existed for at least 10 million years. One such species is the llama (*Lama glama*), which developed efficient protective mechanisms to avoid maladaptation resulting from chronic hypoxia, such as a decreased hormonal vasoconstrictor response, an increased blood hemoglobin concentration, decreased cerebral O_2 consumption, and increased Lactate Dehydrogenase activity (Llanos et al., 2003; Ebensperger et al., 2005). The llama possesses an attenuated cardiovascular response to hypoxia, which prevents the development of pulmonary hypertension and arteriolar muscle remodeling (Harris et al., 1982; Moraga et al., 2011). Contrary to llamas, newborn sheep gestated and born at high altitude have marked pulmonary hypertension compared to their counterparts (Llanos et al., 2011a).

Additionally, different models of hypertension can arise as a result of changes in endothelial function (Panza, 1997; Landmesser and Drexler, 2007). One of the most common causes of dysregulated endothelial vasodilator function is an alteration to the biochemical pathway that produces nitric oxide (NO) (Ignarro, 2002). Different models of hypertension are associated with down-regulation of the NO synthetic pathway and an increase in the plasma levels of asymmetric dimethylarginine (ADMA) and homocysteine. ADMA and homocysteine are inhibitors of nitric oxide synthase (NOS) which contributes to the pathogenesis of pulmonary hypertension (Arrigoni et al., 2003; Millatt et al., 2003; Wierzbicki, 2007; Lüneburg et al., 2016). Additionally, it has been reported that dimethyl-aminohydrolase (DDAH-2) (an enzyme that regulates the degradation of ADMA) and cystathionine β-synthase (CBS) (an enzyme that regulated the degradation of homocysteine) are target molecules due to the existence of polymorphisms in their genes that induce the dysregulation of their metabolism and, therefore, increase the risk of developing cardiovascular diseases (Zhang et al., 2014; Xuan et al., 2016).

NO production can be regulated by plasma levels of L-arginine as a result of the competition between NOS and arginase (Böger, 2004; Pernow and Jung, 2013). It has been suggested that arginase activity plays an important role in the pathogenesis of various pulmonary disorders (Maarsingh et al., 2008; Durante, 2013). For instance, an increase in arginase activity has been associated with several pulmonary and systemic hypertension models (Johnson et al., 2005; López et al., 2009; Chu et al., 2016). Nevertheless, there is no information available about the basal levels of ADMA and homocysteine in animals genetically adapted to life in high altitudes and, therefore, resistant to the development of pulmonary hypertension, such as the llama (*Lama glama*). Also, there is no information regarding the participation of the arginase signaling pathway and its regulation by ADMA and homocysteine in this model. Therefore, the aim of this study was to determine the baseline concentrations of ADMA and homocysteine in an animal model resistant to the development of pulmonary hypertension induced by hypoxia. We also evaluated the effect of ADMA and homocysteine on the arginase pathway and their involvement in the resistance to the development of altitude-induced pulmonary hypertension. We used sheep (Ovis aries) as a non-genetically adapted control group.

MATERIALS AND METHODS

Bioethics Committee

All animal care, maintenance, procedures, and experimentation were performed in accordance with the United Kingdom's Animals (Scientific Procedures) Act 1986, and the American Physiological Society's Guiding Principles for Research Involving Animals and Human Being (American Physiologycal Society, 2002) and were reviewed and approved by the Faculty of Medicine Ethics Committee of the University of Chile.

Animals

Lowland and highland newborn sheep (Ovis aries, $n = 6$) and llamas (*Lama glama*, $n = 5$) were studied near sea level (Santiago, 580 m, 710 mmHg barometric pressure. Lowland) and at high altitude (Putre, 3,600 m, 480 mmHg barometric pressure. Highland).

Determination of Arterial Blood Gases in Lowland and Highland Newborn Sheep and Llamas

Newborns were submitted to a surgical procedure at 4–5 days old and studied at 7–10 days old. Animals were placed under general anesthesia with ketamine-diazepam association (10 mg kg^{-1} i.m. ketostop, Drag Pharma-Invectec, Santiago, Chile: 0.1–0.5 mg kg^{-1} i.m Diazepam, Laboratorio Biosano, Santiago, Chile) and additional local infiltration of 2% lidocaine (Dimecaíne, Laboratorio Beta, Santiago, Chile), polyvinyl catheters (1.2 mm i.d) were placed in the descending aorta and inferior vena cava via hindlimb artery and vein, exteriorized subcutaneously through the animal flank and kept in a pouch sewn onto the skin. Also, a Swan-Ganz catheter (Edwards Swan-Ganz 5 French, Baxter Healthcare Corporation, Irvine, CA, USA) was inserted into the pulmonary artery via an external jugular vein, exteriorized, and placed in a pouch around the neck of the animal. All vascular catheters were filled with a heparinized saline solution (500 IU heparin mL^{-1} in 0.9% NaCl) and plugged with a copper pin. Ampicillin 10 mg kg^{-1} i.v (Ampicilina, Laboratorio Best-Pharma, Santiago, Chile) was administered every 12 h while the animals were catheterized. The experiments commenced 3 days after surgery.

Determination of Arterio-Pulmonary Pressure

Pulmonary arterial pressure (PAP), systemic arterial pressure (SAP), and heart rate (HR) were recorded via a data acquisition system (PowerLab/8SP System and LabChart v7.0 Software; ADInstruments) connected to a computer. Cardiac output (CO) was determined with the thermodilution method by the injection of 3 ml of chilled (0°C) 0.9% NaCl into the pulmonary artery through the Swan-Ganz catheter connected to a CO computer (COM-2 model, Baxter). Mean PAP (mPAP), mean SAP (mSAP), and pulmonary (PVR) vascular resistances were calculated as described previously, Herrera et al. (2007).

Determination of ADMA and Homocysteine Plasma Concentrations

Plasma levels of ADMA (Enzo Life Sciences, Farmingdale, New York, USA) and homocysteine (Alpco Diagnostics, Salem, New Hampshire, USA) were measured by enzyme-linked immunosorbent assay (ELISA) according to the manufacturer's instructions.

Enzyme Preparations

The lungs were excised and frozen using liquid nitrogen and stored at −80°C until further use. The heart tissue was homogenized in a solution comprising of 10 mM Tris-HCl (pH 7.5), 0.1 mM PMSF, 1 mM DTT and 5 mM EDTA, and centrifuged at 5,000 g for 10 min at 4°C. The homogenates were centrifuged for 30 min at 5,000 g and 4°C and the supernatant was collected. Subsequently, the enzyme solution (supernatant) was separated by chromatography on a DEAE-cellulose column equilibrated with 5 mM Tris-HCl pH 7.5. The active fractions eluted with the washings of the column corresponded to arginase I, and the active fractions eluted at 0.10–0.15 M corresponded to arginase II (Venkatakrishnan et al., 2003).

The presence of arginase I and II, in the washing fraction and the eluted fraction, respectively, was confirmed by Western Blot. Finally, the active fractions were pooled and stored at −20°C.

Extraction and Quantification of DDAH-2 and Arginase Type II mRNA Level by qRT-PCR

Total RNA was isolated using TRIZOL reagent (Invitrogen Corp., Carlsbad, CA, USA). RNA concentration and purity were assessed by Ultra Violet (UV) spectrophotometry (1.8 < A260/A280 < 2.0). RNA integrity was evaluated using electrophoresis. Reverse transcription reaction was carried out using 4 μg of total RNA and the First Strand complementary DNA (cDNA) Synthesis kit (Thermo Scientific, Boston, MA, USA).

To make standard curves, 1 μL of first-strand cDNA was amplified with AffinityScript cDNA Synthesis Kit and quantification of Polymerase Chain Reaction (PCR) products were used for plotting standard curves.

Quantitative real-time PCR was carried out using a HT-7500 thermo- cycler (Applied Biosystems) and using Brilliant III Ultra-Fast SYBR® Green QPCR Master Mix. program PCR was of 95°C for 3 min, followed by 40 cycles of 95°C for 30 s and 60°C for 30 s. GAPDH was used as an internal control.

DDAH-2, CBS and eNOS mRNA level was normalized with GAPDH (Gliceraldehído-3-fosfato deshidrogenasa) mRNA to compensate for variations in initial RNA amounts. Normalization was carried out by dividing the logarithmic value of DDAH- 2, CBS and eNOS by the logarithmic value of GAPDH.

Arginase Activity Measurements

Specific arginase activity was determined in lung tissues based on urea production from L-arginine using a colorimetric method with α-isonitrosopropiopheonone (Archibald, 1957). Briefly, 50 μl of the fractions obtained from DEAE-cellulose were incubated in 30 mM Tris-HCl (pH 7.5) containing 100 mM L-arginine at 37°C for 10 min. The reaction was stopped by the addition of 1 ml of an acid mixture containing 9% (v/v) of H_3PO_4 and 23% (v/v) of H_2PO_4. To evaluate the effect of homocysteine and ADMA on arginase activity, a specific arginase activity assay was performed in the presence of physiological concentrations of ADMA and homocysteine (0.5, 1.0, 3.0, 6.0, and 10.0 μM) in a 50 mM Tris-HCl solution (pH 7.5).

TABLE 1 | Arterial blood gases in lowland and highland newborn sheep and llamas ($n = 5$).

Sheep		Llamas	
Lowland	**Highland**	**Lowland**	**Highland**
$PaCO_2$ (mmHg)			
37 ± 1	*32 ± 2	37 ± 1	*32 ± 2
PaO_2 (mmHg)			
78 ± 3	*41 ± 4	94 ± 3	52 ± 4
SaO_2 (%)			
95 ± 1	*66 ± 4	97 ± 2	92 ± 2

Values represent the mean ± SE ($n = 5$ per group). $p < 0.01$.

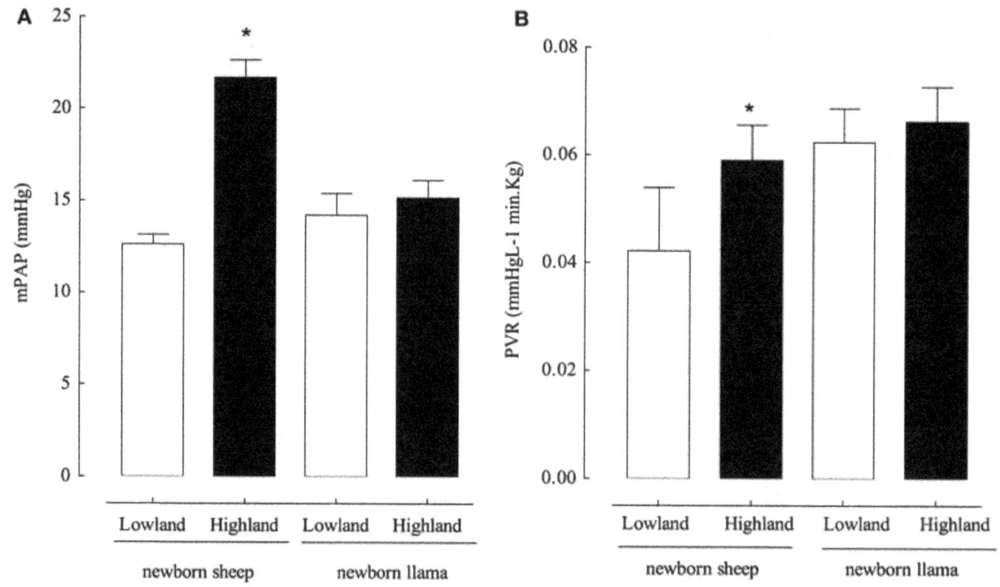

FIGURE 1 | Pulmonary arterial pressure (PAP) and pulmonary vascular resistance (PVR) in newborn sheep and llamas. **(A)** A significant difference was found between the PAP of lowland newborn sheep vs. highland newborn sheep (*$p < 0.01$). No significant differences were observed in the PAP of llamas between these two conditions (n.s). **(B)** A significant difference was found between the PVR of lowland newborn sheep vs. highland newborn sheep (*$p < 0.01$). No significant differences were observed in the PVR between newborn llamas in these two conditions (n.s). *(Llama $n = 5$; sheep $n = 6$).

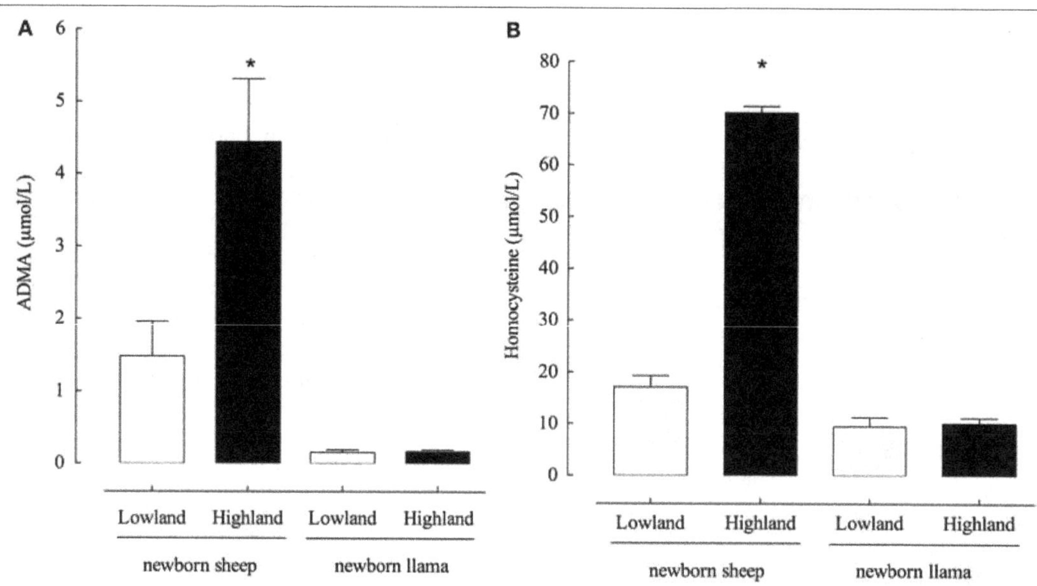

FIGURE 2 | Plasma concentrations of ADMA and homocysteine in newborn llamas and sheep. **(A)** Plasma concentration of ADMA. A significant difference was found between lowland and highland newborn sheep (*$p < 0.01$). **(B)** Plasma concentration of Homocysteine. A significant difference was found between lowland and highland newborn sheep (*$p < 0.01$). No significant differences were observed between ADMA and homocisteine concentrations was found between lowland and highland newborn llama (n.s).

Data Analysis and Statistics

All statistical analyses were performed using GraphPad Prism 5.0 software. The mean values and standard error (SE) were calculated for each parameter. The normality of quantitative variables was established using the Kolmogorov–Smirnov test. The statistical validity of the difference across all testing conditions was established using analysis of variance (ANOVA) of one factor, and ANOVA for repeated measures was performed for differences within the group. Pearson's correlation was also performed. Linear regression analysis was carried out to establish the association between arginase activity (dependent variable) and the other variables. The significance level was established at $p < 0.05$.

RESULTS

A decrease in $PaCO_2$, PaO_2, and SaO_2 values was observed at high altitude conditions in both sheep and llamas. However, newborn llama SaO_2 values were higher at high altitude (**Table 1**). The biggest difference observed between the two species was the higher hemoglobin oxygen saturation in newborn llama compared to newborn sheep at high altitude. This difference is explained by the higher hemoglobin oxygen affinity of llamas compared to sheep (Moraga et al., 1996).

Newborn llamas Are Resistant to the Development of Hypoxia-Induced Pulmonary Hypertension

Newborn llamas do not present significant differences in mPAP (14 ± 1 and 15 ± 0.5 mmHg) between lowland and highland conditions (**Figure 1A**). No modifications were observed in PVR in newborn llamas at lowland vs. highland (**Figure 1B**). On the contrary, newborn sheep had an increased mPAP (12 ± 0.6 mmHg) at lowland compared to highland levels (21 ± 2.0 mmHg) (**Figure 1A**). Additionally, highland newborn sheep exhibited increased PVR values compared to lowland newborn sheep (**Figure 1B**). No significant difference were observed in PVR between both species at lowland and highland ($p > 0.05$).

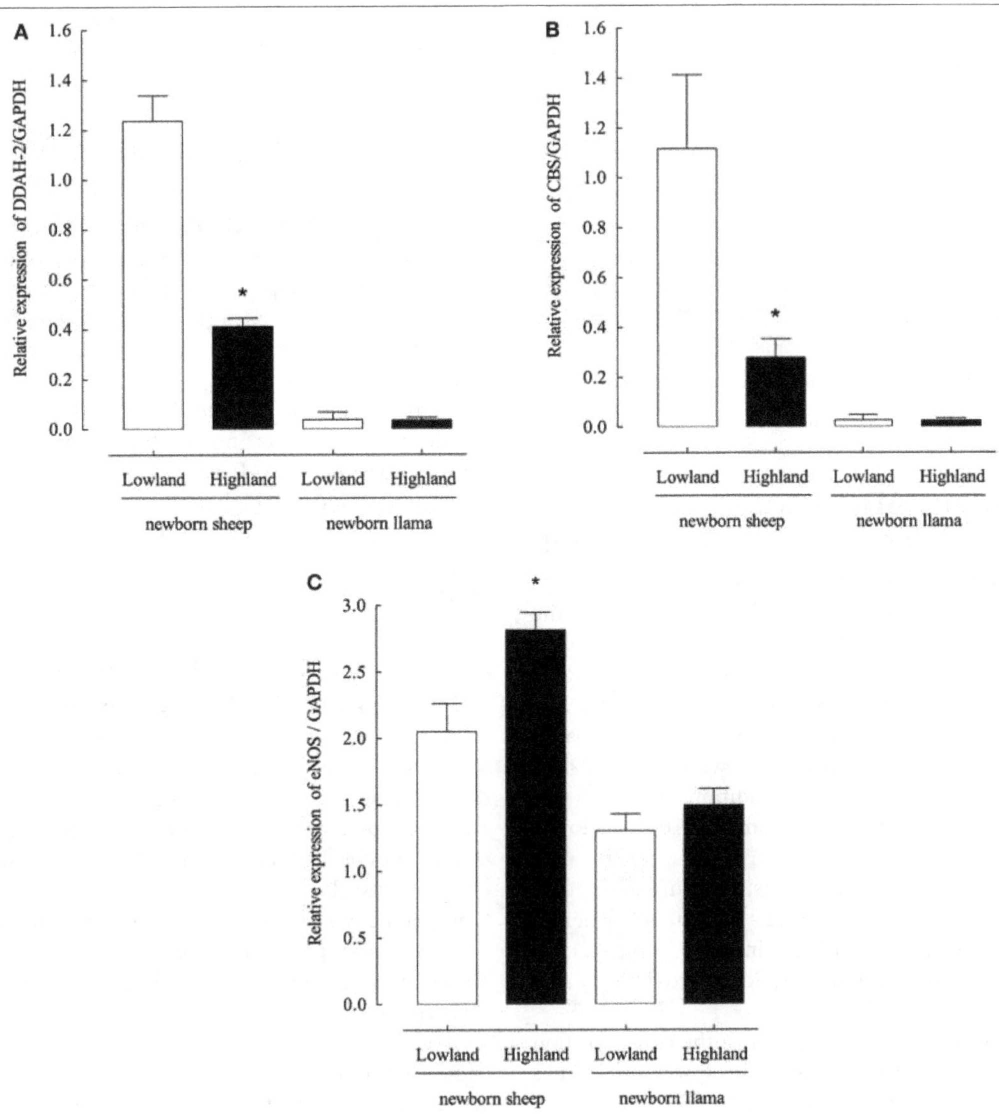

FIGURE 3 | Expression of DDAH-2, CBS and eNOS genes from the lung parenchyma of newborn llamas and sheep. **(A)** Quantitative PCR of DDAH-2 **(B)** Quantitative PCR of CBS **(C)** Quantitative PCR of eNOS. Gene expression was measured by real-time PCR; data were normalized to GAPDH levels. ($n = 6$ per group, $^*p < 0.001$ group).

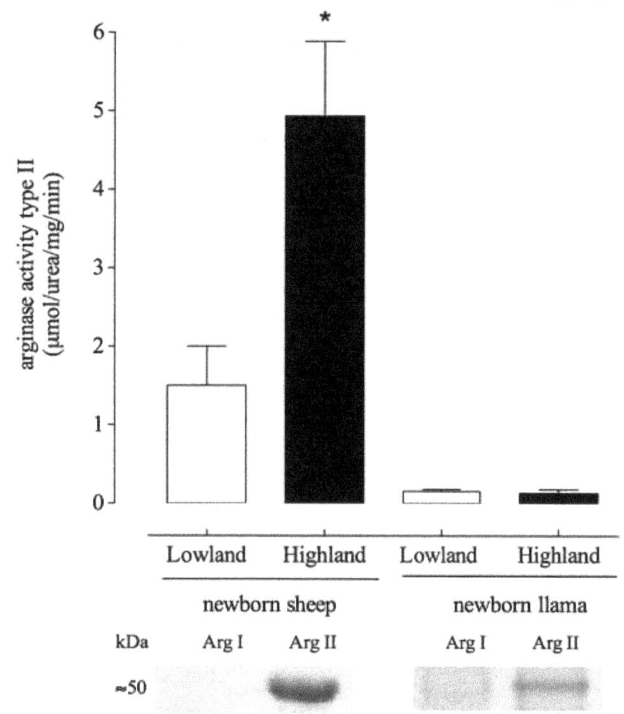

FIGURE 4 | Arginase type II activity from lung parenchyma of newborn llamas and sheep. A significant difference was found between newborn sheep in highland vs. lowland conditions. (* $p < 0.01$). No significant differences were observed in arginase activity between these two conditions in llamas (n.s). (The western blots correspond to the eluted fraction of DEAE-cellulose chromatography).

Llamas Have Low ADMA and Homocysteine Concentrations That do not Increase When Exposed to Hypoxia

To evaluate the role of ADMA and homocysteine in the development of pulmonary hypertension, we measured the basal concentrations of ADMA and homocysteine in the plasma of lowland and highland newborn sheep and llamas. Llamas had significantly lower plasmatic ADMA concentrations compared to sheep, both in lowland and highland newborn animals. In fact, ADMA concentrations in lowland conditions were 1.48 µM in sheep and 0.153 µM in llamas, approximately 10 times lower (**Figure 2A**).

On the contrary to the expected results, exposure to hypoxia did not increase ADMA concentrations in llamas, whereas hypoxic conditions induced a significant increase in the ADMA concentration in sheep, from 1.4 to 4.45 µM (approximately a 4x increase) (**Figure 2A**).

The same phenomenon was observed with the concentration of homocysteine which was significantly lower in llamas compared to sheep, and hypoxia was incapable of producing an increase (**Figure 2B**). In fact, sheep had higher concentrations of homocysteine and hypoxia significantly increased the concentration from 17.32 to 70.4 µM (approximately a 4x increase).

Llamas Have Low DDAH-2 and CBS Expression Levels and Which Are Unaffected by Hypoxia

To evaluate the relationship between the observed concentrations of ADMA and homocysteine and the expression levels DDAH-2 (dimethylarginione dimethyaminohydrolase-1) and CBS (cystathionine-β-synthase), enzymes responsible for the regulation of the endogenous concentrations of ADMA and homocysteine, respectively, the expression levels of DDAH-2 and CBS mRNAs from the lung parenchyma were measured. Low concentrations of DDAH-2 and CBS mRNA from llama lung parenchyma were detected under conditions of normoxia and hypoxia (**Figures 3A,B**), unlike sheep, a significant decrease in expression levels of both genes was observed during hypoxia.

The expression levels of endothelial NOS were also evaluated and it was determined that in the llama there is not significant increase in eNOS expression levels during hypoxia conditions (**Figure 3C**).

Llamas Have Low Levels of Type II Arginase Activity Which Is Not Up-Regulated During Hypoxia

An increase in the expression and activity of arginase has been related to the development of hypertension in different models. Therefore, we measured arginase type II activity in homogenized lungs from newborn sheep and llamas at lowland and highland (**Figure 4**).

Llamas exhibited 10 times less arginase II activity compared to sheep which was not induced by hypoxia (**Figure 4**). Furthermore, arginase II activity remained at similar levels in llamas at lowland and highland.

Additionally, hypoxia induced a significant increase of arginase type II activity by approximately 5 times in newborn sheep.

Arginase Type II in Llamas Is Insensitive to Activation by Homocysteine

ADMA and homocysteine have been described as markers for cardiovascular risk and previous results have shown that ADMA and homocysteine have an activation effect on arginase type II from hypoxia-induced hypertensive rats (López et al., unpublished data). Therefore, we evaluated the effect of these metabolites on arginase type II activity from the lung parenchyma of newborn llamas and sheep (**Figures 5**, **6**). ADMA was a poor inhibitor of arginase type II activity in newborn llamas and sheep at lowland (**Figure 5A**) and highland (**Figure 5B**). However, increased inhibition of arginase type II activity by ADMA was observed in hypoxic conditions in llamas, demonstrating an inhibition of approximately 25% at physiological concentrations of ADMA (1 µM) and reaching a maximum inhibition level of 40% at higher concentrations (10 µM). Additionally, arginase type II activity of newborn llamas in normoxic conditions was not affected by ADMA (**Figures 5A,B**).

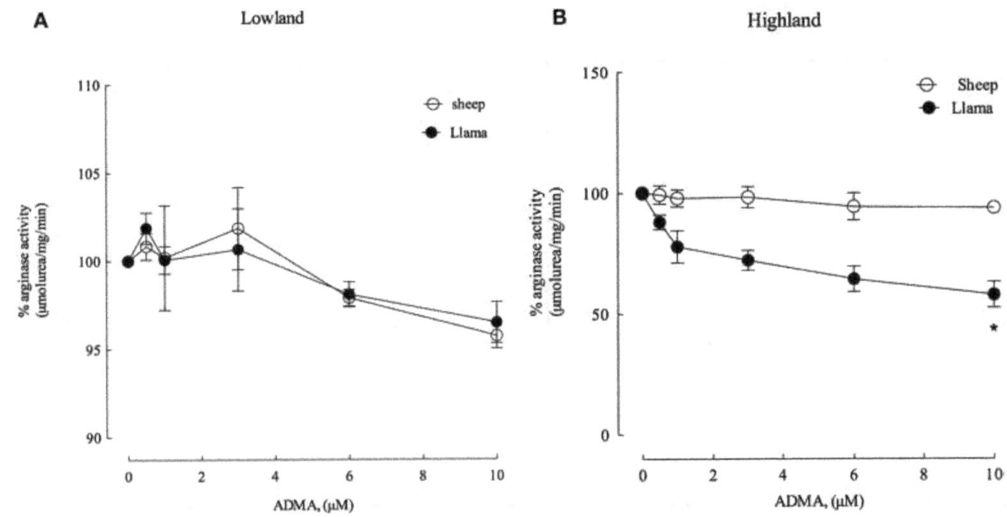

FIGURE 5 | Effect of increasing ADMA concentrations on arginase type II activity from lung parenchyma in newborn llamas and sheep. **(A)** The effect of ADMA on arginase type II activity in lowland conditions. No significant differences were observed in arginase activity between sheep and llamas. **(B)** The effect of ADMA on arginase type II activity in Highland conditions. A significant difference was found between newborn sheep and llamas. *Values represent the mean ±SE ($n = 5$ per group). *$p < 0.01$, Llamas vs. sheep.

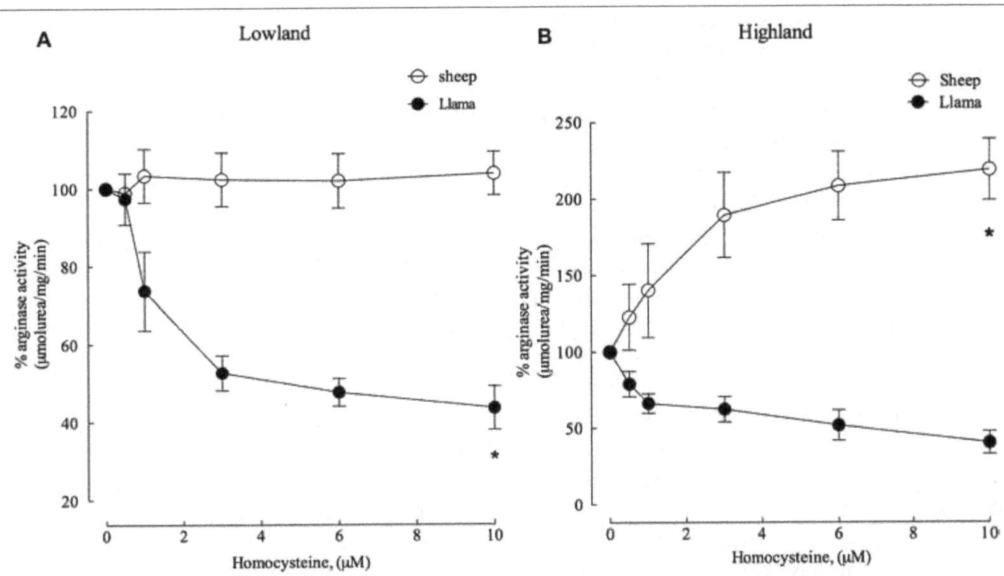

FIGURE 6 | Effect of increasing homocysteine concentrations on arginase type II activity from lung parenchyma in newborn llamas and sheep. **(A)** The effect of homocysteine on arginase type II activity in lowland conditions. A significant difference was observed in arginase activity between sheep and llamas. **(B)** The effect of homocysteine on arginase type II activity in Highland conditions. A significant difference was found in between newborn sheep and llamas. *Values represent the mean ±SE ($n = 5$ per group). *$p < 0.01$, Llamas vs. sheep.

Experiments with homocysteine demonstrated that arginase type II activity in sheep was not affected at lowland. However, homocysteine (4 µM) was an important inhibitor and reduced enzyme activity by approximately 50% (**Figure 6A**) in llamas.

In highland conditions, homocysteine was an important activator of arginase type II in sheep, increasing its activity with increasing concentrations. On the contrary, arginase type II was inhibited in llamas by approximately 50% with 6 µM homocysteine (**Figure 6B**).

DISCUSSION

Llamas are genetically adapted to live in hypobaric hypoxia conditions at high altitudes. Among the physiological adaptations of the adult llama that allow it to live under conditions of oxygen limitation at altitude are: an increased blood hemoglobin concentration, low P_{50}, high muscle myoglobin concentration, a more efficient O_2 extraction at tissue levels, and high lactic dehydrogenase activity. Furthermore,

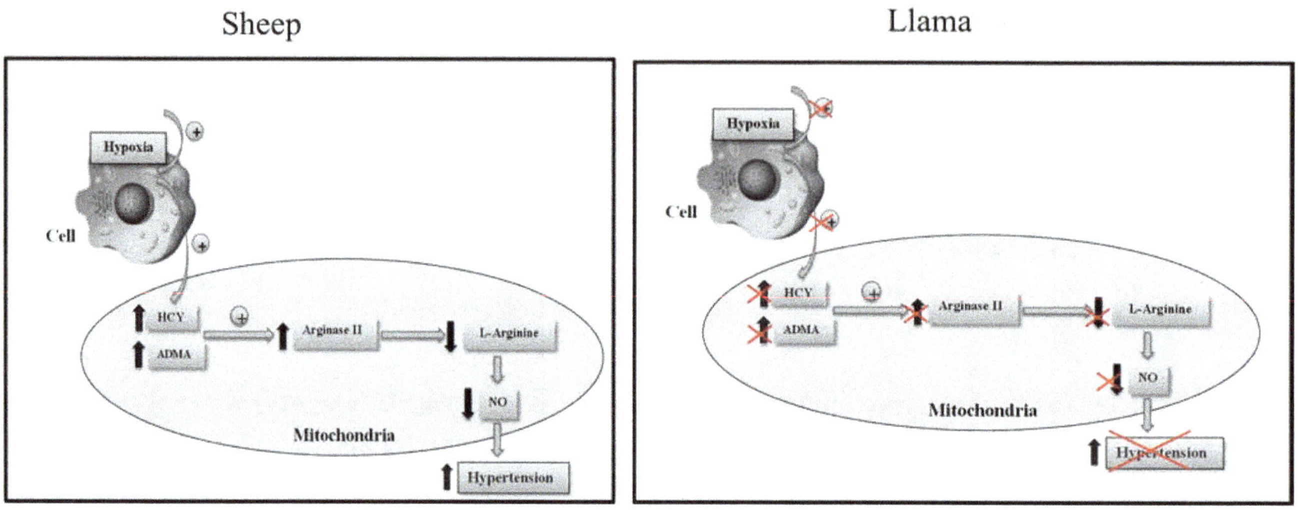

FIGURE 7 | Proposed mechanism for the participation of ADMA, homocysteine and arginase type II in regulating the development of hypoxia-induced hypertension in llamas.

the adult llama avoids pulmonary arterial hypertension and cardiac remodeling, among other adverse effects, by having less muscularized pulmonary arterioles than the adult sheep (Llanos et al., 2011b). Together, these adaptations allow the llama to adapt to life at high altitudes. In agreement with the adaptations of the pulmonary circulatory system previously described, ours results showed that newborn llama at lowland or highland do not show hypertension in pulmonary arteries when calculating the PVR using Ohm's law (Herrera et al., 2007). We observed that the lack of PVR modifications in newborn llama is explained by the maintenance in the cardiac output, similar to that described by Herrera et al. (2008). In contrast, in newborn sheep the higher mPAP and PVR observed at high altitude is explained by an increased cardiac output in newborn sheep. The unaltered PVR in newborn llamas can be explained by their lack of hypertrophic pulmonary vascular remodeling and pulmonary hypertension (Llanos et al., 2011b) by a proposed blunting in this response.

Additionally, studies performed by Herrera et al. (2008) showed that there is an increased pulmonary CO production compared to NO production in newborn llamas. CO is an alternative vasodilator synthesized by the HO- carbon monoxide system that is activated during chronic hypoxia because the relative increase in NO production is not sufficient to counteract the increase in PAP at high altitude. Thus, these authors proposed that activation of the HO-carbon monoxide system induces an adaptation mechanism in these animals during birth that would protect their vascular musculature against the effects of chronic hypoxia and would explain their resistance to the development of pulmonary hypertension. In contrast, the newborn sheep present pulmonary vascular remodeling (Llanos et al., 2011b) and produce hypoxic pulmonary constrictor responses. These observations support our results, since we did not observe a significant increase in eNOS levels in llamas (**Figure 3C**), which would indicate an insufficient amount of NO concentrations and, therefore, reinforce the importance of the activation of the HO-carbon monoxide system in these animals.

In this study, we determined the concentrations of ADMA and homocysteine for the first time in an animal genetically adapted to live at high altitudes. Data showed that llamas had a lower ADMA and homocysteine concentration compared to sheep and other described species (Böger et al., 2000; Lüneburg et al., 2016; **Figure 2A**). It is widely known that ADMA and homocysteine are risk factors for cardiovascular diseases (Wierzbicki, 2007; Böger et al., 2009). We have recently described that hypoxia induces an increase in the concentration of homocysteine and ADMA in hypoxia-induced hypertensive rats (López et al., unpublished). Therefore, based on our study, we hypothesize that low concentrations of ADMA and homocysteine ensure a baseline level of NO synthesis, which together with activation of CO production, results in an adaptation system that allows llamas to live in hypobaric hypoxia conditions without developing pulmonary hypertension.

One explanation for the low levels of ADMA and homocysteine found in llamas could be due to the low expression of key enzymes for the regulation of their synthesis. According to currently available literature, key enzymes in the metabolism of methionine, and therefore in the production of ADMA and homocysteine, have been described as "target molecules" due to the presence of polymorphisms that lead to a deregulation in their metabolism and to the development of cardiovascular diseases. Among these enzymes are cystathionine β-synthase (CBS) (Zhang et al., 2014), methylenetetrahydrofolate reductase (MTHFR) (Yang et al., 2014; Heifetz and Birk, 2015) and dimethyl-aminohydrolase (DDAH-2) (Xuan et al., 2016). The expression and activity levels of these enzymes in llamas and whether they play an important role as therapeutic targets in the hypertensive processes induced by hypoxia remains unknown. Our results show that low expression levels of arginase type II mRNA, associated to the low concentrations of ADMA and Hcy found in llamas, suggest that the NO-arginase pathway is not involved in the resistance to the development of altitude- induced pulmonary hypertension (**Figures 2, 3**).

Additionally, hypoxia did not increase ADMA concentrations which could suggest that, unlike other species, the gene for dimethyl-aminohydrolase-2 (DDAH-2) in llamas does not contain hypoxia response elements such as the hypoxia-inducible factor (HIF-1α) (Pekarova et al., 2015). Contrary to what could be expected in llamas, we found a significant reduction in DDAH-2 expression in rats intolerant to the development of hypoxia-induced hypertension, which could explain the observed increase in ADMA.

Newborn llamas express at least 10 times less arginase type II which is not activated by hypoxia (**Figure 3**). It is widely known that one of the causes of endothelial dysfunction is decreased NO synthesis, which could be explained by a reduction in the concentration of L-arginine required for its synthesis. For this reason, it was shown that an increase in the expression of arginase would be involved in the development of hypertension, since it would compete with eNOS for the use of L- arginine (Durante et al., 2007; Pernow and Jung, 2013). Based on our results, we propose that the lower arginase type II levels leads to greater bioavailability of L-arginine for the synthesis of NO (**Figure 4**) which would explain the resistance to the development of hypertension induced by hypoxia in newborn llamas. In other words, the lower expression of arginase type II in these animals may constitute a mechanism for adaptation at geographical altitudes.

Finally, both ADMA and homocysteine are inhibitors of arginase type II in llamas in both lowland and highland conditions (**Figures 5, 6**). On the contrary, homocysteine from sheep is an activator of arginase (**Figure 6B**). In agreement with previous studies, we found that homocysteine has the same activating effect on arginase II from hypoxia-induced hypertensive rats (López et al., unpublished data). Therefore, the inability of homocysteine and ADMA to activate arginase type II in llamas could represent a protection mechanism in llamas, which would prevent the increased expression of arginase type II in hypoxic conditions in these animals (**Figure 6B**).

Based on our results, we propose that low concentrations of ADMA and homocysteine found in llamas, and also the low arginase type II levels, could constitute an adaptation mechanism that these animals present when faced with hypoxic conditions by impeding the reduction in L-arginine, and thus ensuring baseline synthesis of NO during hypoxia (**Figure 7**).

AUTHOR CONTRIBUTIONS

EU supervises the overall the study. Contributed to sample and data collections. The authors drafted the report. All authors contributed to the interpretation of the results, critical revision of the manuscript and approved the final manuscript.

FUNDING

The research leading to these results has been supported by FONDECYT 11075096 and 1140647.

REFERENCES

American Physiologycal Society (2002). Guiding principles for research in-volving animals and human beings. *Am. J. Physiol. Regul. Integr. Comp. Physiol.* 283, R281–R283. doi: 10.1152/ajpregu.00279.2002

Archibald, R. M. (1957). Colorimetric measurement of uric acid. *Clin. Chem.* 3, 102–105.

Arrigoni, F. I., Vallance, P., Haworth, S. G., and Leiper, J. M. (2003). Metabolism of asymmetric dimethylarginines is regulated in the lung developmentally and with pulmonary hypertension induced by hypobaric hypoxia. *Circulation* 107, 1195–1201. doi: 10.1161/01.CIR.0000051466.00227.13

Böger, R. H. (2004). Asymmetric dimethylarginine, an endogenous inhibitor of nitric oxide synthase, explains the "L-arginine paradox" and acts as a novel cardiovascular risk factor. *J. Nutr.* 134, 2842S–2847S. doi: 10.1093/jn/134.10.2842S

Böger, R. H., Bode-Böger, S. M., Sydow, K., Heistad, D. D., and Lentz, S. R. (2000). Plasma concentration of asymmetric dimethylarginine, an endogenous inhibitor of nitric oxide synthase, is elevated in monkeys with hyperhomocyst(e)inemia or hypercholesterolemia. *Arterioscler. Thromb. Vasc. Biol.* 20, 1557–1564. doi: 10.1161/01.ATV.20.6.1557

Böger, R. H., Sullivan, L. M., Schwedhelm, E., Wang, T. J., Maas, R., Benjamin, E. J., et al. (2009). Plasma asymmetric dimethylarginine and incidence of cardiovascular disease and death in the community. *Circulation* 119, 1592–1600. doi: 10.1161/CIRCULATIONAHA.108.838268

Chu, Y., XiangLi, X., Niu, H., Wang, H., Jia, P., Gong, W., et al. (2016). Arginase inhibitor attenuates pulmonary artery hypertension induced by hypoxia. *Mol. Cell. Biochem.* 412, 91–99. doi: 10.1007/s11010-015-2611-z

Durante, W. (2013). Role of arginase in vessel wall remodeling. *Front. Immunol.* 4:111. doi: 10.3389/fimmu.2013.00111

Durante, W., Johnson, F. K., and Johnson, R. A. (2007). Arginase: a critical regulator of nitric oxide synthesis and vascular function. *Clin. Exp. Pharmacol. Physiol.* 34, 906–911. doi: 10.1111/j.1440-1681.2007.04638.x

Ebensperger, G., Ebensperger, R., Herrera, E. A., Riquelme, R. A., Sanhueza, E. M., Lesage, F., et al. (2005). Fetal brain hypometabolism during prolonged hypoxaemia in the llama. *J. Physiol.* 567(Pt 3), 963–975. doi: 10.1113/jphysiol.2005.094524

Giordano, F. J. (2005). Oxygen, oxidative stress, hypoxia, and heart failure. *J. Clin. Invest.*115, 500–508. doi: 10.1172/JCI200524408

Harris, P., Heath, D., Smith, P., Williams, D. R., Ramirez, A., Krüger, H., et al. (1982). Pulmonary circulation of the llama at high and low altitudes. *Thorax* 37, 38–45. doi: 10.1136/thx.37.1.38

Heifetz, E. M., and Birk, R. Z. (2015). MTHFR C677T polymorphism affects normotensive diastolic blood pressure independently of blood lipids. *Am. J. Hypertens.* 28, 387–392. doi: 10.1093/ajh/hpu152

Herrera, E. A., Pulgar, V. M., Riquelme, R. A., Sanhueza, E. M., Reyes, R. V., Ebensperger, G., et al. (2007). High- altitude chronic hypoxia during gestation and after birth modifies cardiovascular responses in newborn sheep. *Am. J. Physiol. Regul. Integr. Comp. Physiol.* 292, R2234–R2240. doi: 10.1152/ajpregu.00909.2006

Herrera, E. A., Reyes, R. V., Giussani, D. A., Riquelme, R. A., Sanhueza, E. M., Ebensperger, G., et al. (2008). Carbon monoxide: a novel pulmonary artery vasodilator in neonatal llamas of the Andean altiplano. *Cardiovasc. Res.* 77, 197–201. doi: 10.1093/cvr/cvm013

Ignarro, L. J. (2002). Nitric oxide as a unique signaling molecule in the vascular system: a historical overview. *J. Physiol. Pharmacol.* 53(4 Pt 1), 503–514.

Johnson, F. K., Johnson, R. A., Peyton, K. J., and Durante, W. (2005). Arginase inhibition restores arteriolar endothelial function in Dahl rats with salt-induced hypertension. *Am. J. Physiol. Regul. Integr. Comp. Physiol.* 288, R1057–R1062. doi: 10.1152/ajpregu.00758.2004

Landmesser, U., and Drexler, H. (2007). Endothelial function and hypertension. *Curr. Opin. Cardiol.* 22, 316–332. doi: 10.1097/HCO.0b013e3281ca710d

Llanos, A. J., Ebensperger, G., Herrera, E. A., Reyes, R. V., Moraga, F. A., Parer, J. T., et al. (2011a). Counterpoint: high altitude is not for the birds! *J. Appl. Physiol.* 111, 1515–1518. doi: 10.1152/japplphysiol.00821.2011a

Llanos, A. J., Ebensperger, G., Herrera, E. A., Reyes, R. V., Pulgar, V. M., Serón-Ferré, M., et al. (2011b). Fetal and postnatal pulmonary circulation in the Alto Andino. *Placenta* 32(Suppl. 2), S100–S103. doi: 10.1016/j.placenta.2011.01.001

Llanos, A. J., Riquelme, R. A., Sanhueza, E. M., Hanson, M. A., Blanco, C. E., Parer, J. T., et al. (2003). The fetal llama versus the fetal sheep: different strategies to withstand hypoxia. *High Alt. Med. Biol.* 4, 193–202. doi: 10.1089/152702903322022794

Lopez, V., Siques, P., Brito, J., Vallejos, C., and Naveas, N. Carvallo C. (2009). Upregulation of arginase expression and activity in hypertensive rats exposed to chronic intermittent hypobaric hypoxia. *High Alt. Med. Biol.* 10, 373–381. doi: 10.1089/ham.2008.1072

Lüneburg, N., Siques, P., Brito, J., Arriaza, K., Pena, E., Klose, H., et al. (2016). Long-term chronic intermittent hypobaric hypoxia in rats causes an imbalance in the asymmetric dimethylarginine/nitric oxide pathway and ROS activity: a possible synergistic mechanism for altitude pulmonary hypertension? *Pulm. Med.* 16:6578578. doi: 10.1155/2016/6578578

Maarsingh, H., Pera, T., and Meurs, H. (2008). Arginase and pulmonary diseases. *Naunyn Schmiedebergs. Arch. Pharmacol.* 378, 171–184. doi: 10.1007/s00210-008-0286-7

Millatt, L. J., Whitley, G. S., Li, D., Leiper, J. M., Siragy, H. M., Carey, R. M., et al. (2003). Evidence for dysregulation of dimethylarginine dimethylaminohydrolase I in chronic hypoxia-induced pulmonary hypertension. *Circulation* 108, 1493–1498. doi: 10.1161/01.CIR.0000089087.25930.FF

Moraga, F. A., Reyes, R. V., Herrera, E. A., Riquelme, R. A., Ebensperger, G., Pulgar, V. M., et al. (2011). Role of the α-adrenergic system in femoral vascular reactivity in neonatal llamas and sheep: a comparative study between highland and lowland species. *Am. J. Physiol. Regul. Integr. Comp. Physiol.* 301, R1153–R1160. doi: 10.1152/ajpregu.00124.2010

Moraga, F., Monge, C., Riquelme, R., and Llanos, A. J. (1996). Fetal and maternal blood oxygen affinity: a comparative study in llamas and sheep. *Comp. Biochem. Physiol. A Physiol.* 115, 111–115.

Panza, J. A. (1997). Endothelial dysfunction in essential hypertension. *Clin. Cardiol.* 20(11Suppl. 2), II-26–II-33.

Penaloza, D. (2012). Effects of high-altitude exposure on the pulmonary circulation. *Rev. Esp. Cardiol.* 65, 1075–1078. doi: 10.1016/j.rec.2012.06.017

Pekarova, M., Koudelka, A., Kolarova, H., Ambrozova, G., Klinke, A., Cerna, A., et al. (2015). Asymmetric dimethyl arginine induces pulmonary vascular dysfunction via activation of signal transducer and activator of transcription 3 and stabilization of hypoxia-inducible factor 1-alpha. *Vascul. Pharmacol.* 73, 138–148. doi: 10.1016/j.vph.2015.06.005

Pernow, J., and Jung, C. (2013). Arginase as a potential target in the treatment of cardiovascular disease: reversal of arginine steal? *Cardiovasc. Res.* 98, 334–343. doi: 10.1093/cvr/cvt036

Venkatakrishnan, G., Shankar, V., and Reddy, S. R. (2003). Microheterogeneity of molecular forms of arginase in mammalian tissues. *Indian J. Biochem. Biophys.* 40, 400–408.

Wierzbicki, A. S. (2007). Homocysteine and cardiovascular disease: a review of the evidence. *Diab. Vasc. Dis. Res.* 4, 143–150. doi: 10.3132/dvdr.2007.033

Xuan, C., Xu, L. Q., Tian, Q. W., Li, H., Wang, Q., He, G. W., et al. (2016). Dimethylarginine dimethylaminohydrolase 2 (DDAH 2) gene polymorphism, asymmetric dimethylarginine (ADMA) concentrations, and risk of coronary artery disease: a case-control study. *Sci Rep.* 6:33934. doi: 10.1038/srep33934

Yang, K. M., Jia, J., Mao, L. N., Men, C., Tang, K. T., Li, Y. Y., et al. (2014). Methylenetetrahydrofolate reductase C677T gene polymorphism and essential hypertension: a meta-analysis of 10,415 subjects. *Biomed. Rep.* 2, 699–708. doi: 10.3892/br.2014.302

Zhang, Y., Wang, H., Sun, H. W., Chen, Y. L., Ouyang, J. Y., Wang, Y., et al. (2014). Correlation between cystathionine β-synthase T883C genetic polymorphism and primary hypertension. *Exp. Ther. Med.* 8, 713–718. doi: 10.3892/etm.2014.1799

8

Receptor–Receptor Interactions of G Protein-Coupled Receptors in the Carotid Body: A Working Hypothesis

Andrea Porzionato[1*†], Elena Stocco[1†], Diego Guidolin[1], Luigi Agnati[2], Veronica Macchi[1] and Raffaele De Caro[1]

[1] Department of Neuroscience, University of Padua, Padua, Italy, [2] Department of Diagnostic, Clinical Medicine and Public Health, University of Modena and Reggio Emilia, Modena, Italy

***Correspondence:**
Andrea Porzionato
andrea.porzionato@unipd.it

† These authors have contributed equally to this work.

In the carotid body (CB), a wide series of neurotransmitters and neuromodulators have been identified. They are mainly produced and released by type I cells and act on many different ionotropic and metabotropic receptors located in afferent nerve fibers, type I and II cells. Most metabotropic receptors are G protein-coupled receptors (GPCRs). In other transfected or native cells, GPCRs have been demonstrated to establish physical receptor–receptor interactions (RRIs) with formation of homo/hetero-complexes (dimers or receptor mosaics) in a dynamic monomer/oligomer equilibrium. RRIs modulate ligand binding, signaling, and internalization of GPCR protomers and they are considered of relevance for physiology, pharmacology, and pathology of the nervous system. We hypothesize that RRI may also occur in the different structural elements of the CB (type I cells, type II cells, and afferent fibers), with potential implications in chemoreception, neuromodulation, and tissue plasticity. This 'working hypothesis' is supported by literature data reporting the contemporary expression, in type I cells, type II cells, or afferent terminals, of GPCRs which are able to physically interact with each other to form homo/hetero-complexes. Functional data about cross-talks in the CB between different neurotransmitters/neuromodulators also support the hypothesis. On the basis of the above findings, the most significant homo/hetero-complexes which could be postulated in the CB include receptors for dopamine, adenosine, ATP, opioids, histamine, serotonin, endothelin, galanin, GABA, cannabinoids, angiotensin, neurotensin, and melatonin. From a methodological point of view, future studies should demonstrate the colocalization in close proximity (less than 10 nm) of the above receptors, through biophysical (i.e., bioluminescence/fluorescence resonance energy transfer, protein-fragment complementation assay, total internal reflection fluorescence microscopy, fluorescence correlation spectroscopy and photoactivated localization microscopy, X-ray crystallography) or biochemical (co-immunoprecipitation, *in situ* proximity ligation assay) methods. Moreover, functional approaches will be able to show if ligand binding to one receptor produces changes in the biochemical characteristics (ligand recognition, decoding, and trafficking processes) of the other(s). Plasticity aspects would be also of interest, as development and environmental stimuli (chronic continuous or intermittent hypoxia) produce changes in the expression of certain receptors which could potentially invest the dynamic monomer/oligomer equilibrium of homo/hetero-complexes and the correlated functional implications.

Keywords: carotid body, GPCRs, heteromers, receptor mosaics, hypoxia, adenosine, dopamine, plasticity

INTRODUCTION

The carotid body (CB) is a small polymodal peripheral chemoreceptor standing out for its basic role in case of hypoxia, hypercapnia, acidosis, low glucose; in these circumstances, it promotes an adequate respiratory and cardiovascular response as well as other less studied stimuli (Atanasova and Lazarov, 2014; Ortega-Sáenz et al., 2015). Two cell types can be distinguished in the CB, the 'neuron-like' chemosensitive type I cells and the 'glial-like' supportive type II cells. Type I cells synthetize and release many different neurotransmitters and neuromodulators, such as dopamine, acetylcholine, serotonin, histamine, ATP, glutamate, GABA, and substance P. Neurotransmitters and neuromodulators released by type I cells in great measure exert their activity on the afferent endings of the carotid sinus nerve (Porzionato et al., 2018), conveying the stimulation through the glossopharyngeal nerve and petrosal ganglion. The main excitatory stimuli are considered acetylcholine and ATP, binding to the ionotropic nicotinic and $P2X_2/P2X_3$ receptors, respectively. However, autocrine/paracrine modulation of type I cells is also of particular importance and is mainly performed through a series of metabotropic G protein-coupled receptors (GPCRs), such as A_{2A}, $D_{1/2}$, $H_{1/2/3}$, $M_{1/2}$, 5-HT_{2A}, and others (for comprehensive reviews on neurotransmitters in the CB, see Iturriaga and Alcayaga, 2004; Bairam and Carroll, 2005; Nurse, 2005, 2014). Conversely, metabotropic GPCRs are also present in afferent nerve endings and type II cells, where they play a role in neuromodulation of signaling between type I cells and afferent fibers (Tse et al., 2012; Nurse et al., 2018). Many authors have emphasized the absolute peculiarity of the CB, characterized by "a plethora of neurotransmitters and neuromodulators, as well as an even broader spectrum of their receptors" (Nurse, 2014). Apart from the above sensory innervation, the CB also shows sensory innervation from jugular and nodose ganglia, post-ganglionic sympathetic nerve fibers from the superior cervical ganglion, and preganglionic parasympathetic and sympathetic fibers reaching ganglion cells in the CB. Efferent parasympathetic and sympathetic innervation of the CB plays a pivotal role in modulation of blood flow (De Caro et al., 2013).

The CB also shows a high level of structural plasticity, undergoing structural and functional changes during development (e.g., Porzionato et al., 2008a,b; De Caro et al., 2013), aging (e.g., Di Giulio et al., 2012; Zara et al., 2013) and as a consequence of environmental stimuli, such as chronic continuous hypoxia, taking place during acclimation to high altitude (e.g., Wang and Bisgard, 2002). In response to chronic hypoxia, type II cells can act in a stem cell-like manner, differentiating into precursors of neural cells that originate mature glomus cells (Pardal et al., 2007; Platero-Luengo et al., 2014).

The GPCR family involves about 800 human receptors that are organized into five subfamilies, namely classes A (the largest group), B, C, frizzled, and adhesion (Foord, 2002; Guidolin et al., 2018). Considering the structure, GPCRs have a similar conformation showing a peculiar seven TM (7TM) α-helical region, an extracellular amino-terminal segment and an intracellular carboxy-terminal tail (Tuteja, 2009). While the domain that is localized in the extracellular portion allows the ligand(s) – receptor interaction, the TM region is subject to a conformational change when the binding with a ligand occurs; this change is then transmitted to the intracellular region of the GPCR responsible for activating the signaling cascade (Schonenbach et al., 2015; Stockert and Devi, 2015).

According to evidences from *in vitro* and *in vivo* studies, GPCR monomers can recognize/decode signals (Bayburt et al., 2007; Whorton et al., 2007; Kuszak et al., 2009; Lohse, 2010; Guidolin et al., 2018); in particular, an intrinsic plasticity characterizes GPCR monomers signaling, in fact GPCR activation can determine the onset of different signal transduction patterns, like the G proteins and/or arrestin pathways (Zidar et al., 2009; Guidolin et al., 2018). Furthermore, it is established that GPCRs can functionally interact by sharing signaling pathways or by mechanisms of transactivation (see Köse, 2017; Guidolin et al., 2018). In the 1980s, however, Agnati et al. (2005) provided evidence suggesting that GPCRs could also establish structural receptor–receptor interactions (RRIs; see Guidolin et al., 2015, 2018 for recent reviews), in which they can associate with themselves (homodimerization) or with other proteins of the same family (heterodimerization). This concept was later confirmed in transfected mammalian cell systems but also in many different native tissues (i.e., central nervous system; mammary gland; liver; cancer tissues) (see Ferré et al., 2014; Guidolin et al., 2015). It is a fact that class C GPCRs form constitutive homomers or heteromers (Kniazeff et al., 2011; Guidolin et al., 2018). An example is represented by the metabotropic receptor for gamma-aminobutyric acid b ($GABA_B$), that, in the central nervous system, constitutes the major inhibitory neurotransmitter (Calver et al., 2000; Pontier et al., 2006). The receptor for $GABA_B$, which is formed by the subunits $GABA_{B1}$ and $GABA_{B2}$, represents the typical example of constitutive heterodimer (Lohse, 2010). Only $GABA_{B1}$ can bind GABA; however, $GABA_{B2}$, even if alone is not functional, is required as $GABA_{B1}$ as such is considered immature due to the presence of a carboxy-terminal ER retention motif (Galvez et al., 2001; Kamal and Jockers, 2011). Hence, after co-expression, the heterodimerization is the prerequisite to permit the masking of the retention domain and the subsequent translation of the active protein to the plasma-membrane (Terrillon and Bouvier, 2004). The oligomerization process in class A GPCR is a broadly debated topic of interest (see Franco et al., 2016; Guidolin et al., 2018). However, according to the consistent results obtained through multiple approaches, the possibility of class A GPCR complexes is strongly supported (Bouvier and Hébert, 2014; Guidolin et al., 2018). In this respect, studies highlighting the occurrence of a specific and dynamic monomer/oligomer equilibrium in class A homodimers and heterodimers are of particular interest (Kroeger et al., 2003; Palczewski, 2010; Kleinau et al., 2016; Farran, 2017). In fact, according to their half-lives (determined by the association and dissociation rates) class A GPCR dimers are demonstrated to be often transient (Gurevich and Gurevich, 2008). This may contribute in explaining the opposing views regarding the role of class A GPCR monomers versus oligomers (Guidolin et al., 2018).

The amount of data proving the existence of GPCR heteromers showed a huge increase similarly to both development and diffusion of biophysical techniques able to detect the spatial proximity of protein molecules (Guidolin et al., 2015). They involve resonance energy transfer methods including bioluminescence and fluorescence resonance energy transfer (BRET and FRET, respectively), fluorescence complementation, total internal fluorescence microscopy, fluorescence correlation spectroscopy, assays based on bivalent ligands and proximity ligation assays (PLAs).

The basic molecular mechanism leading to the formation of the receptor assemblies are allosteric interactions (Kenakin et al., 2010; Fuxe et al., 2012a). As recently outlined by Changeux and Christopoulos (2016), the cooperativity that emerges in the action of orthosteric and allosteric ligands of the GPCR forming the complex provides the cell decoding apparatus with sophisticated dynamics in terms of recognition and signaling (George et al., 2002; Guidolin et al., 2018). It has been shown, for instance, that GPCR heterodimerization exerts effects by altering or fine-tuning ligand binding, signaling, as well as internalization of GPCR protomers (Bulenger et al., 2005; Satake et al., 2013; Gomes et al., 2016; Guidolin et al., 2018). Angiotensin II receptor (AT_1) – bradykinin receptor (B_2) heterodimer (detected in smooth muscle, omental vessel, and platelets) provides an example: angiotensin II triggers inositol triphosphate (IP3) accumulation in a manner that is much more potent and effective than in the cells showing the expression of AT_1 alone; conversely, IP3 accumulation sustained by bradykinin is slightly weaker in cells expressing the AT_1–B_2 heterodimer with respect to the cells expressing only B_2 (Satake et al., 2013).

Many evidences highlight that dimers may be formed by different mechanisms (Guidolin et al., 2018). Receptor complexes can arise in plasma membrane under the action of hydrophobic forces (Gahbauer and Böckmann, 2016). Receptor assembly may also occur in the endoplasmic reticulum (ER) before trafficking to the plasma membrane. ER is responsible of the structural quality of the synthetized receptors. Thus, only correctly folded receptors are allowed to exit while degradation occur for unfolded or misfolded proteins (Terrillon and Bouvier, 2004). Finally, recent data showed that GPCRs can be safely transferred by microvesicles from a source to a target cell where they become capable of recognizing and decoding their signal (Guescini et al., 2012).

Since GPCRs are implicated in several human diseases and represent major pharmacological targets, GPCR oligomerization process, determining variations in the processes of agonist recognition, signaling, and trafficking of participating receptors via allosteric mechanisms (Fuxe et al., 2012a), is of potential great importance for physiology and pharmacology, and new therapeutic strategies considering GPCR attitude to underwent toward several levels of receptor organization are under study (Farran, 2017).

Therefore, in a scenario where GPCR proteins are demonstrated to be present as monomer, the assumption that they may multimerize represents an interesting aspect to investigate. The purpose of the present article is to highlight indirect evidence of this with regard to the CB. In this tissue, indeed, the presence of multimeric GPCRs has not yet been consistently investigated. Thus, the main focus of the paper will be on possible homo-/heterodimers or mosaic receptors (already confirmed in other cell types) that could be present in the CB (type I and II cells, carotid sinus nerve afferents), with possible functional implications. The 'working hypothesis' of this paper could represent an interesting field of investigation aiming to clarify some aspects of chemoreception, neuromodulation and plasticity in the CB.

INVESTIGATIVE APPROACHES TO GPCR COMPLEXES

As briefly discussed before, the term RRI emphasizes the occurrence of an interaction needing a direct physical contact between the involved receptor proteins responsible for the formation of multimeric assemblies of receptors (dimers or high-order oligomers) at the cell membrane level, acting as integrative input units of membrane-associated molecular circuits (Guidolin et al., 2018). Considerable efforts are currently being directed toward the identification of the most adequate strategy to discover such a supramolecular organization of GPCRs, but no single method is free from limitations giving rise to some discrepancy between various studies (Mackie, 2005; Lambert and Javitch, 2014). Thus, evidence obtained through multiple approaches with consistent results is needed to identify receptor complexes (Bouvier and Hébert, 2014).

In particular, an operational definition of RRI (Fuxe et al., 2010) can be exploited to devise experimental procedures fulfilling the following two measurable conditions:

1. The binding of a ligand to one receptor determines a detectable change in the biochemical features of another receptor, that includes ligand recognition, decoding, and trafficking processes;

2. Involved protomers have not only to be colocalized, but also in close proximity to each other (less than 10 nm), as indicated by specific techniques.

To explore the second point, biophysical and biochemical methods are presently available (see Kaczor and Selent, 2011 for a review).

Biophysical Strategies

Biophysical methods may be divided into three macro-groups that are fluorescence/luminescence-based techniques, specialized microscopic techniques and X-ray crystallography.

As far as fluorescence/luminescence-based techniques are concerned, bioluminescence resonance energy transfer (BRET) and fluorescence resonance energy transfer (FRET) were among the earliest proximity-based assays of this type that were used in studying GPCR heteromerization (Fernández-Dueñas et al., 2012). Both techniques exploit the transfer of energy from a donor to an acceptor in a non-radiative manner (as a result of dipole–dipole coupling). If the donor is a fluorescent molecule with emission characteristics suitable to excite the acceptor, when they are in close proximity (~10 nm) the result will be light emission from the acceptor fluorophore enabling the visualization of the subcellular location of specific receptor complexes.

Protein-fragment complementation assays have also been used to analyze GPCR heteromerization in living cells (Gandia et al., 2008). In this approach, cells are transfected with one GPCR fused to a fragment of fluorophore and another GPCR fused to a complementary fragment. Reconstitution of the active fluorophore would occur only if the two receptors were in close proximity. It is noteworthy that a combination of this technique with BRET or FRET can be devised to demonstrate the presence of GPCR trimers or tetramers (Gandia et al., 2008). In this respect, a specialized microscopic technique, namely atomic force microscopy, has also been explored to demonstrate the existence of GPCR complexes (Agnati et al., 2010).

However, all the mentioned techniques show limitations in answering questions concerning the dynamic nature of receptor complexes. Thus, more recently, the details of the spatial and temporal organization of GPCR complexes have been addressed by using specialized microscopic techniques allowing the direct observation of the state and behavior of individual proteins in living cells. They include total internal reflection fluorescence microscopy (Hern et al., 2010; Guidolin et al., 2018), fluorescence correlation spectroscopy (Chen et al., 2003; Guidolin et al., 2018) and photoactivated localization microscopy (PALM; Jonas et al., 2016).

X-ray crystallography represents a further significant experimental approach in the field. During the last years, crystallization techniques have been object of interest (Grisshammer, 2017), determining important consequences for the analysis of GPCR complexes as well as an increase of the number of experimentally assessed structures (Guidolin et al., 2018).

Biochemical Strategies

Spatial and temporal co-expression of GPCRs in cells and tissues is a necessary condition for the formation of more complex systems. This aspect can be investigated following biochemical approaches. The abundance of a specific mRNA can be detected by Northern-blot analysis, *in situ* hybridization, RT-PCR or microarray analysis. Immunohistochemistry and co-localization analysis (Agnati et al., 2005) can be performed to detect GPCR co-expression and co-localization at protein level. The practical limit of this technique regards the necessity for high-quality antibodies also due to low GPCRs expression levels.

To identify possible complex formation, it is mandatory for biochemical studies extracting GPCRs from the membrane by use of detergent, although shielding their native conformation in detergent is not a trivial task (Park et al., 2004).

Radiation inactivation technique (or target size method) take advantage of gamma rays or high energy electrons to disrupt polypeptides in order to identify the molecular weight of singular components. It is based on the inverse relationship existing between the size of a macromolecule and its dose-dependent inactivation. Hence, the probability to destroy a molecule increases along with its mass: larger is a protein and lower is the energy required to destroy it (Rios et al., 2001). For what it concerns GPCRs, the main limitation of the method is that this variation may be related to interaction with other proteins instead of oligomerization.

To overcome this limitation, co-immunoprecipitation can be used (Skieterska et al., 2013). Interestingly, this method in combination with confocal microscopy and FRET was used to detect homooligomerization of the 5-HT_{2C} receptors as well as the 5-HT_4 homodimerization in combination with BRET (Kaczor and Selent, 2011).

More recently, evidence of heteroreceptor complexes in native tissues has been provided by *in situ* PLA (Trifilieff et al., 2011). This technique could be adequate to highlight evidences regarding the presence of GPCR heteromers in tissue, giving new insights about basic biological mechanisms, heteroreceptor levels as well as their location. Thus, it allows to study the localization and modulation of heteroreceptor complexes, as formalin fixed tissue is used.

Cross-linking experiments are a further promising approach. They involve the use of assays based on bivalent ligands (agonists, antagonists, heteromer-selective antibodies, cross-linking reagents) allowing a direct targeting of the receptor complex (Yekkirala et al., 2013) in cells and tissues.

HOMO- OR HETERO-DIMERS BETWEEN A_1 AND/OR A_{2A} RECEPTORS

Adenosine receptor A_1 homodimers have been identified in brain cortex of pigs by radioligand binding experiments (Ciruela et al., 1995). The capability of A_1 receptors to form homodimers has also been demonstrated in Chinese hamster ovary (CHO) cells transfected with human A_1 receptors (Gracia et al., 2008) and in transfected human embryonic kidney (HEK-293T) cells expressing similar levels of A_1 receptor as the native tissue (Gracia et al., 2013). In bovine cortex, the existence of homomers was also shown through PLA (Gracia et al., 2013).

The effects of homodimerization on the receptor function can be inferred from ligand binding assays. A_1 receptor activation inhibits adenylate cyclase and decreases cAMP concentration. Caffeine is a non-selective adenosine receptor antagonist. In case of low caffeine concentrations (when caffeine only binds to one protomer of the empty homodimer), it determines an increase of the agonist affinity for the other protomer in the A_1 receptor homodimer; whereas, at high concentrations (when caffeine highly saturates both protomers of the homodimer) caffeine behaves like an A_1 antagonist with a reduction of the agonist binding to the receptors. Thus, caffeine modulates A_1 agonist-induced cAMP decrease in a biphasic manner. Interestingly, this is a particular behavior for a classical adenosine receptor antagonist like caffeine and is a pharmacological behavior explanation-lacking without taking into account receptor dimers as a minimal quaternary structure. Moreover, this pharmacological ability can also give explanations about the biphasic effects exerted at low and high concentration of caffeine on locomotor activity (Gracia et al., 2013).

As it regards the CB, adenosine is a well-known neurotransmitter produced in response to acute hypoxia. It can be directly released from type I cells, through an equilibrative nucleoside transporter, or it can be indirectly produced through breakdown of released ATP by ecto-5′-nucleotidase (Conde et al., 2012). Adenosine may act pre- and post-synaptically in the modulation of type I and afferents function. It enhances the firing pattern in the carotid sinus afferents through A_{2A} receptors (Conde et al., 2009a,b; Piskuric and Nurse, 2013). Some discrepancies between studies have been reported about A_1 localization into the CB structures (Bairam et al., 2009). Rocher et al. (1999) described the presence of A_1 in rabbit type I cells, through functional studies on cell cultures. Conversely, in the rat, post-synaptic localization has mainly been suggested as A_1 receptors are significantly expressed in the cytoplasm of nodous and petrosal ganglia (Bairam and Carroll, 2005; Gauda et al., 2006) and immunostaining of whole CB did not permit to specifically localize immunoreaction in type I cells (Bae et al., 2005). Possible species-related differences have been suggested and further analyses also on human material would be necessary. However, to reassume, A_1 homodimerization may be hypothesized in nerve fibers and probably in those species expressing A_1 receptors in type I cells.

A_{2A} homodimerization has also been assessed in the plasma membrane of transfected HEK-293T cells by BRET, FRET, time-resolved BRET and immunoblotting and biotinylating experiments. Evidences highlight that more of 90% of A_{2A} receptors are present as homodimers. In intracellular areas, the presence of a certain amount of monomeric species has been highlighted, suggesting that that they assemble into dimers before reaching cell surface (Canals et al., 2004; Lukasiewicz et al., 2007).

In particular, Canals et al. (2004) demonstrated that A_{2A} homodimers are the functional species at the cell surface. Even though A_{2A} homodimerization is quite constitutive, it is further influenced by specific ligands: agonists (i.e., CGS 21680) and antagonists (i.e., SCH 58261; caffeine) increase and decrease it, respectively (Lukasiewicz et al., 2007).

Various authors confirmed the presence of A_{2A} receptor in the rat type I cells through several different techniques (RT-PCR studies, *in situ* hybridization analysis and immunohistochemistry) (e.g., Gauda, 2000; Kobayashi et al., 2000). Bairam et al. (2009) also demonstrated by Western-blot analysis the tendency of A_{2A} receptor to form homodimer in the CB similarly to the superior cervical ganglion and nucleus tractus solitarius. This is one of the few specific references about receptor dimerization in the CB.

However, there are not studies addressing the issue of how agonist/antagonists may modulate dimerization of adenosine receptors in the nerve fibers and/or type I cells or, conversely, how dimerization may play a role in their pharmacological actions. It must also be considered that environmental conditions (hypoxia, etc.) may modulate receptor expression as well as types of dimerization, potentially modulating pharmacological effects.

Apart from the above homodimers, the ability of A_1 receptors to heterodimerize with A_{2A} receptors was also demonstrated in transfected cells by Ferré et al. (2008). Heterodimerization of these two protomers was assessed *in vitro* and *in vivo* by Ciruela et al. (2006), who confirmed the A_1/A_{2A} heterodimer formation in rat striatal glutamatergic nerve terminals by immunogold detection and co-immunoprecipitation. Recently it has been shown that at the presynaptic membrane of cortico-thalamic glutamatergic terminals A_1 receptors co-localizes and interacts with A_{2A} receptors, forming functional receptor heterodimer in the striatum (Fernández-Dueñas et al., 2017).

The eventual demonstration of A_1/A_{2A} heterodimers in type I cells and/or nerve fibers would be of particular interest in terms of modulation of the glutamatergic transmission. In fact, heterodimerization between the adenosine receptors A_1 and A_{2A}, which are responsible for opposite signaling pathways (inhibitory and excitatory actions, respectively) (Stockwell et al., 2016), has been suggested to exert a function in fine-tuning modulation of striatal glutamatergic neurotransmission by adenosine. Since A_1 receptor shows higher affinity for adenosine than A_{2A}, but A_1 agonist affinity decreases when A_{2A} is activated, the possibility exists that glutamate release may be inhibited or stimulated by a switch mechanism depending on low and high concentrations of adenosine, respectively (Ciruela et al., 2006; Doyle et al., 2012).

HETERO-DIMERS BETWEEN ADENOSINE (A_1 AND A_{2A}) AND PURINERGIC ($P2Y_1$, $P2Y_2$, $P2Y_{12}$) RECEPTORS

$P2Y_1$ (Xu et al., 2005; Tse et al., 2012) and $P2Y_{12}$ (Carroll et al., 2012) receptors have been demonstrated in type I cells, where they inhibit the hypoxia-induced rise in intracellular Ca^{2+}. Conversely, in type II cells, $P2Y_2$ receptors have been demonstrated (Xu et al., 2003), which produces a rise in intracellular Ca^{2+}.

Purinergic receptors have also been reported to form homodimers and hetero-dimers with other purinergic and adenosine receptors (e.g., Schicker et al., 2009). As previously detailed, A_{2A} receptors are expressed in type I cells (Gauda, 2000; Kobayashi et al., 2000) and A1 receptors have been reported in the type I cells of some species (rabbit) (Rocher et al., 1999), although not confirmed in others (rat) (Gauda et al., 2000, 2006). Thus, in type I cells, many RRIs can be hypothesized: $P2Y_1/P2Y_1$, $P2Y_1/P2Y_{12}$, $P2Y_{12}/P2Y_{12}$, $P2Y_1/A_1$, $P2Y_1/A_{2A}$, $P2Y_{12}/A_1$, $P2Y_{12}/A_{2A}$ (e.g., Yoshioka et al., 2001; Nakata et al., 2005, 2010; Schicker et al., 2009). Physical interactions between A_1 and $P2Y_1$ receptors, for instance, produce a conformational change in the A_1 binding pocket with acquisition of $P2Y_1$-like agonistic pharmacology, i.e., a $P2Y_1$ agonist may bind to the A_1 receptor and produce an inhibition of adenylate cyclase which is prevented by A_1 antagonist (Fuxe et al., 2008). All the above RRIs would be particularly intriguing as they would represent other ways of reciprocal modulation between purinergic and adenosine neurotransmission both in type I and II cells.

HOMO- AND HETERO-DIMERS BETWEEN DOPAMINE RECEPTORS (D_1 AND D_2)

According to co-immunoprecipitation data gathered from both rat brain and cells showing co-expression of the D_1

and D_2 receptors, occurs the idea they may constitute the same heteromeric protein complex; moreover, according to immunohistochemistry studies, these receptors are convincingly co-expressed and co-localized within neurons of human and rat brain (Lee et al., 2004). For instance, a significant neuronal subpopulation in rat nucleus accumbens co-expresses D_1 and D_2 receptors, which can form a D_1/D_2 receptor complex (Hopf et al., 2003; Hasbi et al., 2018). Rashid et al. (2007) also provided evidences concerning their co-expression in human embryonic kidney cells. In parallel, Rashid et al. (2007) and Hasbi et al. (2018) demonstrated the ability of D_1 and D_2 receptors to oligomerize *in vivo* in rodent and monkey striata, respectively, through *in situ* PLA, *in situ* FRET and co-immunoprecipitation.

D_1 and D_2 monomers are coupled to G_s and G_i proteins, respectively, and they are usually considered to exert opposite effects at the cellular level (Hopf et al., 2003). Conversely, the heterodimer D_1/D_2 is coupled to $G_{q/11}$. In the nucleus accumbens, the activation of this heterodimer-specific pathway determines an increase of calcium/calmodulin-dependent protein kinase IIα in contrast with the effect produced by the activation of the Gs-D_1 receptor (Rashid et al., 2007).

Numerous studies documented the presence of D_1 receptor in the CB of various animals through Northern blot analysis, RT-PCR and pharmacological studies, although the precise location has not been verified (Almaraz et al., 1991; Bairam et al., 1998, 2003; Schlenker, 2008). Almaraz et al. (1991) suggested expression in blood vessels. Bairam et al. (1998) suggested that D_1 receptor could be expressed in nerve terminals (sensitive and sympathetic). Conversely, D_1 receptors were identified in hamster type I cells through immunohistochemistry (Schlenker and Schultz, 2011). D_2 has been demonstrated in type I cells and nerve fibers of the rat CB by double immunofluorescence (Wakai et al., 2015) and its expression is higher than D_1 (Bairam et al., 1998). The contemporary presence of D_1 and D_2 in type I cells and nerve fibers would support the hypothesis of heterodimerization in these structures. Exogenous dopamine may also inhibit Ca^{2+} responses in type II cells, supporting the presence of corresponding receptors (Leonard and Nurse, 2017; Leonard et al., 2018) and of possible dimerization.

Huey and Powell (2000) explored the consequences of chronic hypoxia on D_2 receptor expression in the arterial chemoreflex pathway. As regards the CB, the authors observed that the regulation of D_2-receptor mRNA expression is time-dependent. Briefly, an initial increase of D_2 receptor mRNA levels was observed after 6 and 12 h, with a subsequent decrease (24, 48 h) and a final significant increase after 168 h of hypoxia. In a noteworthy and analog study, Bairam et al. (2003) considered the effects induced by hypoxia on the expression levels of both D_1 and D_2 receptor mRNAs. The authors highlighted that in 1-day-old rabbits hypoxia affects the expression of D_2- or D_1-receptors mRNA in a manner that is age-dependent. D_2- and D_1-receptors transcript levels increased and decreased after exposure to moderate (15% O_2) and severe (8% O_2) hypoxia, respectively. Conversely, D_2- and D_1-transcript levels decreased independently of hypoxia intensities in adult rabbits. Unlike D_1 receptors, changes in D_2 receptor mRNA levels were independent on exposure time. The D_2 role in the CB has been suggested not to be key under normal conditions, but rather in situations of chronic hypoxia, where D_1 and D_2 receptors density tends to change as previously discussed (Bairam et al., 2003).

The above changes in the expression of the different dopamine receptors after hypoxia suggest the possibility of consequent changes in the amount of D_1/D_2 heterodimers. It is intriguing the idea that D_1/D_2 heterodimer formation may be under the influence of environmental stimuli, mainly hypoxia but possibly others, in the CB.

HETERO-DIMERS BETWEEN ADENOSINE (A_1 AND A_{2A}) AND DOPAMINE (D_1 AND D_2) RECEPTORS

The co-localization of A_1 and D_2 receptors has been showed by immunofluorescence in rat cerebral cortex neurons (Gines et al., 2000). Moreover, the presence of A_1/D_1 complexes was detected in mouse fibroblast Ltk-cells, transfected with human A_1, D_1, and D_2. While the formation of A_1/D_1 heteromers was confirmed by coimmunoprecipitation, A_1 did not seem to form heterodimers with D_2. A_1 and D_1 receptors, separately, also tend to form homodimers; however, the preferred form of dimerization for these two receptors still needs to be elucidated (Agnati et al., 2003). Additionally, A_1/D_1 dimerization was also confirmed by FRET in HEK-293T cells (Shen et al., 2013).

Due to the possible presence of both A_1 and D_1 receptors in type I cells, a role by A_1/D_1 dimerization may be also be supposed. In particular, A_1/D_1 dimerization could represent a way of integration between agonists and/or antagonists for the two different monomers. For instance, Gines et al. (2000) suggested that A_1/D_1 heteromerization may have a role in the antagonistic modulation of D_1 receptor in the brain, thus having an impact on desensitization mechanism of D_1 and receptor trafficking.

A_{2A}/D_2 heterodimers have also been demonstrated both in transfected SH-SY5Y (Hillion et al., 2002; Xie et al., 2010) and HEK-293T cells (Navarro et al., 2014), by immunoprecipitation followed by Western-blotting (SH-SY5Y) and BRET (HEK-293T). In addition, A_{2A}/D_2 heterodimers were identified in neuronal primary cultures of rat striatum by PLA (Navarro et al., 2014) and cAMP accumulation experiments (Hillion et al., 2002). A_{2A}/D_2 heterodimers have also been demonstrated in the mammalian striatum, with particular reference to the striatal enkephalin-containing GABAergic neurons that project to the globus pallidus and comprise the so-called indirect pathway (Fink et al., 1992; Fuxe et al., 1998; Schiffmann et al., 2003; Trifilieff et al., 2011; Doyle et al., 2012; Atack et al., 2014). Thus, A_{2A}/D_2 heterodimers play an important role in the modulation of GABAergic striato-pallidal neuronal function (Bonaventura et al., 2015). In particular, antagonistic A_{2A}-D_2 RRIs occur in the heterodimer, as demonstrated in striatal membrane preparations after incubation with the A_{2A}

agonist CGS21680, leading to a decrease of the affinity of the high affinity D_2 agonist-binding site (Fuxe et al., 1998; Guidolin et al., 2018). Relationships between A_{2A} and D_2 and adenosine/dopamine cross-talks have been proposed as possible new therapeutic approaches for Parkinson's disease, schizophrenia, and drug addiction (Canals et al., 2003; Guidolin et al., 2015).

As previously discussed, both A_{2A} and D_2 are expressed in type I cells of the CB, supporting the hypothesis of A_{2A}/D_2 heterodimer formation also in these cells. The reciprocal influences of the two receptor monomers in the A_{2A}/D_2 complex would be particularly intriguing, as adenosine and dopamine are among the main excitatory and inhibitory neurotransmitters in the CB. Some authors have proposed a functional interaction between A_{2B} and D_2 receptors. In particular, if adenosine levels would become too high, activation of the low affinity A_{2B} would lead to increased dopamine secretion from type I cells (Conde et al., 2006; Livermore and Nurse, 2013) and inhibition of sensory discharge through pre- and post-synaptic D_2 receptors (Conde et al., 2009a,b, 2012; Zhang et al., 2017; Nurse et al., 2018). RRI between A_{2A} and D_2 could represent an opposite way of neuromodulation, increasing signaling efficiency in the presence of low adenosine levels, through allosteric receptor–receptor inhibition of D_2 signaling.

In rat type I cells, Conde et al. (2008, 2009b) also proposed a A_{2B}-D_2 receptor interactions on the basis of *in vitro* pharmacological experiments, although they did not demonstrate if physical RRI occur but only demonstrated an interaction at the adenylyl cyclase level. In particular, they showed that D_2 agonists decrease catecholamine release and inhibit cAMP production in the CB and that these effects are prevented by A_{2B} agonists; conversely, D_2 antagonists increase the release of catecholamines, this phenomenon being also prevented by A_{2B} antagonists. A_{2B}-D_2 RRI, however, have not yet been demonstrated to date in any cell type.

HOMO- AND HETERO-DIMERS BETWEEN OPIOID RECEPTORS (μOR AND δOR)

μOR forms homodimers (Lopez and Salome, 2009) with an elevated stability, as demonstrated in transfected HEK-293 cells by BRET and radioligand binding assays (Wang et al., 2005). μOR/μOR homodimerization occurs prior of transportation to the cell membrane. Sarkar et al. (2012) also proved μOR homodimerization in rat NK cells through Western-blot analysis and immunoprecipitation as well as immunohistochemistry and immunofluorescence.

Also δOR homodimerization was confirmed by Western-blotting and co-immunoprecipitation in different transfected cellular systems, such as CHO cells and COS cells (Cvejic and Devi, 1997). Data obtained by cross-linking experiments in CHO cells indicated that homodimerization does not depend on the expression level of the receptor. Subsequently, the occurrence of homodimers was also assessed in HEK-293T cells by BRET (Johnston et al., 2011) and in rat NK cells by Western-blot assays, immunoprecipitation, immunohistochemistry, and immunofluorescence (Sarkar et al., 2012).

δOR/μOR heterodimers have also been demonstrated (George et al., 2000; Gomes et al., 2002; Sarkar et al., 2012). The heteroreceptor complexes exhibit distinct pharmacological properties from that of the monomers. Low non-signaling doses of δ- or μ-ligands potentiate the binding and signaling of the receptors and the affinity of endomorphin-1 and δ-selective agonists is increased in the heteroreceptor complex, when compared to monomers (Kabli et al., 2010). These properties appeared linked to changes in the signaling pathways activated by the heteroreceptor complexes as compared to individual receptors (Gomes et al., 2013). In NK cells, in which δOR and μOR proteins exist as homo- and heterodimers, differences in cell function were observed depending on the prevalent type of receptor dimerization (Sarkar et al., 2012).

As suggested by Cvejic and Devi (1997) the dimerization also plays an important role in the internalization of the δOR receptor which in its monomeric form may not be internalized. This could be related to the mechanism that takes place after long-term exposure to opioid ligands. Dimerization of δOR receptors seems to be agonist dependent.

As it regards the CB, both μOR and δOR are expressed in type I cells (Ichikawa et al., 2005; Ricker et al., 2015). The expression of both receptors in type I cells suggests the occurrence of homo- and hetero-dimerization, with possible pharmacological implications. Perivascular nerve fibers have also been reported to express δOR (Ichikawa et al., 2005) although further studies will be necessary for detection of other opioid receptor types.

HETERO-DIMERS BETWEEN DOPAMINE (D_1) AND OPIOID (μOR) RECEPTORS

Co-immunoprecipitation, BRET and cross-antagonism assays demonstrated the existence of D_1/μOR heterodimers in both transfected HEK-293 cells and ventral striatum (Tao et al., 2017). D_1 receptor antagonist can antagonize μOR-mediated signaling and function in a dopamine-independent manner, mostly likely via allosteric interactions through the D_1/μOR heteromer. D_1 antagonist (SCH23390) prevented opiate-induced activation of G-protein, inhibition of adenylyl cyclase, phosphorylation of ERK 1/2 and expression of c-fos in transfected cells expressing both receptors and in striatal tissues from wild type, but not DR KO, mice. The ability of an antagonist to inhibit signals originated by stimulation of the partner receptor is a biochemical characteristic that has been described for receptor heterodimers (cross-antagonism) (Tao et al., 2017).

As discussed above, D_1 receptor and μOR were both assessed in the CB, supporting the hypothesis of corresponding RRI. Moreover, changes in the dynamic monomer/oligomer equilibrium may be postulated on the basis of environmental stimuli, as D_1 expression levels, for instance, decrease in hypoxia conditions and along with exposure time (Bairam et al., 2003).

HETERO-DIMERS BETWEEN DOPAMINE (D_1 AND D_2) AND HISTAMINE (H_3) RECEPTORS

Koerner et al. (2004) assessed the presence of histamine receptors (H_1, H_2, H_3) in the CB through RT-PCR studies. In particular, H_3 has been detected in rat type I cells by immunohistochemistry (Lazarov et al., 2009; Del Rio et al., 2009; Thompson et al., 2010). H_3 antagonism results in increased chemosensory activity (Del Rio et al., 2009) and H3 activation inhibits the intracellular Ca^{2+} signaling mediated by activation of muscarinic receptors in type I cells (Thompson et al., 2010). On the basis of the above and following findings, histamine receptors could also be included in the series of GPCRs with potential oligomerization in the CB.

In fact, Ferrada et al. (2009) demonstrated the D_1–H_3 receptor heteromerization in mammalian transfected cells (HEK-293) by BRET and binding assays as well as in the neuronal cell model SK-N-MC by radioligand experiments. The presence of this heteromer in the brain (striatum) was then also proved by Moreno et al. (2011).

An antagonist acting on one of the receptor units that constitute the D_1–H_3 receptor heteromer can cause changes in conformation of the other receptor unit, thus, blocking specific signals that originate in the heteromer. This mechanism could be responsible for unsuspected GPCR antagonists-related therapeutic potentials (Ferrada et al., 2009). D_1/H_3 receptor heteromers work as processors integrating dopamine- as well as histamine-related signals involved in controlling the function of striatal neurons of the direct striatal pathway (Moreno et al., 2011).

A strong and selective heteromeric interaction between D_2 and H_3 was also assessed by radioligand binding experiments in striatal membrane preparations and in co-transfected HEK-293 cells by BRET (Ferrada et al., 2008). According to agonist/antagonist competition experiments, a significant decrease of D_2 receptors affinity for the agonist was encountered after stimulation of H_3 receptors with several H_3 agonists (Ferrada et al., 2008).

HETERO-DIMERS BETWEEN DOPAMINE (D_2) AND SEROTONIN (5-HT_{2A}) RECEPTORS

5-HT_{2A}/D_2 heteroreceptor complexes were demonstrated by PLA and immunofluorescence in co-transfected HEK-293T cells (Lukasiewicz et al., 2010; Borroto-Escuela et al., 2014), as well as in discrete regions of the ventral and dorsal striatum and nucleus accumbens (Borroto-Escuela et al., 2014), medial prefrontal cortex as well as in the pars reticulate of the substantia nigra in rat (Lukasiewicz et al., 2010).

The functional properties of this complex are not yet completely clear (Lukasiewicz et al., 2010). However, ligands with high 5-HT_{2A}/D_2 selectivity and partial agonistic activity on D_2 have been recently identified as new antipsychotic drugs which do not significantly induce extrapyramidal side effects (Möller et al., 2015).

Serotonin is released by type I cells and it acts in a autocrine/paracrine manner on 5-HT_2 receptors which are localized in type I cells, as proved by immunofluorescence and pharmacological/functional studies in the rat CB (Zhang et al., 2003; Jacono et al., 2005; Liu et al., 2011; Yokoyama et al., 2015). Possible expression of 5-HT_{2A} in carotid sinus nerve terminals has also been reported (Nurse et al., 2018). Serotonin is also considered to be involved in long-term facilitation of CB sensory discharge due to chronic intermittent hypoxia (Peng et al., 2009; Prabhakar, 2011). The presence of 5-HT_{2A} and D_2 in type I cells suggests the possibility of heterodimer formation, with functional roles to be investigated. 5-HT_{2A} and D_2 mediate excitatory and inhibitory effects on type I cells and the role of dimerization in the modulation of the two response types is particularly intriguing.

HETERO-DIMERS BETWEEN DOPAMINE (D_2) AND NEUROTENSIN (NTS_1) RECEPTORS

Among CB receptors possibly interacting with D_2 receptor there is also the neurotensin receptor 1 (NTS_1), which has been demonstrated by immunohistochemistry in rat and human type I cells (Porzionato et al., 2009). D_2-NTS_1 complexes have also been highlighted in living HEK293T cells by BRET technology (Borroto-Escuela et al., 2013b). Through these RRI neurotensin reduces dopamine binding and function at D_2 receptor, moving dopamine transmission toward D_1 receptor, which is not antagonized by NTS_1 (Borroto-Escuela and Fuxe, 2017).

HOMO- AND HETERO-DIMERS BETWEEN MELATONIN RECEPTORS (MT_1 AND MT_2)

MT_2 receptors have the ability to form homodimers, as first demonstrated in HEK-293T transfected cells through BRET approaches (including single-cell BRET experiments), as well as Western-blotting and co-immunoprecipitation assays (Ayoub et al., 2002). However, it has also been observed that MT_2 receptors tend to preferentially form heterodimers with MT_1, as proved by BRET techniques (BRET donor saturation assay) in the same cell model (Ayoub et al., 2004).

The homodimerization of MT_2 receptors is not modulated by ligands as it can exist in a constitutive manner in living cells. However, the speculated role of MT_2 dimers is that they are required for explicating biological functions of cells being considered functional signaling units. Modulation of the signaling and trafficking occurs similarly to the $GABA_B$ receptors (Ayoub et al., 2002).

As regards the presence of MT receptors in the CB, an *in situ* hybridization study showed MT_2 expression in the rat type I cells whereas there are not yet data about MT_1 (Tjong et al., 2004).

Thus, to date, we can suppose MT_2 homodimerization in type I cells although further analyses could be of interest for MT_1 detection.

GALANIN RECEPTOR (Gal_1, Gal_2) HETEROMERS

Galanin (Mazzatenta et al., 2014) and galanin receptors 1 (Gal_1) and 2 (Gal_2), but not 3 (Gal_3), (Porzionato et al., 2010) have been demonstrated by immunohistochemistry in rat type I cells. Galanin is known to regulate the differentiation of neural stem cells and plasticity responses in the nervous system (e.g., Cordeo-Llana et al., 2014) and it has been suggested that galanin expression in chemoreceptor cells could provide a signal for neurogenesis and chemoreceptor cell differentiation (Di Giulio et al., 2015; Mazzatenta et al., 2016).

As it concerns this paper, galanin receptors are particularly intriguing because evidence is given about the possibility of Gal_1-Gal_2, D1-Gal_1, Gal-NPY_{Y1}, Gal_1-Gal_2-NPY_{Y2} or Gal_1-Gal_2-AT_1 heteromers, which can be postulated in type I cells (reviewed in Fuxe et al., 2012b).

Although there are not specific data about the expression of the different NPY receptor types in the CB, NPY immunoreactivity has been identified in nerve fibers as well as type I cells of dog, monkey and rat CB (Oomori et al., 1991, 2002). In the rat CB, a reduction in NPY-immunoreactive type I cells was observed from postnatal week 2 onward; conversely, NPY-immunoreactive fibers mainly increase since week 2 after birth (Oomori et al., 2002).

The local renin-angiotensin system in the CB has been extensively studied in the past years (e.g., Fung et al., 2002; Fung, 2014; Lam et al., 2014) and angiotensin II receptor type 1 (AT_1) has been identified in rat type I (Fung et al., 2001; Atanasova et al., 2018) and type II (Murali et al., 2014) cells. In the rat, AT_1 receptors are also up-regulated in response to hypoxia (Fung et al., 2002).

HOMO- AND HETERO-DIMERS BETWEEN ENDOTHELIN RECEPTORS (ET_A AND ET_B)

Endothelin 1 (ET-1) receptors type A (ET_A) and B (ET_B) may form homo- and heterodimers, although the functional implications of different dimerization are still largely unknown. Their behavior was studied after expression in transfected HEK-293T cells by immunoprecipitation, immunoblotting and FRET (Evans and Walker, 2008). These results confirmed the previous data by Gregan et al. (2004) who adopted FRET too, co-localizing ET-1 receptors at the plasma membrane. Furthermore, the latter speculated that ET-1-receptors homodimerization (as well as homo-oligomerization) is constitutive and ligand-independent (Evans and Walker, 2008).

Type I cells synthetize and release ET-1, which may act in autocrine/paracrine manner on the same type I cells through both the above receptors. Chronic continuous hypoxia upregulates ET-1 and ET_A receptor, suggesting a critical role in chronic hypoxia-induced increased chemosensitivity in the rat CB (Chen et al., 2002). Chronic intermittent hypoxia is also known to enhance the CB chemosensory and ventilatory responses to acute hypoxia and produce long-term sensory potentiation of chemosensory discharges (e.g., Peng et al., 2003, 2013; Rey et al., 2004; Pawar et al., 2009). Chronic intermittent hypoxia has been reported to determine an upregulation of ET-1 and ET_B receptor, but not of ET_A receptor, in adult cats (Rey et al., 2007); conversely, upregulation of ET-1 and ET_A receptor, but not ET_B receptor, have been reported in neonatal (Pawar et al., 2009) and adult (Peng et al., 2013) rats.

Endothelin rise intracellular Ca^{2+} in cultured type II cells (Murali et al., 2015). Stimulation of ET_B receptors by ET-1 has been reported to play a role in proliferation of stem cells derived from type II cells and CB hyperplasia following chronic hypoxia (Platero-Luengo et al., 2014).

Thus, RRIs between ET-1 receptors can be hypothesized in type I and II cells. Hypoxia-induced changes in the expression of two different receptor types, together with the involvement of ET-1 in functional/structural modifications, suggests the idea that changes in the monomer/(homo/hetero)-dimer equilibrium may also play a role.

ET_B receptor has also been reported to undergo physical interactions with AT_1 receptor located in the cells of renal proximal tubule (Zeng et al., 2005). RRI between the two receptors would be particularly intriguing in the CB, due to their roles in hypoxia responses.

HETERO-DIMERS BETWEEN GABA ($GABA_{B2}$) AND MUSCARINIC (M_2) RECEPTORS

Boyer et al. (2009) demonstrated by FRET that $GABA_{B2}$ is co-localized and directly associates with M_2 receptor in neuronal PC12 cells. In parallel, the authors observed that in another cell model, i.e., HEK-293T, $GABA_{B1}$ is also required for $GABA_{B2}/M_2$ heterodimerization, contrary to what was observed in PC12. Moreover, through co-immunoprecipitation and immunostaining experiments, the authors supported that signaling complexes $GABA_{B2}/M_2$ exist also *in vivo* in the brain cortex. The association seems to be specific since $GABA_{B2}$ did not associate closely with other related muscarinic receptors (M_1) or with a different GPCR (μOR).

The findings that M_2 and $GABA_{B2}$ are co-localized and associate in cortical neurons, which overlap with brain regions that receive cholinergic projections, suggest that the heterodimer is involved in a novel mechanism for enhancing cholinergic signaling in the brain. In fact, expression of $GABA_{B2}$ in M_2-expressing neurons would allow some neurons to maintain muscarinic signaling during elevated or chronic agonist exposure (Boyer et al., 2009).

Type I cells of the CB express both $GABA_{B1}$ and $GABA_{B2}$ subunits, as confirmed by RT-PCR studies. In addition to molecular biology evidences, localization of $GABA_{B2}$

receptor subunits in sections of the CB was also assayed by immunofluorescence which assessed positive immunoreactivity for the receptor subunit in type I clusters (Fearon et al., 2003). Shirahata et al. (2004) demonstrated the expression of M_2 mRNA and the presence of the receptor protein, by RT-PCR and immunohistochemistry, respectively. In particular, regarding localization, immunohistochemical analysis highlighted M_2 presence in type I cells and petrosal afferent terminals. GABA and acetylcholine (Dasso et al., 1997) show inhibitory and excitatory actions, respectively, on type I cells. The possible occurrence of dimerization may have a role in the reciprocal modulation of actions of the two neurotransmitters.

Muscarinic receptors are also present in type II cells, as muscarinic agonists elicit an increase of intracellular Ca^{2+} levels in these cells (Tse et al., 2012; Murali et al., 2015), but there are not data about the possible expression of GABA receptors too.

CANNABINOID RECEPTOR (CB1) HETEROMERS

The CB_1 receptor was found to be expressed in the CB by techniques such as RT-PCR, immunohistochemistry and *in situ* hybridization, although its levels were relatively low (McLemore, 2004). These findings suggest that endocannabinoids may have an impact on blood flow regulation in the CB, therefore affecting the oxygen pressure and respiratory control. However, the CB_1 function in CB needs to be further investigated, as data present in another study on CB_1 were somewhat discording (Roy et al., 2012).

The CB_1 can form heterodimers with many other different GPCRs which are also assessed to be present in the CB; among these δOR, μOR, A_{2A} and D_2 receptors. In particular, the ability of CB_1 and D_2 receptors to form heterodimers was demonstrated in co-transfected cells (HEK-293T) through co-immunoprecipitation and FRET techniques (Kearn, 2005; Marcellino et al., 2008). It is noteworthy that the activation of CB_1-D_2 receptor heterodimer can have completely opposite effects than activation of the individual receptors.

The above receptors have also been demonstrated to oligomerize in receptor mosaics so that the presence of these complexes may also be postulated for the CB. In particular, the existence of a CB_1-D_2-A_{2A} receptor mosaic has been demonstrated, where CB_1 receptor activation removes the D_2 inhibition of the A_{2A} receptor signaling (Fuxe et al., 2008; Marcellino et al., 2008). The above receptor mosaicism could represent a further way of subtle reciprocal modulation between different neurotransmitters.

HETEROCOMPLEXES BETWEEN GPCR AND OTHER RECEPTOR TYPES

G protein-coupled receptors may undergo direct interactions with other membrane receptors, such as ion channel receptors or receptor tyrosine kinases (Borroto-Escuela et al., 2016). Some of these complexes can be postulated in the CB, with possible roles in modulation of neurotransmission and plasticity.

For instance, NMDA receptor subunits 1, 2A and 2B have been detected in CB, through RT-PCR, and type I cells, through immunohistochemistry. Chronic intermittent hypoxia also increases the expression of $NMDA_1$ and $NMDA_{2B}$ receptors (Liu et al., 2009). It is noteworthy that D_1 receptors can regulate the function of the NMDA receptor by means of direct protein–protein interactions between the carboxyl terminals of D_1 receptor and $NMDA_1$ and $NMDA_{2A}$ (Lee et al., 2002; Li et al., 2010), stimulating NMDA receptor-mediated long-term potentiation (Nai et al., 2010).

FGF receptor 1, which is a tyrosine kinases receptor, has been reported to undergo direct RRI with A_{2A} receptor (Flajolet et al., 2008; Borroto-Escuela et al., 2013a). In particular, as demonstrated in PC12 cells (showing a series of similar properties with type I cells), contemporary activation of the two receptors, but not the single ones, induces activation of the MAPK/ERK pathway, differentiation and neurite extension (Flajolet et al., 2008). The majority of human CB's type I cells have shown a weak to moderate cytoplasmic immunostaining for FGF_1 receptor (Douwes Dekker et al., 2007). In particular, FGF_1 receptor immunoreactivity was shown in type I cells in postnatal rat CB cultures, in both normoxic and hypoxic conditions, as well as in bFGF presence or absence (Paciga and Nurse, 2001). bFGF increased both inward Na^+ and outward K^+ currents after 2 days of treatment on cultured type I cells from E18-19 rat pups (Zhong and Nurse, 1995). In cultures from rat E17-E19 CB, bFGF increases survival and BrdU incorporation; in postnatal P1-P3 cultures, bFGF still stimulates DNA synthesis but does not affect survival. In fetal rat glomus cells, bFGF stimulates neuronal differentiation, producing neurite outgrowth and inducing neurofilament immunoreactivity; these changes can no longer be detected in postnatal cultures (Nurse and Vollmer, 1997). Given the concomitant expression of A_{2A} receptors in type I cells, an heterocomplex could be hypothesized. Moreover, the above developmental changes in the FGF action could partially derive by changes in the monomer–heteromer equilibrium. It is known, for instance, that the expression of A_{2A} receptors in the rat type I cells decreases by PN14 (Gauda et al., 2000).

It is noteworthy that A_{2A}-D_2-FGF receptor mosaic has also been highlighted in other cell types (Fuxe et al., 2010) and could represent a further way of integration between neuromodulation and plasticity mechanisms.

CONCLUSION AND FUTURE PERSPECTIVES

The CB is characterized by the production and release of many different neurotransmitters and neuromodulators which act on various receptor types identifiable on type I and II cells and nerve fibers. Although the main receptors involved in conveying excitatory stimuli from type I cells to afferent nerve fibers are ionotropic (nicotinic, $P2X_2/P2X_3$), a wide series of GPCRs is also expressed in the various structures involved in chemoreception, exerting modulation of neurotransmission.

In other transfected and native cell types, experimental evidence has been provided about the existence of RRIs between GPCRs, with production of homodimers, heterodimers or high-order complexes (receptor mosaics) which may modify ligand binding, signaling and internalization of the protomers. In the present paper, we have reviewed most literature data reporting the contemporary expression in type I cells, type II cells or afferents of GPCRs which are able to physically interact with each other to form homo/hetero-complexes. This is a prerequisite for postulating dimerization and/or oligomerization in the CB. RRIs are particularly intriguing to be hypothesized in the CB, where *in vitro/in vivo* pharmacological/functional data are available about cross-talks between different neurotransmitters/neuromodulators or 'paradoxical' response changes with different concentrations/doses. At least in some cases, such findings could be interpreted through the existence of direct RRIs. Nevertheless, few authors have considered the possibility of di/oligo-merization in the CB (Conde et al., 2008, 2009b) and to the best of our knowledge there are not studies addressing this aspect through up-to-date methodology (see corresponding paragraph). The literature data reviewed in the present paper support the possibility of RRI in the CB and stress the potential implications of di/oligomerization for chemoreception, neuromodulation and plasticity. It is known, in fact, that the expression of certain receptors varies in response to development or environmental stimuli (hypoxia, hyperoxia, etc.); changes in the dynamic monomer/oligomer equilibrium may be the consequence, with correlated functional implications.

In the present paper, we have collected indirect evidence of our 'working hypothesis,' identifying the most significant homo/hetero-complexes which would be worthwhile to be studied in the CB. The direct identification of homo/hetero-complexes in type I, type II and afferent terminations and the characterization of their functional role and relevance in the chemoreception could represent an exciting field of investigation. As previously stated, demonstration of RRIs in the CB should include (1) assessment of colocalization in "close proximity" of two or more receptors and (2) detectable biochemical/functional change in one receptor induced by the binding of a ligand to another receptor. We have here revised literature data highlighting colocalization of different receptors in the various elements of the CB (i.e., type I and II cells, nerve terminals). In addition, colocalization of other receptors could be preliminarily investigated through double immunofluorescence or *in situ* hybridization, both in CB tissue samples and cell cultures.

However, colocalization is just a necessary condition to have direct RRIs and the demonstration of close proximity (i.e., a distance lower than 10 nm) between receptor molecules must be provided. To date, many methods of both biochemical and biophysical nature are available to accomplish this task and most of them could be applied to CB cell cultures. In particular, BRET, FRET or atomic force microscopy could be considered the most useful approaches. Interestingly, *in vitro* models allow to detect changes in cultured CB cells as a response to external pharmacological or environmental (hypoxia, hyperoxia, etc.) stimuli; we have hypothesized that RRIs may increase or decrease in response to external actions. Dynamic modifications of RRIs could also be analyzed in living cells through experimental techniques such as total internal reflection fluorescence microscopy, fluorescence correlation spectroscopy and PALM. Apart from cell cultures, heterocomplexes could be identified in native formalin-fixed CBs through *in situ* PLA, an approach that would even permit the identification of eventual changes in RRIs with respect to experimental conditions of *in vivo* models.

Once demonstrated physical RRIs, functional approaches in cell cultures would have to verify how the agonist/antagonist to one receptor may modify the response of the other receptor(s) toward the corresponding agonists/antagonists.

In conclusion, many *in vitro* and *in vivo* models are available, for research in CB structure/function, which represent adequate material for the application of consistent methods of analysis of potential RRIs.

AUTHOR CONTRIBUTIONS

All the authors contributed to the revision of the literature and discussion of the hypothesis proposed. All the authors read and approved the final version of the manuscript.

REFERENCES

Agnati, L. F., Ferré, S., Lluis, C., Franco, R., and Fuxe, K. (2003). Molecular mechanisms and therapeutical implications of intramembrane receptor/receptor interactions among heptahelical receptors with examples from the striatopallidal GABA neurons. *Pharmacol. Rev.* 55, 509–550. doi: 10.1124/pr.55.3.2

Agnati, L. F., Fuxe, K., Torvinen, M., Genedani, S., Franco, R., Watson, S., et al. (2005). New methods to evaluate colocalization of fluorophores in immunocytochemical preparations as exemplified by a study on A2A and D2 receptors in Chinese hamster ovary cells. *J. Histochem. Cytochem.* 53, 941–953. doi: 10.1369/jhc.4A6355.2005

Agnati, L. F., Guidolin, D., Leo, G., Carone, C., Genedani, S., and Fuxe, K. (2010). Receptor-receptor interactions: a novel concept in brain integration. *Prog. Neurobiol.* 90, 157–175. doi: 10.1016/j.pneurobio.2009.10.004

Almaraz, L., Perez-Garcia, M. T., and Gonzalez, C. (1991). Presence of D1 receptors in the rabbit carotid body. *Neurosci. Lett.* 132, 259–262. doi: 10.1016/0304-3940(91)90315-K

Atack, J. R., Shook, B. C., Rassnick, S., Jackson, P. F., Rhodes, K., Drinkenburg, W. H., et al. (2014). JNJ-40255293, a novel adenosine A2A/A1 antagonist with efficacy in preclinical models of Parkinson's disease. *ACS Chem. Neurosci.* 5, 1005–1019. doi: 10.1021/cn5001606

Atanasova, D. Y., Dandov, A. D., Dimitrov, N. D., and Lazarov, N. E. (2018). Immunohistochemical localization of angiotensin AT1 receptors in the rat carotid body. *Acta Histochem.* 120, 154–158. doi: 10.1016/j.acthis.2018.01.005

Atanasova, D. Y., and Lazarov, N. E. (2014). Expression of neurotrophic factors and their receptors in the carotid body of spontaneously hypertensive rats. *Respir. Physiol. Neurobiol.* 202, 6–15. doi: 10.1016/j.resp.2014.06.016

Ayoub, M. A., Couturier, C., Lucas-Meunier, E., Angers, S., Fossier, P., Bouvier, M., et al. (2002). Monitoring of ligand-independent dimerization and ligand-induced conformational changes of melatonin receptors in living cells by bioluminescence resonance energy transfer. *J. Biol. Chem.* 277, 21522–21528. doi: 10.1074/jbc.M200729200

Ayoub, M. A., Delagrange, P., and Jockers, R. (2004). Preferential formation of MT 1 / MT 2 melatonin receptor heterodimers with distinct ligand interaction properties. *Mol. Pharmacol.* 66, 312–321. doi: 10.1124/mol.104.000398.reasonable

Bae, H., Nantwi, K. D., and Goshgarian, H. G. (2005). Recovery of respiratory function following C2 hemi and carotid body denervation in adult rats: influence of peripheral adenosine receptors. *Exp. Neurol.* 191, 94–103. doi: 10.1016/j.expneurol.2004.09.007

Bairam, A., and Carroll, J. L. (2005). Neurotransmitters in carotid body development. *Respir. Physiol. Neurobiol.* 149, 217–232. doi: 10.1016/j.resp.2005.04.017

Bairam, A., Carroll, J. L., Labelle, Y., and Khandjian, E. W. (2003). Differential changes in dopamine D2- and D1-receptor mRNA levels induced by hypoxia in the arterial chemoreflex pathway organs in one-day-old and adult rabbits. *Biol. Neonate* 84, 222–231. doi: 10.1159/000072306

Bairam, A., Frenette, J., Dauphin, C., Carroll, J. L., and Khandjian, E. W. (1998). Expression of dopamine D1-receptor mRNA in the carotid body of adult rabbits, cats and rats. *Neurosci. Res.* 31, 147–154. doi: 10.1016/S0168-0102(98)00033-39

Bairam, A., Joseph, V., Lajeunesse, Y., and Kinkead, R. (2009). Altered expression of adenosine A1 and A2Areceptors in the carotid body and nucleus tractus solitarius of adult male and female rats following neonatal caffeine treatment. *Brain Res.* 1287, 74–83. doi: 10.1016/j.brainres.2009.06.064

Bayburt, T. H., Leitz, A. J., Xie, G., Oprian, D. D., and Sligar, S. G. (2007). Transducin activation by nanoscale lipid bilayers containing one and two rhodopsins. *J. Biol. Chem.* 282, 14875–14881. doi: 10.1074/jbc.M701433200

Bonaventura, J., Navarro, G., Casadó-Anguera, V., Azdad, K., Rea, W., Moreno, E., et al. (2015). Allosteric interactions between agonists and antagonists within the adenosine A_{2A} receptor-dopamine D_2 receptor heterotetramer. *Proc. Natl. Acad. Sci.* 112, E3609–E3618. doi: 10.1073/pnas.1507704112

Borroto-Escuela, D. O., Flajolet, M., Agnati, L. F., Greengard, P., and Fuxe, K. (2013a). Bioluminescence resonance energy transfer methods to study G protein-coupled receptor-receptor tyrosine kinase heteroreceptor complexes. *Methods Cell Biol.* 117, 141–164. doi: 10.1016/B978-0-12-408143-7.00008-6

Borroto-Escuela, D. O., Ravani, A., Tarakanov, A. O., Brito, I., Narvaez, M., Romero-Fernandez, W., et al. (2013b). Dopamine D2 receptor signaling dynamics of dopamine D2-neurotensin 1 receptor heteromers. *Biochem. Biophys. Res. Commun.* 435, 140–146. doi: 10.1016/j.bbrc.2013.04.058

Borroto-Escuela, D. O., and Fuxe, K. (2017). Diversity and bias through dopamine D2R heteroreceptor complexes. *Curr. Opin. Pharmacol.* 32, 16–22. doi: 10.1016/j.coph.2016.10.004

Borroto-Escuela, D. O., Romero-Fernandez, W., Narvaez, M., Oflijan, J., Agnati, L. F., and Fuxe, K. (2014). Hallucinogenic 5-HT2AR agonists LSD and DOI enhance dopamine D2R protomer recognition and signaling of D2-5-HT2A heteroreceptor complexes. *Biochem. Biophys. Res. Commun.* 443, 278–284. doi: 10.1016/j.bbrc.2013.11.104

Borroto-Escuela, D. O., Wydra, K., Pintsuk, J., Narvaez, M., Corrales, F., Zaniewska, M., et al. (2016). Understanding the functional plasticity in neural networks of the basal ganglia in cocaine use disorder: a role for allosteric receptor-receptor interactions in A2A-D2 heteroreceptor complexes. *Neural Plast.* 2016:4827268. doi: 10.1155/2016/4827268

Bouvier, M., and Hébert, T. E. (2014). CrossTalk proposal: Weighing the evidence for Class A GPCR dimers, the evidence favours dimers. *J. Physiol.* 592, 2439–2441. doi: 10.1113/jphysiol.2014.272252

Boyer, S. B., Clancy, S. M., Terunuma, M., Revilla-Sanchez, R., Thomas, S. M., Moss, S. J., et al. (2009). Direct interaction of GABAB receptors with M2 muscarinic receptors enhances muscarinic signaling. *J. Neurosci.* 29, 15796–15809. doi: 10.1523/JNEUROSCI.4103-09.2009

Bulenger, S., Marullo, S., and Bouvier, M. (2005). Emerging role of homo- and heterodimerization in G-protein-coupled receptor biosynthesis and maturation. *Trends Pharmacol. Sci.* 26, 131–137. doi: 10.1016/j.tips.2005.01.004

Calver, A. R., Medhurst, A. D., Robbins, M. J., Charles, K. J., Evans, M. L., Harrison, D. C., et al. (2000). The expression of GABA(B1) and GABA(B2) receptor subunits in the cNS differs from that in peripheral tissues. *Neuroscience* 100, 155–170. doi: 10.1016/S0306-4522(00)00262-1

Canals, M., Burgueño, J., Marcellino, D., Cabello, N., Canela, E. I., Mallol, J., et al. (2004). Homodimerization of adenosine A2A receptors: qualitative and quantitative assessment by fluorescence and bioluminescence energy transfer. *J. Neurochem.* 88, 726–734. doi: 10.1046/j.1471-4159.2003.02200.x

Canals, M., Marcellino, D., Fanelli, F., Ciruela, F., de Benedetti, P., Goldberg, S. R., et al. (2003). Adenosine A2A-dopamine D2 receptor-receptor heteromerization: qualitative and quantitative assessment by fluorescence and bioluminescence energy transfer. *J. Biol. Chem.* 278, 46741–46749. doi: 10.1074/jbc.M306451200

Carroll, J. L., Agarwal, A., Donnelly, D. F., and Kim, I. (2012). Purinergic modulation of carotid body glomus cell hypoxia response during postnatal maturation in rats. *Adv. Exp. Med. Biol.* 758, 249–253. doi: 10.1007/978-94-007-4584-1_34

Changeux, J. P., and Christopoulos, A. (2016). Allosteric modulation as a unifying mechanism for receptor function and modulation. *Cell* 166, 1084–1102. doi: 10.1016/j.cell.2016.08.015

Chen, J., He, L., Dinger, B., Stensaas, L., and Fidone, S. (2002). Role of endothelin and endothelin A-type receptor in adaptation of the carotid body to chronic hypoxia. *Am. J. Physiol. Lung Cell. Mol. Physiol.* 282, L1314–L1323. doi: 10.1152/ajplung.00454.2001

Chen, Y., Wei, L. N., and Müller, J. D. (2003). Probing protein oligomerization in living cells with fluorescence fluctuation spectroscopy. *Proc. Natl. Acad. Sci. U.S.A.* 100, 15492–15497. doi: 10.1073/pnas.2533045100

Ciruela, F., Casadó, V., Mallol, J., Canela, E. I., Lluis, C., and Franco, R. (1995). Immunological identification of A1 adenosine receptors in brain cortex. *J. Neurosci. Res.* 42, 818–828. doi: 10.1002/jnr.490420610

Ciruela, F., Ferre, S., Casado, V., Cortes, A., Cunha, R. A., Lluis, C., et al. (2006). Heterodimeric adenosine receptors: a device to regulate neurotransmitter release. *Cell. Mol. Life Sci.* 63, 2427–2431. doi: 10.1007/s00018-006-6216-2

Conde, S. V., Gonzalez, C., Batuca, J. R., Monteiro, E. C., and Obeso, A. (2008). An antagonistic interaction between A2B adenosine and D2 dopamine receptors modulates the function of rat carotid body chemoreceptor cells. *J. Neurochem.* 107, 1369–1381. doi: 10.1111/j.1471-4159.2008.05704.x

Conde, S. V., Monteiro, E. C., Obeso, A., and Gonzalez, C. (2009a). Adenosine in peripheral chemoreception: new insights into a historically overlooked molecule. *Adv. Exp. Med. Biol.* 648, 145–159. doi: 10.1007/978-90-481-2259-2_17

Conde, S. V., Obeso, A., Monteiro, E. C., and Gonzalez, C. (2009b). The A(2B)-D(2) receptor interaction that controls carotid body catecholamines release locates between the last two steps of hypoxic transduction cascade. *Adv. Exp. Med. Biol.* 648, 161–168. doi: 10.1007/978-90-481-2259-2_18

Conde, S. V., Monteiro, E. C., Rigual, R., Obeso, A., and Gonzalez, C. (2012). Hypoxic intensity: a determinant for the contribution of ATP and adenosine to the genesis of carotid body chemosensory activity. *J. Appl. Physiol.* 112, 2002–2010. doi: 10.1152/japplphysiol.01617.2011

Conde, S. V., Obeso, A., Vicario, I., Rigual, R., Rocher, A., and Gonzalez, C. (2006). Caffeine inhibition of rat carotid body chemoreceptors is mediated by A2A and A2B adenosine receptors. *J. Neurochem.* 98, 616–628. doi: 10.1111/j.1471-4159.2006.03912.x

Cordeo-Llana, O., Rinaldi, F., Brennan, P. A., Wynick, D., and Caldwell, M. A. (2014). Galanin promotes neuronal differentiation from neuronal progenitor cells in vitro and contributes to the generation of new olfactory neurons in the adult mouse brain. *Exp. Neurol.* 256, 93–104. doi: 10.1016/j.expneurol.2014.04.001

Cvejic, S., and Devi, L. A. (1997). Dimerization of the delta opioid receptor: implication for a role in receptor internalization. *J. Biol. Chem.* 272, 26959–26964. doi: 10.1074/jbc.272.43.26959

Dasso, L. L., Buckler, K. J., and Vaughan-Jones, R. D. (1997). Muscarinic and nicotinic receptors raise intracellular Ca2+ levels in rat carotid body type I cells. *J. Physiol.* 498, 327–338. doi: 10.1113/jphysiol.1997.sp021861

De Caro, R., Macchi, V., Sfriso, M. M., and Porzionato, A. (2013). Structural and neurochemical changes in the maturation of the carotid body. *Respir. Physiol. Neurobiol.* 185, 9–19. doi: 10.1016/j.resp.2012.06.012

Del Rio, R., Moya, E. A., Alcayaga, J., and Iturriaga, R. (2009). Evidence for histamine as a new modulator of carotid body chemoreception. *Adv. Exp. Med. Biol.* 648, 177–184. doi: 10.1007/978-90-481-2259-2_20

Di Giulio, C., Marconi, G. D., Zara, S., Di Tano, A., Porzionato, A., Pokorski, M., et al. (2015). Selective expression of galanin in neuronal-like cells of the human carotid body. *Adv. Exp. Med. Biol.* 860, 315–323. doi: 10.1007/978-3-319-18440-1_36

Di Giulio, C., Zara, S., Cataldi, A., Porzionato, A., Pokorski, M., and De Caro, R. (2012). Human carotid body HIF and NGB expression during human development and aging. *Adv. Exp. Med. Biol.* 758, 265–271. doi: 10.1007/978-94-007-4584-1_36

Douwes Dekker, P. B., Kuipers-Dijkshoornb, N. J., Baelde, H. J., van der Mey, A. G. L., Hogendoorn, P. C. W., and Cornelisse, C. J. (2007). Basic fibroblast growth factor and fibroblastic growth factor receptor–1 may contribute to head and neck paraganglioma development by an autocrine or paracrine mechanism. *Hum. Pathol.* 38, 79–85. doi: 10.1016/j.humpath.2006.06.013

Doyle, S. E., Breslin, F. J., Rieger, J. M., Beauglehole, A., and Lynch, W. J. (2012). Time and sex-dependent effects of an adenosine A2A/A1 receptor antagonist on motivation to self-administer cocaine in rats. *Pharmacol. Biochem. Behav.* 102, 257–263. doi: 10.1016/j.pbb.2012.05.001

Evans, N. J., and Walker, J. W. (2008). Endothelin receptor dimers evaluated by FRET, ligand binding, and calcium mobilization. *Biophys. J.* 95, 483–492. doi: 10.1529/biophysj.107.119206

Farran, B. (2017). An update on the physiological and therapeutic relevance of GPCR oligomers. *Pharmacol. Res.* 117, 303–327. doi: 10.1016/j.phrs.2017.01.008

Fearon, I. M., Zhang, M., Vollmer, C., and Nurse, C. A. (2003). GABA mediates autoreceptor feedback inhibition in the rat carotid body via presynaptic GABA B receptors and TASK-1. *J. Physiol.* 553, 83–94. doi: 10.1113/jphysiol.2003.048298

Fernández-Dueñas, V., Llorente, J., Gandía, J., Borroto-Escuela, D. O., Agnati, L. F., Tasca, C. I., et al. (2012). Fluorescence resonance energy transfer-based technologies in the study of protein-protein interactions at the cell surface. *Methods* 57, 467–472. doi: 10.1016/j.ymeth.2012.05.007

Fernández-Dueñas, V., Pérez-Arévalo, A., Altafaj, X., Ferré, S., and Ciruela, F. (2017). Adenosine A1-A2A receptor heteromer as a possible target for early-onset Parkinson's disease. *Front. Neurosci.* 11:652. doi: 10.3389/fnins.2017.00652

Ferrada, C., Ferre, S., Casado, V., Cortes, A., Justinova, Z., Barnes, C., et al. (2008). Interactions between histamine H3 and dopamine D2 receptors and the implications for striatal function. *Neuropharmacology* 55, 190–197. doi: 10.1016/j.neuropharm.2008.05.008

Ferrada, C., Moreno, E., Casadó, V., Bongers, G., Cortés, A., Mallol, J., et al. (2009). Marked changes in signal transduction upon heteromerization of dopamine D1and histamine H3receptors. *Br. J. Pharmacol.* 157, 64–75. doi: 10.1111/j.1476-5381.2009.00152.x

Ferré, S., Casado, V., Devi, L. A., Filizola, M., Jockers, R., Lohse, M. J., et al. (2014). G protein-coupled receptor oligomerization revisited: functional and pharmacological perspectives. *Pharmacol. Rev.* 66, 413–434. doi: 10.1124/pr.113.008052

Ferré, S., Ciruela, F., Borycz, J., Solinas, M., Quarta, D., Antoniou, K., et al. (2008). Adenosine A1-A2A receptor heteromers: new targets for caffeine in the brain. *Front. Biosci.* 13, 2391–2399. doi: 10.2741/2852

Fink, J. S., Weaver, D. R., Rivkees, S. A., Peterfreund, R. A., Pollack, A. E., Adler, E. M., et al. (1992). Molecular cloning of the rat A2 adenosine receptor: selective co-expression with D2 dopamine receptors in rat striatum. *Brain Res. Mol. Brain Res.* 14, 186–195. doi: 10.1016/0169-328X(92)90173-9

Flajolet, M., Wang, Z., Futter, M., Shen, W., Nuangchamnong, N., Bendor, J., et al. (2008). FGF acts as a co-transmitter through adenosine A(2A) receptor to regulate synaptic plasticity. *Nat. Neurosci.* 11, 1402–1409. doi: 10.1038/nn.2216

Foord, S. M. (2002). Receptor classification: post genome. *Curr. Opin. Pharmacol.* 2, 561–566. doi: 10.1016/S1471-4892(02)00214-X

Franco, R., Martínez-Pinilla, E., Lanciego, J. L., and Navarro, G. (2016). Basic pharmacological and structural evidence for class A G-protein-coupled receptor heteromerization. *Front. Pharmacol.* 7:76. doi: 10.3389/fphar.2016.00076

Fung, M. L. (2014). The role of local renin-angiotensin system in arterial chemoreceptors in sleep-breathing disorders. *Front. Physiol.* 5:336. doi: 10.3389/fphys.2014.00336

Fung, M. L., Lam, S. Y., Chen, Y., Dong, X., and Leung, P. S. (2001). Functional expression of angiotensin II receptors in type-I cells of the rat carotid body. *Pflugers. Arch.* 441, 474–480. doi: 10.1007/s004240000445

Fung, M. L., Lam, S. Y., Dong, X., Chen, Y., and Leung, P. S. (2002). Postnatal hypoxemia increases angiotensin II sensitivity and up-regulates AT1a angiotensin receptors in rat carotid body chemoreceptors. *J. Endocrinol.* 173, 305–313. doi: 10.1677/joe.0.1730305

Fuxe, K., Borroto-Escuela, D. O., Marcellino, D., Romero-Fernandez, W., Frankowska, M., Guidolin, D., et al. (2012a). GPCR heteromers and their allosteric receptor-receptor interactions. *Curr. Med. Chem.* 19, 356–363. doi: 10.2174/092986712803414259

Fuxe, K., Borroto-Escuela, D. O., Romero-Fernandez, W., Tarakanov, A. O., Calvo, F., Garriga, P., et al. (2012b). On the existence and function of galanin receptor heteromers in the central nervous system. *Front. Endocrinol.* 3:127. doi: 10.3389/fendo.2012.00127

Fuxe, K., Ferré, S., Zoli, M., and Agnati, L. F. (1998). Integrated events in central dopamine transmission as analyzed at multiple levels. Evidence for intramembrane adenosine A2A/dopamine D2 and adenosine A1/dopamine D1 receptor interactions in the basal ganglia. *Brain Res. Brain Res. Rev.* 26, 258–273. doi: 10.1016/S0165-0173(97)00049-0

Fuxe, K., Marcellino, D., Borroto-Escuela, D. O., Frankowska, M., Ferraro, L., Guidolin, D., et al. (2010). The changing world of G protein-coupled receptors: from monomers to dimers and receptor mosaics with allosteric receptor-receptor interactions. *J. Recept. Signal Transduct. Res.* 30, 272–283. doi: 10.3109/10799893.2010.506191

Fuxe, K., Marcellino, D., Guidolin, D., Woods, A. S., and Agnati, L. F. (2008). Heterodimers and receptor mosaics of different types of G-protein-coupled receptors. *Physiology* 23, 322–332. doi: 10.1152/physiol.00028.2008

Gahbauer, S., and Böckmann, R. A. (2016). Membrane-mediated oligomerization of G protein coupled receptors and its implication for GPCR function. *Front. Physiol.* 7:494. doi: 10.3389/fphys.2016.00494

Galvez, T., Duthey, B., Kniazeff, J., Blahos, J., Rovelli, G., Bettler, B., et al. (2001). Allosteric interactions between GB1 and GB2 subunits are required for optimal GABA(B) receptor function. *EMBO J.* 20, 2152–2159. doi: 10.1093/emboj/20.9.2152

Gandia, J., Galino, J., Amaral, O. B., Soriano, A., Lluís, C., Franco, R., et al. (2008). Detection of higher-order G protein-coupled receptor oligomers by a combined BRET-BiFC technique. *FEBS Lett.* 582, 2979–2984. doi: 10.1016/j.febslet.2008.07.045

Gauda, E. B. (2000). Expression and localization of A2a and A1-adenosine receptor genes in the rat carotid body and petrosal ganglia. A2a and A1-adenosine receptor mRNAs in the rat carotid body. *Adv. Exp. Med. Biol.* 475, 549–558.

Gauda, E. B., Cooper, R. Z., Donnelly, D. F., Mason, A., and McLemore, G. L. (2006). The effect of development on the pattern of A1 and A2a-adenosine receptor gene and protein expression in rat peripheral arterial chemoreceptors. *Adv. Exp. Med. Biol.* 580, 121–129. doi: 10.1007/0-387-31311-7_19

Gauda, E. B., Northington, F. J., Linden, J., and Rosin, D. L. (2000). Differential expression of a(2a), A(1)-adenosine and D(2)-dopamine receptor genes in rat peripheral arterial chemoreceptors during postnatal development. *Brain Res.* 872, 1–10. doi: 10.1016/S0006-8993(00)02314-2313

George, S. R., Fan, T., Xie, Z., Tse, R., Tam, V., Varghese, G., et al. (2000). Oligomerization of mu- and delta-opioid receptors. Generation of novel functional properties. *J. Biol. Chem.* 275, 26128–26135. doi: 10.1074/jbc.M000345200

George, S. R., O'Dowd, B. F., and Lee, S. P. (2002). G-protein-coupled receptor oligomerization and its potential for drug discovery. *Nat. Rev. Drug Discov.* 1, 808–820. doi: 10.1038/nrd913

Gines, S., Hillion, J., Torvinen, M., Le Crom, S., Casado, V., Canela, E. I., et al. (2000). Dopamine D1 and adenosine A1 receptors form functionally interacting heteromeric complexes. *Proc. Natl. Acad. Sci.* 97, 8606–8611. doi: 10.1073/pnas.150241097

Gomes, I., Ayoub, M. A., Fujita, W., Jaeger, W. C., Pfleger, K. D., and Devi, L. A. (2016). G protein-coupled receptor heteromers. *Annu. Rev. Pharmacol. Toxicol.* 56, 403–425. doi: 10.1146/annurev-pharmtox-011613-135952

Gomes, I., Filipovska, J., Jordan, B. A., and Devi, L. A. (2002). Oligomerization of opioid receptors. *Methods* 27, 358–365. doi: 10.1016/S1046-2023(02)00094-4

Gomes, I., Fujita, W., Chandrakala, M. V., and Devi, L. A. (2013). Disease-specific heteromerization of G-protein-coupled receptors that target drugs of abuse. *Prog. Mol. Biol. Transl. Sci.* 117, 207–265. doi: 10.1016/B978-0-12-386931-9.00009-X

Gracia, E., Cortés, A., Meana, J. J., García-Sevilla, J., Herhsfield, M. S., Canel, E. I., et al. (2008). Human adenosine deaminase as an allosteric modulator of human A1 adenosine receptor: abolishment of negative cooperativity for $[^3H]$(R)-pia binding to the caudate nucleus. *J. Neurochem.* 107, 161–170. doi: 10.1111/j.1471-4159.2008.05602.x

Gracia, E., Moreno, E., Cortés, A., Lluís, C., Mallol, J., McCormick, P. J., et al. (2013). Homodimerization of adenosine A1 receptors in brain cortex explains the biphasic effects of caffeine. *Neuropharmacology* 71, 56–69. doi: 10.1016/j.neuropharm.2013.03.005

Gregan, B., Schaefer, M., Rosenthal, W., and Oksche, A. (2004). Fluorescence resonance energy transfer analysis reveals the existence of endothelin-A and endothelin-B receptor homodimers. *J. Cardiovasc. Pharmacol.* 44, 30–33. doi: 10.1097/01.fjc.0000166218.35168.79

Grisshammer, R. (2017). New approaches towards the understanding of integral membrane proteins: a structural perspective on G protein-coupled receptors. *Protein Sci.* 26, 1493–1504. doi: 10.1002/pro.3200

Guescini, M., Leo, G., Genedani, S., Carone, C., Pederzoli, F., Ciruela, F., et al. (2012). Microvesicle and tunneling nanotube mediated intercellular transfer of G-protein coupled receptors in cell cultures. *Exp. Cell Res.* 318, 603–613. doi: 10.1016/j.yexcr.2012.01.005

Guidolin, D., Agnati, L. F., Marcoli, M., Borroto-Escuela, D., and Fuxe, K. (2015). G-protein-coupled receptor type A heteromers as an emerging therapeutic target. *Expert Opin. Ther. Targets* 19, 265–283. doi: 10.1517/14728222.2014.981155

Guidolin, D., Marcoli, M., Tortorella, C., Maura, G., and Agnati, L. F. (2018). G protein-coupled receptor-receptor interactions give integrative dynamics to intercellular communication. *Rev. Neurosci.* doi: 10.1515/revneuro-2017-0087 [Epub ahead of print].

Gurevich, V. V., and Gurevich, E. V. (2008). How and why do GPCRs dimerize? *Trends Pharmacol. Sci.* 29, 234–240. doi: 10.1016/j.tips.2008.02.004

Hasbi, A., Perreault, M. L., Shen, M. Y. F., Fan, T., Nguyen, T., Alijaniaram, M., et al. (2018). Activation of dopamine D1-D2 receptor complex attenuates cocaine reward and reinstatement of cocaine-seeking through inhibition of DARPP-32, ERK, and ΔFosB. *Front. Pharmacol.* 8:924. doi: 10.3389/fphar.2017.00924

Hern, J. A., Baig, A. H., Mashanov, G. I., Birdsall, B., Corrie, J. E., Lazareno, S., et al. (2010). Formation and dissociation of M1 muscarinic receptor dimers seen by total internal reflection fluorescence imaging of single molecules. *Proc. Natl. Acad. Sci. U.S.A.* 107, 2693–2698. doi: 10.1073/pnas.0907915107

Hillion, J., Canals, M., Torvinen, M., Casadó, V., Scott, R., Terasmaa, A., et al. (2002). Coaggregation, cointernalization, and codesensitization of adenosine A2A receptors and dopamine D2 receptors. *J. Biol. Chem.* 277, 18091–18097. doi: 10.1074/jbc.M107731200

Hopf, F. W., Cascini, M. G., Gordon, A. S., Diamond, I., and Bonci, A. (2003). Cooperative activation of dopamine D1 and D2 receptors increases spike firing of nucleus accumbens neurons via G-protein betagamma subunits. *J. Neurosci.* 23, 5079–5087. doi: 10.1523/JNEUROSCI.23-12-05079.2003

Huey, K. A., and Powell, F. L. (2000). Time-dependent changes in dopamine D2-receptor mRNA in the arterial chemoreflex pathway with chronic hypoxia. *Mol. Brain Res.* 75, 264–270. doi: 10.1016/S0169-328X(99)00321-6

Ichikawa, H., Schulz, S., Höllt, V., and Sugimoto, T. (2005). Delta-opioid receptor-immunoreactive neurons in the rat cranial sensory ganglia. *Brain Res.* 1043, 225–230. doi: 10.1016/j.brainres.2005.02.041

Iturriaga, R., and Alcayaga, J. (2004). Neurotransmission in the carotid body: transmitters and modulators between glomus cells and petrosal ganglion nerve terminals. *Brain Res. Brain Res. Rev.* 47, 46–53. doi: 10.1016/j.brainresrev.2004.05.007

Jacono, F. J., Peng, Y. J., Kumar, G. K., and Prabhakar, N. R. (2005). Modulation of the hypoxic sensory response of the carotid body by 5-hydroxytryptamine: role of the 5-HT2 receptor. *Respir. Physiol. Neurobiol.* 145, 135–142. doi: 10.1016/j.resp.2004.10.002

Johnston, J. M., Aburi, M., Provasi, D., Bortolato, A., Urizar, E., Lambert, N. A., et al. (2011). Making structural sense of dimerization interfaces of delta opioid receptor homodimers. *Biochemistry* 50, 1682–1690. doi: 10.1021/bi101474v

Jonas, K. C., Huhtaniemi, I., and Hanyaloglu, A. C. (2016). Single-molecule resolution of G protein-coupled receptor (GPCR) complexes. *Methods Cell Biol.* 132, 55–72. doi: 10.1016/bs.mcb.2015.11.005-

Kabli, N., Martin, N., Fan, T., Nguyen, T., Hasbi, A., Balboni, G., et al. (2010). Agonists at the δ-opioid receptor modify the binding of μ-receptor agonists to the μ-δ receptor hetero-oligomer. *Br. J. Pharmacol.* 161, 1122–1136. doi: 10.1111/j.1476-5381.2010.00944.x

Kaczor, A. A., and Selent, J. (2011). Oligomerization of G protein-coupled receptors: biochemical and biophysical methods. *Curr. Med. Chem.* 18, 4606–4634. doi: 10.2174/092986711797379285

Kamal, M., and Jockers, R. (2011). Biological significance of GPCR heteromerization in the neuro-endocrine system. *Front. Endocrinol.* 2:2. doi: 10.3389/fendo.2011.00002

Kearn, C. S. (2005). Concurrent stimulation of cannabinoid CB1 and dopamine D2 receptors enhances heterodimer formation: a mechanism for receptor cross-talk? *Mol. Pharmacol.* 67, 1697–1704. doi: 10.1124/mol.104.006882

Kenakin, T., Agnati, L. F., Caron, M., Fredholm, B., Guidolin, D., Kobilka, B., et al. (2010). International workshop at the Nobel Forum, Karolinska Institutet on G protein-coupled receptors: finding the words to describe monomers, oligomers, and their molecular mechanisms and defining their meaning. Can a consensus be reached? *J. Recep. Signal Transduct. Res.* 30, 284–286. doi: 10.3109/10799893.2010.512438

Kleinau, G., Muller, A., and Biebermann, H. (2016). Oligomerization of GPCRs involved in endocrine regulation. *J. Mol. Endocrinol.* 57, R59–R80. doi: 10.1530/JME-16-0049

Kniazeff, J., Prezeau, L., Rondard, P., Pin, J. P., and Goudet, C. (2011). Dimers and beyond: the functional puzzles of class C GPCRs. *Pharmacol. Ther.* 130, 9–25. doi: 10.1016/j.pharmthera.2011.01.006

Kobayashi, S., Conforti, L., and Millhorn, D. E. (2000). Gene expression and function of adenosine A(2A) receptor in the rat carotid body. *Am. J. Physiol. Lung Cell. Mol. Physiol.* 279, L273–L282. doi: 10.1152/ajplung.2000.279.2.L273

Koerner, P., Hesslinger, C., Schaefermeyer, A., Prinz, C., and Gratzl, M. (2004). Evidence for histamine as a transmitter in rat carotid body sensor cells. *J. Neurochem.* 91, 493–500. doi: 10.1111/j.14714159.2004.02740.x

Köse, M. (2017). GPCRs and EGFR – cross-talk of membrane receptors in cancer. *Bioorg. Med. Chem. Lett.* 27, 3611–3620. doi: 10.1016/j.bmcl.2017.07.002

Kroeger, K. M., Pfleger, K. D. G., and Eidne, K. A. (2003). G-protein coupled receptor oligomerization in neuroendocrine pathways. *Front. Neuroendocrinol.* 24, 254–278. doi: 10.1016/j.yfrne.2003.10.002

Kuszak, A. J., Pitchiaya, S., Anand, J. P., Mosberg, H. I., Walter, N. G., and Sunahara, R. K. (2009). Purification and functional reconstitution of monomeric μ-opioid receptors: allosteric modulation of agonist binding by Gi2. *J. Biol. Chem.* 284, 26732–26741. doi: 10.1074/jbc.M109.026922

Lam, S. Y., Liu, Y., Ng, K. M., Liong, E. C., Tipoe, G. L., Leung, P. S., et al. (2014). Upregulation of a local renin-angiotensin system in the rat carotid body during chronic intermittent hypoxia. *Exp. Physiol.* 99, 220–231. doi: 10.1113/expphysiol.2013.074591

Lambert, N. A., and Javitch, J. A. (2014). CrossTalk opposing view: weighing the evidence for class A GPCR dimers, the jury is still out. *J. Physiol.* 592, 2443–2445. doi: 10.1113/jphysiol.2014.272997

Lazarov, N. E., Reindl, S., Fischer, F., and Gratzl, M. (2009). Histaminergic and dopaminergic traits in the human carotid body. *Respir. Physiol. Neurobiol.* 165, 131–136. doi: 10.1016/j.resp.2008.10.016

Lee, F. J., Xue, S., Pei, L., Vukusic, B., Chéry, N., Wang, Y., et al. (2002). Dual regulation of NMDA receptor functions by direct protein-protein interactions with the dopamine D1 receptor. *Cell* 111, 219–230. doi: 10.1016/S0092-8674(02)00962-5

Lee, S. P., So, C. H., Rashid, A. J., Varghese, G., Cheng, R., Lança, A. J., et al. (2004). Dopamine D1 and D2 receptor co-activation generates a novel phospholipase C-mediated calcium signal. *J. Biol. Chem.* 279, 35671–35678. doi: 10.1074/jbc.M401923200

Leonard, E. M., and Nurse, C. A. (2017). "Evidence for dopaminergic inhibitory cell-cell interactions in the rat carotid body," in *XXth Meeting of the International Society of Arterial Chemoreception (ISAC)*, (Baltimore, MD).

Leonard, E. M., Salman, S., and Nurse, C. A. (2018). Sensory processing and integration at the carotid body tripartite synapse: neurotransmitter functions and effects of chronic hypoxia. *Front. Physiol.* 9:225. doi: 10.3389/fphys.2018.00225

Li, Y. C., Liu, G., Hu, J. L., Gao, W. J., and Huang, Y. Q. (2010). Dopamine D(1) receptor-mediated enhancement of NMDA receptor trafficking requires rapid PKC-dependent synaptic insertion in the prefrontal neurons. *J. Neurochem.* 114, 62–73. doi: 10.1111/j.14714159.2010.06720.x

Liu, J., Wei, X., Zhao, C., Hu, S., Duan, J., Ju, G., et al. (2011). 5-HT induces enhanced phrenic nerve activity via 5-HT2Areceptor/PKC mechanism in anesthetized rats. *Eur. J. Pharmacol.* 657, 67–75. doi: 10.1016/j.ejphar.2011.01.048

Liu, Y., Ji, E. S., Xiang, S., Tamisier, R., Tong, J., Huang, J., et al. (2009). Exposure to cyclic intermittent hypoxia increases expression of functional NMDA receptors in the rat carotid body. *J. Appl. Physiol.* 106, 259–267. doi: 10.1152/japplphysiol.90626.2008

Livermore, S., and Nurse, C. A. (2013). Enhanced adenosine A2b receptor signaling facilitates stimulus-induced catecholamine secretion in chronically hypoxic carotid body type I cells. *Am. J. Physiol. Cell Physiol.* 305, C739–C750. doi: 10.1152/ajpcell.00137

Lohse, M. J. (2010). Dimerization in GPCR mobility and signaling. *Curr. Opin. Pharmacol.* 10, 53–58. doi: 10.1016/j.coph.2009.10.007

Lopez, A., and Salome, L. (2009). Membrane functional organisation and dynamic of mu-opioid receptors. *Cell. Mol. Life Sci.* 66, 2093–2108. doi: 10.1007/s00018-009-0008-4

Lukasiewicz, S., Blasiak, E., Faron-Gorecka, A., Polit, A., Tworzydlo, M., Gorecki, A., et al. (2007). Fluorescence studies of homooligomerization of adenosine A2A and serotonin 5-HT1A receptors reveal the specificity of receptor interactions in the plasma membrane. *Pharmacol. Rep.* 59, 379–392.

Lukasiewicz, S., Polit, A., Kedracka-Krok, S., Wedzony, K., Mackowiak, M., and Dziedzicka-Wasylewska, M. (2010). Hetero-dimerization of serotonin 5-HT(2A) and dopamine D(2) receptors. *Biochim. Biophys. Acta* 1803, 1347–1358. doi: 10.1016/j.bbamcr.2010.08.010

Mackie, K. (2005). Cannabinoid receptor homo- and heterodimerization. *Life Sci.* 77, 1667–1673. doi: 10.1016/j.lfs.2005.05.011

Marcellino, D., Carriba, P., Filip, M., Borgkvist, A., Frankowska, M., Bellido, I., et al. (2008). Antagonistic cannabinoid CB1/dopamine D2receptor interactions in striatal CB1/D2heteromers. A combined neurochemical and behavioral analysis. *Neuropharmacology* 54, 815–823. doi: 10.1016/j.neuropharm.2007.12.011

Mazzatenta, A., Marconi, G. D., Macchi, V., Porzionato, A., Cataldi, A., Di Giulio, C., et al. (2016). Coexpression of galanin and nestin in the chemoreceptor cells of the human carotid body. *Adv. Exp. Med. Biol.* 885, 77–82. doi: 10.1007/5584_2015_189

Mazzatenta, A., Marconi, G. D., Zara, S., Cataldi, A., Porzionato, A., and Di Giulio, C. (2014). In the carotid body, galanin is a signal for neurogenesis in young, and for neurodegeneration in the old and in drug-addicted subjects. *Front. Physiol.* 5:427. doi: 10.3389/fphys.2014.00427

McLemore, G. L. (2004). Cannabinoid receptor expression in peripheral arterial chemoreceptors during postnatal development. *J. Appl. Physiol.* 97, 1486–1495. doi: 10.1152/japplphysiol.00378.2004

Möller, D., Salama, I., Kling, R. C., Hubner, H., and Gmeiner, P. (2015). 1,4-Disubstituted aromatic piperazines with high 5-HT2A/D2 selectivity: quantitative structure-selectivity investigations, docking, synthesis and biological evaluation. *Bioorg. Med. Chem.* 23, 6195–6209. doi: 10.1016/j.bmc.2015.07.050

Moreno, E., Hoffmann, H., Gonzalez-Sepulveda, M., Navarro, G., Casado, V., Cortes, A., et al. (2011). Dopamine D1-histamine H3 receptor heteromers provide a selective link to MAPK signaling in GABAergic neurons of the direct striatal pathway. *J. Biol. Chem.* 286, 5846–5854. doi: 10.1074/jbc.M110.161489

Murali, S., Zhang, M., and Nurse, C. A. (2014). Angiotensin II mobilizes intracellular calcium and activates pannexin-1 channels in rat carotid body type II cells via AT1 receptors. *J. Physiol.* 592, 4747–4762. doi: 10.1113/jphysiol.2014.279299

Murali, S., Zhang, M., and Nurse, C. A. (2015). Paracrine signaling in glial-like type II cells of the rat carotid body. *Adv. Exp. Med. Biol.* 860, 41–47. doi: 10.1007/978-3-319-18440-1_5

Nai, Q., Li, S., Wang, S. H., Liu, J., Lee, F. J., Frankland, P. W., et al. (2010). Uncoupling the D1-N-methyl-D-aspartate (NMDA) receptor complex promotes NMDA-dependent long-term potentiation and working memory. *Biol. Psychiatry* 67, 246–254. doi: 10.1016/j.biopsych.2009.08.011

Nakata, H., Suzuki, T., Namba, K., and Oyanagi, K. (2010). Dimerization of G protein-coupled purinergic receptors: increasing the diversity of purinergic receptor signal responses and receptor functions. *J. Recept. Signal Transduct. Res.* 30, 337–346. doi: 10.3109/10799893.2010.509729

Nakata, H., Yoshioka, K., Kamiya, T., Tsuga, H., and Oyanagi, K. (2005). Functions of heteromeric association between adenosine and P2Y receptors. *J. Mol. Neurosci* 26, 233–238. doi: 10.1385/JMN

Navarro, G., Aguinaga, D., Moreno, E., Hradsky, J., Reddy, P. P., Cortés, A., et al. (2014). Intracellular calcium levels determine differential modulation of allosteric interactions within G protein-coupled receptor heteromers. *Chem. Biol.* 21, 1546–1566. doi: 10.1016/j.chembiol.2014.10.004

Nurse, C. A. (2005). Neurotransmission and neuromodulation in the chemosensory carotid body. *Auton. Neurosci.* 120, 1–9. doi: 10.1016/j.autneu.2005.04.008

Nurse, C. A. (2014). Synaptic and paracrine mechanisms at carotid body arterial chemoreceptors. *J. Physiol.* 592, 3419–3426. doi: 10.1113/jphysiol.2013.269829

Nurse, C. A., Leonard, E. M., and Salman, S. (2018). The role of glial-like type II cells as paracrine modulators of carotid body chemoreception. *Physiol. Genomics.* 50, 255–262. doi: 10.1152/physiolgenomics.00142.2017

Nurse, C. A., and Vollmer, C. (1997). Role of basic FGF and oxygen in control of proliferation, survival, and neuronal differentiation in carotid body chromaffin cells. *Dev. Biol.* 184, 197–206. doi: 10.1006/dbio.1997.8539

Oomori, Y., Ishikawa, K., Satho, Y., Matsuda, M., and Ono, K. (1991). Neuropeptide-Y-immunoreactive chief cells in the carotid body of young rats. *Acta Anat.* 140, 120–123. doi: 10.1159/000147046

Oomori, Y., Murabayashi, H., Ishikawa, K., Miyakawa, K., Nakaya, K., and Tanaka, H. (2002). Neuropeptide Y- and catecholamine-synthesizing enzymes: immunoreactivities in the rat carotid body during postnatal development. *Anat. Embryol.* 206, 37–47. doi: 10.1007/s00429-002-0275-4

Ortega-Sáenz, P., Villadiego, J., Pardal, R., Toledo-Aral, J. J., and Lopez-Barneo, J. (2015). Neurotrophic properties, chemosensory responses and neurogenic niche of the human carotid body. *Adv. Exp. Med. Biol.* 860, 139–152. doi: 10.1007/978-3-319-18440-1_16

Paciga, M., and Nurse, C. A. (2001). Basic FGF localization in rat carotid body: paracrine role in O2-chemoreceptor survival. *Neuroreport* 12, 3287–3291. doi: 10.1097/00001756-200110290-00028

Palczewski, K. (2010). Oligomeric forms of G protein-coupled receptors (GPCRs). *Trends Biochem. Sci.* 35, 595–600. doi: 10.1016/j.tibs.2010.05.002

Pardal, R., Ortega-Sàenz, P., Duràn, R., and Lòpez-Barneo, J. (2007). Glia-like stem cells sustain physiologic neurogenesis in the adult mammalian carotid body. *Cell* 131, 364–377. doi: 10.1016/j.cell.2007.07.043

Park, P. S. H., Filipek, S., Wells, J. W., and Palczewski, K. (2004). Oligomerization of G protein-coupled receptors: past, present, and future. *Biochemistry* 43, 15643–15656. doi: 10.1021/bi047907k

Pawar, A., Nanduri, J., Yuan, G., Khan, S. A., Wang, N., Kumar, G. K., et al. (2009). Reactive oxygen species-dependent endothelin signaling is required for augmented hypoxic sensory response of the neonatal carotid body by intermittent hypoxia. *Am. J. Physiol. Regul. Integr. Comp. Physiol.* 296, R735–R742. doi: 10.1152/ajpregu.90490.2008

Peng, Y. J., Nanduri, J., Raghuraman, G., Wang, N., Kumar, G. K., and Prabhakar, N. R. (2013). Role of oxidative stress-induced endothelin-converting enzyme activity in the alteration of carotid body function by chronic intermittent hypoxia. *Exp. Physiol.* 98, 1620–1630. doi: 10.1113/expphysiol.2013.073700

Peng, Y. J., Nanduri, J., Yuan, G., Wang, N., Deneris, E., Pendyala, S., et al. (2009). NADPH oxidase is required for the sensory plasticity of the carotid body by chronic intermittent hypoxia. *J. Neurosci.* 29, 4903–4910. doi: 10.1523/JNEUROSCI.4768-08.2009

Peng, Y. J., Overholt, J. L., Kline, D., Kumar, G. K., and Prabhakar, N. R. (2003). Induction of sensory long-term facilitation in the carotid body by intermittent hypoxia: implications for recurrent apneas. *Proc. Natl. Acad. Sci. U.S.A.* 100, 10073–10078. doi: 10.1073/pnas.1734109100

Piskuric, N. A., and Nurse, C. A. (2013). Expanding role of ATP as a versatile messenger at carotid and aortic body chemoreceptors. *J. Physiol.* 591, 415–422. doi: 10.1113/jphysiol.2012.234377

Platero-Luengo, A., González-Granero, S., Durán, R., Díaz-Castro, B., Piruat, J. I., García-Verdugo, J. M., et al. (2014). An O2-sensitive glomus cell-stem cell synapse induces carotid body growth in chronic hypoxia. *Cell* 156, 291–303. doi: 10.1016/j.cell.2013.12.013

Pontier, S. M., Lahaie, N., Ginham, R., St-Gelais, F., Bonin, H., Bell, D. J., et al. (2006). Coordinated action of NSF and PKC regulates GABAB receptor signaling efficacy. *EMBO J.* 25, 2698–2709. doi: 10.1038/sj.emboj.7601157

Porzionato, A., Macchi, V., Amagliani, A., Castagliuolo, I., Parenti, A., and De Caro, R. (2009). Neurotensin receptor 1 immunoreactivity in the peripheral ganglia and carotid body. *Eur. J. Histochem.* 53, 135–142. doi: 10.4081/ejh.2009.e16

Porzionato, A., Macchi, V., Barzon, L., Masi, G., Belloni, A., Parenti, A., et al. (2010). Expression and distribution of galanin receptor subtypes in the rat carotid body. *Mol. Med. Rep.* 3, 37–41. doi: 10.3892/mmr_00000215

Porzionato, A., Macchi, V., Parenti, A., Matturri, L., and De Caro, R. (2008a). Peripheral chemoreceptors: postnatal development and cytochemical findings in Sudden Infant Death Syndrome. *Histol. Histopathol.* 23, 351–365. doi: 10.14670/HH-23.351

Porzionato, A., Macchi, V., Parenti, A., and De Caro, R. (2008b). Trophic factors in the carotid body. *Int. Rev. Cell Mol. Biol.* 269, 1–58. doi: 10.1016/S1937-6448(08)01001-0

Porzionato, A., Macchi, V., Stecco, C., and De Caro, R. (2018). The carotid sinus nerve - structure, function and clinical implications. *Anat. Rec.* doi: 10.1002/ar.23829 [Epub ahead of print].

Prabhakar, N. R. (2011). Sensory plasticity of the carotid body: role of reactive oxygen species and physiological significance. *Respir. Physiol. Neurobiol.* 178, 375–380. doi: 10.1016/j.resp.2011.05.012

Rashid, A. J., So, C. H., Kong, M. M. C., Furtak, T., El-Ghundi, M., Cheng, R., et al. (2007). D1-D2 dopamine receptor heterooligomers with unique pharmacology are coupled to rapid activation of Gq/11 in the striatum. *Proc. Natl. Acad. Sci. U.S.A.* 104, 654–659. doi: 10.1073/pnas.0604049104

Rey, S., Corthorn, J., Chacón, C., and Iturriaga, R. (2007). Expression and immunolocalization of endothelin peptides and its receptors, ETA and ETB, in the carotid body exposed to chronic intermittent hypoxia. *J. Histochem. Cytochem.* 55, 167–174. doi: 10.1369/jhc.6A7079.2006

Rey, S., Del Rio, R., Alcayaga, J., and Iturriaga, R. (2004). Chronic intermittent hypoxia enhances cat chemosensory and ventilatory responses to hypoxia. *J. Physiol.* 560, 577–586. doi: 10.1113/jphysiol.2004.072033

Ricker, E. M., Pye, R. L., Barr, B. L., and Wyatt, C. N. (2015). Selective mu and kappa opioid agonists inhibit voltage-gated Ca2+ entry in isolated neonatal rat carotid body type I cells. *Adv. Exp. Med. Biol.* 860, 49–54. doi: 10.1007/978-3-319-18440-1_6

Rios, C. D., Jordan, B. A., Gomes, I., and Devi, L. A. (2001). G-protein-coupled receptor dimerization: modulation of receptor function. *Pharmacol. Ther.* 92, 71–87. doi: 10.1016/S0163-7258(01)00160-7

Rocher, A., Gonzalez, C., and Almaraz, L. (1999). Adenosine inhibits L-type Ca2+ current and catecholamine release in the rabbit carotid body chemoreceptor cells. *Eur. J. Neurosci.* 11, 673–681. doi: 10.1046/j.1460-9568.1999.00470.x

Roy, A., Mandadi, S., Fiamma, M.-N., Rodikova, E., Ferguson, E. V., Whelan, P. J., et al. (2012). Anandamide modulates carotid sinus nerve afferent activity via TRPV1 receptors increasing responses to heat. *J. Appl. Physiol.* 112, 212–224. doi: 10.1152/japplphysiol.01303.2010

Sarkar, D. K., Sengupta, A., Zhang, C., Boyadjieva, N., and Murugan, S. (2012). Opiate antagonist prevents μ- and δ-opiate receptor dimerization to facilitate ability of agonist to control ethanol-altered natural killer cell functions and mammary tumor growth. *J. Biol. Chem.* 287, 16734–16747. doi: 10.1074/jbc.M112.347583

Satake, H., Matsubara, S., Aoyama, M., Kawada, T., and Sakai, T. (2013). GPCR heterodimerization in the reproductive system: functional regulation and implication for biodiversity. *Front. Endocrinol. (Lausanne).* 4:100. doi: 10.3389/fendo.2013.00100

Schicker, K., Hussl, S., Chandaka, G. K., Kosenburger, K., Yang, J. W., Waldhoer, M., et al. (2009). A membrane network of receptors and enzymes for adenine nucleotides and nucleosides. *Biochim. Biophys. Acta* 1793, 325–334. doi: 10.1016/j.bbamcr.2008.09.014

Schiffmann, S. N., Dassesse, D., d'Alcantara, P., Ledent, C., Swillens, S., and Zoli, M. (2003). A2A receptor and striatal cellular functions: regulation of gene expression, currents, and synaptic transmission. *Neurology* 61, S24–S29. doi: 10.1212/01.WNL.0000095207.66853.0D

Schlenker, E. H. (2008). In hamsters the D1 receptor antagonist SCH 23390 depresses ventilation during hypoxia. *Brain Res.* 1187, 146–153. doi: 10.1016/j.brainres.2007.10.058

Schlenker, E. H., and Schultz, H. D. (2011). Hypothyroidism attenuates SCH 23390-mediated depression of breathing and decreases D1 receptor expression in carotid bodies, PVN and striatum of hamsters. *Brain Res.* 1401, 40–51. doi: 10.1016/j.brainres.2011.05.034

Schonenbach, N. S., Hussain, S., and O'Malley, M. A. (2015). Structure and function of G protein-coupled receptor oligomers: implications for drug discovery. *Wiley Interdiscip. Rev. Nanomed. Nanobiotechnol.* 7, 408–427. doi: 10.1002/wnan.1319

Shen, J., Zhang, L., Song, W., Meng, T., Wang, X., Chen, L., et al. (2013). Design, synthesis and biological evaluation of bivalent ligands against A1-D1 receptor heteromers. *Acta Pharmacol. Sin.* 34, 441–452. doi: 10.1038/aps.2012.151

Shirahata, M., Hirasawa, S., Okumura, M., Mendoza, J. A., Okumura, A., Balbir, A., et al. (2004). Identification of M1 and M2 muscarinic acetylcholine receptors in the cat carotid body chemosensory system. *Neuroscience* 128, 635–644. doi: 10.1016/j.neuroscience.2004.06.068

Skieterska, K., Duchou, J., Lintermans, B., and Van Craenenbroeck, K. (2013). Detection of G protein-coupled receptor (GPCR) dimerization by coimmunoprecipitation. *Methods Cell Biol.* 117, 323–340. doi: 10.1016/B978-0-12-408143-7.00017-7

Stockert, J. A., and Devi, L. A. (2015). Advancements in therapeutically targeting orphan GPCRs. *Front. Pharmacol.* 6:100. doi: 10.3389/fphar.2015.00100

Stockwell, J., Chen, Z., Niazi, M., Nosib, S., and Cayabyab, F. S. (2016). Protein phosphatase role in adenosine A1 receptor-induced AMPA receptor trafficking and rat hippocampal neuronal damage in hypoxia/reperfusion injury. *Neuropharmacology* 102, 254–265. doi: 10.1016/j.neuropharm.2015.11.018

Tao, Y., Yu, C., Wang, W., Hou, Y., Xu, X., Chi, Z., et al. (2017). Heteromers of μ opioid and dopamine D1 receptors modulate opioid-induced locomotor sensitization in a dopamine-independent manner. *Br. J. Pharmacol.* 174, 2842–2861. doi: 10.1111/bph.13908

Terrillon, S., and Bouvier, M. (2004). Roles of G-protein-coupled receptor dimerization. *EMBO Rep.* 5, 30–34. doi: 10.1038/sj.embor.7400052

Thompson, C. M., Troche, K., Jordan, H. L., Barr, B. L., and Wyatt, C. N. (2010). Evidence for functional, inhibitory, histamine H3 receptors in rat carotid body type I cells. *Neurosci. Lett.* 471, 15–19. doi: 10.1016/j.neulet.2009.12.077

Tjong, Y. W., Chen, Y., Liong, E. C., Ip, S. F., Tipoe, G. L., and Fung, M. L. (2004). Melatonin attenuates rat carotid chemoreceptor response to hypercapnic acidosis. *J. Pineal Res.* 36, 49–57. doi: 10.1046/j.1600-079X.2003.00094.x

Trifilieff, P., Rives, M.-L., Urizar, E., Piskorowski, R. A., Vishwasrao, H. D., Castrillon, J., et al. (2011). Detection of antigen interactions ex vivo by proximity ligation assay: endogenous dopamine D2-adenosine A2A receptor complexes in the striatum. *Biotechniques* 51, 111–118. doi: 10.2144/000113719

Tse, A., Yan, L., Lee, A. K., and Tse, F. W. (2012). Autocrine and paracrine actions of ATP in rat carotid body. *Can. J. Physiol. Pharmacol.* 90, 705–711. doi: 10.1139/y2012-054

Tuteja, N. (2009). Signaling through G protein coupled receptors. *Plant Signal. Behav.* 4, 942–947. doi: 10.4161/psb.4.10.9530

Wakai, J., Takayama, A., Yokoyama, T., Nakamuta, N., Kusakabe, T., and Yamamoto, Y. (2015). Immunohistochemical localization of dopamine D2 receptor in the rat carotid body. *Acta Histochem.* 117, 784–789. doi: 10.1016/j.acthis.2015.07.007

Wang, D., Sun, X., Bohn, L., and Sadee, W. (2005). Opioid receptor homo-and heterodimerization in living cells by quantitative bioluminescence resonance energy transfer. *Mol. Pharmacol.* 67, 2173–2184. doi: 10.1124/mol.104.010272.cept

Wang, Z. Y., and Bisgard, G. E. (2002). Chronic hypoxia-induced morphological and neurochemical changes in the carotid body. *Microsc. Res. Tech.* 59, 168–177. doi: 10.1002/jemt.10191

Whorton, M. R., Bokoch, M. P., Rasmussen, S. G., Huang, B., Zare, R. N., Kobilka, B., et al. (2007). A monomeric G protein-coupled receptor isolated in a high-density lipoprotein particle efficiently activates its G protein. *Proc. Natl. Acad. Sci. U.S.A.* 104, 7682–7687. doi: 10.1073/pnas.0611448104

Xie, H., Hu, L., and Li, G. (2010). SH-SY5Y human neuroblastoma cell line: in vitro cell model of dopaminergic neurons in Parkinson's disease. *Chin. Med. J. (Engl).* 123, 1086–1092.

Xu, J., Tse, F. W., and Tse, A. (2003). ATP triggers intracellular Ca2+ release in type II cells of the rat carotid body. *J. Physiol.* 549, 739–747. doi: 10.1113/jphysiol.2003.039735

Xu, J., Xu, F., Tse, F. W., and Tse, A. (2005). ATP inhibits the hypoxia response in type I cells of rat carotid bodies. *J. Neurochem.* 92, 1419–1430. doi: 10.1111/j.1471-4159.2004.02978.x

Yekkirala, A. S., Kalyuzhny, A. E., and Portoghese, P. S. (2013). An immunocytochemical-derived correlate for evaluating the bridging of heteromeric mu-delta opioid protomers by bivalent ligands. *ACS Chem. Biol.* 8, 1412–1416. doi: 10.1021/cb400113d

Yokoyama, T., Nakamuta, N., Kusakabe, T., and Yamamoto, Y. (2015). Serotonin-mediated modulation of hypoxia-induced intracellular calcium responses in glomus cells isolated from rat carotid body. *Neurosci. Lett.* 597, 149–153. doi: 10.1016/j.neulet.2015.04.044

Yoshioka, K., Saitoh, O., and Nakata, H. (2001). Heteromeric association creates a P2Y-like adenosine receptor. *Proc. Natl. Acad. Sci. U.S.A.* 98, 7617–7622. doi: 10.1073/pnas.121587098

Zara, S., Pokorski, M., Cataldi, A., Porzionato, A., De Caro, R., Antosiewicz, J., et al. (2013). Development and aging are oxygen-dependent and correlate with VEGF and NOS along life span. *Adv. Exp. Med. Biol.* 756, 223–228. doi: 10.1007/978-94-007-4549-0_28

Zeng, C., Wang, Z., Asico, L. D., Hopfer, U., Eisner, G. M., Felder, R. A., et al. (2005). Aberrant ETB receptor regulation of AT_1 receptors in immortalized renal proximal tubule cells of spontaneously hypertensive rats. *Kidney Int.* 68, 623–631. doi: 10.1111/j.1523-1755.2005.00440.x

Zhang, M., Fearon, I. M., Zhong, H., and Nurse, C. A. (2003). Presynaptic modulation of rat arterial chemoreceptor function by 5-HT: role of K+ channel inhibition via protein kinase C. *J. Physiol.* 551, 825–842. doi: 10.1113/jphysiol.2002.038489

Zhang, M., Vollmer, C., and Nurse, C. A. (2017). Adenosine and dopamine oppositely modulate a hyperpolarization-activated current Ih in chemosensory neurons of the rat carotid body in co-culture. *J. Physiol.* doi: 10.1113/JP274743 [Epub ahead of print].

Zhong, H., and Nurse, C. (1995). Basic fibroblast growth factor regulates ionic currents and excitability of fetal rat carotid body chemoreceptors. *Neurosci. Lett.* 202, 41–44. doi: 10.1016/0304-3940(95)12200-1

Zidar, D. A., Violin, J. D., Whalen, E. J., and Lefkowitz, R. J. (2009). Selective engagement of G protein coupled receptor kinases (GRKs) encodes distinct functions of biased ligands. *Proc. Natl. Acad. Sci. U.S.A.* 106, 9649–9654. doi: 10.1073/pnas.0904361106

9

Long-Term Chronic Intermittent Hypobaric Hypoxia Induces Glucose Transporter (GLUT4) Translocation Through AMP-Activated Protein Kinase (AMPK) in the Soleus Muscle in Lean Rats

Patricia Siques[1]*, Julio Brito[1], Karen Flores[1], Stefany Ordenes[1], Karem Arriaza[1], Eduardo Pena[1], Fabiola León-Velarde[2], Ángel L. López de Pablo[3], M. C. Gonzalez[3] and Silvia Arribas[3]

[1] Institute of Health Studies, University Arturo Prat, Iquique, Chile, [2] Department of Biological and Physiological Sciences, Facultad de Ciencias y Filosofía/IIA, Cayetano Heredia University, Lima, Peru, [3] Department of Physiology, Faculty of Medicine, University Autonoma of Madrid, Madrid, Spain

****Correspondence:***
Patricia Siques
psiques@tie.cl

Background: In chronic hypoxia (CH) and short-term chronic intermittent hypoxia (CIH) exposure, glycemia and insulin levels decrease and insulin sensitivity increases, which can be explained by changes in glucose transport at skeletal muscles involving GLUT1, GLUT4, Akt, and AMPK, as well as GLUT4 translocation to cell membranes. However, during long-term CIH, there is no information regarding whether these changes occur similarly or differently than in other types of hypoxia exposure. This study evaluated the levels of AMPK and Akt and the location of GLUT4 in the soleus muscles of lean rats exposed to long-term CIH, CH, and normoxia (NX) and compared the findings.

Methods: Thirty male adult rats were randomly assigned to three groups: a NX (760 Torr) group (n = 10), a CIH group (2 days hypoxia/2 days NX; n = 10) and a CH group (n = 10). Rats were exposed to hypoxia for 30 days in a hypobaric chamber set at 428 Torr (4,600 m). Feeding (10 g daily) and fasting times were accurately controlled. Measurements included food intake (every 4 days), weight, hematocrit, hemoglobin, glycemia, serum insulin (by ELISA), and insulin sensitivity at days 0 and 30. GLUT1, GLUT4, AMPK levels and Akt activation in rat soleus muscles were determined by western blot. GLUT4 translocation was measured with confocal microscopy at day 30.

Results: (1) Weight loss and increases in hematocrit and hemoglobin were found in both hypoxic groups ($p < 0.05$). (2) A moderate decrease in glycemia and plasma insulin was found. (3) Insulin sensitivity was greater in the CIH group ($p < 0.05$). (4) There were no changes in GLUT1, GLUT4 levels or in Akt activation. (5) The level of activated AMPK was increased only in the CIH group ($p < 0.05$). (6) Increased GLUT4 translocation to the plasma membrane of soleus muscle cells was observed in the CIH group ($p < 0.05$).

Conclusion: In lean rats experiencing long-term CIH, glycemia and insulin levels decrease and insulin sensitivity increases. Interestingly, there is no increase of GLUT1 or GLUT4 levels or in Akt activation. Therefore, cellular regulation of glucose seems to primarily involve GLUT4 translocation to the cell membrane in response to hypoxia-mediated AMPK activation.

Keywords: altitude, chronic intermittent hypoxia, insulin sensitivity, GLUT4, AMPK and Akt

INTRODUCTION

Glucose metabolism has been suggested to be improved under different types of hypoxic conditions. In fact, several studies have shown that under chronic hypoxia (CH) and short-term chronic intermittent hypoxia (CIH), glycemia and insulin levels decrease and insulin sensitivity increases in humans (Woolcott et al., 2015) and murine models (Chiu et al., 2004; Chen et al., 2010; Gamboa et al., 2011). However, the changes in long-term CIH have rarely been studied. The definitions of short- and long-term CIH vary. Short-term CIH includes minutes or hours of hypoxia during a brief period, while long-term CIH includes several days of hypoxia over a longer period of time (Siques et al., 2006).

Hypoxia exposure induces an adaptation process to replenish ATP in the cells that generate changes in glucose metabolism (Xia et al., 1997; Gamboa et al., 2011). There are several mechanisms involved in glucose regulation under hypoxic conditions, with the most important role played by glucose transporters (GLUTs) (Chiu et al., 2004; Castrejón et al., 2007; Manolescu et al., 2007). Cellular glucose uptake is mainly accomplished via facilitated transport mediated by a family of GLUTs: GLUT1 is responsible for basal glucose uptake, and GLUT4 is an insulin-regulated GLUT; both transporters are present in skeletal muscles (Scheepers et al., 2004). Insulin and energetic stress increase GLUT4 membrane translocation in skeletal muscles by different signaling mechanisms. Each stimulus, alone and in combination, results in the translocation of intracellular GLUT4 from vesicles to the cell membrane (Thong et al., 2005; Mackenzie and Watt, 2016). One of the mechanisms involved is the insulin pathway, which activates the PI3K/Akt pathway, acting as a metabolic sensor that responds to insulin stimulation and incorporates GLUT4 into the plasma membrane (Kohn et al., 1996). However, under stressful conditions, such as exercise or hypoxia, glucose transport in skeletal muscles occurs via the insulin-independent AMP-activated protein kinase (AMPK) pathway (Hayashi et al., 2000).

Under hypoxic conditions, the AMPK pathway participates in skeletal muscle glucose uptake. When intracellular ATP levels decrease, AMPK switches off ATP-consuming pathways and switches on alternative pathways for ATP regeneration, altering the AMP/ATP ratio (Hayashi et al., 2000; Carling, 2004). It appears that under hypoxic conditions, AMPK can increase glucose transport into muscle cells but also increases the rate of fat utilization by muscles (Fisher, 2006). In contrast, in mice with CH exposure, the Akt and AMPK pathways are not activated, and GLUT4 levels are unchanged (Gamboa et al., 2011). Studies in murine models under short-term CIH have shown an increase in AMPK and GLUT4 levels in skeletal muscles, though these results are controversial (Chiu et al., 2004; Li et al., 2015; Wang et al., 2015).

To our knowledge, information about the AMPK pathway and GLUT4 translocation under long-term CIH in rats is scarce. This new exposure model involves days at hypobaric hypoxia followed by days at normoxia (sea level) over a long period of time. Therefore, many pathophysiological aspects of this condition remain poorly understood or controversial, such as glucose homeostasis.

It is hypothesized that in lean rats exposed to this model of hypoxia (long-term CIH), which combines normoxic and hypoxic periods, the pathways involved in GLUT4 translocation in the soleus muscle are activated resulting in changes in glucose and insulin levels. Thus, an experimental study was designed to evaluate differences in the levels of AMPK, Akt and GLUT4 and the cellular location of GLUT4 in soleus muscles of lean rats exposed to long-term CIH compared to those in CH and normoxia (NX) rats.

MATERIALS AND METHODS

Experimental Model and Study Groups

In this study, 30 male adult Wistar rats (3 months old; body weight 251.6 ± 1.9 g) were obtained from the animal facility of the Institute of Health Studies of Arturo Prat University, Iquique, Chile. The rats were placed in individual cages at a temperature of 22 ± 2°C and a circadian rhythm of 12 h of light and 12 h of dark. Feeding consisted of 10 g/day of food that contained 22.0% crude protein, 5.0% crude fat, 5.0% crude fiber, 9.0% ash, and 12% moisture (5POO®, LabDiet ®, Prolab RMH3000) and water *ad libitum*. Food intake was measured every 4 days by determining the amount of residual food. Movement inside the cage was not restricted, but no exercise was performed.

The rats were randomly distributed into three experimental groups, as follows: normobaric normoxia (NX), which served as a sea level control (n = 10); chronic intermittent hypobaric hypoxia (CIH), with 2 days of exposure to hypobaric hypoxia alternating with 2 days of exposure to NX (n = 10); and chronic hypobaric hypoxia (CH), which involved permanent exposure to hypoxia (n = 10). The exposure time of each group was 30 days, and the hypobaric hypoxia was simulated in a chamber at 428 Torr, which is equivalent to an altitude of 4,600 m above sea level. Chamber conditions were as follows: internal flow of 3.14 L/min of air and humidity between 21 and 30%. The time of ascension from sea level to 428 Torr was 60 min. NX rats were located in the same room at sea level (760 Torr) and housed under the same chamber conditions as the groups exposed to hypoxia. At the end of the exposure period (day 30), the rats were euthanized with an overdose of ketamine (0.9 mg/kg of weight), organs were collected, and specific variables were measured. These experiments were performed at Arturo Prat University.

The animal protocol and experimental model were in accordance with Chilean law N° 20380 regarding animal experimentation and were approved by the Research Ethics Committee of Arturo Prat University, Iquique, Chile.

Body Weight, Glucose and Insulin Measurements

Blood extraction (1 mL) for biochemical measurements was performed after 12 h of fasting via cardiac puncture under anesthesia (0.3 mg/kg body weight). Both biochemical and physiological parameters in all the study groups were performed at day 0 (under basal normoxic conditions) and after 30 days (immediately after descending from the chamber). The hematocrit (Hct) and hemoglobin (Hb) values were measured. Serum insulin was measured using a commercial kit (Rat Insulin ELISA Kit®, ALPCO, Salem, VT, United States), and glucose was measured using a glucometer (CarenSensN®). The HOMA2 model was used to calculate the sensitivity (HOMA2%S) index with the HOMA2 calculator version 2.2 (Diabetes Trial Unit, University of Oxford), and body weight and residual food were measured every 4 days using an electronic scale (Acculab V-1200®, IL, United States).

Western Blot Analysis

In this study, 100 mg of skeletal muscle was obtained from each rat. Protein extraction was started by tissue homogenization (Stir-Pak®, Barrington, IL, United States) with 1 mL RIPA lysis buffer, which contains a cocktail of phosphatase and protease inhibitors (4 mM PMSF, 10 μM leupeptin, 1 mM EDTA, 1 mM EGTA, 20 mM NaF, 20 mM HEPES, and 1 mM DTT). Then, the homogenates were centrifuged (5804 R Eppendorf AG®, Hamburg, Germany) at 12,000 rpm for 20 min at 4°C, and the supernatant was extracted. For quantification of the total protein extracted, the Bradford reaction was used (Bradford, 1976) with a BioPhotometer (Eppendorf AG®, Hamburg, Germany) at 590 nm, and samples were then stored at −80°C. For western blotting, the samples were previously diluted with Laemmli 2X [0.125 M Tris-HCl, 4% SDS (p/v), 20% glycerol (v/v), 0.004% bromophenol blue, 10% β-mercaptoethanol (pH 6.8)]. The proteins were separated according to their molecular weight (MW) under an electric field via sodium dodecyl sulfate-polyacrylamide gel electrophoresis (SDS-PAGE) (30% bis-acrylamide (v/v), 150 mM Tris (pH 6.8 and 8.8), 1.0% TEMED (w/v), H_2O). Electrophoretic separation was initiated with the application of direct current to 150 V over 80 min with a power supply (PolySience®, EPS-300, Taipei, Taiwan, China), and the proteins were then transferred from the SDS-PAGE gel to a polyvinylidene fluoride (PVDF) membrane at 180 mA for 90 min with a semi-dry electroblotting system (OWLTM Separation systems, Panther semi-dry Electroblotters, Thomas Scientific®, Barrington, IL, United States).

To avoid non-specific antibody binding, the membrane was blocked with bovine serum albumin (BSA) at a concentration range of 3–5% in TBS-T solution containing 10 mM HCl, 150 mM NaCl, 0.05% Tween-20 at pH 7.4. The blocking time was 1 h at room temperature.

Once the PVDF membrane was blocked, it was incubated with the corresponding primary antibody [GLUT4 (sc-1608), GLUT1 (sc-7903) AMPKα1/2 (sc-25792), p-AMPKα1/2 (sc-101630), Akt1/2/3 (sc-8312), p-Akt1/2/3 (sc-33437), and β-actin (sc-130657)] at a dilution of 1:500 (Santa Cruz Biotechnology®, CA, United States) and incubated overnight at 4°C. Finally, the membrane was incubated with secondary antibodies (anti-goat and anti-rabbit antibodies, Santa Cruz Biotechnology®, CA, United States) at a dilution 1:2000 in 3% BSA for 1 h at room temperature and then washed with TBS-T and imaged in a dark room with a chemiluminescence kit (Chemiluminescence West Pico®, Super Signal Substrate, Thermo Scientific®, Rockford, IL, United States). The density of the bands was measured with ImageJ and normalized according to β-actin expression.

Confocal Microscopy

The presence of GLUT4 in the plasma membrane of soleus muscle cells was determined by immunofluorescence using confocal microscopy. After euthanasia, the soleus muscle was detached completely and immersed in 4% paraformaldehyde and embedded in paraffin. Muscles were cut transversally in relation to the direction of the muscle fibers. Slices (3 μm thick) were deparaffinized and then hydrated by incubating them in xylene three times for 5 min and in 100% ethanol and then 95% two times for 10 min. Subsequently, the sections were washed with distilled water two times for 5 min. Antigens were unmasked with citrate in a pascal pot at 95°C for 20 min and then incubated in a permeabilization buffer (0.4% TRITON X-100 in PBS) for 30 min. Then, the sections were blocked with 5% BSA and incubated in 0.4% TRITON X-100 in PBS for 1.5 h. For the detection of GLUT4, the secondary antibody Alexa Fluor® 647 (A-21244) was used, and the nuclei were labeled with 4,6-diamidino-2-phenylindole (DAPI). The plasma membrane was labeled with WGA (L4895, SIGMA®, San Luis, MO, United States). The samples were visualized in a mounting medium (Citifluor, Aname, Spain) with a Leica TCS SP2 confocal system (Leica® Microsystems, Wetzlar, Germany) at University Autonoma of Madrid, Spain, using an emission wavelength of 405 nm for DAPI and an emission wavelength of 633 nm for Alexa Fluor® 647 and 488 nm for WGA. Serial images were 1 μm thick (12 μm in total) and were captured with a 63x objective at a zoom factor of 1–4 in randomly chosen areas under identical conditions of brightness, contrast, and laser power for all of the experimental groups. MetaMorph® image analysis software (Universal Imaging Co., United Kingdom) was used for quantification of the total number of cells and the intensity of GLUT4 fluorescence, which was used to calculate the amount of GLUT4 present in the plasma membrane by subtracting the total intensity of the cells from the intensity of the cytoplasm.

Data Analysis

All data recorded were included into a database and analyzed using the SPSS program (IBM SPSS® V.21.0®, Armonk, NY, United States). The normality of the variables was established by the Kolmogorov-Smirnov test, and all variables had a normal distribution. The means, standard errors (SEs) and confidence intervals (CIs) were calculated for all variables. To determine differences in the measured variables over time, in each group, a paired-sample Student's T test was performed. To assess the magnitude of change in variables, between days 30 and 0, the means difference and 95% CIs were calculated for each variable. After obtaining these values the means differences between groups were also calculated using paired and independent sample Student's T test, respectively. Equal variances were assumed according to F value. To establish the inter-group differences, one-way analysis of variance (ANOVA) with the least significant difference (LSD) *post hoc* test was performed. The level of significance was established at the 95% confidence level, with $p < 0.05$ being considered significant.

RESULTS

General Variables

At day 30 under both hypoxic conditions (CIH and CH) rats showed an increase in Hct ($p < 0.001$) compared to the NX group, with a higher value in the CH group ($p < 0.01$) than in the CIH group. Likewise, Hb was increased in both hypoxic conditions, with the CH group showing a non-significant trend toward higher levels than in the CIH group. Body weight was lower in both hypoxia-exposed groups (CIH and CH), without a difference between these two groups. It is important to note that food intake was 100% in the CH and NX groups, whereas in the CIH group, 60% of the rats ate only 70% of the food inside the chamber during periods of hypoxia, although during periods of NX, food intake was normal in the CIH group (**Table 1**). Means difference for day 30–0 between groups: for hematocrit NX vs CIH: −18.26 (−24.33, −12.18) and body weight NX vs CIH: −24.75 (−36.03, −13.46) were found.

Glycemia, Insulin and HOMA2%S

Both hypoxia-exposed groups (CIH and CH) exhibited a decrease in blood glucose levels at day 30 and CH showed levels lower than those in the CIH group ($p < 0.05$). There was a decrease in serum insulin levels under both hypoxic conditions, but unexpectedly, the level of insulin was lower in the CIH group than in the CH group ($p < 0.05$). The insulin sensitivity index (HOMA2%S) increased more in the CIH group than in the NX and CH groups ($p < 0.05$), and the difference was proportional to the insulin level (**Figure 1**).

Protein Measurements: GLUTs, AMPK and Akt

The protein expression of GLUT1 and 4 was not different among groups (**Figures 2A–C**). AMPK activation, measured as the p-AMPK/total AMPK ratio, surprisingly, showed an

TABLE 1 | General characteristics.

	NX	CIH	CH	CH vs CIH means difference
Hematocrit(%)				
Day 0	45.56 ± 1.17	44.54 ± 2.48	43.04 ± 1.40	
Day 30	46.30 ± 1.72	63.54 ± 1.16*#†	70.58 ± 0.69*#	
Mean difference 30–0	0.74 (−3.25, 4.73)	19.0 (13.81, 24.18)	27.54 (23.50, 31.57)	8.54 (2.43, 14.64)
Hemoglobin(mg/dL)				
Day 0	14.18 ± 0.30	14.36 ± 0.30	14.5 ± 0.19	
Day 30	15.37 ± 0.70	19.77 ± 0.59*#	20.64 ± 0.36*#	
Means difference 30–0	1.19 (−0.76, 3.14)	5.41 (3.90, 6.91)	6.14 (5.04, 7.23)	1.04 (−0.92, 3.00)
Body weight (g)				
Day 0	251.80 ± 1.9	251.09 ± 2.8	251.50 ± 1.1	
Day 30	260.80 ± 3.8	235.40 ± 5.8*#	233.10 ± 2.9*#	
Means difference 30–0	9.08 (2.74, 15.41)	−15.67 (−26.03, −5.30)	−18.37 (−25.19, −11.54)	−2.70 (−14.22, 8.82)
Food intake (g)				
Day 0	10.0 ± 0.0	10.0 ± 0.0	10.0 ± 0.0	
Day 30	10.0 ± 0.0	7.8 ± 0.79*#†	10.0 ± 0.0	
Means difference 30–0	-	−2.15 (−3.94, −0.35)	-	2.15 (0.48, 3.81)

*Variables measured in the normoxic group (NX; n = 10), chronic intermittent hypoxia group (CIH; n = 10), and chronic hypoxia group (CH; n = 10). Values are means ($\bar{X}$) ± standard error (SEs) for hematocrit, hemoglobin, body weight and food intake; measured at day 0 and 30. *p < 0.001: hypoxia-exposed group vs NX; †p < 0.01: CIH vs CH; #p < 0.001: day 0 vs day 30. Means difference and confidence intervals (95% CI) between days 30 and 0 for each variable are shown. Means difference and confidence intervals (95% CI) of these changes between groups CH vs. CIH (days 30 to 0) are also presented.*

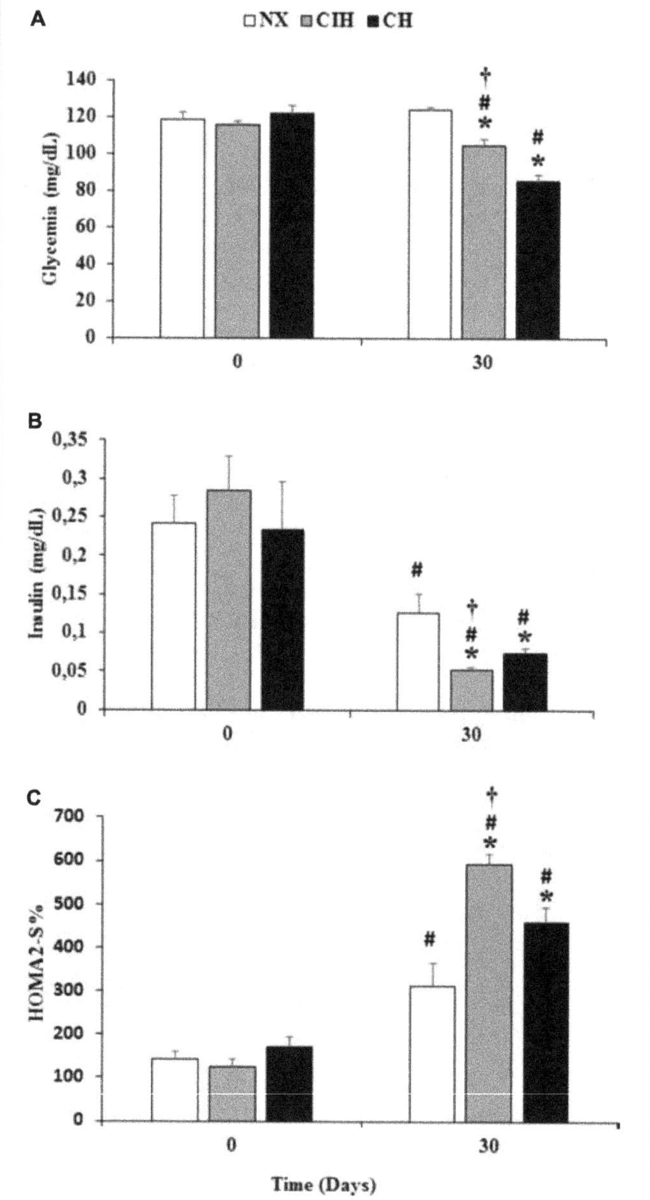

FIGURE 1 | Biochemical variables. Measured in the normoxic group (NX; $n = 10$), chronic intermittent hypoxia group (CIH; $n = 10$), and chronic hypoxia group (CH; $n = 10$). Comparisons of **(A)** glycemia, **(B)** insulin level and **(C)** homeostatic model assessment 2 values (HOMA2%S) at day 0 and 30. Values are means ($\bar{X}$) ± standard error (SE). $^*p < 0.001$: hypoxia-exposed group vs. NX; $^\dagger p < 0.05$: CIH vs. CH; $^\# p < 0.001$: day 0 vs. day 30.

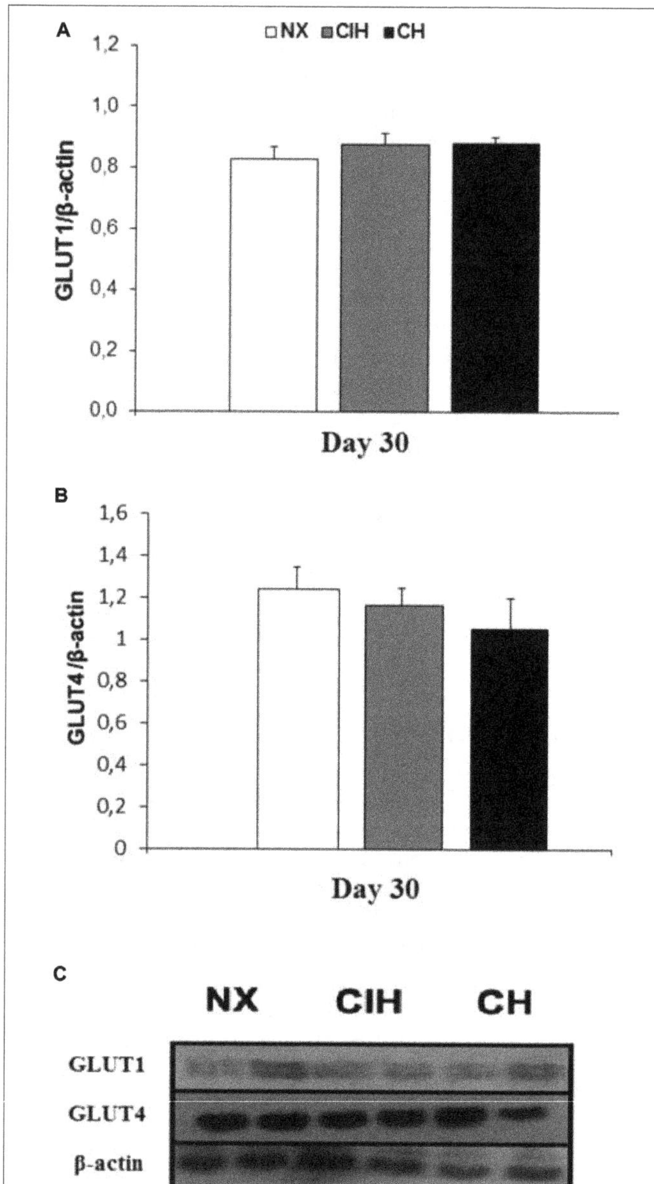

FIGURE 2 | Proteins expressions levels of glucose transporters. GLUT1 and GLUT4 protein levels in soleus muscles of lean rats in the normoxic group (NX; $n = 10$), chronic intermittent hypoxia group (CIH; $n = 10$), and chronic hypoxia group (CH; $n = 10$). **(A)** GLUT1 protein levels, normalized by β-actin; **(B)** GLUT4 protein levels, normalized by β-actin; and **(C)** representative bands for GLUT1, GLUT4 and β-actin. Values in **(A)** and **(B)** are means ($\bar{X}$) ± standard errors (SEs).

increase in the CIH group ($p < 0.05$), whereas the CH and NX groups showed no differences (**Figures 3A,C**). Conversely, Akt activation, measured as the p-Akt/total Akt ratio, showed no difference among the studied groups (**Figures 3B,C**).

GLUT4 Translocation

It is worth noting that the results showed a remarkable increase in the translocation of GLUT4 from vesicles to the plasma membrane in rat soleus muscles only in the CIH group ($p < 0.05$) (**Figure 4A**). These differences are also shown in representative images (**Figure 4B**).

DISCUSSION

This research in lean rats exposed to long-term CIH showed the following with respect to the CH and NX groups: (1) different patterns in glucose regulation, (2) lower blood glucose and

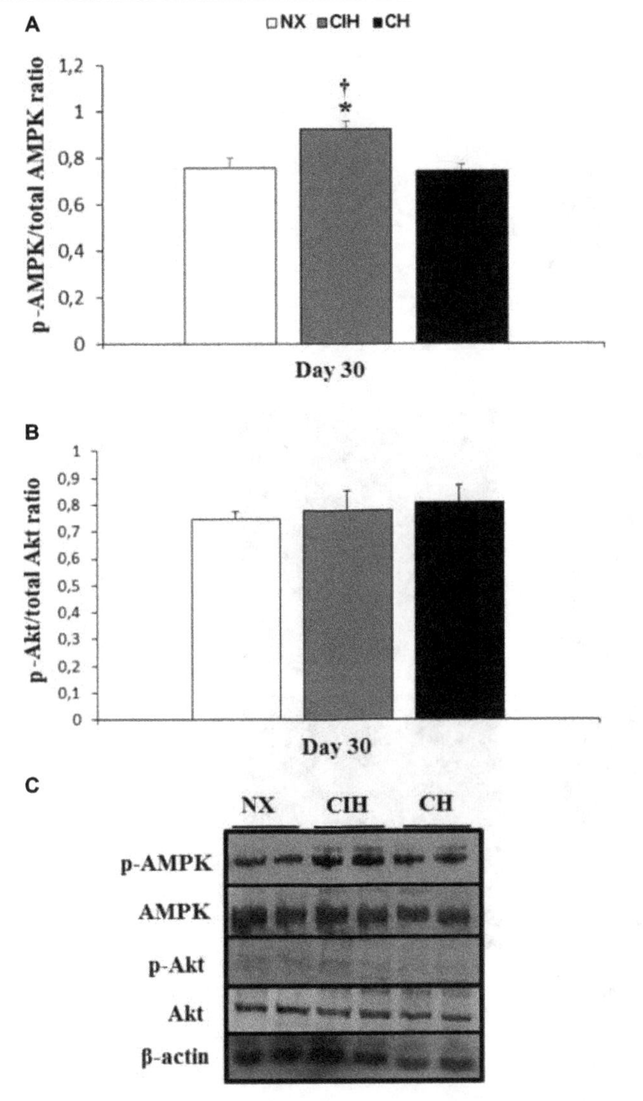

FIGURE 3 | Activation of AMPK and Akt. Measured in the soleus muscles of lean rats in the normoxic group (NX; $n = 10$), chronic intermittent hypoxia group (CIH; $n = 10$), and chronic hypoxia group (CH; $n = 10$). **(A)** Comparison of p-AMPK/total AMPK ratio, normalized by β-actin; **(B)** comparison of p-Akt/total Akt ratio, normalized by β-actin; and **(C)** representative bands for activated AMPK (p-AMPK), total AMPK, activated Akt (p-Akt), total Akt and β-actin. Values in **(A)** and **(B)** are means ($\bar{X}$) ± standard errors (SEs).*$p < 0.05$: hypoxia-exposed group vs. NX; †$p < 0.05$: CIH vs. CH.

plasma insulin levels and an increase in insulin sensitivity, (3) hypoxia-induced AMPK pathway activation, but not insulin-dependent Akt pathway activation and (4) an increase in GLUT4 translocation to plasma membranes in rat soleus muscle cells.

General Findings

As expected in this model, Hb and Hct increased in the CIH group but to a lesser extent than in the CH group. These results are in agreement with those of other studies using this model, both in humans (Richalet et al., 2002) and rats (Siques et al., 2006; Brito et al., 2015). The body weight decreases observed in this study are also in agreement with previous reports in rats (Siques et al., 2006; Lüneburg et al., 2016). This latter effect could have ancillary influences on glucose metabolism, since body weight is highly correlated with insulin sensitivity (Evans et al., 1984). Nevertheless, high-altitude-induced CH leads to an inexorable loss of skeletal muscle mass as a consequence of an increase in protein degradation, which could explain the weight loss observed in this study (Chaudhary et al., 2012). Under CIH, this loss could also be attributed to a loss of appetite in rats (Bigard et al., 1996), as rats left some food uneaten during hypoxia exposure in the current study. Therefore, both mechanisms could contribute to the effect.

Blood Glucose and Serum Insulin Levels

Previous altitude-based studies have shown that glucose homeostasis is influenced by acute or CH exposure in humans (Brooks et al., 1991; Kelly et al., 2010) and by CH exposure in mice (Gamboa et al., 2011). The current study shows that under long-term CIH, rats show improved glucose uptake, lower fasting glucose and insulin levels and increased insulin sensitivity, which also would occur under other types of hypoxia. Thus, the same phenomena have been shown in rats under short-term CIH, normobaric hypoxia and hypoxic regimen lasting hours (Chiu et al., 2004; Chen et al., 2011; Faramoushi et al., 2016), excluding obstructive sleep apnea syndrome studied in humans (Kim et al., 2013) and mice (Thomas et al., 2017). Although, controversially, some reports show no changes in glucose metabolism in rats exposed to CIH (Wang et al., 2015; Li et al., 2016). Likewise, exposure to cyclic hypobaric hypoxia in humans for 10 weeks demonstrated a decrease in glucose but no influence on insulin (Marquez et al., 2013). When drawing conclusions and making comparisons from some of the differences found in the literature regarding these effects, it must be considered that the regimen and the degree of hypoxia will lead to variation in the results (Debevec and Millet, 1985); however, most of these studies tend to agree in showing that under hypoxia, glucose regulation is improved in both rats and humans (Sawhney et al., 1986; Larsen et al., 1997; Woolcott et al., 2015; Sacramento et al., 2016). Moreover, this glucose improvement under different regimens of hypoxia would take some time and reach a plateau in the long term, resulting in rather normal value as observed in human studies (Woolcott et al., 2015; Żebrowska et al., 2018) and in rats (Chen et al., 2016). Therefore, the improved glucose regulation in rats under long-term CIH in this study supports the contribution of hypoxia to these phenomena and, to our knowledge, has not been previously reported.

GLUT, AMPK and Akt in Soleus Muscle

Skeletal muscle is the most important regulator of glucose homeostasis and uptake (Mas et al., 2006; Gamboa et al., 2011). Glucose uptake in skeletal muscle is normally regulated by insulin-related pathways, where Akt can play a role as an insulin-stimulated signal leading to GLUT4 translocation to the cell membrane under physiological conditions (Huang and Czech, 2007). However, under exercise- and hypoxia-induced stress, the AMP/ATP ratio is increased, activating an alternative pathway: insulin-independent AMPK signaling (Hayashi et al., 2000).

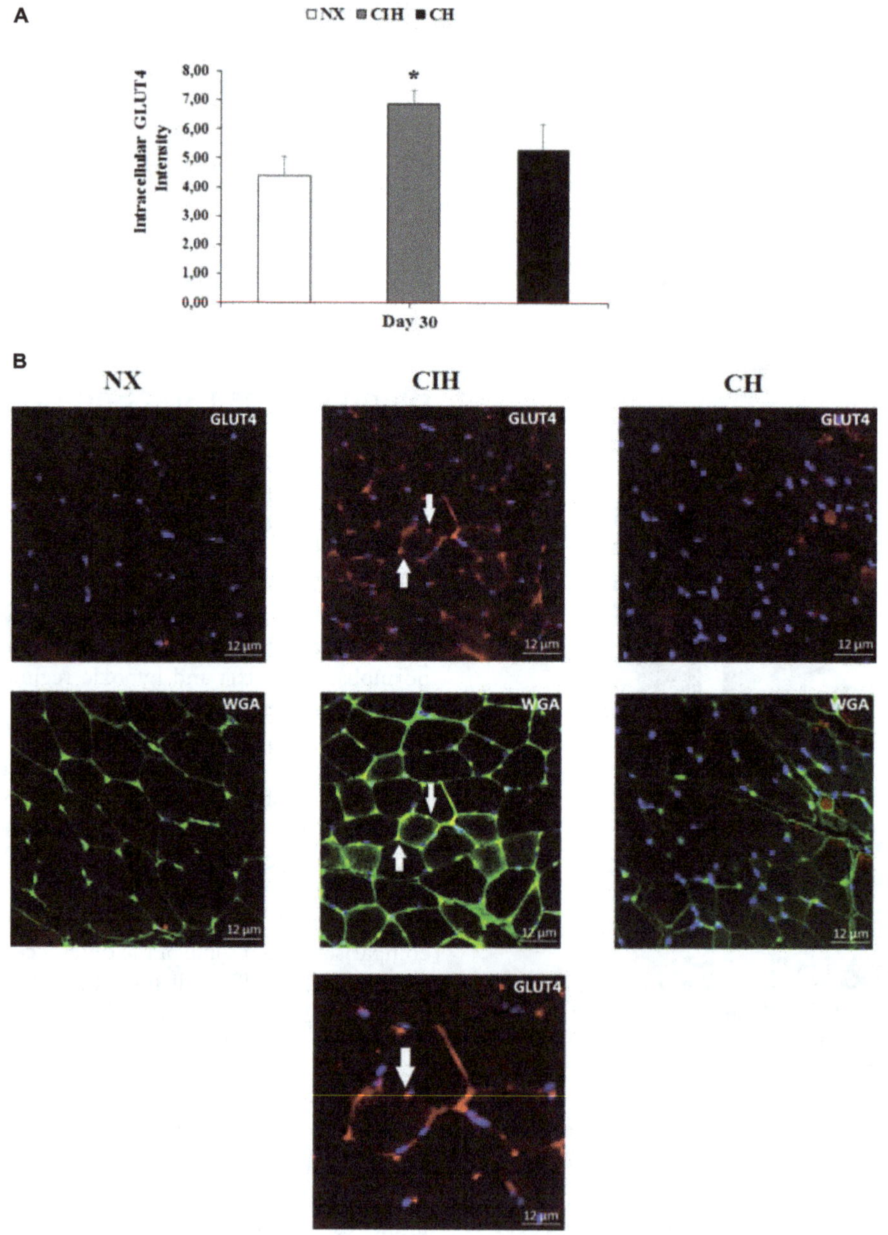

FIGURE 4 | Comparison of GLUT4 location. Measured in the normoxic group (NX; $n = 10$), chronic intermittent hypoxia group (CIH; $n = 10$), and chronic hypoxia group (CH; $n = 10$). **(A)** Quantitative analysis of the intensity of GLUT4 in soleus muscles from all groups and **(B)** representative examples GLUT4 measurements obtained by confocal microscopy (x63, zoom 1). Values in **(A)** are means ($\bar{X}$) ± standard errors (SEs). *$p < 0.05$: hypoxia-exposed group vs NX. White arrow indicates GLUT4 localized in the plasma membrane of muscle. DAPI staining (first row); WGA staining (second row) and an amplified CIH cell at the third row (x63, zoom 2).

It is well known that skeletal muscle has two main GLUT transporters: the constitutive GLUT1 and the insulin-dependent GLUT4, with the latter being the most relevant. In acute exposure to hypoxia GLUT4 levels increase in rats (Dill et al., 2001), and obese rats (Zucker) under short-term CIH and in response to altitude training showed increased GLUT4 levels (Chen et al., 2011), whereas under CH, no increase in GLUT4 occurs in rats and mice (Chiu et al., 2004; Gamboa et al., 2011). According to our results from long-term CIH exposure, both GLUT1 and GLUT4 levels showed no changes, similarly to what has been reported under CH. However, there was an increase in intracellular translocation of GLUT4 to the membrane. This trafficking could be considered as a compensatory mechanism to increase glucose uptake instead the increasing protein levels (Chen et al., 2008; Jørgensen et al., 2009; Gamboa et al., 2011). Interestingly, this translocation has not been previously reported in a long-term CIH model.

Additionally, Gamboa et al. (2011) found that in normobaric CH (during fasting), no activation of the Akt pathway occurs, which is consistent with the results of this study. Likewise, controversial findings indicating that chronic stress induced by reactive oxygen species (ROS) can also decrease the stimulatory effect of insulin on the Akt pathway and that glucose uptake could be mediated by the intrinsic activity of GLUT4 under hypoxic conditions have been reported (Ding et al., 2016). A role for ROS in the effect of insulin under hypoxia is a promising theory because high levels of ROS have been consistently found in humans with both acute and chronic exposure to hypobaric hypoxia (Jefferson et al., 2004) and in rats exposed to long-term CIH (Siques et al., 2014; Lüneburg et al., 2016).

The increase in GLUT4 translocation seen in this study could be explained on the basis of other pathways involved in the regulation of plasma glucose levels under energetic stress, including the AMPK pathway, as previously reported (Bradley et al., 2015). Activated AMPK acts downstream by phosphorylating and activating AS160 (Akt substrate 160), which is the main regulatory protein of the trafficking of intracellular GLUT4 (Kramer et al., 2006). It has also been shown that activated AMPK can increase the sensitivity to insulin in rats (Fisher et al., 2002). Our results support a role of AMPK but not of Akt, as the activation of AMPK was found to be increased under long-term CIH. Moreover, recent studies suggest that higher levels of insulin downregulate AMPK activity via Ser485/491 phosphorylation of the AMPK-α subunit. In this case, a lower blood insulin concentration might induce AMPK signal activation in rats (Kido et al., 2017), which would be another way of increasing AMPK activation; however, this idea needs further experimental support.

It has been observed that AMPK is activated in mice exposed to acute hypoxia (Viganò et al., 2011). This could explain the greater level of activated AMPK under CIH than under CH because, as described previously, this model involves intermittent and acute episodes of hypoxia, which results in a turn-on–turn-off regime for biological responses (Powell and Garcia, 2000). In this context, under CIH and during hypoxic training in humans, HIF-1α has been observed to be upregulated (Hoppeler and Vogt, 2001), and HIF-1α accumulation has been reported in muscle cell culture (Kubis et al., 2005). Moreover, HIF-1α could have a critical role in maintaining the GLUT4 transporter translocation in skeletal muscle cells (Sakagami et al., 2014). Since AMPK activation is consistent with the increased translocation of GLUT4 observed in this study, it could be surmised that this effect in the soleus muscle is mediated via upregulation of p-AMPK and that p-Akt does not play a role under the conditions studied here. Thus, the increases in translocation of GLUT4 to the cell membrane and AMPK activation in long-term CIH are novel findings.

Interestingly, age could play a role in GLUT regulation. Xia et al. (1997) showed that adult rats under CH exposure show slight increases in GLUT protein expression, whereas immature rats show great increases because immature tissues are more sensitive to oxygen deprivation. This latter report is almost coincident with our results regarding scarce or no GLUT4 protein increase in adult rats, although the current study is in CIH. Thus, this current study might give support to the hypothesis that in adult rats, GLUT regulation would occur not at the protein level but by GLUT translocation, resulting in increased glucose utilization.

This study in lean rats suggests that long-term CIH might have a beneficial effect in improving insulin sensitivity and glucose tolerance as has been suggested for rats exposed to short-term CIH lasting hours (Tian et al., 2016). However, several considerations must be taken into account: the hypoxia regimen and exposure duration (Xia et al., 1997); the existence of several confounding factors such as vitamin D, pollution, ozone, and diet (Woolcott et al., 2015); the differences in response to hypoxia among rat's strain where Wistar is more intolerant to altitude (Ou and Smith, 1983; Hayward et al., 1999); and whether results from animal models can be fully extrapolated to clinical settings. Additionally, it is important to contrast the present findings with those from another model of CIH, i.e., obstructive sleep apnea syndrome, where the opposite metabolic patterns occur (Kim et al., 2013; Thomas et al., 2017).

This study has some limitations, such as the use of a very specific experimental animal model (lab rats with long-term CIH) that is more sensitive to hypoxia than human beings and with strict diet and environmental control, which increases the difficulty of comparing different CIH regimens and could prevent a direct translation of these findings into clinical or occupational health. However, this rat species was chosen, due to its known hypoxic intolerance, to assess the maximal effects of hypoxia and to perform preliminary molecular studies that would face ethical and logistic difficulties in humans. Another limitation is the difficulty of comparison given the wide variety of regimes, species, models, and the scarce reports on long-term CIH. However, this latter issue makes our results novel. Therefore, this study may contribute to the understanding of glucose metabolism in long-term CIH, which is poorly understood, and may provide directions for future research in animals and humans.

CONCLUSIONS

Lean rats exposed to long-term CIH show a decrease in glycemia and insulin, along with an increase in insulin sensitivity compared to normoxic exposure. Interestingly, there is no increase in the levels of glucose transporter proteins GLUT1 or GLUT4 nor in the level of activated Akt. Therefore, glucose cell regulation and the relative hypoglycemia observed seem to be primarily a result of increased GLUT4 translocation to the cell membrane elicited by hypoxia-mediated AMPK activation.

AUTHOR CONTRIBUTIONS

PS, JB, KF, and SO conceived and designed the study, performed the experiments, analyzed and interpreted the data, drafted the manuscript, critically revised important intellectual content in the manuscript, and provided overall supervision. FL-V assisted in critical decisions and revision. KA, EP, FL-V, ÁLdP, MG, and SA contributed to the interpretation of the results and critical revisions of the manuscript. All authors approved the final manuscripts and agreed to be accountable for all aspects of the work.

FUNDING

This study was supported by grants from projects GORE FIC-Tarapaca BIP30434827-0 and FIC-Tarapaca BIP30477541-0.

ACKNOWLEDGMENTS

We would like to thanks to Pilar Rodriguez and Gabriela Lamas for their technical assistance in the laboratory.

REFERENCES

Bigard, A. X., Douce, P., Merino, D., Lienhard, F., and Guezennec, C. Y. (1996). Changes in dietary protein intake fail to prevent decrease in muscle growth induced by severe hypoxia in rats. *J. Appl. Physiol.* 80, 208–215. doi: 10.1152/jappl.1996.80.1.208

Bradford, M. (1976). A rapid and sensitive method for the quantitation of microgram quantities of protein utilizing the principle of protein-dye binding. *Anal. Biochem.* 72, 248–254. doi: 10.1016/0003-2697(76)90527-3

Bradley, H., Shaw, C. S., Bendtsen, C., Worthington, P. L., Wilson, O. J., Strauss, J. A., et al. (2015). Visualization and quantitation of GLUT4 translocation in human skeletal muscle following glucose ingestion and exercise. *Physiol. Rep.* 3:e12375. doi: 10.14814/phy2.12375

Brito, J., Siques, P., Arribas, S. M., López de Pablo, A., González, M. C., Naveas, N., et al. (2015). Adventitial alterations are the main features in pulmonary artery remodeling due to long-term chronic intermittent hypobaric hypoxia in rats. *Biomed. Res. Int.* 2015:169841. doi: 10.1155/2015/169841

Brooks, G. A., Butterfield, G. E., Wolfe, R. R., Groves, B. M., Mazzeo, R. S., Sutton, J. R., et al. (1991). Increased dependence on blood glucose after acclimatization to 4,300 m. *J. Appl. Physiol.* 70, 919–927. doi: 10.1152/jappl.1991.70.2.919

Carling, D. (2004). The AMP-activated protein kinase cascade – a unifying system for energy control. *Trends Biochem. Sci.* 29, 18–24. doi: 10.1016/j.tibs.2003.11.005

Castrejón, V., Carbó, R., and Martínez, M. (2007). Mecanismos moleculares que intervienen en el transporte de la glucosa. *REB* 26, 49–57.

Chaudhary, P., Suryakumar, G., Prasad, R., Singh, S. N., Ali, S., and Ilavazhagan, G. (2012). Chronic hypobaric hypoxia mediated skeletal muscle atrophy: role of ubiquitin-proteasome pathway and calpains. *Mol. Cell. Biochem.* 364, 101–113. doi: 10.1007/s11010-011-1210-x

Chen, C.-Y., Tsai, Y. L., Kao, C. L., Lee, S. D., Wu, M. C., Mallikarjuna, K., et al. (2010). Effect of mild intermittent hypoxia on glucose tolerance, muscle morphology and AMPK-PGC-1α signaling. *Chin. J. Physiol.* 53, 62–71. doi: 10.4077/CJP.2010.AMK078

Chen, S., Murphy, J., Toth, R., Campbell, D. G., Morrice, N. A., and Mackintosh, C. (2008). Complementary regulation of TBC1D1 and AS160 by growth factors, insulin and AMPK activators. *Biochem. J.* 409, 449–459. doi: 10.1042/BJ20071114

Chen, X., Zhao, T., Huang, X., Wu, L., Wu, K., Fan, M., et al. (2016). Intermittent hypoxia maintains glycemia in streptozotocin-induced diabetic rats. *Cell Stress Chaperones* 21, 515–522. doi: 10.1007/s12192-016-0679-3

Chen, Y.-C., Lee, S.-D., Ho, L.-T., and Kuo, C.-H. (2011). The effects of altitude training on the AMPK-related glucose transport pathway in the red skeletal muscle of both lean and obese zucker rats. *High Alt. Med. Biol.* 12, 371–378. doi: 10.1089/ham.2010.1088

Chiu, L.-L., Chou, S.-W., Cho, Y.-M., Ho, H.-Y., Ivy, J. L., Hunt, D., et al. (2004). Effect of prolonged intermittent hypoxia and exercise training on glucose tolerance and muscle GLUT4 protein expression in rats. *J. Biomed. Sci.* 11, 838–846.

Debevec, T., and Millet, G. P. (1985). Discerning normobaric and hypobaric hypoxia: significance of exposure duration. *J. Appl. Physiol.* 116:1255. doi: 10.1152/japplphysiol.00873.2013

Dill, R. P., Chadan, S. G., Li, C., and Parkhouse, W. S. (2001). Aging and glucose transporter plasticity in response to hypobaric hypoxia. *Mech. Ageing Dev.* 122, 533–545. doi: 10.1016/S0047-6374(01)00216-0

Ding, H., Heng, B., He, W., Shi, L., Lai, C., Xiao, L., et al. (2016). Chronic reactive oxygen species exposure inhibits glucose uptake and causes insulin resistance in C2C12 myotubes. *Biochem. Biophys. Res. Commun.* 478, 798–803. doi: 10.1016/j.bbrc.2016.08.028

Evans, D. J., Murray, R., and Kissebah, A. H. (1984). Relationship between skeletal muscle insulin resistance, insulin-mediated glucose disposal, and insulin binding. Effects of obesity and body fat topography. *J. Clin. Invest.* 74, 1515–1525. doi: 10.1172/JCI111565

Faramoushi, M., Sasan, R. A., Sarraf, V. S., and Karimi, P. (2016). Cardiac fibrosis and down regulation of GLUT4 in experimental diabetic cardiomyopathy are ameliorated by chronic exposures to intermittent altitude. *J. Cardiovasc. Thorac. Res.* 8, 26–33. doi: 10.15171/jcvtr.2016.05

Fisher, J. S. (2006). Potential role of the AMP-activated protein kinase in regulation of insulin action. *Cellscience* 2, 68–81.

Fisher, J. S., Gao, J., Han, D.-H., Holloszy, J. O., and Nolte, L. A. (2002). Activation of AMP kinase enhances sensitivity of muscle glucose transport to insulin. *Am. J. Physiol. Endocrinol. Metab.* 282, E18–E23. doi: 10.1152/ajpendo.2002.282.1.E18

Gamboa, J. L., Garcia-Cazarin, M. L., and Andrade, F. H. (2011). Chronic hypoxia increases insulin-stimulated glucose uptake in mouse soleus muscle. *Am. J. Physiol. Regul. Integr. Comp. Physiol.* 300, R85–R91. doi: 10.1152/ajpregu.00078.2010

Hayashi, T., Hirshman, M. F., Fujii, N., Habinowski, S. A., Witters, L. A., and Goodyear, L. J. (2000). Metabolic stress and altered glucose transport: activation of AMP-activated protein kinase as a unifying coupling mechanism. *Diabetes* 49, 527–531. doi: 10.2337/diabetes.49.4.527

Hayward, L. F., Johnson, A. K., and Felder, R. B. (1999). Arterial chemoreflex in conscious normotensive and hypertensive adult rats. *Am. J. Physiol.* 276(4 Pt 2), H1215–H1222.

Hoppeler, H., and Vogt, M. (2001). Muscle tissue adaptations to hypoxia. *J. Exp. Biol.* 204, 3133–3139.

Huang, S., and Czech, M. P. (2007). The GLUT4 glucose transporter. *Cell Metab.* 5, 237–252. doi: 10.1016/j.cmet.2007.03.006

Jefferson, J. A., Simoni, J., Escudero, E., Hurtado, M.-E., Swenson, E. R., Wesson, D. E., et al. (2004). Increased oxidative stress following acute and chronic high altitude exposure. *High Alt. Med. Biol.* 5, 61–69. doi: 10.1089/152702904322963690

Jørgensen, S. B., Honeyman, J., Oakhill, J. S., Fazakerley, D., Stöckli, J., Kemp, B. E., et al. (2009). Oligomeric resistin impairs insulin and AICAR-stimulated glucose uptake in mouse skeletal muscle by inhibiting GLUT4 translocation. *Am. J. Physiol. Endocrinol. Metab.* 297, E57–E66. doi: 10.1152/ajpendo.90744.2008

Kelly, K. R., Williamson, D. L., Fealy, C. E., Kriz, D. A., Krishnan, R. K., Huang, H., et al. (2010). Acute altitude-induced hypoxia suppresses plasma glucose and leptin in healthy humans. *Metab. Clin. Exp.* 59, 200–205. doi: 10.1016/j.metabol.2009.07.014

Kido, K., Yokokawa, T., Ato, S., Sato, K., and Fujita, S. (2017). Effect of resistance exercise under conditions of reduced blood insulin on AMPKα Ser485/491 inhibitory phosphorylation and AMPK pathway activation. *Am. J. Physiol. Regul. Integr. Comp. Physiol.* 313, R110–R119. doi: 10.1152/ajpregu.00063.2017

Kim, N. H., Cho, N. H., Yun, C. H., Lee, S. K., Yoon, D. W., Cho, H. J., et al. (2013). Association of obstructive sleep apnea and glucose metabolism in subjects with or without obesity. *Diabetes Care* 36, 3909–3915. doi: 10.2337/dc13-0375

Kohn, A. D., Summers, S. A., Birnbaum, M. J., and Roth, R. A. (1996). Expression of a constitutively active Akt Ser/Thr kinase in 3T3-L1 adipocytes stimulates glucose uptake and glucose transporter 4 translocation. *J. Biol. Chem.* 271, 31372–31378. doi: 10.1074/jbc.271.49.31372

Kramer, H. F., Witczak, C. A., Fujii, N., Jessen, N., Taylor, E. B., Arnolds, D. E., et al. (2006). Distinct signals regulate AS160 phosphorylation in response to insulin, AICAR, and contraction in mouse skeletal muscle. *Diabetes* 55, 2067–2076. doi: 10.2337/db06-0150

Kubis, H. P., Hanke, N., Scheibe, R. J., and Gros, G. (2005). Accumulation and nuclear import of HIF1 alpha during high and low oxygen concentration in skeletal muscle cells in primary culture. *Biochim. Biophys. Acta* 1745, 187–195.

Larsen, J. J., Hansen, J. M., Olsen, N. V., Galbo, H., and Dela, F. (1997). The effect of altitude hypoxia on glucose homeostasis in men. *J. Physiol.* 504, 241–249. doi: 10.1111/j.1469-7793.1997.241bf.x

Li, G., Wang, J., Ye, J., Zhang, Y., and Zhang, Y. (2015). PPARα protein expression was increased by four weeks of intermittent hypoxic training via AMPKα2-dependent manner in mouse skeletal muscle. *PLoS One* 10:e0122593. doi: 10.1371/journal.pone.0122593

Li, X., Liu, Y., Ma, H., Guan, Y., Cao, Y., Tian, Y., et al. (2016). Enhancement of glucose metabolism via PGC-1α participates in the cardioprotection of chronic intermittent hypobaric hypoxia. *Front. Physiol.* 8:219. doi: 10.3389/fphys.2016.00219

Lüneburg, N., Siques, P., Brito, J., Arriaza, K., Pena, E., Klose, H., et al. (2016). Long-term chronic intermittent hypobaric hypoxia in rats causes an imbalance in the asymmetric dimethylarginine/nitric oxide pathway and ROS activity: a possible synergistic mechanism for altitude pulmonary hypertension? *Pulm. Med.* 2016, 1–9. doi: 10.1155/2016/6578578

Mackenzie, R. W., and Watt, P. A. (2016). Molecular and whole body insight of the mechanisms surrounding glucose disposal and insulin resistance with hypoxic treatment in skeletal muscle. *J. Diabetes Res.* 2016:6934937. doi: 10.1155/2016/6934937

Manolescu, A. R., Witkowska, K., Kinnaird, A., Cessford, T., and Cheeseman, C. (2007). Facilitated hexose transporters: new perspectives on form and function. *Physiology* 22, 234–240. doi: 10.1152/physiol.00011.2007

Marquez, J. L., Rubinstein, S., Fattor, J. A., Shah, O., Hoffman, A. R., and Friedlander, A. L. (2013). Cyclic hypobaric hypoxia improves markers of glucose metabolism in middle-aged men. *High Alt. Med. Biol.* 14, 263–272. doi: 10.1089/ham.2012.1057

Mas, A., Montane, J., Anguela, X. M., Munoz, S., Douar, A. M., Riu, E., et al. (2006). Reversal of type 1 diabetes by engineering a glucose sensor in skeletal muscle. *Diabetes* 55, 1546–1553. doi: 10.2337/db05-1615

Ou, L. C., and Smith, R. P. (1983). Probable strain differences of rats in susceptibilities and cardiopulmonary responses to chronic hypoxia. *Respir. Physiol.* 53, 367–377.

Powell, F. L., and Garcia, N. (2000). Physiological effects of intermittent hypoxia. *High Alt. Med. Biol.* 1, 125–136. doi: 10.1089/15270290050074279

Richalet, J.-P., Donoso, M. V., Jiménez, D., Antezana, A.-M., Hudson, C., Cortès, G., et al. (2002). Chilean miners commuting from sea level to 4500 m: a prospective study. *High Alt. Med. Biol.* 3, 159–166. doi: 10.1089/15270290260131894

Sacramento, J. F., Ribeiro, M. J., Rodrigues, T., Guarino, M. P., Diogo, L. N., Seiça, R., et al. (2016). Insulin resistance is associated with tissue-specific regulation of HIF-1α and HIF-2α during mild chronic intermittent hypoxia. *Respir. Physiol. Neurobiol.* 228, 30–38. doi: 10.1016/j.resp.2016.03.007

Sakagami, H., Makino, Y., Mizumoto, K., Isoe, T., Takeda, Y., Watanabe, J., et al. (2014). Loss of HIF-1α impairs GLUT4 translocation and glucose uptake by the skeletal muscle cells. *Am. J. Physiol. Endocrinol. Metab.* 306, E1065–E1076. doi: 10.1152/ajpendo.00597.2012

Sawhney, R. C., Malhotra, A. S., Singh, T., Rai, R. M., and Sinha, K. C. (1986). Insulin secretion at high altitude in man. *Int. J. Biometeorol.* 30, 231–238.

Scheepers, A., Joost, H. G., and Schurmann, A. (2004). The glucose transporter families SGLT and GLUT: molecular basis of normal and aberrant function. *J. Parenter. Enteral. Nutr.* 28, 364–371. doi: 10.1177/0148607104028005364

Siques, P., Brito, J., León-Velarde, F., Barrios, L., Cruz, J. J. D. L., López, V., et al. (2006). Time course of cardiovascular and hematological responses in rats exposed to chronic intermittent hypobaric hypoxia (4600 m). *High Alt. Med. Biol.* 7, 72–80. doi: 10.1089/ham.2006.7.72

Siques, P., Brito, J., Naveas, N., Pulido, R., Cruz, J. J. D. L., Mamani, M., et al. (2014). Plasma and liver lipid profiles in rats exposed to chronic hypobaric hypoxia: changes in metabolic pathways. *High Alt. Med. Biol.* 15, 388–395. doi: 10.1089/ham.2013.1134

Thomas, A., Belaidi, E., Moulin, S., Horman, S., van der Zon, G. C., Viollet, B., et al. (2017). Chronic intermittent hypoxia impairs insulin sensitivity but improves whole-body glucose tolerance by activating skeletal muscle AMPK. *Diabetes* 66, 2942–2951. doi: 10.2337/db17-0186

Thong, F. S. L., Dugani, C. B., and Klip, A. (2005). Turning signals on and off: GLUT4 traffic in the insulin-signaling highway. *Physiology* 20, 271–284. doi: 10.1152/physiol.00017.2005

Tian, Y.-M., Liu, Y., Wang, S., Dong, Y., Su, T., Ma, H.-J., et al. (2016). Anti-diabetes effect of chronic intermittent hypobaric hypoxia through improving liver insulin resistance in diabetic rats. *Life Sci.* 150, 1–7. doi: 10.1016/j.lfs.2016.02.053

Viganò, A., Vasso, M., Caretti, A., Bravatà, V., Terraneo, L., Fania, C., et al. (2011). Protein modulation in mouse heart under acute and chronic hypoxia. *Proteomics* 11, 4202–4217. doi: 10.1002/pmic.201000804

Wang, X., Yu, Q., Yue, H., Zeng, S., and Cui, F. (2015). Effect of intermittent hypoxia and rimonabant on glucose metabolism in rats: involvement of expression of GLUT4 in skeletal muscle. *Med. Sci. Monit.* 21, 3252–3260. doi: 10.12659/MSM.896039

Woolcott, O. O., Ader, M., and Bergman, R. N. (2015). Glucose homeostasis during short-term and prolonged exposure to high altitudes. *Endocr. Rev.* 36, 149–173. doi: 10.1210/er.2014-1063

Xia, Y., Warshaw, J. B., and Haddad, G. G. (1997). Effect of chronic hypoxia on glucose transporters in heart and skeletal muscle of immature and adult rats. *Am. J. Physiol. Regul. Integr. Comp. Physiol.* 273, R1734–R1741. doi: 10.1152/ajpregu.1997.273.5.R1734

Żebrowska, A., Hall, B., Kochańska-Dziurowicz, A., and Janikowska, G. (2018). The effect of high intensity physical exercise and hypoxia on glycemia, angiogenic biomarkers and cardiorespiratory function in patients with type 1 diabetes. *Adv. Clin. Exp. Med.* 27, 207–216. doi: 10.17219/acem/66354

10

Serotonin and Adenosine G-Protein Coupled Receptor Signaling for Ventilatory Acclimatization to Sustained Hypoxia

Esteban A. Moya and Frank L. Powell*

Division of Physiology, Department of Medicine, University of California, San Diego, La Jolla, CA, United States

***Correspondence:**
Esteban A. Moya
eamoya@ucsd.edu

Different patterns of hypoxia evoke different forms of plasticity in the neural control of ventilation. For example, acute intermittent hypoxia produces long term facilitation (LTF) of ventilation, while chronic sustained hypoxia (CH) causes ventilatory acclimatization to hypoxia (VAH). In both LTF and VAH, ventilation in normoxia is greater than normal after the hypoxic stimulus is removed and the acute hypoxic ventilatory response can increase. However, the mechanisms of LTF and VAH are thought to be different based on previous results showing serotonin $5HT_2$ receptors, which are G protein coupled receptors (GPCR) that activate G_Q signaling, contribute to LTF but not VAH. Newer results show that a different GPCR, namely adenosine A_{2A} receptors and the G_S signaling pathway, cause LTF with more severe intermittent hypoxia, i.e., PaO_2 = 25–30 Torr for G_S versus 35–45 Torr for LTF with the G_Q signaling pathway. We hypothesized adenosine A_{2A} receptors and G_S signaling are involved in establishing VAH with longer term moderate CH and tested this in adult male rats by measuring ventilatory responses to O_2 and CO_2 with barometric pressure plethysmography after administering MSX-3 or ketanserin (A_{2A} and $5HT_2$ antagonists, respectively, both 1 mg/Kg i.p.) during CH for 7 days. Blocking G_S or G_Q signals throughout CH exposure, significantly decreased VAH. After VAH was established, G_Q blockade did not affect ventilation while G_S blockade increased VAH. Similar to LTF, data support roles for both G_Q and G_S pathways in the development of VAH but after VAH has been established, the G_S pathway inhibits VAH.

Keywords: hypoxia, control of breathing, ventilatory acclimatization, serotonin, adenosine, neuroplasticity

INTRODUCTION

Exposure to chronic sustained hypoxia (CH) produces (1) an increase in ventilation that persists after normoxia is restored and (2) an increase in the acute hypoxic ventilatory response (HVR). This is called ventilatory acclimatization to hypoxia (VAH) and it depends on plasticity in both carotid body chemoreceptors and medullary respiratory control circuits (Pamenter and Powell, 2016). Plasticity in ventilatory control circuits can also be produced by other patterns of hypoxia with similar results. For example, acute intermittent hypoxia produces long term facilitation (LTF) with increases in ventilation and phrenic nerve activity that persist in normoxia after the hypoxia protocol, and increases in the HVR to successive bouts of intermittent hypoxia [reviewed by Dale-Nagle et al. (2010), Pamenter and Powell (2016), and Turner et al. (2017)]. Despite similar physiological changes in LTF and VAH, several lines of evidence have been used to argue that the signaling mechanisms for LTF do not explain VAH. For example, LTF is well-known to require activation of serotonin receptors (Bach and Mitchell, 1996; Baker-Herman and Mitchell, 2002) but serotonin receptor blockade does not reverse VAH after 4 h of hypoxia in goats (Herman et al., 1999), and whole-body serotonin depletion in rats does not block VAH after 1 day of sustained hypoxia (Olson, 1987). Also, exposure to sustained hypoxia for 25 min (i.e., a continuous exposure equal to the total duration of hypoxia in an intermittent hypoxia protocol that causes LTF) does not cause LTF (Devinney et al., 2013). Effects of longer exposure to hypoxia, such as 7 days used to show plasticity in CNS respiratory centers (Pamenter and Powell, 2016), have not been studied though.

More recently, a second mechanism for LTF that depends on adenosine receptors and more severe levels of intermittent hypoxia has been described (Nichols et al., 2012; reviewed in Pamenter and Powell, 2013). Exposure to moderate levels of intermittent hypoxia (arterial P_{O2} = 45–55 mm Hg) induces LTF by a serotonin-dependent pathway but exposure to more severe intermittent hypoxia (arterial P_{O2} = 25–35 mm Hg) also activated an adenosine-dependent pathway to induce LTF (Nichols et al., 2012). Increased phrenic nerve activity does not strictly depend on intermittent hypoxia *per se* and can be induced by direct pharmacological activation of serotonin 5-HT_2 receptors (MacFarlane and Mitchell, 2009) or adenosine A_{2A} receptors (Golder et al., 2008). Both of these pathways depend on G-protein coupled receptor (GPCR) signaling but they involve different GPCR pathways. The serotonergic or "Q pathway" depends on activation of G_Q protein, increased levels of BDNF and phosphorylation of ERK protein to induce phrenic LTF (Satriotomo et al., 2012). The adenosine or "S pathway" depends on activation of G_S protein, PKA and phosphorylation of AKT (Devinney et al., 2013). Since the blocking of one these pathways can increase LTF, G_S and G_Q signaling interact via cross-talk inhibition (Dale-Nagle et al., 2010; Devinney et al., 2013; Navarrete-Opazo and Mitchell, 2014).

The role of adenosine-dependent G_S mechanisms in VAH, and the contribution serotonin-dependent G_Q mechanisms to exposures to sustained hypoxia longer than 1 day have not been studied. We hypothesized that longer exposure to moderate hypoxia could activate the adenosine-G_S pathway described for LTF in severe intermittent hypoxia and contribute to VAH. To test this, we measured the hypoxic and hypercapnic ventilatory response in rats exposed to 7 days of CH with chronic blockade of adenosine A_{2A} receptors during CH. We also tested the effects of chronic serotonin 5-HT_2 receptor blockade during 7 days of CH, and the effects of acute A_{2A} and 5-HT_2 receptor blockade after VAH was established, to compare signaling mechanisms during VAH and LTF.

MATERIALS AND METHODS

Animals

Experiments were performed in male Sprague-Dawley rats (Harlan) weighing 250–300 g housed in 12:12 h light dark cycle and fed with standard diet *at libitum* except during measurements in the plethysmograph. All the experimental procedures were approved by the Institutional Animal Care and Use Committee of the University of California, San Diego.

Chronic Hypoxia

The rats were exposed to CH in a hypobaric chamber for 7 days (barometric pressure = 380 Torr, P_{IO2} = 70 Torr, temperature 21°C and 40% humidity), and normoxic control rats were housed in the same conditions in the room outside the chamber. The chamber was opened every other day for cage cleaning, and replacement of food and water.

Plethysmography

Ventilatory responses to hypoxia and hypercapnia were measured in unrestrained rats using a whole body barometric plethysmograph (7 L) modified for continuous flow (Reid et al., 2005; Pamenter et al., 2014a). Briefly, flow was maintained constant through the chamber while a pressure transducer (mMP45 with 2 cmH2O diaphragm, Validyne) recorded the changes attributable to warming and expansion of inhaled gasses. On the experimental day, the rats were weighed and sealed into the plethysmograph chamber along with a temperature and humidity probe (Thermalert TH5, Physitemp). A constant gas flow (3 l/min) was delivered with a mass flow controller and gas mixer (MFC-4 Sable Systems) upstream of the chamber. Gasses exited the chamber through a valve and into a vacuum pump (Model 25, Precision Scientific) to isolate pressure changes from breathing in the chamber during constant flow with high input and output impedances. This also allowed us to maintain chamber pressure near-atmospheric pressure and reference pressure measurements in the chamber to atmosphere. Inspired and expired carbon dioxide fractions were measured with an O2/CO2 analyzer (FOXBOX Field Analysis system, Sable Systems) sampling from the chamber.

Ventilatory Response Measurements

We measured the HVR and the hypercapnic ventilatory response (HCVR) with the following protocols. For normoxic control animals, we put rats in the plethysmograph for 45 min of acclimation to 21% O_2, followed by 5 min of exposure to 10% O_2 to further acclimate rats to the experimental conditions, i.e., changes in inspired gasses. Then we returned rats to 21% O_2 for 15 min for the first measure of ventilation in baseline conditions (normoxia in this case). Rats were exposed to 10% O_2 for 15 min, returned to baseline conditions for 15 min, exposed to 7%CO_2/21%O_2 for 15 min, and finally returned to baseline conditions for 15 min. The protocol was similar but opposite for CH rats. In this case, the baseline condition was 10% O_2 and they were acclimated to changes in inspired gas by exposure to 21% O_2 for 5 min. The HVR in CH rats was measured by exposing them to 21% O_2 for 15 min after a baseline breathing 10% O_2.

All ventilatory parameters were recorded on an analog-digital acquisition system (PowerLab 8SP, AD Instruments) and analyzed with the LabChart 8-Pro Software, sampling at a rate of 1 kHz. We analyzed a minimum of 30 s between 10 and 15 min after changing gas concentrations for respiratory frequency (f_R), tidal volume (V_T) and their product, inspired ventilation ($\dot{V}_I$), which was normalized to body mass [ml/(min·kg)] using 0.2-ml calibration pulses (Drorbaugh and Fenn, 1955; Jacky, 1978).

Serotonin and Adenosine Receptor Antagonist Administration

We designed two studies to determine the effects of serotonin and adenosine on VAH using ketanserin (an antagonist of serotonin $5HT_2$ receptors) and MSX-3 (an antagonist adenosine A_{2A} receptors). Firstly, to test the role of $5HT_2$ and A_{2A} receptors on VAH during CH exposure, we administered ketanserin tartrate (Tocris, Minneapolis, MN, United States) or MSX-3 hydrate (Sigma–Aldrich, St. Louis, MO, United States) continuously using osmotic pumps (1 mg/Kg/day for both). Rats were initially anesthetized with isofluorane (initially 5% and maintained with 1–2% in 100% O_2) and we implanted mini osmotic pumps (Model 2002, Alzet Osmotic Pumps, Cupertino, CA, United States) filled with ketanserin or MSX-3 dissolved in 40% DMSO/Saline subcutaneously 1 day before start the CH exposure. Vehicle control rats were implanted with osmotic pumps filled with 40% DMSO/Saline (Vehicle). After surgery, rats were administrated with bupenophirine (0.03 mg/Kg, i.p.) and enrofloxacin (4 mg/Kg, i.p.).

Secondly, to assess the effect of $5HT_2$ (Ketanserin) or A_{2A} (MSX-3) antagonists on VAH after it was established by CH, we studied a different group of rats and measured ventilatory responses in the same individuals before and after exposure to CH (7 days). Then we injected Ketanserin or MSX-3 (1 mg/Kg i.p.) and returned the rats to hypobaric CH for an additional day. The next day, we injected the rats with antagonists again and repeated the ventilatory measurements.

Statistics

Data was expressed as mean ± SEM. Statistical analysis was performed using two-way ANOVA between drug and CH effect or repeated measurement ANOVA test followed by Bonferroni *post hoc* analysis (GraphPad Prism, 5.0, United States). $p < 0.05$ was set as the level of statistical significance.

RESULTS

Chronic Serotonin $5HT_2$ Receptor Blockade During CH Decreased Ventilatory Acclimatization to Hypoxia

To determine the contribution of serotonin receptors on VAH we studied the effect of the $5HT_2$ receptor antagonist ketanserin administrated continuously in rats during exposure to CH. $\dot{V}_I$ increased with acute hypoxia (10% O_2) and CH as expected for a normal HVR and VAH (**Figure 1**). In rats breathing 21% O_2, there was a significant interaction for $\dot{V}_I$ between chronic O_2 level and ketanserin ($p = 0.0001$). *Post hoc* analysis showed $\dot{V}_I$ was significantly decreased by ketanserin after CH (**Figure 1B**) but not in normoxic control conditions (**Figure 1A**). In rats breathing 21% O_2, the decrease in $\dot{V}_I$ was explained by a significant decrease in V_T, which showed a significant interaction between chronic O_2 and drug ($p = 0.01$) (**Figures 1E,F**) while f_R no longer showed a significant increase with drug after CH, which had been observed in normoxic controls (**Figures 1C,D**); the interaction of chronic O_2 level and ketanserin on f_R was significant ($p = 0.0292$).

The effects of ketanserin in rats breathing 10% O_2 were similar to those observed when breathing 21% O_2 (**Figure 1**). $\dot{V}_I$ showed a significant interaction between chronic O_2 level and ketanserin ($p < 0.0001$) with ketanserin significantly decreasing $\dot{V}_I$ in 10% O_2 after CH, in contrast to significantly increasing it in normoxic control rats (**Figures 1A,B**). Ketanserin significantly increased f_R in normoxic control rats during acute hypoxia while changes in f_R with ketanserin were not significant in acute hypoxia after CH (**Figures 1C,D**). The interaction for chronic O_2 level and ketanserin were not significant for V_T breathing 10% O_2 although it tended to decrease with ketanserin after CH (**Figures 1E,F**).

Table 1 shows no significant effect of ketanserin on $\dot{V}_I$ in rats breathing 7% CO_2 before or after CH. $\dot{V}_I$ increased during hypercapnia after CH in all cases, as expected for acclimatization. Hence, differences observed in $\dot{V}_I$ and the HVR with ketanserin after CH are not explained by hypercapnic responses or general changes in ventilatory drive. **Table 2** shows metabolic rates (CO_2 production, $\dot{V}_{CO2}$) were not significantly different between normoxic control and CH rats [23.2 ± 0.6 and 26.2 ± 2.0 (ml/(kg min))], with vehicle or ketanserin breathing 21 or 10% O_2. Hence, the differences in $\dot{V}_I$ found between conditions are not explained by differences in the effects of metabolism on ventilatory drive.

Summarizing, $5HT_2$ receptor blockade during CH blunted the increase in $\dot{V}_I$ in 10% O_2 that normally occurs with VAH and decreased $\dot{V}_I$ in 21% O_2 by a similar amount, i.e., there was a parallel downward shift of the HVR curve ($\dot{V}_I$ versus inspired O_2). This was mainly due to an effect of ketanserin on V_T. Ketanserin increased f_R in 21% and 10% O_2 in normoxic control but not CH rats, which had a higher f_R that was similar to the elevated level caused by ketanserin in the normoxic controls.

Chronic Adenosine A_{2A} Receptor Blockade During CH Exposure Decreased Ventilatory Acclimatization to Hypoxia

Figure 2 shows that the general pattern of changes in ventilation after CH with the A_{2A} antagonist MSX-3 were similar to those described above for effects of $5HT_2$ receptor blockade. $\dot{V}_I$ increases with acute hypoxia and CH as expected for a normal HVR and VAH (**Figures 2A,B**). $\dot{V}_I$ breathing 21% O_2 showed a significant interaction between chronic O_2 level and MSX-3 ($p = 0.0005$) as MSX-3 tended to increase $\dot{V}_I$ in normoxic control rats (**Figure 2A**) and significantly decreased it in CH rats (**Figure 2B**). We observed similar patterns of change in f_R and V_T with a significant interaction between chronic O_2 level and MSX-3 for V_T ($p = 0.0002$) and f_R ($p < 0.0001$) (**Figures 2C–F**). The effects of MSX-3 during 10% O_2 breathing was similar; there was a significant interaction between chronic O_2 level and MSX-3 for $\dot{V}_I$ ($p < 0.0011$) so $\dot{V}_I$ was significantly decreased by MSX-3

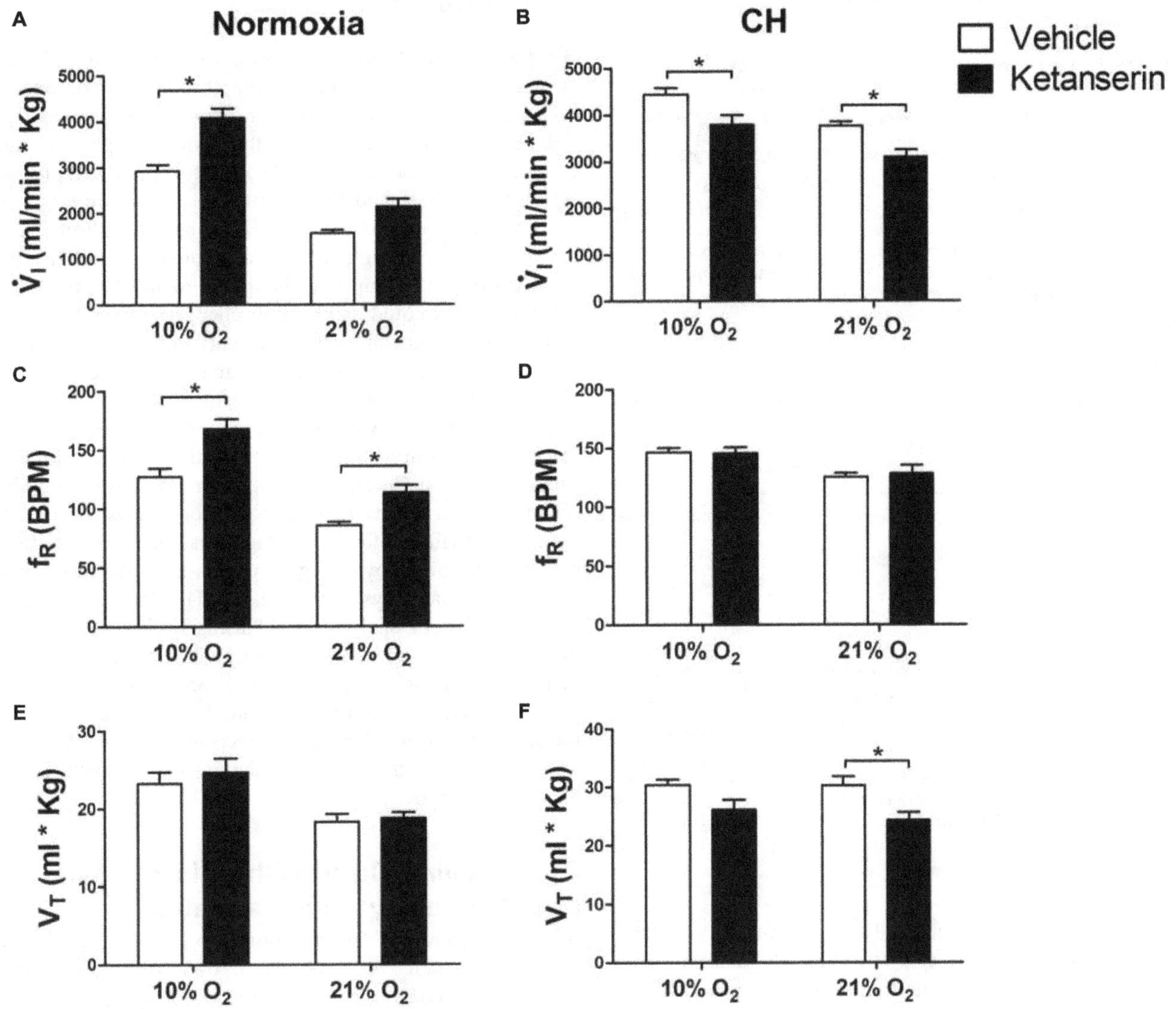

FIGURE 1 | Effect of $5HT_2$ antagonist on ventilation in control (Normoxic) rats and rats acclimatized to chronic hypoxia (CH). **(A)** Blocking $5HT_2$ receptors with ketanserin in Normoxic rats increased ventilation ($\dot{V}_I$) in acute hypoxia (10% O_2) and had no significant effect during normoxia (21% O_2). **(B)** CH significantly increased $\dot{V}_I$ with vehicle; ketanserin significantly decreased $\dot{V}_I$ in CH rats during acute hypoxia and normoxia, in contrast to normoxic controls. **(C–F)** $\dot{V}_I$ increased with ketanserin in Normoxic rats because of frequency (f_R) but it decreased with ketanserin in CH rats because of tidal volume (V_T). *$p < 0.05$, Bonferroni after two-way ANOVA, $n = 6$ rats per group.

after CH ($p < 0.05$) in contrast to a significant increase ($p < 0.05$) in the normoxic control rats.

Table 1 shows that these changes in $\dot{V}_I$ with MSX-3 treatment were not due to changes in the ventilatory response to CO_2, which was not significantly different between vehicle and drug. $\dot{V}_I$ increased during hypercapnia after CH in all cases, as expected for acclimatization. Also, $\dot{V}_{CO2}$ was not significantly different between normoxic control and CH rats with vehicle or MSX-3 breathing 21 or 10% (**Table 2**). Hence, the differences in $\dot{V}_I$ found between conditions are not explained by differences in the effects of metabolism on ventilatory drive.

Summarizing, A_{2A} receptor blockade during CH blunted the increase in $\dot{V}_I$ in 10 and 21% O_2 that normally occur with VAH by a similar amount so there was a parallel downward shift of the HVR curve ($\dot{V}_I$ comparing acute O_2 level, 21 versus 10% O_2). This was due effects of MSX-3 on both f_R and V_T.

Acute Administration of Ketanserin After CH Did Not Reverse VAH

To test if $5HT_2$ receptor blockade affects ventilatory responses after VAH is already established, we measured the ventilation in the same rats (1) before and (2) after 7 days of CH, and (3) after 2 more days of CH with two acute doses of ketanserin (1 mg i.p./kg daily). CH caused a significant increase of $\dot{V}_I$ during 21 or 10% O_2 breathing (**Figure 3A**). Ketanserin administered for 2 days more

TABLE 1 | Responses to hypercapnia in rats treated with $5HT_2$ and A_{2A} receptor antagonists during CH exposure.

$\dot{V}_I$ (mL/min*Kg)	Normoxia		CH	
	0% CO_2	7% CO_2	0% CO_2	7% O_2
Vehicle	1560 ± 68	4008 ± 364	3764 ± 87	7958 ± 859*
Ketanserin	1983 ± 219	4594 ± 429	3097 ± 157	8150 ± 627*
MSX-3	1983 ± 151	4962 ± 425	2961 ± 157	7647 ± 871*

*Ketanserin or MSX-3 administered during chronic hypoxia (CH) did not affect the ventilation ($\dot{V}_I$) during hypercapnia (7% CO_2). *$p < 0.05$ versus Normoxia group breathing 7% CO_2. Bonferroni's test after two-way ANOVA comparing the effects of Drug and CH during 7% CO_2, n = 5–6 rats for all groups.*

TABLE 2 | Metabolic rates in rats treated with $5HT_2$ and A_{2A} receptor antagonists during CH exposure.

Group	O_2 (%)	$\dot{V}_{CO2}$ [mL/(in*Kg)]	
		Ketanserin (η = 6)	MSX-3 (η = 5–6)
Normoxia vehicle	21	23.2 ± 0.6	23.2 ± 0.6
Normoxia drug		21.2 ± 0.8	25.8 ± 1.5
CH vehicle		26.2 ± 2.0	26.4 ± 2.3
CH drug		20.9 ± 0.5	25.3 ± 2.3
Normoxia vehicle	10	21.8 ± 0.6	21.8 ± 0.6
Normoxia drug		21.3 ± 0.4	23.8 ± 0.9
CH vehicle		22.6 ± 1.8	22.4 ± 1.5
CH drug		22.4 ± 1.3	22.5 ± 1.5

CO_2 production ($\dot{V}_{CO2}$) of rats treated with ketanserin and MSX-3 or vehicle during normoxic or chronic hypoxia (CH). No significant differences between conditions. Bonferroni's test after two-way ANOVA, n = 5–6.

of CH did not cause any significant difference in the HVR versus CH alone (**Figure 3A**). However, $\dot{V}_I$ in 21% O_2 breathing after CH + ketanserin resulted from a significantly decreased f_R and increased V_T (**Figures 3B,C**). Ketanserin did not affect neither $\dot{V}_I$ in 7% CO_2 (**Table 3**) nor metabolic rates (**Table 4**) after VAH was established.

Acute Administration of MSX-3 After CH Increased Ventilation

To test if the A_{2A} receptor blockade had an effect after VAH was established, we measured ventilatory responses using repeated measurements in rats during (1) normoxic control conditions, (2) after 7 days of CH, and (3) after 2 additional days of CH with acute injections of MSX-3 (1 mg/kg i.p. daily). Exposure to CH produced a significant increase of $\dot{V}_I$ in rats breathing 21 or 10% O_2 (**Figure 4A**). MSX-3 produced additional increases of $\dot{V}_I$ in both, 21 and 10% O_2 breathing (**Figure 4A**). This was due to significant effects of MSX-3 on f_R and V_T during 21% O_2 breathing and on non-significant increases of f_R and V_T during 10% O_2 breathing (**Figures 4B,C**). MSX-3 administration after VAH was established by CH did not have significant effects on CH-induced increases in ventilation during 7% CO_2 breathing (**Table 3**) nor produce changes in metabolic rate (**Table 4**).

DISCUSSION

We found that chronic inhibition of either serotonin $5HT_2$ or adenosine A_{2A} receptors *during* chronic hypoxia decreased VAH: $\dot{V}_I$ breathing normoxic or hypoxic gas increased with CH plus drug significantly less than with CH plus vehicle. In contrast, acute blockade of $5HT_2$ receptors *after* VAH had been established by CH had no effect on $\dot{V}_I$ and acute blockade of adenosine A_{2A} receptors after VAH had been established actually increased $\dot{V}_I$ breathing normoxic or hypoxic gas (relative to CH without drug). We found no changes in metabolic rates between conditions that could cause other changes in ventilatory drive. Also we found no differences in ventilatory responses to CO_2 with drug treatments indicating that the effects of drugs were specific to hypoxic responses and any increases or decreases in $\dot{V}_I$ observed with drugs were not generalized increases in ventilatory drive or ventilatory limitations, respectively. Hence our results support a role for G_Q and G_S signaling in establishing ventilatory acclimatization to sustained hypoxia for 7 days. Furthermore, the different effects of GPCR antagonists during versus after CH might be explained by changes in cross-talk inhibition between G_Q and G_S pathways, activated by $5HT_2$ and A_{2A} receptors respectively. Both of these mechanisms have been shown to be important for chemoreflex plasticity with intermittent hypoxia in LTF but this is the first evidence for them with VAH from CH. However, it is important to note that we have not identified the site of action for these drug effects and we have not actually tested elements of the specific signaling pathways being activated by these receptors.

G_Q Signaling During Chronic Hypoxia and Ventilatory Acclimatization

In normoxic control rats, we found no effect of chronic $5HT_2$ receptor blockade with ketanserin on $\dot{V}_I$ during normoxia. In normoxic control rats breathing 10% O_2 or 21% O_2 f_R and $\dot{V}_I$ significantly increased (**Figure 1**). Similar increases in phrenic nerve responses to acute hypoxia following acute administration of ketanserin to anesthetized normoxic control rats have been reported, although f_R increased more than V_T in those experiments (Kinkead and Mitchell, 1999).

As expected, CH increased $\dot{V}_I$, in rats breathing 21 or 10% O_2 but chronic ketanserin during CH significantly decreased $\dot{V}_I$ at both levels of inspired O_2, mainly by effects of V_T (**Figure 1**). These effects of blocking serotonin receptors and presumably G_Q signaling on $\dot{V}_I$ in CH rats breathing normoxic gas are similar to those found for ventilatory and phrenic long term facilitation (vLTF and pLTF, respectively). Methysergide (a general 5HT receptor antagonist) administered before moderate acute intermittent hypoxia (IH), prevents phrenic LTF and specifically increased amplitude in integrated phrenic activity for 30–90 min after intermittent hypoxia (Bach and Mitchell, 1996). Also, administering ketanserin 20 min before moderate IH prevents the development of phrenic LTF (Kinkead and Mitchell, 1999; Fuller et al., 2001) and ketanserin 1 day before additional to immediately before moderate IH blocks ventilatory LTF (McGuire et al., 2004).

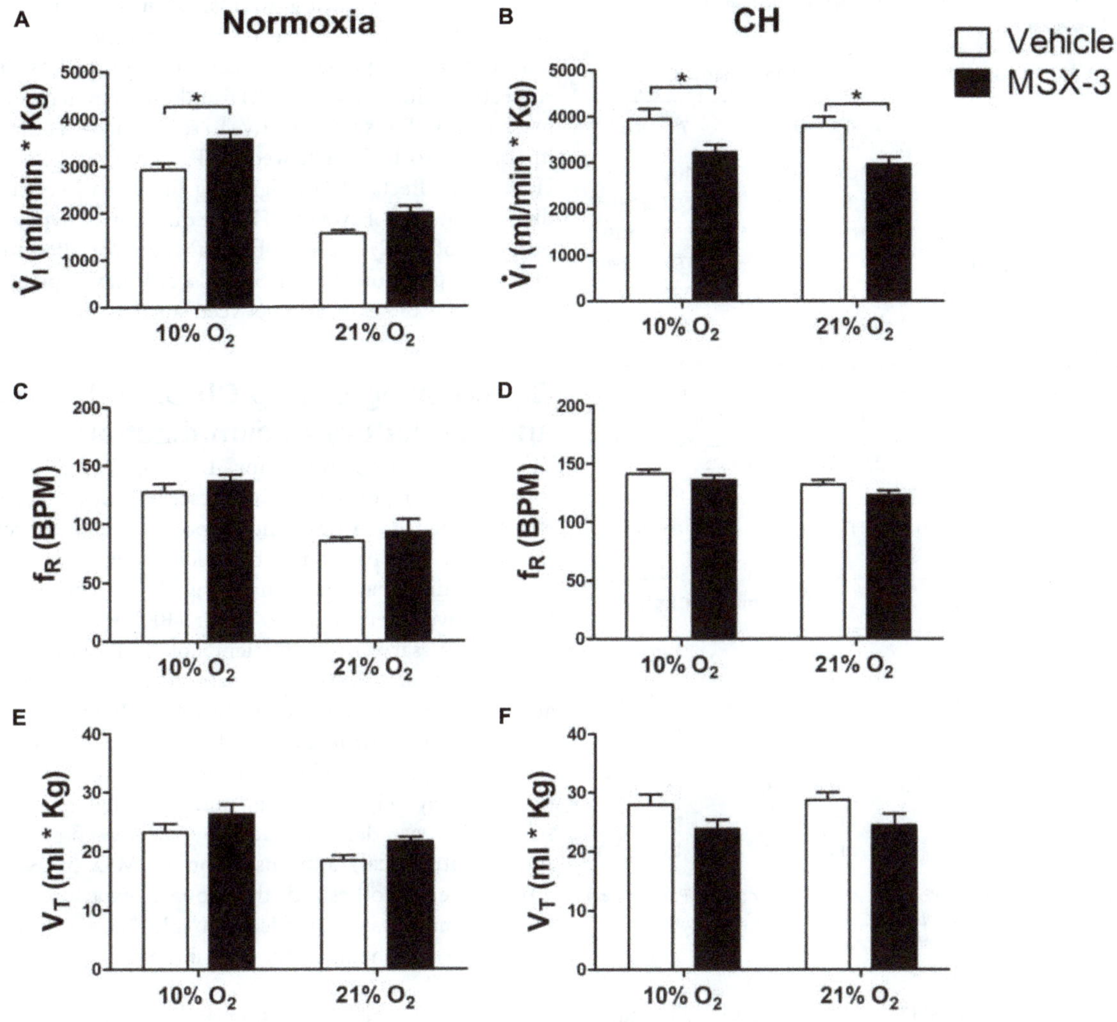

FIGURE 2 | Effect of A_{2A} antagonist on ventilation in control (Normoxic) rats and rats acclimatized to chronic hypoxia (CH). **(A)** Blocking A_{2A} receptors with MSX-3 in Normoxic rats increased ventilation ($\dot{V}_I$) in acute hypoxia (10% O_2) and had no significant effect during normoxia (21% O_2). **(B)** CH significantly increased $\dot{V}_I$ with vehicle but MSX-3 significantly decreased $\dot{V}_I$ in CH rats during acute hypoxia and normoxia, in contrast to normoxic controls. **(C–F)** There were no significant effects of MSX-3 on respiratory frequency (f_R) or tidal volume (V_T). *$p < 0.05$, Bonferroni after two-way ANOVA, $n = 6$ rats per group.

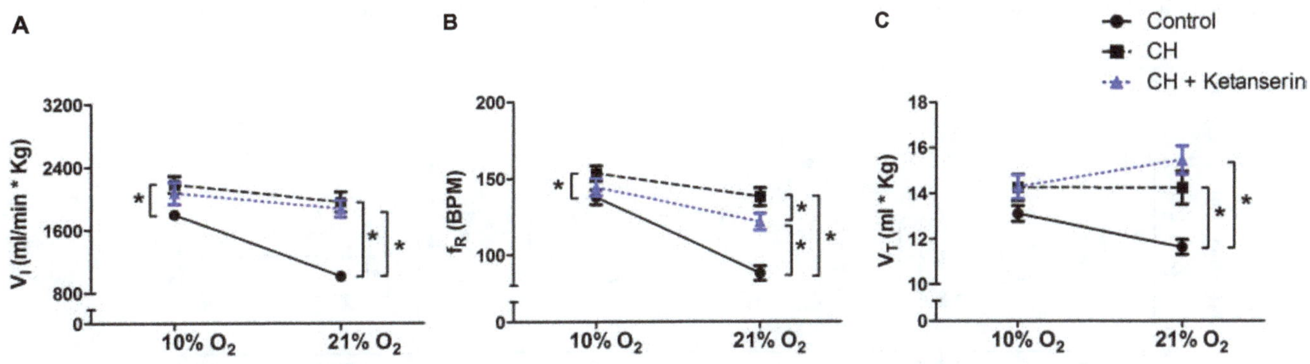

FIGURE 3 | Repeated measurements blocking $5HT_2$ receptors after VAH was established. Blocking $5HT_2$ receptors with ketanserin after chronic sustained hypoxia (CH) has no effect on ventilation ($\dot{V}_I$, **A**), respiratory frequency (f_R, **B**) or tidal volume (V_T, **C**) during normoxia (21% O_2) or acute hypoxia (10% O_2). *$p < 0.05$, Bonferroni after repeated measurements two-way ANOVA, $n = 10$ rats.

TABLE 3 | Responses to hypercapnia in rats treated with $5HT_2$ and A_{2A} receptor antagonists after CH exposure.

Drug	Group	$\dot{V}_I$ (mL/min*Kg)	
		0% CO_2	7% CO_2
Ketanserin (η = 10)	Control	1013 ± 47	4195 ± 573
	CH	1959 ± 128	7683 ± 1186*
	CH + Drug	1871 ± 107	6824 ± 1010*
MSX-3 (η = 9)	Control	1163 ± 79	4791 ± 654
	CH	1777 ± 118	6624 ± 778*
	CH + Drug	2396 ± 90	7340 ± 969*

*Chronic hypoxia (CH) increased $\dot{V}_I$ in normoxia (0% CO_2, 21%O_2) and the ventilatory response to hypercapnia (7% CO_2); this was not affected by ketanserin or MSX-3 administered after acclimatization was established by CH. *$p < 0.05$ versus 7% CO_2 Control, Bonferroni's test after repeated measures two-way ANOVA, n = 10 rats for ketanserin and n = 9 for MSX-3 treated rats.*

TABLE 4 | Metabolic rates in rats treated with $5HT_2$ and A_{2A} receptor antagonists after CH exposure.

Drug	Group	$\dot{V}_{CO2}$ [mL/(min*Kg)]	
		21% O_2	10% O_2
Ketanserin (η = 10)	Control	8.6 ± 1.0	11.4 ± 0.9
	CH	12.8 ± 1.5	13.2 ± 1.0
	CH + Drug	15.7 ± 1.5	15.7 ± 1.5
MSX-3 (η = 9)	Control	11.2 ± 0.5	12.6 ± 0.5
	CH	13.4 ± 1.3	13.9 ± 1.4
	CH + Drug	14.4 ± 1.2	15.0 ± 0.9

CO_2 production ($\dot{V}_{CO2}$) was not affected by CH, inspired O_2 or drug with ketanserin or MSX-3 administered after acclimatization to CH. Bonferroni's test after repeated measures two-way ANOVA, n = 9–10 rats per group.

The effects of blocking $5HT_2$ receptors and presumably G_Q signaling on $\dot{V}_I$ in rats breathing hypoxic gas appears to be different after IH versus CH. However, we found chronic ketanserin decreased the normal increase in $\dot{V}_I$, during 10% O_2 breathing with CH, thereby blunting the increase in acute HVR that occurs with VAH. This can be compared to the effects of ketanserin on progressive augmentation (PA), which is observed in studies of LTF with IH protocols as increases in ventilation or phrenic activity during successive bouts of hypoxia (Pamenter and Powell, 2016). The effects of IH on ventilatory drive during normoxia and hypoxia have been distinguished as LTF and PA, respectively, in part because LTF and PA seem to involve different mechanisms; PA is not sensitive to serotonin receptor antagonists in contrast to LTF [reviewed by Pamenter and Powell (2016)]. Hence the effects of G_Q signaling on $\dot{V}_I$ in hypoxia appear to differ following CH versus IH. The duration of hypoxic exposure, duration of $5HT_2$ receptor blockade, and/or effects of blocking $5HT_2$ receptors outside the spinal cord may explain differences in the effects of ketanserin between studies.

G_S Signaling During Chronic Hypoxia and Ventilatory Acclimatization

The second mechanism for LTF operative during severe intermittent hypoxia was first described in a pharmacological study designed to test the hypothesis that phrenic motor facilitation (pMF) could be elicited by direct stimulation of a signaling pathways involving A_{2A} receptors, mimicking brain derived neurotrophic factor (BDNF), which was known to be necessary and sufficient for LTF with moderate IH (Golder et al., 2008). The study found activating spinal adenosine A_{2A} receptors produced pMF in anesthetized rats and increased normoxic ventilatory drive in conscious rats. Subsequently, this adenosine mechanism has been shown to work by G_S signaling and contributes to LTF with severe IH as demonstrated by decreased LTF following spinal (intrathecal) administration of MSX-3 (Nichols et al., 2012). We hypothesized that longer exposure to moderate hypoxia may result in a comparable "dose" of hypoxia and evoke this mechanism to contribute to VAH with days of CH.

In normoxic control rats, chronic systemic blockade of A_{2A} receptors and presumably G_S signaling with MSX-3 did not affect $\dot{V}_I$ breathing 21% O_2 but it did increase $\dot{V}_I$ breathing 10% O_2 (**Figure 2A**). Spinal MSX-3 has no effect on phrenic nerve activity during normoxia in anesthetized rats using severe IH for LTF studies (Nichols et al., 2012), which agrees with our results in normoxic controls breathing 21% O_2. However, MSX-3 did not affect PA in the LTF study (Nichols et al., 2012),

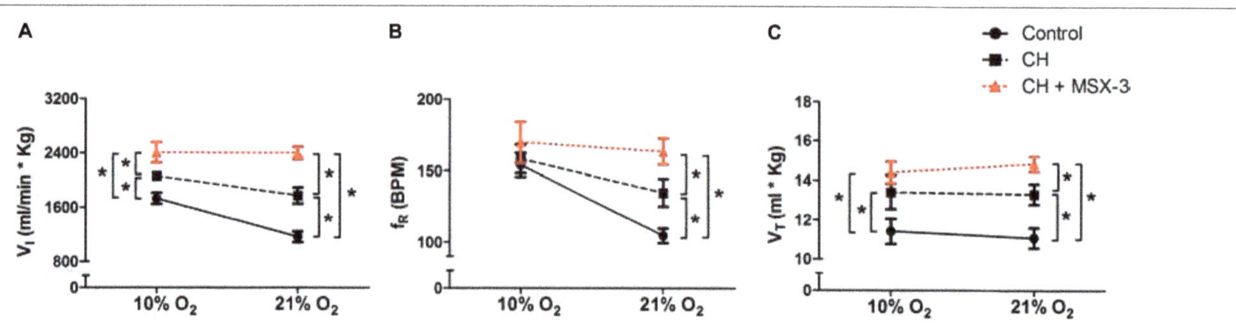

FIGURE 4 | Repeated measurements blocking A_{2A} receptors after VAH was established. Blocking A_{2A} receptors with MSX-3 after CH increased ventilation ($\dot{V}_I$, **A**), more than CH alone in acute hypoxia or normoxia. This was caused by significant increases in respiratory frequency (f_R, **B**) and tidal volume (V_T, **C**) in normoxia (21% O_2) that were not observed in acute hypoxia (10% O_2). *$p < 0.05$, Bonferroni after repeated measurement two-way ANOVA, *n* = 9 rats.

in contrast to the increase we would predict from effects we observed in acute hypoxia (**Figure 2A**). The duration of hypoxic exposure, duration of A_{2A} receptor blockade, effects of A_{2A} receptor blockade in other parts of the reflex pathway outside the spinal cord, and/or wakefulness may explain differences in the effects of MSX-between studies.

Effects of Blocking G_S and G_Q Signaling After Ventilatory Acclimatization Is Established

Acute administration of ketanserin after VAH was established by CH did not change $\dot{V}_I$ in rats breathing 21 or 10% O_2 (**Figure 3**). These results agree with experiments done in goats were administration of ketanserin did not produce significant changes after sustained hypoxia (Herman et al., 2001). In contrast, acute administration of MSX-3 after VAH was established by CH increased $\dot{V}_I$ in rats breathing 21 or 10% O_2 (**Figure 4**). Note that this is opposite the effect of MSX-3 to decrease $\dot{V}_I$ when administered during CH (compare **Figures 2, 4**). This might be explained by cross-talk inhibition between G_S and G_Q signaling that has been demonstrated recently for pMF (Hoffman et al., 2010; Devinney et al., 2013). In a model proposed for such crosstalk (see Figure 6, Devinney et al., 2016), G_S and G_Q signals following moderate acute sustained hypoxia (ASH) cancel each other so pMF is not observed. However, blocking adenosine A_{2A} receptors with MSX-3 disinhibits a 5-HT_2 receptor-dependent mechanism in moderate ASH and reveals pMF (i.e., increases phrenic activity in normoxia after moderate ASH). In contrast, blocking 5-HT_2 receptors in moderate ASH does not increase phrenic activity; the A_{2A} adenosine pathway is disinhibited but it is not sufficiently activated by moderate ASH to cause pMF. *Severe* ASH does activate the A_{2A} adenosine mechanism, however, and 5HT_2 antagonists do increase pMF following severe ASH.

Hence, our results showing increased $\dot{V}_I$ with MSX-3 after CH agree better with plasticity induced in phrenic nerve activity by moderate versus severe ASH. We observed increases in $\dot{V}_I$ after MSX-3 but not ketanserin administered after VAH was established. Also, the increases with MSX-3 after CH were greater in 21 than 10% O_2 breathing (**Figure 4**), similar to the significant effect of MSX-3 after moderate ASH on phrenic activity in normoxia (i.e., pMF) but not on the phrenic response to hypoxia (see Figure 2, Devinney et al., 2016). Together, the data do not support our hypothesis that longer durations of moderate sustained hypoxia act more like shorter exposures to severe hypoxia. However, the level of hypoxia in our awake preparations was intermediate to moderate and severe hypoxia in these other studies (e.g., Devinney et al., 2016) with arterial P_{O2} being measured as 37–42 Torr in other studies of rats breathing 10% O_2 before or after acclimatization (Aaron and Powell, 1993; Popa et al., 2011). A meta-analysis of the effects of different patterns of IH on LTF shows that the physiological consequences (e.g., hypertension versus motor nerve facilitation) depend on both the level of hypoxia and the duration of hypoxia (i.e., total number of IH bouts) (Navarrete-Opazo and Mitchell, 2014). Further study is needed to draw any firm conclusions about the level of P_{O2} necessary to evoke specific mechanisms of plasticity with short versus long-term hypoxia.

Limitations

Our results support both similarities and differences in G_Q and G_S signaling for plasticity in ventilatory control with CH and intermittent hypoxia. However, as noted above, we did not actually study specific signaling mechanisms but the effects of blocking GPCR that initiate these signaling pathways. Also, it is important that the site of action of drug effects in our experiments cannot be localized because drugs were administered systemically. Specifically, we have not studied the effects of receptor or signaling blockade in phrenic or hypoglossal motor neurons, which are primary sites of plasticity for LTF (Bach and Mitchell, 1996; Fuller et al., 2001; Baker-Herman and Mitchell, 2002). The drug effects we studied could be occurring at phrenic motor neurons but also at the at the carotid bodies, which increase O_2-sensitivity with CH (Kumar and Prabhakar, 2012), and/or the nucleus tractus solitarii, which exhibits plasticity contributing to VAH and is the site of the primary synapse from carotid body chemoreceptors is in the CNS (Pamenter and Powell, 2016). While this limits our ability to localize and test precise mechanisms, it also described the physiological consequences of systemic therapeutics acting on these mechanisms as they would occur in a clinical situation without targeted application.

The effects we observed could certainly involve phrenic motor neurons, where G_Q and G_S signaling have been described for LTF (see above). However, the changes in ventilation that we observed with ketanserin could be explained also by serotonin effects at 5-HT_2 receptors in the carotid body, which contribute to increased O_2-sensitivity with chronic intermittent hypoxia [i.e., "sensory LTF," reviewed by Peng et al. (2006) and Kumar and Prabhakar (2012)] and produced a prolonged chemosensory response to hypoxia (Jacono et al., 2005). Similarly, MSX-3 administration could involve effects on the peripheral chemoreceptors, since adenosine is modulating the activity of the carotid bodies acting through A_{2A} receptors (Nurse and Piskuric, 2013; Conde et al., 2017). Kobayashi et al. (2000) proposed that adenosine inhibits voltage-dependent Ca^{2+} currents in the glomus cells, suggesting that activation of A_{2A} receptors have a inhibitory effect on the carotid body activity. On the other hand, a recent publication from Zhang et al. (2017) demonstrated that adenosine A_{2A} receptors have a pre and postsynaptic effects in glomus cell and petrosal ganglion neuron co-cultures, which is consistent with the excitatory effects of adenosine in the carotid bodies observed by other authors (Fitzgerald et al., 2009; Nurse and Piskuric, 2013; Conde et al., 2017).

We have been especially interested in plasticity in the NTS, which is important for VAH as discussed above. Serotonin 5-HT_{2A} receptors have been reported in the NTS and to explain in excitatory postsynaptic currents (Austgen and Kline, 2013). Adenosine A_{2A} receptors in the NTS are reported to attenuate sympathetic reflexes (Minic et al., 2015) but their role in the ventilatory control has not been determined. Further investigation into possible roles for serotonin 5-HT_{2A} and adenosine A_{2A} receptors in the NTS on ventilatory chemoreflexes and testing their potential contribution to plasticity demonstrated for glutamatergic neurotransmission in the NTS with VAH (Pamenter et al., 2014a,b), still need to be investigated. Serotonin acting at central as well as peripheral sites in high altitude adapted pikas modulates the HVR (Bai et al., 2015), so there is a precedent for serotonergic effects in the CNS as well as at the carotid bodies.

CONCLUSION

The effect of manipulating G_Q and G_S signaling by blocking 5HT2 and A2a receptors, respectively, appear more similar for VAH and LTF in rats breathing normoxic versus hypoxic gas, and these effects are different before and after VAH is established. We also found some evidence for cross-talk between G_Q and G_S signaling in VAH but it was not reciprocal as demonstrated for LTF. However, all of these ideas need further research. Most LTF studies do not focus on changes in the hypoxic response like VAH studies do, but rather the long-term changes in normoxic ventilatory drive. Most importantly, we need to determine the neuroanatomical substrate for these effects in VAH and the role of these signaling pathways in chemoreceptors, CNS integrative centers and motor neurons.

AUTHOR CONTRIBUTIONS

EM and FP designed the experiments, interpreted the data, and wrote and reviewed the paper. EM performed the experiments, figures, data analysis, and first draft of the manuscript.

FUNDING

This work was supported by NIH grant R01 HL-081823.

REFERENCES

Aaron, E. A., and Powell, F. L. (1993). Effect of chronic hypoxia on hypoxic ventilatory response in awake rats. *J. Appl. Physiol.* 74, 1635–1640. doi: 10.1152/jappl.1993.74.4.1635

Austgen, J. R., and Kline, D. D. (2013). Endocannabinoids blunt the augmentation of synaptic transmission by serotonin 2A receptors in the nucleus tractus solitarii (nTS). *Brain Res.* 1537, 27–36. doi: 10.1016/j.brainres.2013.09.006

Bach, K. B., and Mitchell, G. S. (1996). Hypoxia-induced long-term facilitation of respiratory activity is serotonin dependent. *Respir. Physiol.* 104, 251–260. doi: 10.1016/0034-5687(96)00017-5

Bai, Z., Voituron, N., Wuren, T., Jeton, F., Jin, G., Marchant, D., et al. (2015). Respiratory physiology & neurobiology role of glutamate and serotonin on the hypoxic ventilatory response in high-altitude-adapted plateau Pika. *Respir. Physiol. Neurobiol.* 214, 39–45. doi: 10.1016/j.resp.2015.03.006

Baker-Herman, T. L., and Mitchell, G. S. (2002). Phrenic long-term facilitation requires spinal serotonin receptor activation and protein synthesis. *J. Neurosci.* 22, 6239–6246.

Conde, S. V., Monteiro, E. C., and Sacramento, J. F. (2017). Purines and carotid body: new roles in pathological conditions. *Front. Pharmacol.* 8:913. doi: 10.3389/fphar.2017.00913

Dale-Nagle, E. A., Hoffman, M. S., MacFarlane, P. M., Satriotomo, I., Lovett-Barr, M. R., Vinit, S., et al. (2010). Spinal plasticity following intermittent hypoxia: implications for spinal injury. *Ann. N. Y. Acad. Sci.* 1198, 252–259. doi: 10.1111/j.1749-6632.2010.05499.x

Devinney, M. J., Huxtable, A. G., Nichols, N. L., and Mitchell, G. S. (2013). Hypoxia-induced phrenic long-term facilitation: emergent properties. *Ann. N. Y. Acad. Sci.* 1279, 143–153. doi: 10.1111/nyas.12085

Devinney, M. J., Nichols, N. L., and Mitchell, G. S. (2016). Sustained hypoxia elicits competing spinal mechanisms of phrenic motor facilitation. *J. Neurosci.* 36, 7877–7885. doi: 10.1523/JNEUROSCI.4122-15.2016

Drorbaugh, J. E., and Fenn, W. O. (1955). A barometric method for measuring ventilation in newborn infants. *Pediatrics* 16, 81–87.

Fitzgerald, R. S., Shirahata, M., and Chang, I. (2009). The impact of adenosine and an A2A adenosine receptor agonist on the ACh-induced increase in intracellular calcium of the glomus cells of the cat carotid body. *Brain Res.* 1301, 20–33. doi: 10.1016/j.brainres.2009.08.100

Fuller, D. D., Zabka, A. G., Baker, T. L., and Mitchell, G. S. (2001). Phrenic long-term facilitation requires 5-HT receptor activation during but not following episodic hypoxia. *J. Appl. Physiol.* 90, 2001–2006; discussion 2000.

Golder, F. J., Ranganathan, L., Satriotomo, I., Hoffman, M., Lovett-Barr, M. R., Watters, J. J., et al. (2008). Spinal adenosine a2a receptor activation elicits long-lasting phrenic motor facilitation. *J. Neurosci.* 28, 2033–2042. doi: 10.1523/JNEUROSCI.3570-07.2008

Herman, J. K., O'Halloran, K. D., and Bisgard, G. E. (2001). Effect of 8-OH DPAT and ketanserin on the ventilatory acclimatization to hypoxia in awake goats. *Respir. Physiol.* 124, 95–104. doi: 10.1016/S0034-5687(00)00191-192

Herman, J. K., O'Halloran, K. D., Mitchell, G. S., and Bisgard, G. E. (1999). Methysergide augments the acute, but not the sustained, hypoxic ventilatory response in goats. *Respir. Physiol.* 118, 25–37. doi: 10.1016/S0034-5687(99)00070-5

Hoffman, M. S., Golder, F. J., Mahamed, S., and Mitchell, G. S. (2010). Spinal adenosine A_{2A} receptor inhibition enhances phrenic long term facilitation following acute intermittent hypoxia. *J. Physiol.* 558, 255–266. doi: 10.1113/jphysiol.2009.180075

Jacky, J. P. (1978). A plethysmograph for long-term measurements of ventilation in unrestrained animals. *J. Appl. Physiol.* 45, 644–647.

Jacono, F. J., Peng, Y. J., Kumar, G. K., and Prabhakar, N. R. (2005). Modulation of the hypoxic sensory response of the carotid body by 5-hydroxytryptamine: role of the 5-HT2receptor. *Respir. Physiol. Neurobiol.* 145, 135–142. doi: 10.1016/j.resp.2004.10.002

Kinkead, R., and Mitchell, G. S. (1999). Time-dependent hypoxic ventilatory responses in rats: effects of ketanserin and 5-carboxamidotryptamine. *Am. J. Physiol.* 277, R658–R666.

Kobayashi, S., Conforti, L., and Millhorn, D. E. (2000). Gene expression and function of adenosine A 2A receptor in the rat carotid body. *Am. J. Physiol. Lung. Cell. Mol. Physiol.* 279, L273–L282. doi: 10.1152/ajplung.2000.279.2.L273

Kumar, P., and Prabhakar, N. R. (2012). Peripheral chemoreceptors: function and plasticity of the carotid body. *Compr. Physiol.* 2, 141–219. doi: 10.1002/cphy.c100069

MacFarlane, P. M., and Mitchell, G. S. (2009). Episodic spinal serotonin receptor activation elicits long-lasting phrenic motor facilitation by an NADPH oxidase-dependent mechanism. *J. Physiol.* 587, 5469–5481. doi: 10.1113/jphysiol.2009.176982

McGuire, M., Zhang, Y., White, D. P., and Ling, L. (2004). Serotonin receptor subtypes required for ventilatory long-term facilitation and its enhancement after chronic intermittent hypoxia in awake rats. *Am. J. Physiol. Regul. Integr. Comp. Physiol.* 286, R334–R341. doi: 10.1152/ajpregu.00463.2003

Minic, Z., O'Leary, D. S., and Scislo, T. J. (2015). NTS adenosine A 2a receptors inhibit the cardiopulmonary chemoreflex control of regional sympathetic outputs via a GABAergic mechanism. *Am. J. Physiol. Heart Circ. Physiol.* 309, H185–H197. doi: 10.1152/ajpheart.00838.2014

Navarrete-Opazo, A., and Mitchell, G. S. (2014). Therapeutic potential of intermittent hypoxia: a matter of dose. *Am. J. Physiol. Regul. Integr. Comp. Physiol.* 307, R1181–R1197. doi: 10.1152/ajpregu.00208.2014

Nichols, N. L., Dale, E. A., and Mitchell, G. S. (2012). Severe acute intermittent hypoxia elicits phrenic long-term facilitation by a novel adenosine-dependent mechanism. *J. Appl. Physiol.* 112, 1678–1688. doi: 10.1152/japplphysiol.00060.2012

Nurse, C. A., and Piskuric, N. A. (2013). Signal processing at mammalian carotid body chemoreceptors. *Semin. Cell Dev. Biol.* 24, 22–30. doi: 10.1016/j.semcdb.2012.09.006

Olson, E. B. J. (1987). Ventilatory adaptation to hypoxia occurs in serotonin-depleted rats. *Respir. Physiol.* 69, 227–235. doi: 10.1016/0034-5687(87)90029-6

Pamenter, M. E., Carr, J. A., Go, A., Fu, Z., Reid, S. G., and Powell, F. L. (2014a). Glutamate receptors in the nucleus tractus solitarius contribute to ventilatory acclimatization to hypoxia in rat. *J. Physiol.* 592, 1839–1856. doi: 10.1113/jphysiol.2013.268706

Pamenter, M. E., Nguyen, J., Carr, J. A., and Powell, F. L. (2014b). The effect of combined glutamate receptor blockade in the NTS on the hypoxic ventilatory response in awake rats differs from the effect of individual glutamate receptor blockade. *Physiol. Rep.* 2:e12092. doi: 10.14814/phy2.12092

Pamenter, M. E., and Powell, F. L. (2013). Signalling mechanisms of long term facilitation of breathing with intermittent hypoxia. *F1000Prime Rep.* 5:23. doi: 10.12703/P5-23

Pamenter, M. E., and Powell, F. L. (2016). Time domains of the hypoxic ventilatory response and their molecular basis. *Compr. Physiol.* 6, 1345–1385. doi: 10.1002/cphy.c150026

Peng, Y. J., Yuan, G., Jacono, F. J., Kumar, G. K., and Prabhakar, N. R. (2006). 5-HT evokes sensory long-term facilitation of rodent carotid body via activation of NADPH oxidase. *J. Physiol.* 576, 289–295. doi: 10.1113/jphysiol.2006.116020

Popa, D., Fu, Z., Go, A., and Powell, F. L. (2011). Ibuprofen blocks time-dependent increases in hypoxic ventilation in rats. *Respir. Physiol. Neurobiol.* 178, 381–386. doi: 10.1016/j.resp.2011.03.024

Reid, S. G., Powell, F. L., and Stephen, G. (2005). Effects of chronic hypoxia on MK-801-induced changes in the acute hypoxic ventilatory response. *J. Appl. Physiol.* 4, 2108–2114. doi: 10.1152/japplphysiol.01205.2004

Satriotomo, I., Dale, E. A., Dahlberg, J. M., and Mitchell, G. S. (2012). Repetitive acute intermittent hypoxia increases expression of proteins associated with plasticity in the phrenic motor nucleus. *Exp. Neurol.* 237, 103–115. doi: 10.1016/j.expneurol.2012.05.020

Turner, A. S., Streeter, K., Greer, J., Gordon, S., and Fuller, D. D. (2017). Pharmacological modulation of hypoxia-induced respiratory neuroplasticity. *Respir. Physiol. Neurobiol.* doi: 10.1016/j.resp.2017.11.008 [Epub ahead of print].

Zhang, M., Vollmer, C., and Nurse, C. A. (2017). Adenosine and dopamine oppositely modulate a hyperpolarization activated current I h in chemosensory neurons of the rat carotid body in co-culture. *J. Physiol.* doi: 10.1113/JP274743 [Epub ahead of print].

11

Effects on Cognitive Functioning of Acute, Subacute and Repeated Exposures to High Altitude

*Matiram Pun[1,2], Veronica Guadagni[1,2,3,4], Kaitlyn M. Bettauer[1,2,5], Lauren L. Drogos[1,2], Julie Aitken[6], Sara E. Hartmann[1,2], Michael Furian[7], Lara Muralt[7], Mona Lichtblau[7], Patrick R. Bader[7], Jean M. Rawling[8], Andrea B. Protzner[2,9], Silvia Ulrich[7], Konrad E. Bloch[7], Barry Giesbrecht[10] and Marc J. Poulin[1,2,3,4,11,12]**

[1] Department of Physiology & Pharmacology, Cumming School of Medicine, University of Calgary, Calgary, AB, Canada, [2] Hotchkiss Brain Institute, Cumming School of Medicine, University of Calgary, Calgary, AB, Canada, [3] Department of Clinical Neuroscience, Cumming School of Medicine, University of Calgary, Calgary, AB, Canada, [4] O'Brien Institute for Public Health, Cumming School of Medicine, University of Calgary, Calgary, AB, Canada, [5] Department of Psychology, Faculty of Science, University of British Columbia, Vancouver, BC, Canada, [6] Biomedical Engineering Graduate Program, University of Calgary, Calgary, AB, Canada, [7] Pulmonary Division, Sleep Disorders Centre and Pulmonary Hypertension Clinic, University Hospital Zürich, Zurich, Switzerland, [8] Department of Family Medicine, Cumming School of Medicine, University of Calgary, Calgary, AB, Canada, [9] Department of Psychology, Faculty of Arts, University of Calgary, Calgary, AB, Canada, [10] Department of Psychological and Brain Sciences, Institute for Collaborative Biotechnologies, University of California, Santa Barbara, Santa Barbara, CA, United States, [11] Libin Cardiovascular Institute of Alberta, Cumming School of Medicine, University of Calgary, Calgary, AB, Canada, [12] Faculty of Kinesiology, University of Calgary, Calgary, AB, Canada

***Correspondence:**
Marc J. Poulin
poulin@ucalgary.ca

Objective: Neurocognitive functions are affected by high altitude, however the altitude effects of acclimatization and repeated exposures are unclear. We investigated the effects of acute, subacute and repeated exposure to 5,050 m on cognition among altitude-naïve participants compared to control subjects tested at low altitude.

Methods: Twenty-one altitude-naïve individuals (25.3 ± 3.8 years, 13 females) were exposed to 5,050 m for 1 week (*Cycle 1)* and re-exposed after a week of rest at sea-level (*Cycle 2*). Baseline (BL, 520 m), acute (Day 1, HA1) and acclimatization (Day 6, HA6, 5,050 m) measurements were taken in both cycles. Seventeen control subjects (24.9 ± 2.6 years, 12 females) were tested over a similar period in Calgary, Canada (1,103 m). The Reaction Time (RTI), Attention Switching Task (AST), Rapid Visual Processing (RVP) and One Touch Stockings of Cambridge (OTS) tasks were administered and outcomes were expressed in milliseconds/frequencies. Lake Louise Score (LLS) and blood oxygen saturation (SpO_2) were recorded.

Results: In both cycles, no significant changes were found with acute exposure on the AST total score, mean latency and SD. Significant changes were found upon acclimatization solely in the altitude group, with improved AST Mean Latency [HA1 (588 ± 92) vs. HA6 (526 ± 91), $p < 0.001$] and Latency SD [HA1 (189 ± 86) vs. HA6 (135 ± 65), $p < 0.001$] compared to acute exposure, in *Cycle 1*. No significant differences were present in the control group. When entering Acute SpO_2 (HA1-BL), Acclimatization SpO_2 (HA6-BL) and LLS score as covariates for both cycles, the effects of acclimatization on AST outcomes disappeared indicating that the changes were partially explained by SpO_2

and LLS. The changes in AST Mean Latency [ΔBL (−61.2 ± 70.2) vs. ΔHA6 (−28.0 ± 58), $p = 0.005$] and the changes in Latency SD [ΔBL (−28.4 ± 41.2) vs. ΔHA6 (−0.2235 ± 34.8), $p = 0.007$] across the two cycles were smaller with acclimatization. However, the percent changes did not differ between cycles. These results indicate independent effects of altitude across repeated exposures.

Conclusions: Selective and sustained attention are impaired at altitude and improves with acclimatization.The observed changes are associated, in part, with AMS score and SpO_2. The gains in cognition with acclimatization during a first exposure are not carried over to repeated exposures.

Keywords: altitude, cognition, hypoxia, brain, CANTAB, AMS/LLS, SpO_2, ALMA

INTRODUCTION

Mountains occupy one fifth of the earth's surface and are popular destinations for a variety of activities such as trekking, climbing, pilgrimages, mining, scientific experiments and celestial observations. Further, more than 140 million people worldwide live at altitudes over >2,500 m, (Penaloza and Arias-Stella, 2007) and many high-altitude dwellers sojourn at lower altitudes. The barometric pressure decreases exponentially with altitude gain and this hypobaric hypoxia leads to reduced inspired partial pressure of oxygen (West, 1996). Unacclimatized lowlanders may suffer from cerebral symptoms such as headache, nausea, vomiting and impaired coordination when exposed to high altitudes (>2,500 m) (Hackett and Roach, 2001; Bärtsch and Swenson, 2013). The brain, particularly the hippocampus and other areas within the limbic system, is very sensitive and vulnerable to hypoxia (Hornbein, 2001; Virués-Ortega et al., 2004; Wilson et al., 2009).

High altitude exposure has a detrimental effect on cognitive functions with slower reaction times and reduced psychomotor vigilance i.e., slower reaction times as a measure of reduced sustained attention (high altitude, 1,500–3,500 m); impaired learning, spatial and working memory (very high altitude, 3,500–5,500 m) and impaired memory retrieval (extreme altitude, >5,500 m) (Virués-Ortega et al., 2004; Wilson et al., 2009; Yan, 2014; Taylor et al., 2016; Bickler et al., 2017; McMorris et al., 2017). The effects of hypoxia on cognitive functions have been previously explored among climbers (Kramer et al., 1993), trekkers (Dykiert et al., 2010), military personnel (Shukitt-Hale et al., 1998), flight crews (Nation et al., 2017), and high altitude residents (Virues-Ortega et al., 2011; Wang et al., 2014). Kramer et al. for example, report impairments in learning and memory processes especially when individuals were required to learn new skills while executing perceptual and semantic memory tasks. Similarly, Shukitt-Hale et al. report deterioration of both mood and performance in military personnel exposed to high-altitude. Futher, high altitude exposure has been shown to increase reaction times and impair memory encoding and retention (McMorris et al., 2017; Nation et al., 2017). However, Dykiert et al. suggest more pronounced changes in mean reaction times only above 4,000 m. Different types of hypoxic exposures such as field (Subudhi et al., 2014; Davranche et al., 2016), simulated hypobaric hypoxia (Hornbein et al., 1989; Asmaro et al., 2013; Malle et al., 2013), normobaric hypoxia (Turner et al., 2015) and intermittent hypoxia (Champod et al., 2013) have been investigated. Davranche et al. showed impaired information processing (speed and accuracy) at high altitude while Hornbein et al. reported impaired visual long-term memory during chamber simulation. With very high altitude exposure (5,260 m), Subudhi et al. found impairments in reaction times and in performance on the code substitution tasks (simultaneous and match to sample) which then improved with acclimatization. In the study by Malle et al., an increased rate of error frequency and worsened working memory were reported while Asmaro et al. observed impairments in cognitive flexibility and attention, short-term and working memory and executive functions. Similarly, Turner et al found that acute normobaric hypoxia affected memory, attention and executive functions. Although the aforementioned studies differ in types of hypoxic exposure, duration, modality and severity, the reported neurocognitive impairments are consistent across studies (Virués-Ortega et al., 2004; McMorris et al., 2017). Regardless, the significant differences across study design and the inadequately powered sample sizes limit the currently available studies and futher research is therefore needed.

A large number of high altitude workers, such as the ones involved in the large mining industry in the Chilean mountains or scientists, engineers and staff at the Atacama Large Millimeter/submillimeter Array (ALMA) scientific observatory, travel periodically to high altitudes for work. The workers at ALMA are periodically exposed to "very high altitude" (i.e., 5,050 m) for an entire week [including sleep periods at "high altitude" (i.e., 2,950 m)] followed by a week of rest at near-sea level (i.e., 520 m). Hypoxia associated with high altitude may impair cognitive performance and therefore it may lead to higher rates of errors (Hornbein et al., 1989; Davranche et al., 2016) and elevated risks of occupational injuries while performing their duties as seen among high altitude miners (Vearrier and Greenberg, 2011). However, there is no study examining the effects of this unique ascent profile and work schedule at very high altitude on cognitive functioning.

Hence, here we investigate the effects of acute, acclimatization, and repeated exposure to very high altitude on cognitive functions in altitude-naïve individuals bringing them to ALMA (5,050 m) with the same schedule that the workers would follow over a month. We hypothesize that acute exposure to high altitude will result in slower reaction times, decreased attention and reduced executive functions (reduced flexibility and ability to shift, greater fixation, reduced executive control and planning ability) which will then be restored with acclimatization. Further, we hypothesize that the positive changes in cognitive function due to acclimatization will be carried over to repeated exposure after a week of rest at low altitude. Finally, we aim to explore the role of AMS and blood oxygen saturation (SpO_2) on changes in cognitive functions.

MATERIALS AND METHODS

Participants

A total of 41 participants (21 altitude-exposed, 20 controls) were recruited. All participants provided written informed consent. Inclusion criteria were currently living at <1,300 m (participants must have been living in Calgary, 1,103 m, for at least 1 year) and no overnight stays at altitudes >1,500 m during the 4 weeks preceding the study. Exclusion criteria included previous history of altitude illnesses at moderate altitude (<3,000 m), current pregnancy, and health impairment that required regular treatment. The screening for the inclusion/exclusion of participants was carried out at the Foothills Medical Center, Cumming School of Medicine, University of Calgary, Calgary, Canada (1,103 m). Twenty-one altitude-naive healthy young adults (age = 25.2 ± 3.7 years, education = 17.1 ± 2.5 years, 13 females, BMI = 24.5 ± 8.1 $kg{\cdot}m^{-2}$) took part in the high-altitude expedition, 18 of whom lived in Calgary and three of whom lived in Zurich and surrounding area (Switzerland, altitude 490 m) and were therefore screened at University Hospital of Zurich, Zurich, Switzerland. Twenty altitude-naive healthy young adults completed the testing sessions at the University of Calgary, Canada (altitude, 1,103 m), and formed the control group. Within the control group, three participants did not complete the cognitive sessions for reasons external to the study, and therefore were excluded from the analyses. Hence, the control group included a total of 17 participants in the final analyses (age = 24.9 ± 2.6 years, education = 16.8 ± 1.8 years, 12 females, BMI = 23.4 ± 2.7 kgm^{-2}). The total final sample included in the analyses (from both Altitude and Control) consisted of 38 participants (age = 25.1 ± 3.2 years, education = 17 ± 2.2 years, 25 females). The study was approved by the University of Calgary Conjoint Health Research Ethics Board (CHREB ID: REB15-2709) and registered as a clinical trial in ClinicalTrials.gov (NCT02738307). The flow of study participants through the Altitude and Control protocols is illustrated in **Figure 1**.

Study Design

The high-altitude exposure schedule spanned over the course of a month with two cycles of high altitude exposure (*Cycle 1* and *Cycle 2*) separated by a week at low altitude (**Figure 2**). The baseline measurements were taken in Santiago, Chile (520 m). The participants then flew to the Calama airport (~2 h) and took a bus (~2 h) to the basecamp at The Atacama Large Millimeter/submillimeter Array (ALMA) Operation Support Facility (ALMA ASF; 2,900 m). The participants traveled to the ALMA Observatory (5,050 m) by motor vehicle (about 45 min). Throughout the 6-day high altitude expedition (*Cycles 1* and *2*), participants spent nights at a support facility (ASF, 2,900 m) and commuted to ALMA Observatory (5,050 m) by motor vehicle to spend 4–8 h each day. According to ALMA policy, the participants were allowed to spend only 4 h at 5,050 m on the first day. Recovery measurements were taken in Santiago, Chile (520 m). The control subjects followed the same testing schedule as the altitude group at the Brain Dynamics Lab, The University of Calgary, Calgary, Canada without changes in altitude (1,103 m). An overview of the cognitive testing schedule is illustrated in **Figure 2** (**Figure 2A** for altitude and **Figure 2B** for control). The first test was a familiarization test in *Cycle 1* while the second test was the baseline (BL). The first measurement at altitude (test 3 on day 1 of altitude exposure) was an acute exposure test (HA1) while test 4 at altitude (on day 6 of altitude exposure) was an acclimatization measurement (HA6). A similar schedule was followed in *Cycle 2*, and the same testing schedule and protocol (i.e., high-altitude protocol) was mirrored in the control group.

Cognitive Test Battery

Cognitive tests assessed three domains of cognitive function: processing speed, sustained attention and executive functions. We created a custom battery with tests available within the Cambridge Neuropsychological Test Automated Battery (CANTAB® Cogntive Assessment Software; Cambridge Cognition, 1994). The CANTAB cognition battery can be administered several times while controlling for learning and repetition effects (Lowe and Rabbitt, 1998; Syväoja et al., 2015). This is achieved by generating random stimuli each time a participant logs in into his/her account for a new testing phase. The tests were administered on iPad Air 1 (model: A1474, dimensions: 9.7 inches retina display, iSO 9.3.1, Apple Inc., Cupertino, CA) and were completed in 30 min. The battery was administered nine times over the course of the expedition and nine times in controls as illustrated in **Figure 2** (**Figure 2A** for altitude and **Figure 2B** for controls). The individual components of the CANTAB battery included the Reaction Time (RTI) task to assess processing speed, the Attention Switching Task (AST) and the Rapid Visual Processing (RVP) task to assess attention and the One Touch Stockings of Cambridge (OTS) to test executive functions. The CANTAB cognition outcome measures, along with their abbreviations,and examples of the tasks, have been illustrated in **Figure 3**.

The RTI task is a measure of motor and processing speed. Participants are required to hold a button at the bottom of the screen (starting position). Circles are presented at the top of the screen (either 1 or 5 circles) and at some point, one of the circles will flash yellow. Participants must then tap the

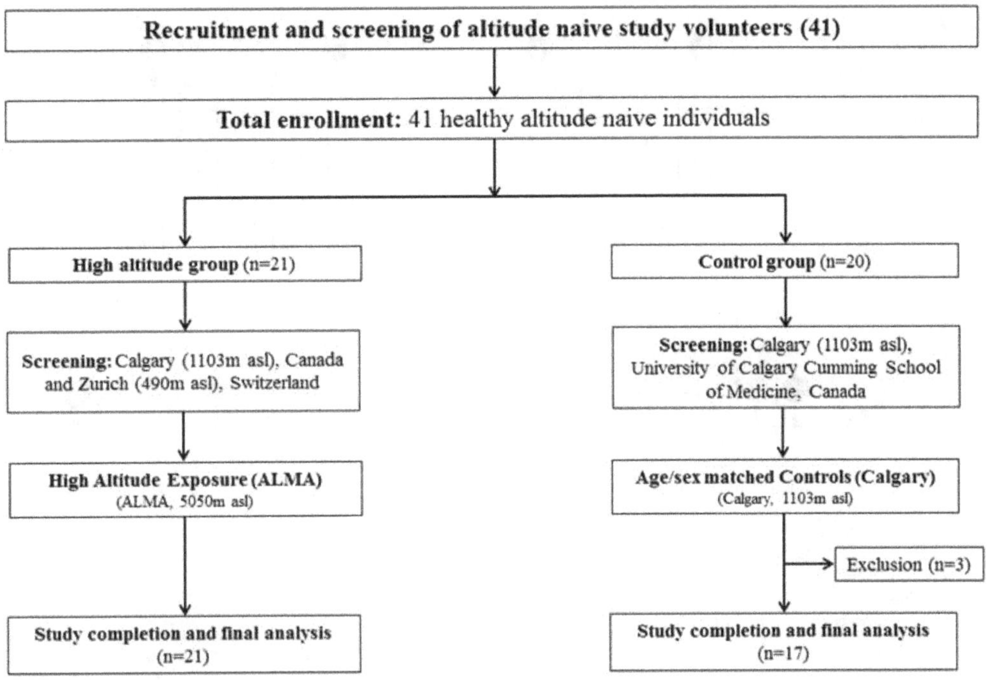

FIGURE 1 | Study flowchart for Altitude and Control group study participants. Figure illustrates participant flow through the experimental protocols (CONSORT diagram) showing the flow of study participants for high altitude protocol (ALMA) and controls (Calgary). n, number; asl, above sea level; m, meter; kg, kilogram; ALMA, the Atacama Large Millimeter Array.

highlighted circle as quickly as possible and then go back to the starting position. The outcome measures that we analyzed for this task are limited to the harder condition including 5 circles. The median reaction time (RTIFMDRT) considers how long it takes for the participants to touch the yellow circle after perceiving the change in color. Movement time (RTIFMMT) instead refers to the interval between the release of the starting position button and contact with the yellow circle. The AST measures individuals' ability to inhibit irrelevant information (selective attention). An arrow appears on the screen either on the left or right portion of the screen, pointing in either direction. Each trial displays a cue prompting the participant to press the left or right button on the screen to evaluate either the position of the arrow in the screen or the direction where the arrow is pointing. The RVP task is a measure of sustained attention. During the test, an array of numbers from 2 to 9 is presented in a pseudo-randomized order in the middle of the screen. The participants are required to press as fast as they can a button at the bottom of the screen when they see a certain array (2-4-6, 4-6-8, and 3-5-7). The OTS task measures executive function and the ability to plan. The participants are shown combinations of three-dimensional (3-D) colored balls and they must indicate in a box at the bottom of the screen, the number of moves (least possible amount) that they think are required to reproduce the same combination from a different starting position. All the CANTAB parameters were measured in milliseconds (ms) except ASTTC and OTSPSFC which represented frequencies (n).

Lake Louise Score (LLS) and SpO_2

AMS was assessed using the Lake Louise Score (LLS) (Roach et al., 1993) and diagnosed when the total LLS score was ≥ 5 (Maggiorini et al., 1998; Dellasanta et al., 2007). The SpO_2 was measured at rest with a finger pulse oximeter placed on the index finger.

Data Analyses

Cognitive outcomes

Cognitive changes over the course of the high-altitude exposure compared to baseline were analyzed with a series of Repeated Measures Mixed Model Analyses of Variance (RM-ANOVAs). We utilized RM-ANOVA to test our *a priori* hypothesis of expected changes in cognitive outcomes from baseline (BL, 520 m) to acute exposure to altitude (HA1) and acclimatization period (HA6) during each cycle. The cognitive outcome measures at BL, HA1 and HA6 were entered as within-subjects factors (altitude exposure*3) while group (Altitude vs. Control) as between-subjects factor in the analysis model. Cognitive outcome measures (RTI, AST, RVP and OTS) for *Cycle 1* and *Cycle 2* were analyzed separately to test the specific hypothesis of carry-over effects due to re exposure to very high altitude. All the analyses were two-tailed, and statistical significance was set at $p < 0.05$. Descriptive data were expressed as mean $\pm$ standard deviation (mean $\pm$ SD) and were assessed for violation of normality. Greenhouse-Geisser (GG) correction was used when sphericity, as measured with the Mauchly's test, was violated. Only significant altitude exposure (BL, HA1, HA6)

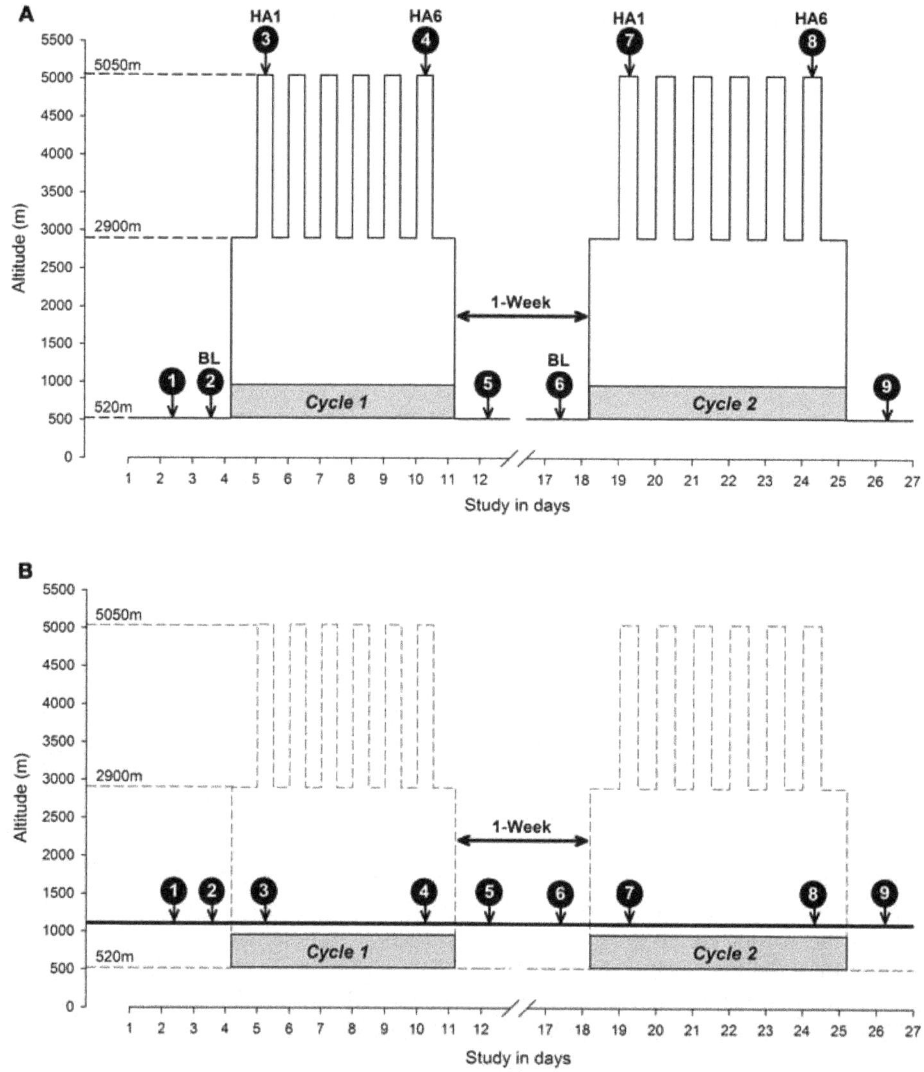

FIGURE 2 | Study design diagram: Altitude vs. Control. **(A)** Altitude study protocol in which study participants were exposed to altitude at ALMA; **(B)** Control study protocol in which data were collected in Calgary. The y-axis depicts altitude in meters and the x-axis depicts the study time in days. The dashed lines connecting to the y-axis indicates altitude as baseline altitude (Santiago, 520 m), sleeping altitude (ALMA Operations Support Facility Center, 2,900 m) and high altitude working station (ALMA, 5,050 m). The downward arrows indicate the nine cognitive function testing sessions over 26 days at corresponding altitude in y-axis and expedition days in x-axis during two cycles of high altitude expedition interspersed with a week of resting at low altitude. The average altitude exposure at ALMA Observatory work station during each day was ~4–8 hrs/day. The remainder of the time was spent at the ALMA base camp of an altitude of 2,900 m to sleep. In the control protocol **(B)**, the high-altitude cycle (expedition) has been depicted as dashed lines but experimental altitude (Calgary, 1,103 m asl) has been depicted as a bold solid line crossing the two cycles with data collection time points (white numbers inside black filled circles with arrows going down to respective days matching high altitude protocol similar to **A**). The solid line with arrows on both sides between two cycles (1-Week) indicates 7 days rest a low altitude separating two cycles in both panels. BL, baseline; HA1, high altitude acute exposure at day 1; HA6, high altitude acclimatization exposure at day 6; 1-Week, one week break between two cycles of expedition in **(A)** and data collection in **(B)**.

* group (altitude, controls) interactions were followed up by using pairwise comparisons with Bonferroni corrections to test within group differencies at each altitude exposure. The statistical analyses were carried out using the Statistical Package for the Social Sciences (SPSS, Version 24, IBM Corporation, New York 10504-1722, USA). The graphical illustration (study design and changes in cognition plots) were genereated using SyStat (SigmaPlot 13.0, Systat Software Inc, San Jose, CA, USA).

Covariates

To examine the contribution of SpO_2 changes and total LLS to changes in cognitive measure due to altitude exposure, we used a Repeated Measures Analyses of Covariance (RM-ANCOVAs) with either SpO_2 changes or LLS as covariates. The changes in SpO_2 with altitude exposure were computed as acute change in SpO_2 (Acute SpO_2 = HA1 – BL), acclimatization change in SpO_2 (Acclimatization SpO_2 = HA6 – BL) and change in SpO_2 at

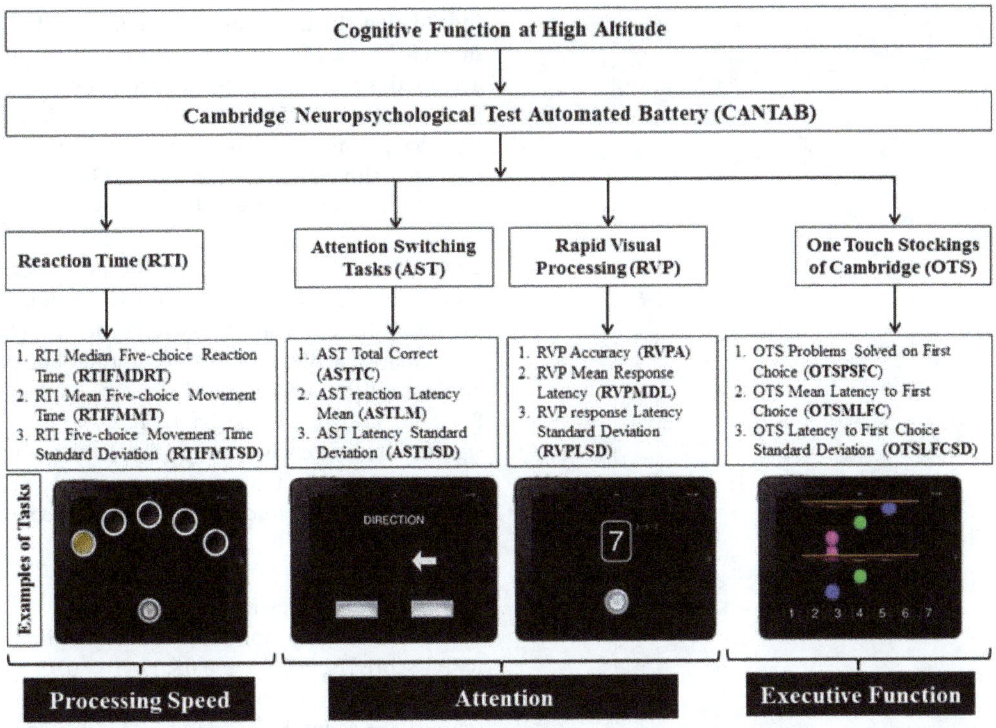

FIGURE 3 | CANTAB battery tests that were incorporated in the study. Reaction time (RTI), attention (AST and RVP) and executive functions (OTS) have been tested. The red boxes indicate the grouping classification of the test batteries i.e. reaction time, attention and executive function. The bottom part of the figure illustrates representative example pictures of respective CANTAB battery/task used in the study (Cambridge Cognition, 1994) from left to right: RTI, AST, RVP, and OTS.

high altitude (Altitude SpO_2 = HA6 - HA1). The changes were calculated for both cycles separately.

Acclimatization carry-over effects over the cycles

We tested the carry-over effects from *Cycle 1* to *Cycle 2* by computing differences in scores at baseline (ΔBL), acute exposure (ΔHA1) and acclimatization (ΔHA6) for each cognitive outcome measures i.e., change (Δ) = *Cycle 2 - Cycle 1* at each data point in two cycles. Another RM-ANOVA was used to analyze persisting differences across the two cycles at different altitude exposures. We further extended our analysis to explore the acclimatization carry-over effects by calculating percent change in the cognitive variables and comparing them between the two cycles with paired t-tests. The acute percent change was calculated as [(BL-HA1)/BL*100] and acclimatization percent change as [(BL-HA6)/BL*100] whereas percent change at high altitude as [(HA1-HA6)/HA1*100] for both cycles.

RESULTS

Details of the analyzed cognitive outcomes (mean ± SD) with RM-ANOVA for the altitude group and control participants are presented in **Table 1**. The more extensive descriptive data for all valid entries across all the sessions for both *Cycle 1* (Familiarization, FL; Baseline, BL; Acute exposure, HA1 and Acclimatization exposure, HA6 and Recovery, REC) and *Cycle 2* (Baseline, BL; Acute exposure, HA1 and Acclimatization exposure, HA6 and Recovery, REC) in both altitude and control groups have been presented in the **Supplemental Table 1**.

High Altitude Exposure: *Cycle 1*

Cognitive Outcomes

Reaction Time (RTI)

There was a significant main effect of altitude exposure (BL = 361.0 ± 37.0, HA1 = 367.1 ± 52.5, HA6 = 353.8 ± 31.8) on the RTIFMTSD [$F_{(1.331,42.590)} = 6.01$, $p = 0.012$ GG, $\eta_p^2 = 0.158$). However, there was no group-by-phase interaction ($p = 0.181$) meaning that there were no differences between the altitude group and controls at different altitude exposures. There was no main effect of altitude or group-by-phase interaction on the RTIFMDRT and the RTIFMMT.

Attention Switching Task (AST)

There was a main effect of altitude exposure [BL = 544.3 ± 94.2, HA1 = 534.7 ± 89.3, HA6 = 503.9 ± 79.9, $F_{(2, 64)} = 11.2$, $p < 0.001$, $\eta_p^2 = 0.259$] and a group by altitude exposure interaction (altitude vs. controls) [$F_{(2, 64)} = 4.6$, $p = 0.013$, $\eta_p^2 = 0.126$] on the ASTLM scores. This means that there were significant differences between the altitude and control groups

TABLE 1 | Cognitive parameters of altitude and control participants at baseline, acute and acclimatization exposures from *Cycle 1* and *Cycle 2*.

	Cycle 1						*Cycle 2*					
	BL		HA1		HA6		BL		HA1		HA6	
	Alt (Sant)	Ctrl (Calg)	Alt (ALMA)	Ctrl (Calg)	Alt (ALMA)	Ctrl (Calg)	Alt (Sant)	Ctrl (Calg)	Alt (ALMA)	Ctrl (Calg)	Alt (ALMA)	Ctrl (Calg)
REACTION TIME (ms)												
RTIFMDRT	365.3 ± 40.2	356.8 ± 34.5	379.4 ± 54.4	354.9 ± 49.1	355.0 ± 33.8	352.8 ± 30.8	362.7 ± 38.5	354.9 ± 32.9	358.5 ± 33.3	350.2 ± 29.4	351.0 ± 41.6	348.7 ± 26.5
RTIFMMT	192.4 ± 76.0	189.9 ± 44.1	242.3 ± 145.2	188.6 ± 43.3	203.5 ± 78.3	190.5 ± 41.5	198.0 ± 85.3	187.5 ± 38.9	203.5 ± 74.6	185.4 ± 39.5	175.8 ± 61.9	184.9 ± 41.0
RTIFMTSD	26.5 ± 10.3	31.3 ± 11.3	48.3 ± 44.0	38.7 ± 22.2	27.7 ± 11.8	34.1 ± 17.8	30.6 ± 15.6	31.9 ± 16.8	35.3 ± 21.2	27.7 ± 11.7	23.1 ± 7.5	36.3 ± 27.4
ATTENTION (ms/*n*)												
ASTTC (*n*)	155.3 ± 7.7	157.8 ± 2.7	151.9 ± 13.2	157.2 ± 2.6	156.4 ± 3.5	157.4 ± 2.3	156.0 ± 3.0	158.0 ± 2.5	152.1 ± 7.3	157.1 ± 2.5	154.8 ± 3.7	156.9 ± 3.3
ASTLM	572.6 ± 98.1	516.0 ± 83.6	574.9 ± 84.3***	494.6 ± 77.0	517.1 ± 81.4***	490.8 ± 78.8	510.1 ± 77.7	469.9 ± 67.8	528.4 ± 96.6*	471.9 ± 70.2	485.2 ± 82.1*	470.7 ± 63.9
ASTLSD	166.3 ± 61.9	131.4 ± 62.9	177.0 ± 78.9***	127.1 ± 46.9	125.8 ± 57.5***	120.6 ± 56.0	137.3 ± 62.0	107.1 ± 41.0	164.3 ± 82.3**	113.1 ± 43.2	122.5 ± 53.4**	115.6 ± 49.0
RVPA	0.96 ± 0.05	0.96 ± 0.07	0.94 ± 0.08	0.97 ± 0.03	0.97 ± 0.04	0.98 ± 0.02	0.97 ± 0.05	0.98 ± 0.02	0.96 ± 0.05	0.99 ± 0.02	0.98 ± 0.04	0.99 ± 0.02
RVPMDL	427.0 ± 41.1	402.9 ± 50.0	467.0 ± 110.7	395.2 ± 44.2	410.1 ± 35.2	391.4 ± 35.1	414.7 ± 46.4	381.5 ± 34.7	414.8 ± 34.8	378.6 ± 34.6	392.9 ± 36.6	394.6 ± 42.2
RVPLSD	109.5 ± 43.0	117.8 ± 123.0	123.0 ± 91.6	95.8 ± 63.4	104.1 ± 67.9	91.4 ± 47.0	103.4 ± 58.3	81.2 ± 44.0	132.7 ± 95.1	85.3 ± 40.0	88.8 ± 44.7	85.6 ± 56.6
EXECUTIVE FUNCTION (ms/*n*)												
OTSPSFC (*n*)	12.4 ± 1.8	12.2 ± 1.8	11.9 ± 1.7	12.5 ± 0.9	12.1 ± 2.0	12.4 ± 1.5	13.1 ± 1.6	12.8 ± 1.9	12.0 ± 2.0	12.9 ± 1.9	12.6 ± 1.7	12.8 ± 1.6
OTSMLFC	14,575.5 ± 5,670.1	13,615.5 ± 5,282.7	11,917.9 ± 5,382.6	14,092.9 ± 5,766.3	10,960.2 ± 7,442.5	10,650.0 ± 4,035.9	11,724.9 ± 14,035.0	10,190.8 ± 4,799.3	9,014.3 ± 5,038.3	10,188.3 ± 4,683.9	6,940 ± 2,141	9,711.0 ± 3,933.1
OTSLFCSD	16,425.9 ± 9,036.1	14,867.7 ± 8,546.1	12,687.6 ± 7,740.9	15,925.1 ± 10,273.4	10,531.6 ± 9,235.8	11,074.2 ± 6,830.9	13,783.4 ± 20,937.9	10,490.0 ± 7,068.4	9,544.1 ± 7,884.5	11,474.9 ± 7,297.5	5,990.2 ± 2,673.6	11,422.2 ± 7,297.2

The mean and SD presented here are from the Repeated Measure ANOVA.

**** <0.001, ** <0.01, * <0.05; The asterisks (*) indicate statistically significant group-by-altitude exposure interaction.*

at different altitudes. Follow-up pairwise comparisons revealed indeed that, in the altitude group, the ASTLM score was not impacted by acute exposure to altitude, but decreased with the acclimatization compared to acute exposure [HA1 (587.9 ± 91.9) vs. HA6 (525.8 ± 91.2), $t_{(19)} = 5.784$, $p < 0.001$]. No significant differences were present in the control group. We observed similar effects for the ASTLSD with a main effect of altitude exposure [BL= 148.8 ± 63.9, HA1 = 152.0 ± 69.0, HA6 = 123.2 ± 55.9, $F_{(2, 64)} = 9.3$, $p < 0.001$, $\eta_p^2 = 0.226$] and a group (altitude *vs* controls) by altitude exposure interaction [$F_{(2, 64)} = 4.8$, $p = 0.011$, $\eta_p^2 = 0.131$]. At follow up comparisons in the altitude group exclusively, the ASTLSD score was not impacted by acute exposure to altitude but decreased with the acclimatization as compared to acute exposure [HA1 (189.4 ± 86.1) vs. HA6 (134.5 ± 64.9); $t_{(19)} = 5.427$, $p < 0.001$]. No significant differences were found in the control group. There was no main effect of altitude exposure, nor group (altitude vs. control) by altitude exposure interaction for the ASTTC score.

Rapid Visual Processing (RVP)

There was a significant main effect of altitude exposure on the RVPA score [BL= 0.95 ± 0.05, HA1 = 0.95 ± 0.06, HA6 = 0.97 ± 0.03; $F_{(2, 64)} = 3.5$, $p = 0.037$, $\eta_p^2 = 0.098$] and on the RVPMDL score [BL= 414.9 ± 46.7, HA1 = 431.1 ± 90.6, HA6 = 400.7 ± 35.8; $F_{(1.376,44.021)} = 3.6$, $p = 0.03$, $\eta_p^2 = 0.1$]. However, the group by altitude exposure interactions showed only a trend (RVPA, $p = 0.162$, $\eta_p^2 = 0.055$ and RVPMDL, $p = 0.064$, $\eta_p^2 = 0.093$). The RVPLSD did not change with altitude or between groups.

One Touch Stockings of Cambridge (OTS)

We observed a main effect of altitude exposure on both OTSMLFC [BL= 12.26 ± 1.78, HA1 = 12.20 ± 1.38, HA6 = 12.24 ± 1.74; $F_{(2, 64)} = 6.861$, $p = 0.002$, $\eta_p^2 = 0.177$] score and OTSLFCSD [BL= 15646.7 ± 8696.2, HA1 = 14306.3 ± 9106.2, HA6 = 10802.8 ± 8003.5; $F_{(2, 64)} = 5.081$, $p = 0.009$, $\eta_p^2 = 0.137$] but no group by altitude exposure interactions. However, there was no main effect of altitude exposure and group by altitude exposure interaction on the OTSPSFC score.

SpO_2 and Lake Louise Score (LLS)

The effect of altitude exposure on ASTLM reported previously during acute and acclimatization visits disappeared when controlling for Acute SpO_2 and Acclimatization SpO_2. However, the effect of altitude exposure on ASTLM persisted when controlling for Altitude SpO_2 [$F_{(2, 30)} = 7.6$, $p = 0.002$, $\eta_p^2 = 0.338$]. Similar observations were found in ASTLSD. The differences in altitude exposure on ASTLSD when controlling for both Acute SpO_2 and Acclimatization SpO_2 disappeared but the altitude exposure effect persisted when controlling for Altitude SpO_2 [$F_{(2, 30)} = 9.2$, $p = 0.001$, $\eta_p^2 = 0.38$]. During acute exposure (HA1), when total LLS was entered as covariate, the changes in ASTLM due to altitude still persisted [$F_{(2, 30)} = 3.6$, $p = 0.039$, $\eta_p^2 = 0.195$]. On the contrary, the effect of altitude exposure on ASTLSD disappeared with LLS as covariate.

High Altitude Exposure: *Cycle 2*

Cognitive Outcomes

Reaction Time (RTI)

The RTIFMTSD score had no main effect of altitude exposure, but a group by altitude exposure interaction [$F_{(2, 70)} = 5.96$, $p = 0.004$, $\eta_p^2 = 0.145$]. The follow up comparisons showed that the RTIFMTSD score was not affected by the acute altitude exposure. However, it decreased after the acclimatization from acute exposure [HA1 (35.2 ± 21.1) vs. HA6 (23 ± 8), $t_{(19)} = 2.590$, $p = 0.018$]. These results, however, did not survive Bonferroni correction for multiple comparisons. The RM-ANOVA on the RTIFMDRT score and on the RTIFMMT score did not show any significant effects of altitude exposure. No significant differences were present in the control group.

Attention Switching Task (AST)

There was a main effect of altitude exposure [BL= 156.8 ± 2.9, HA1 = 154 ± 6, HA6 = 155.7 ± 3.6, $F_{(1.436,50.272)} = 7.6$, $p = 0.004_{GG}$, $\eta_p^2 = 0.178$] on the ASTTC and a group by altitude exposure interaction [$F_{(1.436,50.272)} = 3.6$, $p = 0.034_{GG}$, $\eta_p^2 = 0.092$]. In the follow up comparisons, the ASTTC decreased from baseline to altitude [BL (156 ± 3) vs. HA1 (152.3 ± 7.2), $t_{(20)} = 2.889$, $p = 0.009$] and improved with the acclimatization [HA1 (152.1 ± 7.2) vs. HA6 (154.7 ± 3.6), $t_{(19)} = -2.309$, $p = 0.032$] only in the altitude group. However, the changes did not survive multiple comparisons correction. There was a main effect of altitude exposure (BL = 492 ± 75, HA1 = 502 ± 89, HA6 = 478.5 ± 73.6, $F_{(2, 70)} = 3.471$, $p = 0.037$, $\eta_p^2 = 0.09$] on the ASTLM score and a group by altitude exposure interaction [$F_{(2, 70)} = 3.144$, $p = 0.049$, $\eta_p^2 = 0.082$]. In the follow-up comparisons, ASTLM score slightly increased with acute exposure although this change was not significant. However, ASTLM score significantly decreased with the acclimatization compared to acute exposure [HA1 (528.4 ± 96.6) vs. HA6 (485.2 ± 82.1), $t_{(19)} = 2.879$, $p = 0.010$] in the altitude group and not in the control group. Similarly, we found a main effect of altitude exposure (BL = 123.4 ± 54.8, HA1 = 140.7 ± 71.2, HA6 = 119.3 ± 50.8, $F_{(2, 70)} = 3.6$, $p = 0.032$, $\eta_p^2 = 0.093$] on the ASTLSD score, and a group by altitude exposure interaction [$F_{(2, 70)} = 4.0$, $p = 0.023$, $\eta_p^2 = 0.103$]. On follow-up comparisons, difference in ASTLSD score was only a trend [BL (135 ± 61) vs. HA1 (161.1 ± 81.5), $t_{(20)} = -1.845$, $p = 0.080$]. ASTLSD decreased with the acclimatization compared to acute exposure [HA1 (164.3 ± 82.3) vs. HA6 (122.4 ± 53.3), $t_{(19)} = 3.005$, $p = 0.007$]. The AST variables did not change significantly over different time points in the control group as we observed in the altitude group.

Rapid Visual Processing (RVP)

There was no main effect of altitude exposure nor group by altitude exposure interaction on the RVPA. There was no main effect of altitude exposure on the RVPMDL score, but there was a group by altitude exposure interaction [$F_{(2,70)} = 4.7$, $p = 0.012$, $\eta_p^2 = 0.119$]. However, when directly compared, there was no difference. There was a trend to decrease with acclimatization compared to acute exposure [HA1 (414.8 ± 34.7) vs. HA6 (392.8 ± 36.5), $t_{(19)} = 2.081$, $p = 0.051$] on RVPMDL, however this trend did not survive a correction for multiple comparisons (Bonferroni). The RVPLSD score did not change over time with the exposure to altitude. The RVP variables in control group did not vary significantly over time.

One Touch Stockings of Cambridge (OTS)

There were no significant main effects nor interactions on the OTSPSFC score, OTSMLFC and OTSLFCSD.

SpO_2 and Lake Louise Score (LLS)

The changes in SpO_2 for *Cycle 2* were calculated in a similar manner as in *Cycle 1* and entered as covariates in the RM-ANCOVA analysis to investigate the role of ΔSpO_2 cognitive changes at altitude. The significant changes due to altitude exposure persisted when controlling for Altitude SpO_2 [$F_{(2, 30)} = 3.6$, $p = 0.037$, $\eta_p^2 = 0.167$] on the ASTLM score but disappeared when controlling for Acute ΔSpO_2 and Acclimatization SpO_2. The significant changes on the ASTLSD score due to altitude exposure persisted even after controlling for Altitude SpO_2 [$F_{(2, 30)} = 3.7$, $p = 0.033$, $\eta_p^2 = 0.172$] but there were no significant changes when controlling for Acute SpO_2 and Acclimatization SpO_2. The total LLS was entered as covariate in the ANCOVA to investigate the role of AMS symptoms on the ASTLM and ASTLSD scores relative to HA1. The cognitive changes related to different exposures to altitude disappeared with AMS score as covariate.

Acclimatization Carry-Over Effects Over the Cycles

We explored the carry-over effect across the cycles (*Cycle 1* and *Cycle 2*) with the calculation of changes in cognitive functions i.e. ΔCANTAB = *Cycle 2* - *Cycle 1* at BL, HA1 and HA6 time points. We then ran a RM-ANOVA on the cognitive outcomes change scores at ΔBL, ΔHA1. and ΔHA6. There was a main effect of altitude exposure on ASTLM [$F_{(2, 64)} = 5.8$, $p = 0.005$, $\eta_p^2 = 0.154$] with a smaller change in ASTLM over the acclimatization exposure compared to baseline [ΔBL (−61.2 ± 70.2) vs. HA6 (−28.0 ± 58.0, $p = 0.007$)]. Similarly, we found a main effect of altitude on ASTLSD score [$F_{(2, 64)} = 4.0$, $p = 0.023$, $\eta_p^2 = 0.112$] with a smaller change in ASTLSD over acclimatization exposure compared to baseline [ΔBL (−28.4 ± 41.2) vs. ΔHA6 (−0.2235 ± 34.8), $p = 0.032$]. For both outcomes (ASTLM and ASTLSD), there was no significant group by altitude exposure interaction. There were no significant changes across the two cycles for AST total correct nor other outcomes for the OTS, RVP, and RTI tests. The changes in cognitive function at altitude over two cycles as analyzed with RM-ANOVA have been illustrated in **Figure 4**.

We did not observe any significant differences in the percent changes of AST parameters during acclimatization indicating that the significant changes observed over the acclimatization period in *Cycle 1* are similar in magnitude as the changes observed in *Cycle 2*. Similarly, there were no significant differences in the percent changes at altitude from the baseline between the two cycles.

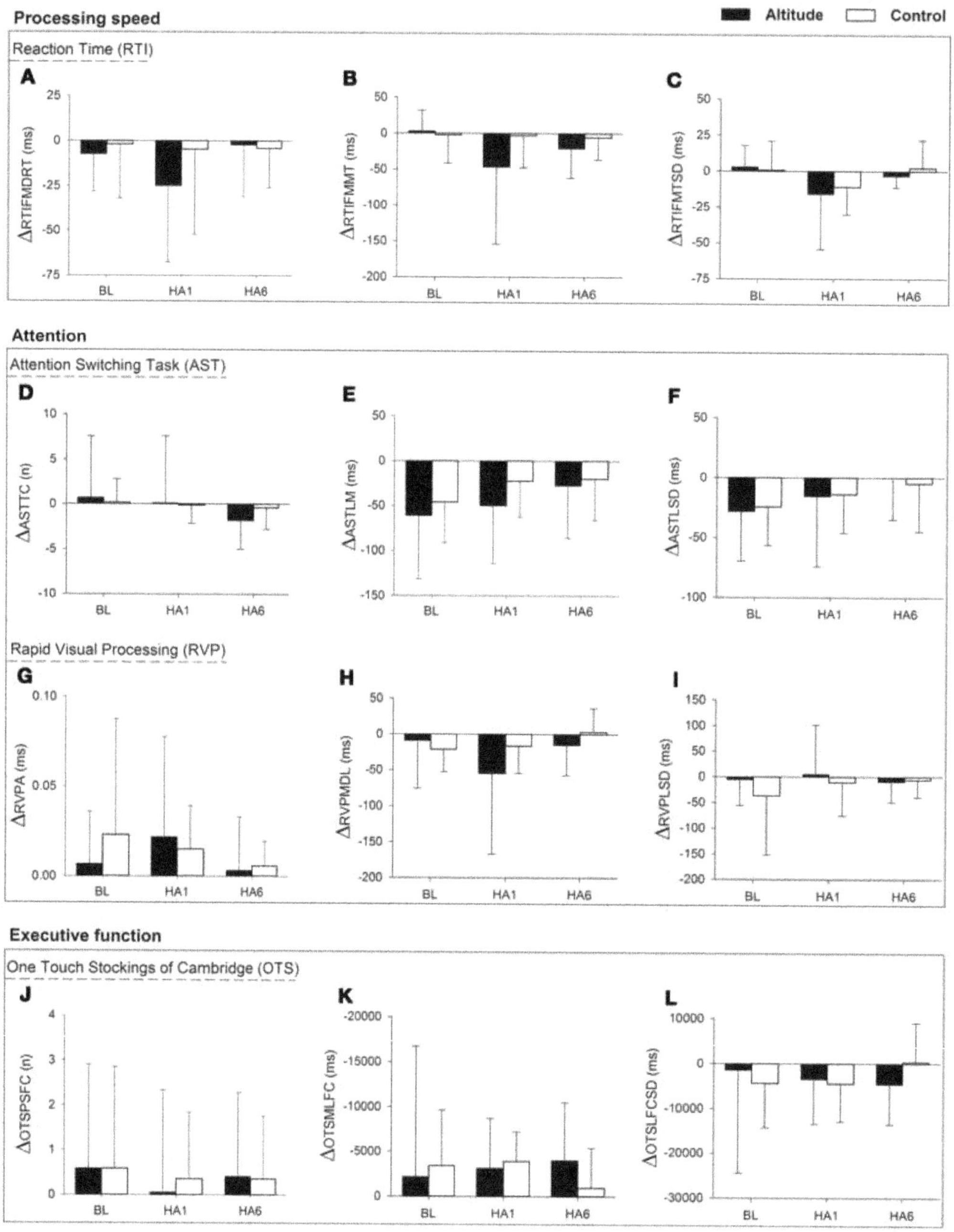

FIGURE 4 | Changes in cognition (CANTAB outcome parameters with RM-ANOVA) over two cycles (ΔCANTAB = *Cycle 2 – Cycle 1*) at very high altitude during acute, subacute and repeated exposure comparing with controls. Figure has three horizontal box panels. The first panel **(A–C)** illustrates "processing speed" i.e., changes in Reaction Time (RTI) parameters (ΔRTIFMDRT, ΔRTIFMMT, and ΔRTIFMTSD), the second box panel contains "attention" in which first panel within the box **(D–F)** shows changes in Attention Switching Task (AST) parameters (ΔASTTC, ΔASTLM, and ΔASTLSD) while the second panel within the second box **(G–I)** shows changes in Rapid Visual Processing (RVP) parameters (ΔRVPA, ΔRVPMDL, and ΔRVPLSD) and the third box panel **(J–L)** shows changes in One Touch Stockings of Cambridge (OTS) parameters (ΔOTSPSFC, ΔOTSMLFC, and ΔOTSLFCSD). The x-axis depicts different time points of data collection for Altitude exposure and Control groups at Baseline (BL), Acute exposure (HA1) and Acclimatization exposure (HA6). The y-axis depicts changes in cognitive parameters as mean ± SD for Altitude and Control group. Symbols: Black filled bars, Altitude group; empty bars, Control group; Δ, Change; ms, milliseconds; n, number. BL, baseline; HA1, acute exposure to altitude (day 1); HA6, acclimatization exposure to altitude (day 6); RTI, Reaction Time; AST, Attention Switching Task; RVP, Rapid Visual Processing; OTS, One Touch Stockings of Cambridge; ΔRTIFMDRT, RTI Median Five-choice Reaction Time; ΔRTIFMMT, RTI Mean Five-choice Movement Time; ΔRTIFMTSD, RTI Five-choice Movement Time Standard Deviation; ΔASTTC, AST Total Correct; ΔASTLM, AST Latency Mean; ΔASTLSD, AST Latency Standard Deviation; ΔRVPA, Rapid Visual Processing Accuracy; ΔRVPMDL, ΔRVP Mean Response Latency; ΔRVPLSD, RVP Response Latency Standard Deviation; ΔOTSPSFC, OTS Problems Solved on First Choice; ΔOTSMLFC, OTS Mean Latency First Choice; ΔOTSLFCSD, OTS Latency to First Choice Standard Deviation.

DISCUSSION

In this study, we investigated the effects of acute exposure, acclimatization and repeated exposure to very high altitude on cognitive functions in altitude-naïve individuals compared to control subjects tested at low altitude. We report four major findings. First, cognitive abilities, particularly sustained attention and inhibition of irrelevant information (selective attention) measured with the AST, significantly improved with acclimatization in both cycles. Second, the improvement gained in cognitive functions during the acclimatization period in *Cycle 1* did not carry over to the repeated exposure in *Cycle 2.* Third, changes in SpO_2 explained changes in ASTLM score and ASTLSD score during acute and acclimatization exposures, but not during altitude stay in both cycles. Finally, the degree of acute mountain sickness, reflected by the LLS, explains in part the changes in AST scores (ASTLSD in *Cycle 1*, and ASTLM and ASTLSD in *Cycle 2*). We did not find any significant changes in reaction times, visual processing and executive functions during acute and acclimatization exposures. The novelty and strengths of this study include a strong experimental design, a robust cognitive battery not previously used in altitude studies and the use of a control group tested at low altitude.

Previous studies have used a variety of cognitive tests to separately assess processing speed, attention and executive functions (Harris et al., 2009; Subudhi et al., 2014; Nation et al., 2017; Phillips et al., 2017). However, none has used a battery to test these cognitive domains concurrently. Here, we used a custom cognitive battery built within the CANTAB (Cambridge Cognition, 1994; Strauss et al., 2006) cognitive test collection, which included tests to assess all three domains simultaneously. Custom batteries assembled within CANTAB have been shown to be robust and well suited for repeated measures testing (Syväoja et al., 2015). Within the analyses, we selected outcomes such as mean response latency, standard deviation, and accuracy for each cognitive domain, variables previously used and validated for neuropsychological assessments in other contexts and clinical populations (Sweeney et al., 2000). We included the RTI task because reaction times have been used as a measure of processing speed in both field (Kramer et al., 1993; Ma et al., 2015; Chen et al., 2017) and laboratory (hypoxic chamber) (Hornbein et al., 1989; Turner et al., 2015; Pramsohler et al., 2017) settings. Further, we chose the Attention Switching Task as a measure of attention and ability to inhibit irrelevant information. High altitude exposure significantly decreases test accuracy and increases reaction time in the "Word-Color Stroop Test," a test that also measures inhibition and attention (Asmaro et al., 2013). Similarly, the choice of Rapid Visual Processing Task was based on the previous studies (Kramer et al., 1993; Finn and McDonald, 2012) in which this task was used due to its sensitivity to both neurological damage (Finn and McDonald, 2012) and high altitude exposure (Kramer et al., 1993). Finally, we chose the One Touch Stockings of Cambridge Test to assess executive functions at altitude in line with previous studies (Asmaro et al., 2013). Similarly, we used problems solved on first choice, Mean Latency and SD of first choice which are the outcomes that CANTAB recommends to assess planning and spatial working memory (Naef et al., 2017). To our knowledge, this is the first time that a CANTAB custom cognitive battery has been used to explore the effects of very high altitude and hypoxia exposure. Cognitive assessments in the altitude literature are often confounded by multiple factors such as mode and rate of ascent, absolute altitude gained, physical exertion or exercise, cold, radiation and individual susceptibility to hypobaric hypoxia (Virués-Ortega et al., 2004; Yan, 2014; Taylor et al., 2016; McMorris et al., 2017). In our study, we controlled these confounding factors by using a design that involved rapid ascent to very high altitude (5,050 m), minimal or no physical activity and lack of exposure to environmental stressors because participants remained inside the ALMA facility during the testing sessions.

Processing Speed

Previous studies have often reported a reduction in reaction times during acute exposure to altitude (Ma et al., 2015; Chen et al., 2017). It is often argued that the reduction in processing speed is a compensatory mechanisms to try to increase test accuracy at the expense of speed (Bahrke and Shukitt-Hale, 1993). Consistently with previous studies (Dykiert et al., 2010; Subudhi et al., 2014), we found that altitude exposure reduced the variability (SD) in the RTI Five-choice Movement Time but that the group-by-altitude interaction was not signficant in *Cycle 1.* During repeated exposure, in *Cycle 2,* altitude exposure had no effect on the RTI Five-time Movement time SD score although there was a group by altitude interaction (i.e., altitude and control subjects have different variances in processing speed at different altitudes). With acclimatization in *Cycle 2,* the RTI Five-time Movement time SD decreased during acclimatization although the significance was lost after *post-hoc* corrections. The lack of significant effects of acute exposure to altitude on reaction times, contrary to findings of other studies (Sharma et al., 1975; Dykiert et al., 2010), could be due to the small sample size and to the fact that participants were exposed to 5,050 m only 6–8 h/day and slept at lower altitude (2,900 m). Further, participants in our study may have benefitted from the specific exposure pattern with sleeping at lower altitude (Richalet et al., 2002; Farias et al., 2006; Vearrier and Greenberg, 2011) compared to other types of expedition/climbing exposure (Cavaletti et al., 1987; Kramer et al., 1993; Abraini et al., 1998). The mean and median five-choice reaction time scores did not vary significantly (neither the main effect of altitude nor the group-by-altitude interaction were significant) during acute, subacute and repeated altitude exposures. It is possible that the RTI task was too simple or not sensitive enough to measure the effects of high altitude exposure as reported previously (Roach et al., 2014). Alternatively, it is possible that complex reaction times are not profoundly affected below 6,000 m altitude (Virués-Ortega et al., 2004).

Attention

In our study, we found that in the AST task both Mean Reaction Latency and Reaction Latency SD were significantly affected by altitude exposure and a group by altitude interaction (i.e., the altitude group and the control group performed differently with different altitude exposures with the only the altitude group showing differences at the three data points). AST Mean

Reaction Latency score and AST Reaction Latency SD score improved over acclimatization compared to acute exposure but were not significantly different from baseline. This suggests that acclimatization plays a crucial role in restoring cognitive functions (Subudhi et al., 2014). The Mean Reaction Latency and SD seem to be more sensitive measures to assess the effects of high altitude exposure as compared to AST Total Correct score. With the repeated exposure in *Cycle 2,* in contrast to *Cycle 1,* there was a main effect of altitude on the AST Total Correct score and a group by altitude interaction. Particularly, the AST Total Correct score decreased during acute exposure and improved with acclimatization. In *Cycle* 2, both AST Mean Latency and AST Latency SD showed a main effect of altitude exposure as well as a group by altitude interaction. Both AST Mean Latency and AST Latency SD improved with acclimatization but only trended to increase (i.e., worse performance) with acute exposure. Interestingly, in both cycles, we did not find significant differences in AST Mean Latency and SD due to acute exposure but we found significant improvements with acclimatization. However, the observed changes did not translate to repeated exposures consistent with previous findings on re-ascent (Subudhi et al., 2014). The intriguing finding, i.e., no effect of acute exposure to altitude, may be due to the passive exposure (the ascent via motorized vehicles) and the lack of physical exertion at altitude. Our study participants were in fact comfortably resting at the ALMA Observatory facility at 5,050 m and measurements were taken a few hours after their arrival. Previous studies either recruited climbers (Cavaletti and Tredici, 1993; Kramer et al., 1993; Bonnon et al., 1999) and trekkers (Harris et al., 2009; Phillips et al., 2017) or simulated altitude by lowering the percentage of Oxygen (FiO_2) and/or pressure in an altitude chamber (Hornbein et al., 1989; Pramsohler et al., 2017). This heterogeneity in the study population and absolute altitude reached makes it harder to compare findings from the different studies. The individual variability in cerebral hypoxia susceptibility during acute high altitude exposure (Cavaletti and Tredici, 1993) may also partially explain our findings. The consistent improvement over acclimatization in both cycles could be in fact due to our unique pattern of high altitude exposure (i.e., ~16 h spent at 2,900 m (sleeping altitude) and ~8 h spent at very high altitude (5,050 m). The pattern of repeated re-oxygenation (2/3 of the 24-h cycle spent at 2,900 vs. 5,050 m) with restful sleep might have significantly increased the beneficial effects of the acclimatization process and thereby improved AST outcomes. The testing schedule used in our study simulates the schedule of the workers at ALMA and other mining industries in the South American Andes (Richalet et al., 2002; Farias et al., 2006; Vearrier and Greenberg, 2011) and therefore differs slightly from the schedules commonly used in the field (Ma et al., 2015; Chen et al., 2017) or in chamber high altitude simulation (Hornbein et al., 1989; Turner et al., 2015). Overall our findings indicate that sustained attention and the ability to inhibit irrelevant information (selective attention) are impacted by acute high altitude exposure. This suggests that precision tasks that require long-term focus might be affected, and therefore, more difficult to execute during high altitude exposure.

We observed only subtle changes in the Rapid Visual Processing outcomes during altitude exposure in both *Cycle 1* and *2.* The significant effects observed were lost on *post-hoc* corrections for multiple comparisons. Our findings regarding RVP are consistent with findings from others who reported that rapid exposure to altitude has little effect on visual and auditory attention as compared to effects on learning and memory (Nation et al., 2017).

Executive Function

A previous study conducted in an altitude chamber with equivalent simulated altitude of 6,096 m (FiO_2 = 10%) demonstrated impairments in cognitive functions including executive functions (Turner et al., 2015). We found a significant main effect of altitude exposure on both OTS Mean Latency to First Choice and SD scores but no group by altitude interaction. We did not find a significant main effect of altitude exposure on the OTS Problems Solved on First Choice score nor group by altitude interaction. Hence, the executive functions, measured with the OTS task, are not impaired by altitude exposure. Similar results were found for *Cycle 2.* The executive functions, as measured with the OTS task, do not seem to be affected by exposure to hypoxia as much as other cognitive domains (McMorris et al., 2017).

Role of SpO_2 and LLS Score on Cognition

SpO_2 on Cognitive Changes

The cognitive changes following cerebral impairment due to altitude hypoxia could be related to changes in SpO_2 (Yan et al., 2011; McMorris et al., 2017). In *Cycle 1,* the significant effects of altitude exposure disappeared when controlling for Acute SpO_2 and Acclimatization SpO_2 for AST Mean Reaction Latency scores and AST reaction Latency SD scores. Hence, the effects seen during acute and acclimatization exposures are primarily driven by hypobaric hypoxia. Interestingly, the significant result persisted when controlling for Altitude SpO_2 in both AST Mean Reaction Latency scores and AST Latency SD scores. During the repeated exposure in *Cycle 2,* we found a similar pattern as in *Cycle 1.* Significant cognitive changes in the AST Mean Reaction Latency scores and AST Reaction Latency SD scores due to altitude exposure persisted when controlling for Altitude SpO_2, but disappeared when controlling for Acute SpO_2 and Acclimatization SpO_2. The altitude effects on AST Mean Latency and AST Latency SD observed in the acclimatization period (HA6-HA1) in both cycles, provide strong evidence of a beneficial effect of acclimatization on cognition. On the other hand, the effects are cycle specific i.e., the effects found in *Cycle* 1 do not carry over to *Cycle 2.* Further, our results sheds light on the important role played by Altitude SpO_2 (HA6-HA1) on cognitive functioning strengthening the idea of using oxygen supplementation at very high altitude to improve safety and work performance among scientists and workers (West, 2003, 2015; Moraga et al., 2018).

Total LLS Score on Cognitive Changes

AMS symptoms are classified as cerebral symptoms (Wilson et al., 2009; Imray et al., 2010) and consequentially, they are expected to be associated with impaired cognitive functions at high altitude (Dykiert et al., 2010) although this relationship is still unclear (Virués-Ortega et al., 2004; Yan, 2014). In *Cycle 1*, the significant changes in AST mean reaction latency scores due to acute altitude exposure (HA1) persisted when including the LLS score as covariate in the model, indicating that the AMS symptoms are not associated with changes in AST Mean Reaction Latency scores. Conversely, the effect of altitude exposure on AST Reaction Latency SD score disappeared with LLS score entered as covariate, which indicates that AMS symptoms may have played a role in changes in cognitive abilities for this outcome. These findings suggest that AMS score could be associated with certain outcomes (AST Latency SD, an index of variability) but not others (AST Mean Latency) during acute altitude exposure. It is noteworthy that recent studies have found that poor sleep quality is not to be associated with AMS (MacInnis et al., 2013; Hall et al., 2014). It is therefore possible that some of the cognitive functions that are altered by sleep disturbances are not sensitive to high altitude exposure or symptoms of AMS. Consistently, Kramer and colleagues did not find any significant correlations between AMS severity and cognitive performance among climbers (Kramer et al., 1993). The rate of ascent, the absolute altitude gained and the physical activity in the field might be responsible for the discrepancy in the findings. With repeated exposure in *Cycle 2*, the cognitive changes related to acute altitude exposure (HA1) disappeared when using total LLS score as a covariate. The AMS symptoms seem to play a role in changes in cognitive abilities for these outcomes even during repeated exposures although the LLS score in the repeated exposure was significantly decreased compared to acute exposure (HA1, *Cycle 1*).

Acclimatization, Repeated Exposure and Carry-Over Effects

The principal reason behind the implementation of such work schedule in the Chilean workers with sleep periods at lower altitude, repeated exposure to 5,050 m, and a week of rest at sea-level is to try to minimize the adverse effects of very high altitude on workers' health and performance (Richalet et al., 2002; Farias et al., 2006; Vearrier and Greenberg, 2011) and allow them to see their families during the week of rest at low altitude. In our study which reproduces this schedule over two work-week cycles, we found a significant main effect of altitude exposure for the AST Mean Reaction Latency and AST Latency SD with a significant decrease in both AST Mean Reaction Latency and SD over the acclimatization exposure compared to baseline and AST Latency SD change across cycles. This indicates that the changes between baseline and acclimatization in *Cycle* 1 are different from the changes happening in *Cycle* 2, confirming that the significant improvement in cognitive functions with acclimatization is not maintained with a week of rest or with repeated exposure. Our findings are consistent with Subudhi and colleagues who reported that cognitive functions improved with acclimatization and the obtained gains are not completely retained upon re-ascent/repeated exposure (Subudhi et al., 2014). It is not entirely clear whether sleep at lower altitude favors this outcome or if this is a consequence of the acclimatization period itself. Further, we did not find any differences when comparing the two cycles in terms of percent change for AST during acute and acclimatization exposures. This means that the magnitude of the changes observed over the acclimatization in *Cycle 1* is not different from the magnitude of the changes observed in *Cycle 2*. Our findings suggest that the acclimatization of cognitive functions at altitude is a dynamic process and it may not reach a plateau within approximately a week, in contrast to other physiological variables such as ventilatory acclimatization (Pamenter and Powell, 2016). One possibility is that cognitive functions may not benefit from high altitude acclimatization (Taylor et al., 2016) unlike other physiological functions such as athletic performance. However, these relationships may be different at higher elevation, with longer durations of stay and increased physical exertion (Shukitt-Hale et al., 1998).

Strengths and Limitations

Strengths

We exposed young healthy altitude-naïve individuals to very high altitude following the same schedule as the ALMA workers. Thus, this study is highly relevant to a significant workforce in Chile and other parts of South America, and could be of interest to governments and policy makers who regulate work at high altitude. We used a custom cognitive battery generated from the Cambridge Neuropsychological Test Automated Battery (CANTAB) test collection, which has not been used previously in high altitude research. The comprehensive cognitive battery tests processing speed, attention and executive function was used to assess the effects of acute exposure, acclimatization exposure and repeated exposure to very high altitude. Participants completed the cognitive assessments at various time points of altitude exposure. Similarly, we recruited a control group at low altitude, to test the between-group differences as well as control for practice effects. The use of this custom testing battery constitutes a strength of the study. The neuropsychological assessment is in fact conducted using portable wireless touch screen tablets and therefore applicable in many remote settings. The data are then stored and can be either wireless transferred or downloaded later. Further we administered the battery in English but it is validated to be administered in multiple languages making it a very flexible assessment tool in a variety of populations and settings. Another strength of the study is the use of a experimental design that controls factors such as environmental stressors and the effects physical exertion. This design allowed us to untangle the effects of hypoxia at high altitude from other confounders.

Limitations

This study has also some limitations. First, it provides only a snapshot of the high-altitude exposure which is hard to compare to the repeated exposures of the high-altitude workers who have been following this schedule for many years. Second, we did not collect cognitive data at sleeping altitude i.e., mid-altitude (2,900 m) where participants (and workers) spend >15 h/day while they only spent ~8 h/day at 5,050 m. Sleeping at lower altitude and increased oxygen levels might have had beneficial effects that counteracted the negative effects of acute high-altitude exposure. These should be areas of further investigation. Third, the findings from the study should be interpreted carefully when generalizing to other types of high altitude exposure or paticipants' groups due to the unique ascent profile, relatively small sample size and the weekly shift-work schedule that was used in our study. Finally, the participants in this study were passively exposed to altitude (via travel by plane from 520 to 2,900 m and by motorized vehicle from 2,900 to 5,050 m) and had minimal physical exertion as opposed to previous studies in climbers and trekkers.

CONCLUSIONS

The findings of our study highlight the importance of acclimatization on restoring cognitive function after acute exposure to very high altitude. However, it is important to consider that the gains in cognitive functions during the acclimatization period in the first exposure are not carried over to repeated exposures. The SpO_2 is associated with cognitive changes during acute and acclimatization exposure and AMS scores might partially explain the cognitive changes. Taken together, our results suggest that the tasks that need sustained focus and high level of precision may be affected during acute exposure and also during repeated exposure or re-ascent. These findings and their implications for the safety and performance of the workers in the mine industry and other high-altitude workers highlight the importance of linking research groups and scientific findings with the organizational strategies of these specialized work sites. The findings would also be helpful for the related organizations and governments in policy formulation aiming at increasing the safety and security of high altitude workers. Future studies should focus on the effects of high altitude on learning and declarative memory, should include data collection at sleeping altitude (2,900 m) and most importantly, should recruit workers who have been working at high altitude for extended periods. The effects of room oxygen enrichment "oxygen conditioning" at high altitude (West, 2016a,b) for newcomers, as well as for high altitude residents, should also be the topic of future investigations.

AUTHOR CONTRIBUTIONS

MP and VG organized the data, carried out the analyses, drafted the manuscript and took the lead of manuscript finalization and submission process. KMB, LD, and JA were involved in the control data collection, export, organization and preliminary analyses. KEB, BG, JR, and MJP were involved in the conceptualization, design, and planning of the study. SH, MF, SU, KEB, and MJP were involved in the field for the data collection, troubleshooting, and manuscript finalization. All authors went through all the versions of the manuscript and approved them.

FUNDING

MJP is supported by a Discovery Grant from the Natural Sciences and Engineering Research Council (NSERC) of Canada (Principal Investigator (PI), MJP; 2014-05554), and a CIHR Operating Grant on the Regulation of cerebral blood flow in OSA (PI: MJP). AP is supported by an NSERC Discovery Grant of Canada (PI, ABP; 2013-418454). JA received support from and NSERC CGS-M scholarship. SH received support from the Dr Chen Fong doctoral scholarship (Hotchkiss Brain Institute). LD is supported by an Alberta Innovates Health Services (AIHS) Postgraduate Fellowship. VG is supported by The Brenda Strafford Centre on Aging, within the O'Brien Institute for Public Health, and the Brenda Strafford Foundation Chair for Alzheimer Research (BSFCAR). MJP holds the BSFCAR. KEB and SU are supported by Lunge Zurich, Swiss National Science Foundation. BG is supported by the Institute for Collaborative Biotechnologies through grant W911NF-09-0001 from the U.S. Army Research Office. The content of the information does not necessarily reflect the position or the policy of the Government, and no official endorsement should be inferred.

ACKNOWLEDGMENTS

We express our sincere thanks to the study participants who took part in the high-altitude expedition to ALMA Observatory, Chile. The research would have been impossible without their involvement and cooperation throughout the expedition. We would also like to acknowledge our Chilean collaborators from the ALMA Head Office in Santiago, Chile and the staff of the ALMA observatory (Ivan Lopez, Daniel Soza, Charlotte Pon, and the health & safety and polyclinic teams), who greatly facilitated the study. Finally, we would like to thank Alicia Morales Soto for helping facilitate the logistics in Santiago.

REFERENCES

Abraini, J. H., Bouquet, C., Joulia, F., Nicolas, M., and Kriem, B. (1998). Cognitive performance during a simulated climb of Mount Everest: implications for brain function and central adaptive processes under chronic hypoxic stress. *Pflugers Arch.* 436, 553–559. doi: 10.1007/s004240050671

Asmaro, D., Mayall, J., and Ferguson, S. (2013). Cognition at altitude: impairment in executive and memory processes under hypoxic conditions. *Aviat. Space Environ. Med.* 84, 1159–1165. doi: 10.3357/ASEM.3661.2013

Bahrke, M. S., and Shukitt-Hale, B. (1993). Effects of altitude on mood, behaviour and cognitive functioning. *Rev. Sports Med.* 16, 97–125.

Bärtsch, P., and Swenson, E. R. (2013). Acute high-altitude illnesses. *N. Engl. J. Med.* 368, 2294–2302. doi: 10.1056/NEJMcp1214870

Bickler, P. E., Feiner, J. R., Lipnick, M. S., Batchelder, P., MacLeod, D. B., and Severinghaus, J. W. (2017). Effects of acute, profound hypoxia on healthy humans: implications for safety of tests evaluating pulse oximetry or tissue oximetry performance. *Anesth. Analg.* 124, 146–153. doi: 10.1213/ane.0000000000001421

Bonnon, M., Noël-Jorand, M. C., and Therme, P. (1999). Criteria for psychological adaptation to high-altitude hypoxia. *Percept. Mot. Skills* 89, 3–18.

Cambridge Cognition, U. o. C. (1994). *Cambridge Neuropsychological Test Automated Battery (CANTAB) [Online]*. Cambridge Cognition - University of Cambridge. Available online at: http://www.cambridgecognition.com/cantab/ (Accessed January, 31 2018).

Cavaletti, G., Moroni, R., Garavaglia, P., and Tredici, G. (1987). Brain damage after high-altitude climbs without oxygen. *Lancet* 1:101.

Cavaletti, G., and Tredici, G. (1993). Long-lasting neuropsychological changes after a single high altitude climb. *Acta Neurol. Scand.* 87, 103–105.

Champod, A. S., Eskes, G. A., Foster, G. E., Hanly, P. J., Pialoux, V., Beaudin, A. E., et al. (2013). Effects of acute intermittent hypoxia on working memory in young healthy adults. *Am. J. Respir. Crit. Care Med.* 187, 1148–1150. doi: 10.1164/rccm.201209-1742LE

Chen, X., Zhang, Q., Wang, J., Liu, J., Zhang, W., Qi, S., et al. (2017). Cognitive and neuroimaging changes in healthy immigrants upon relocation to a high altitude: a panel study. *Hum. Brain. Mapp* 38, 3865–3877. doi: 10.1002/hbm.23635

Davranche, K., Casini, L., Arnal, P. J., Rupp, T., Perrey, S., and Verges, S. (2016). Cognitive functions and cerebral oxygenation changes during acute and prolonged hypoxic exposure. *Physiol. Behav.* 164, 189–197. doi: 10.1016/j.physbeh.2016.06.001

Dellasanta, P., Gaillard, S., Loutan, L., and Kayser, B. (2007). Comparing questionnaires for the assessment of acute mountain sickness. *High. Alt. Med. Biol.* 8, 184–191. doi: 10.1089/ham.2007.8305

Dykiert, D., Hall, D., van Gemeren, N., Benson, R., Der, G., Starr, J. M., et al. (2010). The effects of high altitude on choice reaction time mean and intra-individual variability: Results of the Edinburgh Altitude Research Expedition of 2008. *Neuropsychology* 24, 391–401. doi: 10.1037/a0018502

Farias, J. G., Osorio, J., Soto, G., Brito, J., Siques, P., and Reyes, J. G. (2006). Sustained acclimatization in Chilean mine workers subjected to chronic intermittent hypoxia. *High Alt. Med. Bol.* 7, 302–306. doi: 10.1089/ham.2006.7.302

Finn, M., and McDonald, S. (2012). Computerised cognitive training for older persons with mild cognitive impairment: a pilot study using a randomised controlled trial design. *Brain Impairment* 12, 187–199. doi: 10.1375/brim.12.3.187

Hackett, P. H., and Roach, R. C. (2001). High-altitude illness. *N. Engl. J. Med.* 345, 107–114. doi: 10.1056/NEJM200107123450206

Hall, D. P., MacCormick, I. J., Phythian-Adams, A. T., Rzechorzek, N. M., Hope-Jones, D., Cosens, S., et al. (2014). Network analysis reveals distinct clinical syndromes underlying acute mountain sickness. *PLoS ONE* 9:e81229. doi: 10.1371/journal.pone.0081229

Harris, G. A., Cleland, J., Collie, A., and McCrory, P. (2009). Cognitive assessment of a trekking expedition to 5100 m: a comparison of computerized and written testing methods. *Wilderness Environ. Med.* 20, 261–268. doi: 10.1580/08-weme-or-261r.1

Hornbein, T. F. (2001). The high-altitude brain. *J. Exp. Biol.* 204, 3129–3132. Available online at: http://jeb.biologists.org/content/204/18/3129

Hornbein, T. F., Townes, B. D., Schoene, R. B., Sutton, J. R., and Houston, C. S. (1989). The cost to the central nervous system of climbing to extremely high altitude. *N. Engl. J. Med.* 321, 1714–1719. doi: 10.1056/nejm1989122132 12505

Imray, C., Wright, A., Subudhi, A., and Roach, R. (2010). Acute mountain sickness: pathophysiology, prevention, and treatment. *Prog. Cardiovasc. Dis.* 52, 467–484. doi: 10.1016/j.pcad.2010.02.003

Kramer, A. F., Coyne, J. T., and Strayer, D. L. (1993). Cognitive function at high altitude. *Hum Factors* 35, 329–344. doi: 10.1177/001872089303 500208

Lowe, C., and Rabbitt, P. (1998). Test/re-test reliability of the CANTAB and ISPOCD neuropsychological batteries: theoretical and practical issues. Cambridge neuropsychological test automated battery. International study of post-operative cognitive dysfunction. *Neuropsychologia* 36, 915–923.

Ma, H., Wang, Y., Wu, J., Luo, P., and Han, B. (2015). Long-term exposure to high altitude affects response inhibition in the conflict-monitoring stage. *Sci Rep* 5:13701. doi: 10.1038/srep13701

MacInnis, M. J., Lanting, S. C., Rupert, J. L., and Koehle, M. S. (2013). Is poor sleep quality at high altitude separate from acute mountain sickness? factor structure and internal consistency of the lake Louise score questionnaire. *High Alt. Med. Biol.* 14, 334–337. doi: 10.1089/ham.2013.1030

Maggiorini, M., Müller, A., Hofstetter, D., Bärtsch, P., and Oelz, O. (1998). Assessment of acute mountain sickness by different score protocols in the Swiss Alps. *Aviat. Space. Environ. Med.* 69, 1186–1192.

Malle, C., Quinette, P., Laisney, M., Bourrilhon, C., Boissin, J., Desgranges, B., et al. (2013). Working memory impairment in pilots exposed to acute hypobaric hypoxia. *Aviat. Space. Environ. Med.* 84, 773–779. doi: 10.3357/ASEM.3482.2013

McMorris, T., Hale, B. J., Barwood, M., Costello, J., and Corbett, J. (2017). Effect of acute hypoxia on cognition: a systematic review and meta-regression analysis. *Neurosci. Biobehav. Rev.* 74, 225–232. doi: 10.1016/j.neubiorev.2017.01.019

Moraga, F. A., López, I., Morales, A., Soza, D., and Noack, J. (2018). The effect of oxygen enrichment on cardiorespiratory and neuropsychological responses in workers with chronic intermittent exposure to high altitude (ALMA, 5,050 m). *Front. Physiol.* 9:187. doi: 10.3389/fphys.2018.00187

Naef, M., Müller, U., Linssen, A., Clark, L., Robbins, T. W., and Eisenegger, C. (2017). Effects of dopamine D2/D3 receptor antagonism on human planning and spatial working memory. *Transl. Psychiatry* 7:e1107. doi: 10.1038/tp.2017.56

Nation, D. A., Bondi, M. W., Gayles, E., and Delis, D. C. (2017). Mechanisms of memory dysfunction during high altitude hypoxia training in military aircrew. *J. Int. Neuropsychol. Soc.* 23, 1–10. doi: 10.1017/s1355617716000965

Pamenter, M. E., and Powell, F. L. (2016). Time domains of the hypoxic ventilatory response and their molecular basis. *Compr. Physiol.* 6, 1345–1385. doi: 10.1002/cphy.c150026

Penaloza, D., and Arias-Stella, J. (2007). The heart and pulmonary circulation at high altitudes: healthy highlanders and chronic mountain sickness. *Circulation* 115, 1132–1146. doi: 10.1161/CIRCULATIONAHA.106.62454

Phillips, L., Basnyat, B., Chang, Y., Swenson, E. R., and Harris, N. S. (2017). Findings of cognitive impairment at high altitude: relationships to acetazolamide use and acute mountain sickness. *High Alt. Med. Biol.* 18, 121–127. doi: 10.1089/ham.2016.0001

Pramsohler, S., Wimmer, S., Kopp, M., Gatterer, H., Faulhaber, M., Burtscher, M., et al. (2017). Normobaric hypoxia overnight impairs cognitive reaction time. *BMC Neurosci* 18:43. doi: 10.1186/s12868-017-0362-3

Richalet, J. P., Donoso, M. V., Jiménez, D., Antezana, A. M., Hudson, C., Cortès, G., et al. (2002). Chilean miners commuting from sea level to 4500 m: a prospective study. *High Alt. Med. Biol.* 3, 159–166. doi: 10.1089/15270290260131894

Roach, E. B., Bleiberg, J., Lathan, C. E., Wolpert, L., Tsao, J. W., and Roach, R. C. (2014). AltitudeOmics: decreased reaction time after high altitude cognitive testing is a sensitive metric of hypoxic impairment. *Neuroreport* 25, 814–818. doi: 10.1097/wnr.0000000000000169

Roach, R. C., Bärtsch, P., Hackett, P. H., and Oelz, O. (1993). "The Lake Louise acute mountain sickness scoring system," in *Hypoxia and Molecular Medicine*, eds J. R. Sutton, C. S. Houston and G. Coates (Burlington, VT: Queen City Press), 272–274.

Sharma, V. M., Malhotra, M. S., and Baskaran, A. S. (1975). Variations in psychomotor efficiency during prolonged stay at high altitude. *Ergonomics* 18, 511–516. doi: 10.1080/00140137508931485

Shukitt-Hale, B., Banderet, L. E., and Lieberman, H. R. (1998). Elevation-dependent symptom, mood, and performance changes produced by exposure to hypobaric hypoxia. *Int. J. Aviat. Psychol.* 8, 319–334. doi: 10.1207/s15327108ijap0804_1

Strauss, E., Sherman, E. M., and Spreen, O. (2006). *CANTAB in 'A Compendium of Neuropsychological Tests: Administration, Norms, and Commentary'.* New York, NY: Oxford University Press, Inc. Available online at: https://global.oup.com/academic/product/a-compendium-of-neuropsychological-tests-9780195159578?cc=ca&lang=en&

Subudhi, A. W., Bourdillon, N., Bucher, J., Davis, C., Elliott, J. E., Eutermoster, M., et al. (2014). AltitudeOmics: the integrative physiology of human acclimatization to hypobaric hypoxia and its retention upon reascent. *PLoS ONE* 9:e92191. doi: 10.1371/journal.pone.0092191

Sweeney, J. A., Kmiec, J. A., and Kupfer, D. J. (2000). Neuropsychologic impairments in bipolar and unipolar mood disorders on the CANTAB neurocognitive battery. *Biol. Psychiatry* 48, 674–684. doi: 10.1016/S0006-3223(00)00910-0

Syväoja, H. J., Tammelin, T. H., Ahonen, T., Räsänen, P., Tolvanen, A., Kankaanpää, A., et al. (2015). Internal consistency and stability of the CANTAB neuropsychological test battery in children. *Psychol. Assess.* 27, 698–709. doi: 10.1037/a0038485

Taylor, L., Watkins, S. L., Marshall, H., Dascombe, B. J., and Foster, J. (2016). The impact of different environmental conditions on cognitive function: a focused review. *Front. Physiol.* 6:372. doi: 10.3389/fphys.2015.00372

Turner, C. E., Barker-Collo, S. L., Connell, C. J., and Gant, N. (2015). Acute hypoxic gas breathing severely impairs cognition and task learning in humans. *Physiol. Behav.* 142, 104–110. doi: 10.1016/j.physbeh.2015.02.006

Vearrier, D., and Greenberg, M. I. (2011). Occupational health of miners at altitude: adverse health effects, toxic exposures, pre-placement screening, acclimatization, and worker surveillance. *Clin. Toxicol. (Phila)* 49, 629–640. doi: 10.3109/15563650.2011.607169

Virues-Ortega, J., Bucks, R., Kirkham, F. J., Baldeweg, T., Baya-Botti, A., and Hogan, A. M. (2011). Changing patterns of neuropsychological functioning in children living at high altitude above and below 4000 m: a report from the Bolivian Children Living at Altitude (BoCLA) study. *Dev. Sci.* 14, 1185–1193. doi: 10.1111/j.1467-7687.2011.01064.x

Virués-Ortega, J., Buela-Casal, G., Garrido, E., and Alcázar, B. (2004). Neuropsychological functioning associated with high-altitude exposure. *Neuropsychol. Rev.* 14, 197–224. doi: 10.1007/s11065-004-8159-4

Wang, Y., Ma, H., Fu, S., Guo, S., Yang, X., Luo, P., et al. (2014). Long-term exposure to high altitude affects voluntary spatial attention at early and late processing stages. *Sci. Rep.* 4:4443. doi: 10.1038/srep04443

West, J. B. (1996). Prediction of barometric pressures at high altitude with the use of model atmospheres. *J. Appl. Physiol. (1985)* 81, 1850–1854.

West, J. B. (2003). Improving oxygenation at high altitude: acclimatization and O_2 enrichment. *High Alt. Med. Biol.* 4, 389–398. doi: 10.1089/152702903769192340

West, J. B. (2015). A strategy for oxygen conditioning at high altitude: comparison with air conditioning. *J. Appl. Physiol. (1985)* 119, 719–723. doi: 10.1152/japplphysiol.00421.2015

West, J. B. (2016a). Cognitive impairment of school children at high altitude: the case for oxygen conditioning in schools. *High Alt. Med. Biol.* 17, 203–207. doi: 10.1089/ham.2016.0026

West, J. B. (2016b). Oxygen conditioning: a new technique for improving living and working at high altitude. *Physiology (Bethesda)* 31, 216–222. doi: 10.1152/physiol.00057.2015

Wilson, M. H., Newman, S., and Imray, C. H. (2009). The cerebral effects of ascent to high altitudes. *Lancet Neurol.* 8, 175–191. doi: 10.1016/S1474-4422(09)70014-6

Yan, X. (2014). Cognitive impairments at high altitudes and adaptation. *High Alt. Med. Biol.* 15, 141–145. doi: 10.1089/ham.2014.1009

Yan, X., Zhang, J., Gong, Q., and Weng, X. (2011). Prolonged high-altitude residence impacts verbal working memory: an fMRI study. *Exp. Brain. Res.* 208, 437–445. doi: 10.1007/s00221-010-2494-x

12

Daily Intermittent Normobaric Hypoxia Over 2 Weeks Reduces BDNF Plasma Levels in Young Adults

Andreas Becke[1,2†], Patrick Müller[2†], Milos Dordevic[2], Volkmar Lessmann[3,4], Tanja Brigadski[3,5] and Notger G. Müller[2,4]*

[1] *Institute of Cognitive Neurology and Dementia Research, Otto-von-Guericke-Universität Magdeburg, Magdeburg, Germany,* [2] *Neuroprotection Laboratory, German Center for Neurodegenerative Diseases (DZNE), Magdeburg, Germany,* [3] *Institute of Physiology, Otto-von-Guericke-Universität Magdeburg, Magdeburg, Germany,* [4] *Center for Behavioral Brain Sciences, Magdeburg, Germany,* [5] *Informatics and Microsystem Technology, University of Applied Sciences, Kaiserslautern, Kaiserslautern, Germany*

Correspondence:
Patrick Müller
patrick.mueller@dzne.de

† These authors have contributed equally to this work

Background: The results from animal and human research indicate that acute intermittent hypoxia can enhance brain-derived neurotrophic factor (BDNF) plasma levels and gene expression. As BDNF is known to promote the differentiation of new neurons and the formation of synapses, it has been proposed to mediate adult neuroplasticity. Thus, the present study aimed to analyze the long-term effects of daily intermittent exposure to normobaric hypoxia (simulating high altitude exposure at approximately 4000–5000 m) over 2 weeks on BDNF levels in young adults.

Methods: Twenty-eight young adults (age: 19–33 years) were randomized into a hypoxic intervention group (*N* = 14) or the control group (*N* = 14). Participants in the intervention group breathed intermittent normobaric hypoxic air at resting conditions (5 min intervals, 80–85% SpO_2 measured via a finger pulse oximeter, 12 sessions for 60 min/day for 2 weeks) via a hypoxic generator. BDNF plasma and serum levels were determined at baseline and at 2 weeks after intervention using sandwich ELISAs.

Results: After 2 weeks of daily intermittent hypoxic treatment (IHT), we found a significant group x time interaction effect for BDNF plasma levels based on a significant decrease in BDNF levels in the hypoxia group.

Conclusion: Our results demonstrate that daily intermittent administration of hypoxic air has a significant effect on BDNF regulation in healthy young adults. Contrary to other results reporting an increase in BDNF levels under hypoxic conditions, the present data suggest that hypoxic treatment using intensive IHT can reduce BDNF plasma levels for at least 2 weeks. This finding indicates that the daily application of hypoxic air is too frequent for the aimed physiological response, namely, an increase in BDNF levels.

Keywords: hypoxia, BDNF, neuroplasticity, IHT, adaptation

INTRODUCTION

Hypoxia is defined by a reduced oxygen content in air and can be divided into intermittent and chronic forms. Thereby, intermittent hypoxia applies to a large spectrum of stimuli that range from exercise in high altitude to obstructive sleep apnea (OSA). Intermittent hypoxia treatment (IHT) was first used in sports medicine to enhance human physical performance (erythropoiesis and angiogenesis) (Viscor et al., 2018). During the following years, hypoxic training was increasingly employed for non-pharmacological treatment of several diseases (e.g., bronchial asthma, hypertension, and cardiovascular diseases). IHT can effectively stimulate various metabolic processes (Serebrovskaya et al., 2008) and can have numerous positive health effects similar to cardiovascular physical activity (Enette et al., 2017). IHT may serve as a protective mechanism for the brain by inducing neurogenesis. For instance, histological studies in adult rats have shown that IHT promotes a transient increase in progenitor cell proliferation in the subventricular zone and a long-term increase in the dentate gyrus (Zhu et al., 2005) and has the potential to recover spatial learning deficits after cerebral ischemia by increased hippocampal neurogenesis (Tsai et al., 2011). However, intermittent normobaric hypoxia is not associated with positive effects only *per se*. For example, the clinical syndrome of OSA leads to intermittent hypoxia as well (Burtscher et al., 2009) and is associated with numerous negative effects such as reduced cognitive performance (Yan, 2014; Malle et al., 2016). Hence, based on different characteristics such as the dose and the duration, we can assume that hypoxia induces both protective and pathological effects. It has been proposed that low-dose intermittent hypoxia (9–16% inspired O_2) with short durations can enhance positive physiological processes, whereby high-dose hypoxia (2–8% inspired O_2) is associated with progressively pathological mechanisms (Navarrete-Opazo and Mitchell, 2014).

The results from animal and human research indicate that acute intermittent hypoxia (Vermehren-Schmaedick et al., 2012) and physical activity (Enette et al., 2017) can enhance brain-derived neurotrophic factor (BDNF) blood levels and BDNF gene expression. Such gene expression is explained by an oxygen deficit recognized by the oxygen sensory system (Sharp and Bernaudin, 2004) changing the oxygen-dependent degradation domain of hypoxia-inducible factor (HIF-1), thereby inducing an increase in HIF-1-alpha levels (Wiener et al., 1996). HIF-1-alpha is known to act as a transcription factor to modulate the expression of several genes, such as BDNF growth factor levels (Helan et al., 2014). The BDNF neurotrophin is a member of the nerve growth factor family and is widely expressed in the human brain, especially in the hippocampus, but it is also expressed in peripheral tissues such as the pulmonary vasculature (Aravamudan et al., 2012; Helan et al., 2014). Current research studies indicate BNDF plasma levels as a potential biomarker for reliable diagnosis of neurocognitive disorders (Levada et al., 2016). The protein is secreted in an activity-dependent manner but is also secreted in response to hypoxia (Haubensak et al., 1998; Hartmann et al., 2001; Kohara et al., 2001; Brigadski et al., 2005; Matsuda et al., 2009; Brigadski and Leßmann, 2014; Helan et al., 2014; Edelmann et al., 2015; Hartman et al., 2015). Research results indicate that 75% of the BDNF in the peripheral blood plasma originates from the brain (Krabbe et al., 2007; Rasmussen et al., 2009). Several studies have suggested that BDNF is an important modulator of the CNS and promotes the differentiation of new neurons and synapses (Huang and Reichardt, 2001; Leschik et al., 2013; Park and Poo, 2013; Edelmann et al., 2014). BDNF, therefore, represents one of the major mediators of neuroplasticity (Calabrese et al., 2014). Furthermore, some authors have suggested that BDNF blood levels may serve as a biomarker for the diagnosis of neurodegenerative diseases and psychiatric disorders and can also serve as a surrogate marker for the success of therapies in these disorders (Ruscheweyh et al., 2011). Reduced BDNF blood levels have been reported in Alzheimer's disease (Laske et al., 2007) and mild cognitive impairment (Forlenza et al., 2010).

Regarding the effect of intermittent hypoxia on BDNF blood levels in humans, the status of research is currently unclear. The results from animal and human studies have shown an acute increase in BDNF plasma levels in response to hypoxia. Helan et al. (2014) observed an increase in BDNF levels in 30 healthy volunteers after 72 h of normobaric hypoxia. Schega et al. (2016) reported no effects on BDNF in serum in older adults (N = 34, 66.4 ± 3.3 years) after 4 weeks of intermittent normobaric hypoxia (3× per week for 90 min) in addition to cardiovascular exercise. However, their data indicated that BDNF levels increased in the exercise-intervention group and in the exercise control-group after a compensation period of several weeks. This finding raises the question of whether the delayed effect could have been observed after hypoxic treatment alone, i.e., without concomitant cardiovascular exercise intervention.

Previous studies in animal research indicate an occurrence of neurogenesis in dentate gyrus within 4 weeks subsequent to intermittent hypoxia (Zhu et al., 2005). Based on these results we conducted a feasibility study to test the effects of 2 weeks of daily exposure to hypoxic air, which simulated intermittent hypoxia treatment (IHT), on peripheral BDNF levels. Therefore, we expected an increase in BDNF levels (as a central mediator of neurogenesis).

With respect to previous research on passive IHT methods, a protocol was chosen that has been shown to increase aerobic capacity and exercise tolerance in elderly men (Burtscher et al., 2004). In view of the data from Zhu et al. (2005) and based on recommendations for IHT regimes (Bassovitch and Serebrovskaya, 2009), we estimated the peak long-term effects of IHT to emerge 2 weeks after the intervention. If successful, this process is an easy to administer, low-cost intervention that may have great potential in inducing neuroplasticity and preventing cognitive deficits.

MATERIALS AND METHODS

The study was designed as a two-week randomized, controlled intervention. The ethics committee at the Otto-von-Guericke-Universität Magdeburg, approved the study, and all of the subjects signed a written informed consent form prior to participation. The exclusion criteria were acute or chronic cardiovascular, renal, metabolic, orthopedic and/or neurological diseases.

Twenty-eight young adults (age: 19–33 years) were randomized to a hypoxic intervention group [N = 14 (9 female), mean age 27.78, SD = 2.39] or a control group [N = 14 (5 female), mean age 22.85, SD 2.35] using the website www.randomization.com. The participants in the intervention group breathed intermittent normobaric hypoxic air at resting conditions (5 min intervals at a target of 80–85% SpO_2 via a finger pulse oximeter, 12 sessions for 60 min/day for 2 weeks) generated by a hypoxic generator (b-cat and integra ten). The simulated high altitude was continuously manually adjusted between 4000 and 5000 m to reach the target SpO_2. The control group received no intervention.

Fasting blood samples were taken in the mornings at baseline and at posttest (2 weeks after the last training session). From the blood samples, the plasma and serum concentrations of BDNF were determined using sandwich ELISAs (BDNF DuoSet; R&D Systems, Wiesbaden, Germany) as previously described (Schega et al., 2016).

For the intervention group, the blood samples for the small blood count were taken 4 times at baseline, 1 week after the intervention, at the end of intervention (consecutive day of last intervention session) and 2 weeks after the intervention. Five missing data sets for the second time point and 3 missing data sets for the third time point were reported (subjects did not show up).

Statistical analysis of BDNF plasma levels, BDNF serum levels and small blood count levels were performed with SPSS (SPSS 22 Inc./IBM). The intervention effects for BDNF were tested using repeated-measures ANOVAs with group (IHT and CG) as the between-subject factor and time (pre and post) as the within-subject factor. Age and gender were included as covariates. Additionally, *post hoc* pairwise comparisons were performed to determine the longitudinal changes in the hypoxia and control groups separately. In the case of non-normal distribution of data, we used the Mann-Whitney U-test or the Wilcoxon test instead of t-tests. The effect size was quantified by partial eta squared (η^2). For interaction effects, the percentage changes from baseline to post measures were calculated for BDNF and small blood count values and were then correlated with Pearson's formula.

RESULTS

The plasma and serum levels of BDNF were analyzed in the blood samples before the onset of the intervention as well as after the intervention. A significant group x time interaction effect was observed for the BDNF plasma levels [$F(1,26) = 10.742, p = 0.002, \eta^2 = 0.292$]. *Post hoc* pairwise comparisons showed a significant decrease in BDNF plasma levels only in the hypoxia group from baseline to the posttest period (Wilcoxon-Test, $Z = -3.296$, $p = 0.001$). The intraindividual changes in BDNF plasma levels reached a reduction of 66.34% of the pretreatment period. No significant time × group interactions emerged for BDNF serum levels (see **Table 1** and **Figure 1**).

For the intervention group, blood samples for a small blood count were collected 4 times at baseline, 1 week after the intervention, at the end of the intervention (consecutive day of the last intervention session) and 2 weeks after the intervention. Five missing data sets for the second time point and 3 missing data sets for the third time point were reported (subjects did not show up). Using mixed linear effects to model the effect over time, the red blood cell distribution showed a linear decrease over time ($p < 0.01$; **Table 2**).

Furthermore, an analysis of Pearson correlations between the baseline to post measure changes (%) revealed a close to significant positive correlation (one-tailed) for BDNF plasma and leucocyte counts ($R_{WBC} = 0.446$; $p = 0.055$) and a trend for a negative BDNF and lymphocyte interaction ($R_{lym} = -0.374$; $p = 0.094$).

DISCUSSION

Normobaric hypoxia such as with high-altitude training is generally assumed to have positive effects on physical and cognitive performance. Here, we tested the effect of a daily intermittent normobaric hypoxic training during a period of 2 weeks on the BDNF levels. While we observed the expected effects on blood parameters such as on the mean corpuscular hemoglobin concentration, contrary to our expectation, we found BDNF plasma levels to be significantly reduced 2 weeks after daily intermittent normobaric hypoxia over a period of 2 weeks. Regarding BDNF serum levels, no changes were detected. Research results from Pan et al. (1998) indicate that BDNF can pass the blood brain barrier by a high-capacity, saturable transport system and that 75% of BDNF plasma levels stems from the brain (Krabbe et al., 2007; Rasmussen et al., 2009).

Decreased BDNF levels are typically found in animal research when the animals have previously experienced stress. Various types of stress, including oxidative stress, have been shown to lead to decreased BDNF gene expression in cortical regions, including the hippocampus (Smith, 1996; Smith and Cizza, 1996; Bath et al., 2013; Kwon et al., 2013; Rothman and Mattson, 2013). In humans, a reduction in BDNF levels was seen after muscle damage or with very intensive physical exercise. To avoid such overtraining, successful exercise training is known to require sufficient resting periods (Parra et al., 2000). In rodents, physical activity induces BDNF gene expression in cortical regions, especially in the hippocampus (Neeper et al., 1995; Uysal et al., 2015). Studies on humans have reported an increase in BDNF levels following sportive interventions (Erickson et al., 2012; Müller et al., 2017a,b; Rehfeld et al., 2018). Others, however, failed to show changes in the levels of any of the neurotrophic factors that were assessed (Maass et al., 2016). A current review by Enette et al. (2017) provides a comprehensive analysis of the effects of aerobic training on BDNF plasma and serum levels in older adults. In 11 of the 14 randomized controlled trials that were included, the authors reported significantly increased BDNF plasma and/or serum levels after aerobic intervention.

Together, these findings indicate that our IHT protocol with its daily applications of hypoxic air might have been too intensive

TABLE 1 | Statistics of rANOVA on BDNF plasma and serum levels.

		Time			Group			Interaction (time x group)		
BDNF	***df***	***F***	***P***	η^2	***F***	***p***	η^2	***F***	***p***	η^2
plasma level	1,26	11.52	0.002**	0.307	0.425	0.520	0.016	10.742	0.003**	0.292
Serum level	1,25	2.24	0.147	0.082	10.53	0.003**	0.296	3.68	0.066	0.128

**$p < 0.01$.

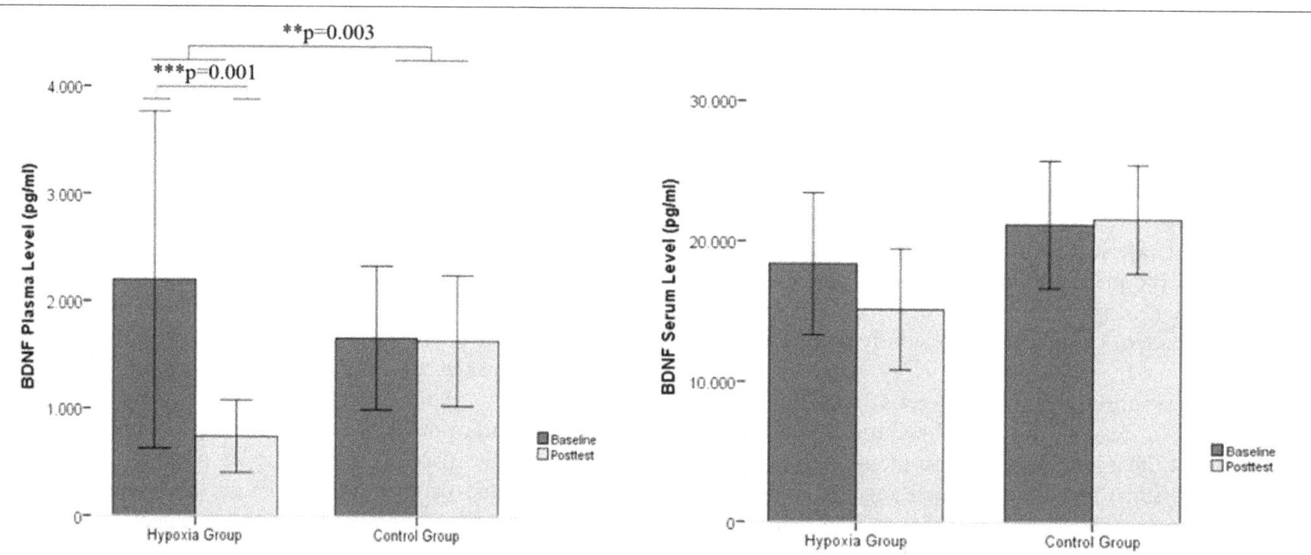

FIGURE 1 | BDNF plasma and serum levels between baseline and post intervention measures in the hypoxia intervention group and the control group (Mean ± SD). **$p < 0.01$ and ***$p < 0.001$.

TABLE 2 | Small blood count for the treatment group.

	Small blood count											
	Baseline (*N* = 14)		**1 week IHT (*N* = 9)**		**2 weeks IHT (*N* = 11)**		**Posttest (*N* = 14)**		**Linear time effect**		**Quadratic time effect**	
	Mean	**SD**	**Mean**	**SD**	**Mean**	**SD**	**Mean**	**SD**	***F***	***p***	***F***	***p***
RBCC ($\times 10^6$/ml)	4.94	0.43	5.00	0.29	4.75	0.36	4.83	0.36	1.066	0.308	0.628	0.539
RDW (%)	13.66	0.90	13.64	0.13	12.70	0.62	12.61	0.59	20.84	0.00**	1.259	0.295
HCT	0.46	0.03	0.44	0.03	0.43	0.03	0.45	0.03	1.852	0.181	1.443	0.248
HBG (mmol/L)	9.07	0.72	9.22	0.81	8.89	0.62	8.74	0.58	2.120	0.153	0.318	0.729
MCH (fmol)	1.84	0.13	1.84	0.08	1.87	0.10	1.81	0.09	0.287	0.595	0.903	0.414
MCHC (mmol/l)	19.79	0.79	21.02	0.55	20.48	0.52	19.70	0.53	0.163	0.689	11.77	0.000**
MCV (fl)	93.14	3.80	87.40	2.79	91.64	4.37	92.07	4.08	0.145	0.705	3.866	0.029*
WBC ($\times 10^3$/ml)	8.22	3.72	7.72	1.80	7.28	0.75	6.21	0.80	5.099	0.030*	0.106	0.899
SumGranul	0.63	0.10	0.66	0.06	0.61	0.06	0.58	0.06	3.369	0.074^t	0.603	0.552
Segs	0.60	0.10	0.63	0.05	0.58	0.07	0.55	0.06	3.839	0.057^t	0.908	0.411
Mono	0.06	0.01	0.07	0.01	0.06	0.02	0.06	0.02	0.071	0.792	0.496	0.613
Thrombocyte ($\times 10^3$/ml)	285.14	78.16	278.80	41.56	271.91	66.43	252.64	42.76	1.883	0.178	0.074	0.929

The mean values and SD for the RBCC, red blood cell count; RDW, red blood cell distribution width; HCT, hematocrit; HBG, hemoglobin; hypEryth, hypochromic erythrocytes; WBC, leukocyte count; MCH, lymphocytes, mean corpuscular/cellular hemoglobin; MCHC, mean corpuscular hemoglobin concentration; MCV, mean corpuscular volume; Mono, absolute monocyte count; Segs, segmented neutrophil granulocytes; SumGranul, sum granulocytes, thrombocytes. **$p < 0.01$ *$p < 0.05$ $^t p < 0.09$.

and, therefore, too stressful for the participants' bodies. In agreement with this finding, we observed a change in blood marker levels that were indicative of inflammation, namely, lymphocytes and granulocytes. Intensive physical exercise also induces inflammatory processes (Brown et al., 2015), and the latter has also been shown to relate to reduced BDNF levels after acute exercise at higher intensities (Nofuji et al., 2012; Cabral-Santos et al., 2016). Other conditions in which a reduction in BDNF levels was observed in the past include sleep apnea (Wang et al., 2012), birth stress associated with psychiatric disease later in life (Cannon et al., 2008), and stroke with low functional outcome (Lasek-Bal et al., 2015). With respect to the present study, the results of Wang et al. (2017) are of special relevance, as sleep apnea is associated with nocturnal intermittent hypoxia. Again, this finding suggests that "overdosing" hypoxia has detrimental effects on BDNF secretion.

The assumption that our IHT protocol was too intense and therefore decreased BDNF levels leads to the crucial question of whether other less stressful IHT protocols could still have a positive effect. In addition, methodological aspects (sampling time and preanalytical variations) could have an influence on the gained results. Indeed, there is an ongoing discussion of what type of hypoxia treatment is most effective (Serebrovskaya and Xi, 2016). A protocol that increases physical fitness at the same time may have negative effects on BDNF (Enette et al., 2017). Indeed, we had used a protocol that, in a former study, had shown positive effects on aerobic capacity.

Metabolic and Cardiovascular Response to Hypoxia

Several field experiments in the mountains and environmental studies in chambers report physiological effects of hypoxia (Heinonen et al., 2016). These experiments show that hypoxia can induce cardiovascular stress, can increase sympathetic neural activation and can alter energy metabolism. The complex metabolic response causes a release of various stress hormones (Kayser and Verges, 2013). Regarding cardiovascular response to normobaric hypoxia Heinonen et al. (2014) reported a significantly increased cardiac output, ejection fraction and tachycardia. Additionally, Heinonen et al. (2014, 2017) discuss hypoxia as a potential trigger for the release of brain natriuretic peptide (BNP) and the hormone apelin.

Limitations and Outlook

This randomized controlled feasibility study has several limitations. First, the sample size was small ($N = 28$). Second, the blood samples were only analyzed at baseline and after 2 weeks of intervention. Another limiting factor in the BDNF blood analyses is the large variances.

Future studies are needed to evaluate the correct dose of normobaric intermittent hypoxia to increase BDNF plasma levels and examine the underlying neurobiological mechanisms. An intensive assessment (neuropsychology, MRI/PET, cortisol, and IGF-1) would be useful to analyze the physiological adaptations to hypoxia.

In addition, BDNF has been suggested to play a mediating role in schizophrenia (Sokoloff et al., 2004; Guillin et al., 2007). Thus, several studies indicate an increase of the BDNF levels and gene expression in patients with schizophrenia (Laske and Eschweiler, 2006). In conclusion, an intermittent normobaric hypoxia regimen that successfully increases the BDNF levels may offer a non-pharmacological treatment to patients with schizophrenia.

AUTHOR CONTRIBUTIONS

AB contributed to study organization, data analysis, paper writing, and paper reviewing. PM contributed to data analysis, paper writing, and paper reviewing. MD reviewed the paper. VL and TB contributed to data analysis and paper reviewing. NM contributed to study organization, paper writing, and paper reviewing.

REFERENCES

Aravamudan, B., Thompson, M., Pabelick, C., and Prakash, Y. S. (2012). Brain-derived neurotrophic factor induces proliferation of human airway smooth muscle cells. *J. Cell Mol. Med.* 16, 812–823. doi: 10.1111/j.1582-4934.2011.01356.x

Bassovitch, O., and Serebrovskaya, T. V. (2009). "Equipment and regimes for intermittent hypoxia therapy," in *Intermittent Hypoxia: From Molecular Mechanismsto Clinical Applications*, eds L. Xi and T. V. Serebrovskaya (New York, NY: Nova Science Publishers).

Bath, K. G., Schilit, A., and Lee, F. S. (2013). Stress effects on BDNF expression: effects of age, sex, and form of stress. *Neuroscience* 239, 149–156. doi: 10.1016/j.neuroscience.2013.01.074

Brigadski, T., Hartmann, M., and Lessmann, V. (2005). Differential vesicular targeting and time course of synaptic secretion of the mammalian neurotrophins. *J. Neurosci.* 25, 7601–7614. doi: 10.1523/JNEUROSCI.1776-05.2005

Brigadski, T., and Leßmann, V. (2014). BDNF: a regulator of learning and memory processes with clinical potential. *e-Neuroforum* 5, 1–11. doi: 10.1007/s13295-014-0053-9

Brown, W. M., Davison, G. W., McClean, C. M., and Murphy, M. H. (2015). A systematic review of the acute effects of exercise on immune and inflammatory indices in untrained adults. *Sports Med. Open* 1:35. doi: 10.1186/s40798-015-0032-x

Burtscher, M., Haider, T., Domej, W., Linser, T., Gatterer, H., and Faulhaber, M. (2009). Intermittent hypoxia increases exercise tolerance in patients at risk for or with mild COPD. *Respir. Physiol. Neurobiol.* 165, 97–103. doi: 10.1016/j.resp.2008.10.012

Burtscher, M., Pachinger, O., Ehrenbourg, I., Mitterbauer, G., Faulhaber, M., Puhringer, R., et al. (2004). Intermittent hypoxia increases exercise tolerance in elderly men with and without coronary artery disease. *Int. J. Cardiol.* 96, 247–254. doi: 10.1016/j.ijcard.2003.07.021

Cabral-Santos, C., Castrillon, C. I., Miranda, R. A., Monteiro, P. A., Inoue, D. S., Campos, E. Z., et al. (2016). Inflammatory cytokines and BDNF response to high-intensity intermittent exercise: effect the exercise volume. *Front. Physiol.* 7:509. doi: 10.3389/fphys.2016.00509

Calabrese, F., Rossetti, A. C., Racagni, G., Gass, P., Riva, M. A., and Molteni, R. (2014). Brain-derived neurotrophic factor: a bridge between inflammation and neuroplasticity. *Front. Cell Neurosci.* 8:430. doi: 10.3389/fncel.2014.00430

Cannon, T. D., Yolken, R., Buka, S., Torrey, E. F., and Collaborative Study Group on the Perinatal Origins of Severe Psychiatric Disorders (2008). Decreased neurotrophic response to birth hypoxia in the etiology of schizophrenia. *Biol. Psychiatry* 64, 797–802. doi: 10.1016/j.biopsych.2008.04.012

Edelmann, E., Cepeda-Prado, E., Franck, M., Lichtenecker, P., Brigadski, T., and Lessmann, V. (2015). Theta burst firing recruits BDNF release and signaling in postsynaptic CA1 neurons in spike-timing-dependent LTP. *Neuron* 86, 1041–1054. doi: 10.1016/j.neuron.2015.04.007

Edelmann, E., Lessmann, V., and Brigadski, T. (2014). Pre- and postsynaptic twists in BDNF secretion and action in synaptic plasticity. *Neuropharmacology* 76(Pt C), 610–627. doi: 10.1016/j.neuropharm.2013.05.043

Enette, L., Vogel, T., Fanon, J. L., and Lang, P. O. (2017). Effect of interval and continuous aerobic training on basal serum and plasma brain-derived neurotrophic factor values in seniors: a systematic review of intervention studies. *Rejuvenation Res.* 20, 473–483. doi: 10.1089/rej.2016.1886

Erickson, K. I., Miller, D. L., and Roecklein, K. A. (2012). The aging hippocampus: interactions between exercise, depression, and BDNF. *Neuroscientist* 18, 82–97. doi: 10.1177/1073858410397054

Forlenza, O. V., Diniz, B. S., Teixeira, A. L., Ojopi, E. B., Talib, L. L., Mendonca, V. A., et al. (2010). Effect of brain-derived neurotrophic factor Val66Met polymorphism and serum levels on the progression of mild cognitive impairment. *World J. Biol. Psychiatry* 11, 774–780. doi: 10.3109/15622971003797241

Guillin, O., Demily, C., and Thibaut, F. (2007). Brain-derived neurotrophic factor in schizophrenia and its relation with dopamine. *Int. Rev. Neurobiol.* 78, 377–395. doi: 10.1016/S0074-7742(06)78012-6

Hartman, W., Helan, M., Smelter, D., Sathish, V., Thompson, M., Pabelick, C. M., et al. (2015). Role of hypoxia-induced brain derived neurotrophic factor in human pulmonary artery smooth muscle. *PLoS One* 10:e0129489. doi: 10.1371/journal.pone.0129489

Hartmann, M., Heumann, R., and Lessmann, V. (2001). Synaptic secretion of BDNF after high-frequency stimulation of glutamatergic synapses. *EMBO J.* 20, 5887–5897. doi: 10.1093/emboj/20.21.5887

Haubensak, W., Narz, F., Heumann, R., and Lessmann, V. (1998). BDNF-GFP containing secretory granules are localized in the vicinity of synaptic junctions of cultured cortical neurons. *J. Cell Sci.* 111(Pt 11), 1483–1493.

Heinonen, I., Luotolahti, M., Vuolteenaho, O., Nikinmaa, M., Saraste, A., Hartiala, J., et al. (2014). Circulating N-terminal brain natriuretic peptide, and cardiac function in response to acute systemic hypoxia in healthy humans. *J. Transl. Med.* 12:189. doi: 10.1186/1479-5876-12-189

Heinonen, I., Vuolteenaho, O., Koskenvuo, J., Arjamaa, O., and Nikinmaa, M. (2017). Systemic hypoxia increases circulating concentration of apelin in humans. *High Alt. Med. Biol.* 18, 292–295. doi: 10.1089/ham.2017.0017

Heinonen, I. H., Boushel, R., and Kalliokoski, K. K. (2016). The circulatory and metabolic responses to hypoxia in humans - with special reference to adipose tissue physiology and obesity. *Front. Endocrinol.* 7:116. doi: 10.3389/fendo.2016.00116

Helan, M., Aravamudan, B., Hartman, W. R., Thompson, M. A., Johnson, B. D., Pabelick, C. M., et al. (2014). BDNF secretion by human pulmonary artery endothelial cells in response to hypoxia. *J. Mol. Cell Cardiol.* 68, 89–97. doi: 10.1016/j.yjmcc.2014.01.006

Huang, E. J., and Reichardt, L. F. (2001). Neurotrophins: roles in neuronal development and function. *Annu. Rev. Neurosci.* 24, 677–736. doi: 10.1146/annurev.neuro.24.1.677

Kayser, B., and Verges, S. (2013). Hypoxia, energy balance and obesity: from pathophysiological mechanisms to new treatment strategies. *Obes. Rev.* 14, 579–592. doi: 10.1111/obr.12034

Kohara, K., Kitamura, A., Morishima, M., and Tsumoto, T. (2001). Activity-dependent transfer of brain-derived neurotrophic factor to postsynaptic neurons. *Science* 291, 2419–2423. doi: 10.1126/science.1057415

Krabbe, K. S., Nielsen, A. R., Krogh-Madsen, R., Plomgaard, P., Rasmussen, P., Erikstrup, C., et al. (2007). Brain-derived neurotrophic factor (BDNF) and type 2 diabetes. *Diabetologia* 50, 431–438. doi: 10.1007/s00125-006-0537-4

Kwon, D. H., Kim, B. S., Chang, H., Kim, Y. I., Jo, S. A., and Leem, Y. H. (2013). Exercise ameliorates cognition impairment due to restraint stress-induced oxidative insult and reduced BDNF level. *Biochem. Biophys. Res. Commun.* 434, 245–251. doi: 10.1016/j.bbrc.2013.02.111

Lasek-Bal, A., Jedrzejowska-Szypulka, H., Rozycka, J., Bal, W., Holecki, M., Dulawa, J., et al. (2015). Low concentration of BDNF in the acute phase of ischemic stroke as a factor in poor prognosis in terms of functional status of patients. *Med. Sci. Monit.* 21, 3900–3905. doi: 10.12659/MSM.895358

Laske, C., and Eschweiler, G. W. (2006). Brain-derived neurotrophic factor. vom nervenwachstumsfaktor zum plastizitätsmodulator bei kognitiven prozessen und psychischen erkrankungen. *Der Nervenarzt* 77, 523–537. doi: 10.1007/s00115-005-1971-0

Laske, C., Stransky, E., Leyhe, T., Eschweiler, G. W., Maetzler, W., Wittorf, A., et al. (2007). BDNF serum and CSF concentrations in Alzheimer's disease, normal pressure hydrocephalus and healthy controls. *J. Psychiatr. Res.* 41, 387–394. doi: 10.1016/j.jpsychires.2006.01.014

Leschik, J., Eckenstaler, R., Nieweg, K., Lichtenecker, P., Brigadski, T., Gottmann, K., et al. (2013). Embryonic stem cells stably expressing BDNF-GFP exhibit a BDNF-release-dependent enhancement of neuronal differentiation. *J. Cell Sci.* 126, 5062–5073. doi: 10.1242/jcs.135384

Levada, O. A., Cherednichenko, N. V., Trailin, A. V., and Troyan, A. S. (2016). Plasma brain-derived neurotrophic factor as a biomarker for the main types of mild neurocognitive disorders and treatment efficacy: a preliminary study. *Dis. Mark.* 2016:4095723. doi: 10.1155/2016/4095723

Maass, A., Duzel, S., Brigadski, T., Goerke, M., Becke, A., Sobieray, U., et al. (2016). Relationships of peripheral IGF-1, VEGF and BDNF levels to exercise-related changes in memory, hippocampal perfusion and volumes in older adults. *Neuroimage* 131, 142–154. doi: 10.1016/j.neuroimage.2015.10.084

Malle, C., Bourrilhon, C., Quinette, P., Laisney, M., Eustache, F., and Pierard, C. (2016). Physiological and cognitive effects of acute normobaric hypoxia and modulations from oxygen breathing. *Aerosp. Med. Hum. Perform.* 87, 3–12. doi: 10.3357/AMHP.4335.2016

Matsuda, N., Lu, H., Fukata, Y., Noritake, J., Gao, H., Mukherjee, S., et al. (2009). Differential activity-dependent secretion of brain-derived neurotrophic factor from axon and dendrite. *J. Neurosci.* 29, 14185–14198. doi: 10.1523/JNEUROSCI.1863-09.2009

Müller, P., Rehfeld, K., Schmicker, M., Hökelmann, A., Dordevic, M., Lessmann, V., et al. (2017a). Evolution of neuroplasticity in response to physical activity in old age: the case for dancing. *Front. Aging Neurosci.* 9:56. doi: 10.3389/fnagi.2017.00056

Müller, P., Schmicker, M., and Müller, N. G. (2017b). Preventive strategies for dementia. *Z. Gerontol. Geriatr.* 50, 89–95. doi: 10.1007/s00391-017-1202-x

Navarrete-Opazo, A., and Mitchell, G. S. (2014). Therapeutic potential of intermittent hypoxia: a matter of dose. *Am. J. Physiol. Regul. Integr. Comp. Physiol.* 307, R1181–R1197. doi: 10.1152/ajpregu.00208.2014

Neeper, S. A., Gomez-Pinilla, F., Choi, J., and Cotman, C. (1995). Exercise and brain neurotrophins. *Nature* 373:109. doi: 10.1038/373109a0

Nofuji, Y., Suwa, M., Sasaki, H., Ichimiya, A., Nishichi, R., and Kumagai, S. (2012). Different circulating brain-derived neurotrophic factor responses to acute exercise between physically active and sedentary subjects. *J. Sports Sci. Med.* 11, 83–88.

Pan, W., Banks, W. A., Fasold, M. B., Bluth, J., and Kastin, A. J. (1998). Transport of brain-derived neurotrophic factor across the blood-brain barrier. *Neuropharmacology* 37, 1553–1561. doi: 10.1016/S0028-3908(98)00141-5

Park, H., and Poo, M. M. (2013). Neurotrophin regulation of neural circuit development and function. *Nat. Rev. Neurosci.* 14, 7–23. doi: 10.1038/nrn3379

Parra, J., Cadefau, J. A., Rodas, G., Amigo, N., and Cusso, R. (2000). The distribution of rest periods affects performance and adaptations of energy metabolism induced by high-intensity training in human muscle. *Acta Physiol. Scand.* 169, 157–165. doi: 10.1046/j.1365-201x.2000.00730.x

Rasmussen, P., Brassard, P., Adser, H., Pedersen, M. V., Leick, L., Hart, E., et al. (2009). Evidence for a release of brain-derived neurotrophic factor from the brain during exercise. *Exp. Physiol.* 94, 1062–1069. doi: 10.1113/expphysiol.2009.048512

Rehfeld, K., Lüders, A., Hökelmann, A., Lessmann, V., Kaufmann, J., Brigadski, T., et al. (2018). Dance training is superior to repetitive physical exercise in inducing brain plasticity in the elderly. *PLoS One* 13:e0196636. doi: 10.1371/journal.pone.0196636

Rothman, S. M., and Mattson, M. P. (2013). Activity-dependent, stress-responsive BDNF signaling and the quest for optimal brain health and resilience throughout the lifespan. *Neuroscience* 239, 228–240. doi: 10.1016/j.neuroscience.2012.10.014

Ruscheweyh, R., Willemer, C., Kruger, K., Duning, T., Warnecke, T., Sommer, J., et al. (2011). Physical activity and memory functions: an interventional study. *Neurobiol. Aging* 32, 1304–1319. doi: 10.1016/j.neurobiolaging.2009.08.001

Schega, L., Peter, B., Brigadski, T., Lessmann, V., Isermann, B., Hamacher, D., et al. (2016). Effect of intermittent normobaric hypoxia on aerobic capacity and cognitive function in older people. *J. Sci. Med. Sport* 19, 941–945. doi: 10.1016/j.jsams.2016.02.012

Serebrovskaya, T. V., Manukhina, E. B., Smith, M. L., Downey, H. F., and Mallet, R. T. (2008). Intermittent hypoxia: cause of or therapy for systemic hypertension? *Exp. Biol. Med.* 233, 627–650. doi: 10.3181/0710-MR-267

Serebrovskaya, T. V., and Xi, L. (2016). Intermittent hypoxia training as non-pharmacologic therapy for cardiovascular diseases: practical analysis on methods and equipment. *Exp. Biol. Med.* 241, 1708–1723. doi: 10.1177/1535370216657614

Sharp, F. R., and Bernaudin, M. (2004). HIF1 and oxygen sensing in the brain. *Nat. Rev. Neurosci.* 5, 437–448. doi: 10.1038/nrn1408

Smith, M. A. (1996). Hippocampal vulnerability to stress and aging: possible role of neurotrophic factors. *Behav. Brain Res.* 78, 25–36. doi: 10.1016/0166-4328(95)00220-0

Smith, M. A., and Cizza, G. (1996). Stress-induced changes in brain-derived neurotrophic factor expression are attenuated in aged Fischer 344/N rats. *Neurobiol. Aging* 17, 859–864. doi: 10.1016/S0197-4580(96)00066-8

Sokoloff, P., Leriche, L., and Diaz, J. (2004). Brain-derived neurotrophic factor (BDNF) bridges the gap between dopamine and glutamate dysfunctions in schizophrenia. *Behav. Pharmacol.* 15, A4–A4. doi: 10.1097/00008877-200409000-00030

Tsai, Y. W., Yang, Y. R., Wang, P. S., and Wang, R. Y. (2011). Intermittent hypoxia after transient focal ischemia induces hippocampal neurogenesis and c-Fos expression and reverses spatial memory deficits in rats. *PLoS One* 6:e24001. doi: 10.1371/journal.pone.0024001

Uysal, N., Kiray, M., Sisman, A. R., Camsari, U. M., Gencoglu, C., Baykara, B., et al. (2015). Effects of voluntary and involuntary exercise on cognitive functions, and VEGF and BDNF levels in adolescent rats. *Biotech. Histochem.* 90, 55–68. doi: 10.3109/10520295.2014.946968

Vermehren-Schmaedick, A., Jenkins, V. K., Knopp, S. J., Balkowiec, A., and Bissonnette, J. M. (2012). Acute intermittent hypoxia-induced expression of brain-derived neurotrophic factor is disrupted in the brainstem of methyl-CpG-binding protein 2 null mice. *Neuroscience* 206, 1–6. doi: 10.1016/j.neuroscience.2012.01.017

Viscor, G., Torrella, J. R., Corral, L., Ricart, A., Javierre, C., Pages, T., et al. (2018). Physiological and biological responses to short-term intermittent hypobaric hypoxia exposure: from sports and mountain medicine to new biomedical applications. *Front. Physiol.* 9:814. doi: 10.3389/fphys.2018.00814

Wang, W. H., He, G. P., Xiao, X. P., Gu, C., and Chen, H. Y. (2012). Relationship between brain-derived neurotrophic factor and cognitive function of obstructive sleep apnea/hypopnea syndrome patients. *Asian Pac. J. Trop. Med.* 5, 906–910. doi: 10.1016/S1995-7645(12)60169-2

Wang, Y., Chai, Y., He, X., Ai, L., Sun, X., Huang, Y., et al. (2017). Intermittent hypoxia simulating obstructive sleep apnea causes pulmonary inflammation and activates the Nrf2/HO-1 pathway. *Exp. Ther. Med.* 14, 3463–3470. doi: 10.3892/etm.2017.4971

Wiener, C. M., Booth, G., and Semenza, G. L. (1996). *In vivo* expression of mRNAs encoding hypoxia-inducible factor 1. *Biochem. Biophys. Res. Commun.* 225, 485–488. doi: 10.1006/bbrc.1996.1199

Yan, X. (2014). Cognitive impairments at high altitudes and adaptation. *High Alt. Med. Biol.* 15, 141–145. doi: 10.1089/ham.2014.1009

Zhu, L. L., Zhao, T., Li, H. S., Zhao, H., Wu, L. Y., Ding, A. S., et al. (2005). Neurogenesis in the adult rat brain after intermittent hypoxia. *Brain Res.* 1055, 1–6. doi: 10.1016/j.brainres.2005.04.075

13

Hemoglobin Changes After Long-Term Intermittent Work at High Altitude

Almaz Akunov[1,2†], Akylbek Sydykov[1,3†], Turgun Toktash[4], Anara Doolotova[4] and Akpay Sarybaev[1,2]*

[1] Department of Mountain and Sleep Medicine and Pulmonary Hypertension, National Center of Cardiology and Internal Medicine, Bishkek, Kyrgyzstan, [2] Kyrgyz Indian Mountain Biomedical Research Center, Bishkek, Kyrgyzstan, [3] Excellence Cluster Cardio-Pulmonary System, Universities of Giessen and Marburg Lung Center, Member of the German Center for Lung Research (DZL), Justus Liebig University Giessen, Giessen, Germany, [4] Medical Department, Kumtor Gold Company, Bishkek, Kyrgyzstan

Correspondence:
Akpay Sarybaev
ak_sar777@mail.ru

† These authors have contributed equally to this work

Chronic high altitude hypoxia leads to an increase in red cell numbers and hemoglobin concentration. However, the effects of long-term intermittent hypoxia on hemoglobin concentration have not fully been studied. The aim of this study was to evaluate hemoglobin levels in workers commuting between an elevation of 3,800 m (2-week working shift) and lowland below 1,700 m (2 weeks of holiday). A total of 266 healthy males, aged from 20 to 69 years (mean age 45.9 ± 0.6 years), were included into this study. The duration of intermittent high altitude exposure ranged from 0 to 21 years. Any cardiac or pulmonary disorder was excluded during annual check-ups including clinical examination, clinical lab work (blood cell count, urine analysis, and biochemistry), ECG, echocardiography, and pulmonary function tests. The mean hemoglobin level in workers was 16.2 ± 0.11 g/dL. Univariate linear regression revealed an association of the hemoglobin levels with the years of exposure. Hemoglobin levels increased 0.068 g/dL [95% CI: 0.037 to 0.099, $p < 0.001$] for every year of intermittent high altitude exposure. Further, after adjusting for other confounding variables (age, living at low or moderate altitude, body mass index, and occupation) using multivariable regression analysis, the magnitude of hemoglobin level changes decreased, but remained statistically significant: 0.046 g/dL [95% CI: 0.005 to 0.086, $p < 0.05$]. Besides that, a weak linear relationship between hemoglobin levels and body mass index was revealed, which was independent of the years of exposure to high altitude (0.065 g/dL [95% CI: 0.006 to 0.124, $p < 0.05$]). We concluded that hemoglobin levels have a linear relationship with the exposure years spent in intermittent hypoxia and body mass index.

Keywords: chronic intermittent hypoxia, high altitude, shift workers, hemoglobin, body mass index

INTRODUCTION

Last decades, the number of people traveling to high altitude is increasing in connection with economic or recreational purposes (West, 2012). High altitude environment poses many challenges, but exposure to alveolar hypoxia is the most prominent among them (Burtscher et al., 2018). The ambient hypoxia triggers a number of physiologic responses including hyperventilation, increased resting heart rate and stimulation of erythrocyte production with the goal of maintaining the oxygen content of arterial blood at or above sea level values (West, 2004). In permanent high altitude residents, exposure to chronic hypoxia leads to an increase in erythrocyte numbers and hemoglobin concentration (Leon-Velarde et al., 2000).

A large group of people, such as workers of mining companies, employees of road construction companies or military divisions in high-altitude border areas are exposed repetitively to high altitude over a long time by commuting between high altitude and lowland (Powell and Garcia, 2000; Richalet et al., 2002; West, 2002; Farias et al., 2013). However, the effects of the long-term exposure to intermittent hypoxia on hemoglobin concentration have been less well studied. Only few studies have assessed hematological changes induced by long-term intermittent high altitude exposure. Some studies reported a marked increase in hemoglobin (or hematocrit) levels in response to long-term exposure to intermittent high altitude (Gunga et al., 1996; Heinicke et al., 2003), whereas others did not find a significant effect (Richalet et al., 2002; Brito et al., 2007, 2018). Therefore, the aim of the current study was to determine the association of long-term intermittent high altitude exposure with hemoglobin levels as well as to explore the nature of this possible relationship.

MATERIALS AND METHODS

Subjects and Study Design

This is a cross-sectional study of mine employees exposed repetitively to high altitude for long periods of time. All of them work at the gold mine run by the Kumtor Gold Company (Centerra Gold Inc., Canada). Mine employees are transported to the mine site by bus, and the ascent lasts 7 h in total.

Every worker undergoes an annual medical checkup in a specially designated clinic in Bishkek (Kyrgyzstan, 760 m), which includes physical examination, clinical lab work (complete blood count, urine analysis, and biochemistry), ECG, echocardiography, exercise testing and spirometry. All the male employees of the Kumtor Gold Company, who had medical checkup during October–December 2016, were enrolled into the study. The inclusion criteria were male sex, uninterrupted working at high altitude in 14×14 shifts (14 days of working at altitude followed by a resting period of 14 days at lowland) and a healthy status without serious cardiopulmonary comorbidities. The exclusion criteria were chronic obstructive pulmonary disease, moderate or severe hypertension, and coronary heart disease.

In total, 266 healthy males (aged 45.9 ± 0.6 years) were included into the study. Subjects were truck drivers, gold mill operators, camp and kitchen staff, security personnel, and engineers. All subjects commuted between high altitude and living place (760 m or 1,600 m) in a 14×14 shift regimen. The miners slept at 3,800 m and worked a 12-h day shift at 3,800 to 4,000 m, only few subjects (operators of drilling rigs) went to 4,500 m.

Written informed consent was obtained from all participants in accordance with the Declaration of Helsinki. This study was approved by the Research Ethics Committee of the National Center of Cardiology and Internal Medicine, Bishkek, Kyrgyzstan.

Measured Variables

Measures were taken once at low altitude in a specially designated clinic in Bishkek during the annual medical check-up. Usually, the annual medical check-up is carried out 1 week after descent. Any cardiac or pulmonary disorder was excluded based on the results of clinical examination, clinical lab work (blood cell count, urine analysis, and biochemistry), ECG, echocardiography, and pulmonary function tests.

General Data

Weight and height measured by means of a digital weight scale and a stadiometer with each participant barefoot and wearing underwear. Body mass index values were calculated as weight in kilograms divided by height in meters squared and rounded to 1 decimal place.

Hematological Measurements

Complete blood count was performed by an automated hematology analyser Mindray BC-2300 (Guangzhou Shihai Medical Equipment Co., Ltd., China) using 15 μm of EDTA whole venous blood according to the manufacturer's instructions. Hematocrit, concentration of hemoglobin, erythrocytes, leukocytes, and platelets were measured. The analyser uses electrical impedance method for cell counting and cyanide free method for hemoglobin detection. Red blood cell indices included hemoglobin concentration and mean corpuscular volume.

Data Analysis

Statistical analysis was performed using SPSS version 23.0 for Windows (IBM, Chicago, IL, United States). Data are expressed as mean ± standard error. The Kolmogorov–Smirnov test was used to assess the normality of distribution of quantitative variables. All quantitative variables were distributed normally. Linearity was assessed through examination of various bivariate scatterplots. Linear regression (univariate and multivariable) analysis was used to check the association between hemoglobin levels and other parameters. Differences between different BMI categories were assessed by one-way ANOVA followed by Tukey's multiple comparisons *post hoc* test. For comparing proportions, we used chi-squared test. For linear trend in quantitative variables we used one-way ANOVA linear contrast method. The values $P < 0.05$ were considered as statistically significant. Statistical power analysis was performed using G*Power 3.1.

RESULTS

Characteristics describing the subjects are provided in **Table 1**. One hundred and eighty-four workers were residents of moderate altitude (1,600 m); the remaining 82 men were residents of low altitude (760 m). The duration of exposure to intermittent high altitude ranged from 0 to 21 years. The average record of service was 10.1 years. The majority of subjects were ethnic Kyrgyz

(92%), but there were some Caucasians too (8%). Prevalence of obesity in the sample was 16.1 ± 2.4%. The mean hemoglobin level in workers was 16.2 ± 0.11 g/dL (**Table 1**). **Table 2** shows higher hemoglobin levels, as well as age and BMI, in subjects with longer duration of high altitude exposure. It is clear that hemoglobin levels are higher when the duration of exposure is longer ($p < 0.001$). Notably, the differences in age and BMI were also statistically significant; therefore, we cannot ascribe the differences in hemoglobin levels to the effects of high altitude alone. Indeed, hemoglobin values were significantly higher in obese subjects compared to those with normal weight (**Figure 1**).

Univariate linear regression revealed an association of the hemoglobin levels with the years of exposure (**Figure 2**). In a univariate regression model, every consecutive year was associated with an increase in hemoglobin of 0.068 g/dL [95% CI: 0.037 to 0.099, $p < 0.001$].

Further, after adjusting for other variables (age, living at low or moderate altitude, BMI, and occupation) using multivariable regression analysis, the magnitude of hemoglobin level changes decreased, but remained statistically significant: 0.046 g/dL [95% CI: 0.005 to 0.086, $p < 0.05$]. Despite a significant association of the hemoglobin levels with age by univariate regression analysis, it failed to prove the significance after adjusting for the rest variables (BMI, years of exposure, altitude of residence (0.006 g/dL [95% CI −0.024 to −0.035]) (**Table 3**). However, BMI and duration of exposure retained to have a weak but significant relationship with hemoglobin levels (0.065 g/dL [95% CI: 0.006 to 0.124] and 0.046 g/dL [95% CI: 0.005 to 0.086], respectively) (**Table 3**).

TABLE 1 | Anthropometric hematological characteristics of the subjects ($n = 266$).

Variables	Mean ± SEM
Age, years	45.9 ± 0.6
Body mass index, kg/m^2	26.8 ± 0.22
Obesity, %	16.1 ± 2.4
Kyrgyz ethnicity, %	91.4 ± 1.7
Job (outdoor vs. indoor)	73.1 ± 2.7
Duration of intermittent high altitude exposure, years	10.1 ± 0.4
Erythrocytes, 10^{12}/L	5.12 ± 0.03
Hemoglobin, g/dL	16.2 ± 0.11
Hematocrit, %	48 ± 0.3
Mean corpuscular volume, fL	93.9 ± 0.3
Leukocytes, 10^9/L	7.28 ± 0.12
Platelets, 10^9/L	245 ± 3.5

DISCUSSION

To our best knowledge, this is the first study performed on a large population of Kyrgyz workers intermittently exposed to high altitude for a very long period up to 21 years. We showed that there is a statistically significant correlation between the hemoglobin levels and the years of exposure. Using multivariable regression analysis, we showed that hemoglobin levels increase by an average of 0.046 g/dL for every consecutive year of intermittent high altitude exposure, after adjusting for other variables (age, living at low or moderate altitude, BMI, and occupation). Interestingly, the residence at low or moderate altitudes did not affect the hemoglobin levels. This may be due to the relatively small difference in the altitude of residence (less than 900 m).

Chronic high altitude hypoxia leads to an increase in red cell numbers and hemoglobin concentration. Previous studies have shown that permanent high altitude residents possess elevated hemoglobin levels and hematocrit values (Leon-Velarde et al., 2000). In sea-level residents, hematocrit and hemoglobin concentration were elevated after exposure to 3,550-m altitude for 8 months; however, none of the parameters reached pathological values (Siques et al., 2007). Only few studies have assessed hematological changes induced by long-term intermittent high altitude exposure in a comprehensive manner. An earlier study in Chilean workers exposed to intermittent high altitude for >5 years revealed hemoglobin values that were comparable to those reported in the literature for high altitude populations (Gunga et al., 1996). Similarly, increased hemoglobin concentration and hematocrit values (15.8 ± 1.2 g/dL and 46.2 ± 3.8%, respectively) were shown in Chilean army officers exposed to intermittent hypoxia for about 22 years after 3 days following descent to sea level (Heinicke et al., 2003). Remarkably, hemoglobin concentration and hematocrit values (16.5 ± 0.9 g/dL and 48.1 ± 2.9%, respectively) measured at high altitude were comparable to those found in permanent high altitude residents (Heinicke et al., 2003). Another study conducted in a group of Chilean army officers exposed to intermittent high altitude for at least 12 years (50% had been >25 years at altitude) reported a smaller increase in hemoglobin

TABLE 2 | Distribution of the hemoglobin levels, age, body mass index, and residence place of the subjects according to the years of high altitude exposure.

Variables	Intermittent high altitude exposure, years					P
	0	1–5	6–10	11–15	>15	
Hb, g/dL	14.9 ± 0.25	15.9 ± 0.27	16.1 ± 0.18	16.5 ± 0.26	16.6 ± 0.2	<0.001
Age, years	37.3 ± 1.6	39.2 ± 1.8	44.4 ± 0.9	50.1 ± 1.3)	53.3 ± 0.8	<0.001
BMI, kg/m^2	24.3 ± 0.9	26.4 ± 0.6	26.7 ± 0.4	27.6 ± 0.5	27.7 ± 0.4	<0.01
Residents of moderate altitude, %	88 ± 8	53 ± 9	68 ± 5	66 ± 8	76 ± 6	NS

Data are presented as mean ± SEM (n = 266). Hb, hemoglobin; BMI, body mass index. p for linearity (hemoglobin, age, BMI) was determined using one-way ANOVA linear contrast analysis; p for trend (residents) was determined using chi^2-criterion.

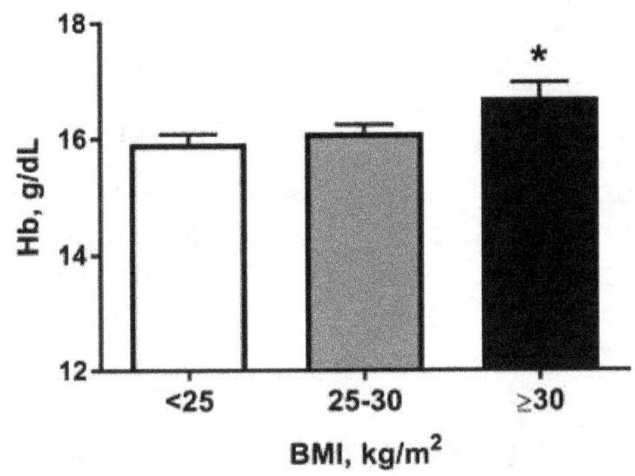

FIGURE 1 | Hemoglobin (Hb) levels in subjects according to their body mass index (BMI) category: normal weight (<25), overweight (25–30), and obese (≥30). $^{*}P < 0.05$ for differences between normal weight and obese subjects. Data presented as mean ± SEM. Statistical analysis was carried out using one-way ANOVA followed by Tukey's multiple comparison test.

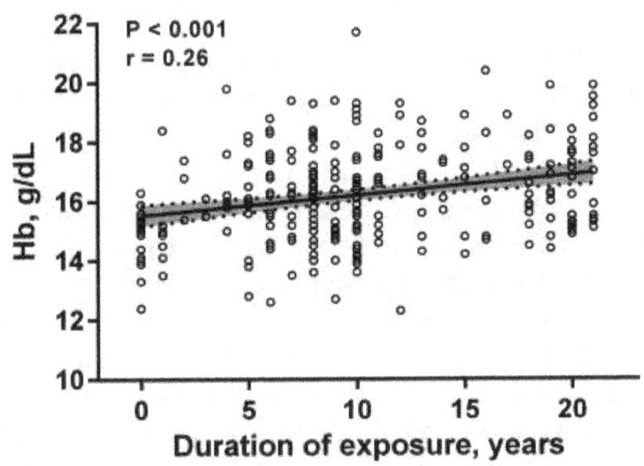

FIGURE 2 | Scatter plot of correlation between the hemoglobin (Hb) levels and the years of exposure to intermittent high altitude. The best-fit line is shown, and the shaded area represents the 95% confidence intervals (n = 266).

concentration and hematocrit values (15.1 ± 1.0 g/dL and 45.02 ± 2.7%, respectively) measured on day 1 following descent to sea level (Brito et al., 2007). Similarly, a period of 2.5-year exposure to intermittent hypoxia induced a significant hematocrit increase in Chilean miners, which was, however, lower than what is observed in permanent high altitude residents (Richalet et al., 2002). A recent cross-sectional study in healthy Chilean male miners working at an altitude of 4,400 or 4,800 m for, on average, 14 years reported mean hematocrit and hemoglobin values of 47.6 ± 0.3% and 16.2 ± 0.1 g/dL, respectively, with none of the subjects having pathological values (Brito et al., 2018). In our study, hemoglobin concentration and hematocrit values in shift workers were higher than those observed in sea level residents, but were lower than values reported in Aymara native residents at 3,800–4,065 m (Beall et al., 1998).

Various factors may be responsible for the discrepancy. A meta-analysis and a Monte Carlo simulation on the extracted data showed that red cell volume expansion for a given duration of exposure is dependent on the altitude (Rasmussen et al., 2013). The authors suggested that, at altitudes above 4,000 m, exposure time must exceed 2 weeks to exert a significant effect and that the magnitude of the erythropoietic response depends on the initial red cell volume (Rasmussen et al., 2013). In addition, hemoglobin mass returns to baseline sea level values in 2–3 weeks following descent to sea level (Wachsmuth et al., 2013). Moreover, the mining companies and military divisions in different countries implement various commuting patterns complicating the interpretation of the hematological changes induced by the long-term intermittent high altitude exposure. The most common shift patterns range from 4×3 days to 28×28 days (Gunga et al., 1996; Richalet et al., 2002; Heinicke et al., 2003; Sarybaev et al., 2003; Brito et al., 2007; Vinnikov et al., 2011). Furthermore, ethnic differences have been shown in hematological responses in high altitude residents (Beall, 2006). If ethnicity affects hematological responses to chronic intermittent high altitude exposure is not known.

Another explanation could be the various duration of stay at high altitude and the elevation achieved in different studies Therefore, a term "hypoxic dose" has recently been introduced as a new metric incorporating both altitude and total exposure time to measure an increase in hemoglobin mass because of intermittent hypoxic training or intermittent hypoxic exposure (Garvican-Lewis et al., 2016a). The models suggest that hypoxic exposure in excess of 250 km h is sufficient to produce an increase in hemoglobin mass (Garvican-Lewis et al., 2016b). In our study, the workers were exposed to the hypoxic dose of about 1,300 km h, which is considered to be sufficient to induce an increase in hemoglobin levels.

Univariate analysis showed a relationship of hemoglobin levels with aging; however, after adjusting for other variables, the value ceased to be significant. These results are in line with the findings from other studies. Thus, no significant hematocrit change over 11.6 years was demonstrated in a recent prospective study (Carallo et al., 2011). In another study, while fibrinogen, another blood viscosity parameter, increased with age, the hemoglobin level on the contrary slightly decreased in the elderly subjects (Coppola et al., 2000). Notably, we revealed a significant relation of hemoglobin levels with the BMI in workers exposed to intermittent high altitude for a long period. It is in accordance with other studies that demonstrated a positive association between hemoglobin and BMI in lowland populations (Micozzi et al., 1989; Skjelbakken et al., 2010). In contrast, no correlation between hemoglobin levels and BMI was reported by others (Ghadiri-Anari et al., 2014). Nevertheless, in a recent prospective study of high-altitude mine workers in Peru, male gender, duration of the intermittent high altitude exposure and BMI were independent predictors of hemoglobin level changes (Mejia et al., 2017). The underlying mechanisms remain poorly understood. However, a negative effect of BMI on oxygen saturation was demonstrated in Chinese Han young males during high altitude acclimatization (Peng et al., 2013). Interestingly, a negative association between BMI and blood oxygenation was also found in healthy high altitude residents in Peru (Pereira-Victorio et al., 2014; Miele et al., 2016). These data

TABLE 3 | Associations between hemoglobin levels and other variables by univariate and multivariable analysis.

Variables	Univariate			Multivariable*		
	b	95% CI	*p*	*b*	95% CI	*p*
Age, years	0.027	0.006–0.048	<0.05	0.006	−0.024 – 0.035	NS
BMI, kg/m^2	0.084	0.027–0.141	<0.01	0.065	0.006 – 0.124	<0.05
Years of intermittent high altitude exposure	0.068	0.037–0.099	<0.001	0.046	0.005 – 0.086	<0.05
Residence at moderate altitude	0.023	−0.39 – 0.44	NS	−0.061	−0.239 – 0.117	NS

*BMI, body mass index. *adjusted for the other variables. R^2 = 0.07.*

suggest that shift workers with higher BMI will have a greater increase in hemoglobin during chronic intermittent high altitude exposure.

It has been shown that borderline polycythemia (hematocrit above 50%) was associated with increased mortality from coronary heart disease (Kunnas et al., 2009). However, the connection between hemoglobin and cardiovascular diseases is complex and is still not clear (Brown et al., 2001; Frackiewicz et al., 2018). We have to admit that prolonged intermittent high altitude hypoxia can provoke cardiovascular events in patients with clinical or subclinical coronary atherosclerosis because of blood rheology changes. Interestingly, accumulating evidence demonstrates that short-term daily sessions of hypoxia alternating with equal durations of normoxia for 2–3 weeks exert beneficial effects on various cardiovascular diseases (Serebrovskaya and Xi, 2016), thus potentially opposing deleterious effects of polycythemia. At the same time, the increase in hemoglobin levels due to chronic intermittent high altitude exposure should not lead to increased probability of cardiovascular events *per se*.

Although the literature on the relation between changes in hemoglobin concentration and cardiovascular disorders in subjects exposed to long-term intermittent high altitude hypoxia is very scarce, we believe that such a small, though statistically significant, increase in hemoglobin concentration represents an adaptive response rather than a risk factor for cardiovascular diseases. An annual increase in hemoglobin level by 0.046 g/dL means that for every 10 years of work at intermittent high altitude hypoxia hemoglobin levels will rise, on average, less than 0.5 g/dL. Indeed, in most of the subjects chronically exposed to intermittent high altitude, hemoglobin concentration and hematocrit reach intermediate values that are higher than those in sea level residents but lower than those in healthy high altitude dwellers (Richalet et al., 2002; Brito et al., 2007). It is unlikely that this rather small increase in hemoglobin levels would have any significant pathological effects (Burtscher, 2014; Corante et al., 2018).

Additionally, another issue related to hemoglobin levels at high-altitude is the change in skeletal muscle mass, since muscles are the main consumer of oxygen in the body. While some studies indicated some decrease in skeletal muscle mass at high-altitude exposure (Hoppeler et al., 1990; MacDougall et al., 1991; Mizuno et al., 2008), the others were not able to show significant loss of muscle mass (Lundby et al., 2004; D'Hulst et al., 2016; Jacobs et al., 2016). Differences in the hypoxic doses may account for this discrepancy. Thus, it has been suggested that a minimum hypoxic exposure of 5,000 km h is required for hypoxia-induced muscle atrophy to develop (D'Hulst and Deldicque, 2017). Although, we have not measured the skeletal muscle fiber cross sectional area changes in the workers, it seems unlikely that the relatively low hypoxic dose in our study can significantly affect the skeletal muscle.

Another kind of intermittent hypoxia which deserves further commentary is obstructive sleep apnea syndrome (OSAS). OSAS is a pathological condition characterized by recurrent or cyclic short periods of isobaric hypoxia and asphyxia during sleep (coupled with oxygen desaturation), often more than 60 times per hour (Neubauer, 2001). Such frequent fluctuations of oxygen saturation lead to sympathetic overactivity, increased oxidative stress, and activation of inflammatory response pathways (Mansukhani et al., 2014; Passali et al., 2015; de Lima et al., 2016). In addition to hypoxemia, these events are associated with significant hypercapnia. Consequently, OSAS is an independent and well-known major risk factor for various cardiovascular diseases, including hypertension, stroke, myocardial infarction, and congestive heart failure (Kendzerska et al., 2014; Drager et al., 2015; Bauters et al., 2016). In contrast, chronic intermittent hypoxic exposure in miners involves prolonged cycles of hypobaric hypoxia alternating with normobaric normoxia. The frequency of high altitude intermittent hypoxia is usually one to four times a month, which does not have such unfavorable effects on the body. Thus, as previously pointed out (Richalet et al., 2002), OSAS is quite different from the chronic intermittent hypoxic exposure in miners.

One of the limitations of this study is its cross-sectional nature. Further, most of the subjects were permanent residents of a moderate altitude, so the difference in altitude between the residence place and working altitude was relatively small. Nevertheless, the strengths of our study include high number of subjects, which provided the high statistical power, and larger duration of intermittent high altitude exposure than in most other studies.

CONCLUSION

In summary, this study adds to the growing body of knowledge concerning the physiology of long-term intermittent high altitude exposure. We defined for the first time hemoglobin levels in Kyrgyz shift workers commuting between high altitude and lowland. Further, our study provides evidence that hemoglobin levels have a linear relationship with years of intermittent high altitude exposure and BMI. Apparently, in chronic intermittent hypoxia exposure even over longer periods, excessive erythrocytosis does not represent a major problem for healthy shift workers. Our findings might have important implications for occupational medical surveillance to monitor health status of the workers exposed to chronic intermittent high altitude. We hope that our study would encourage further research to explore the long-term consequences of this unique biological condition.

AUTHOR CONTRIBUTIONS

AA, AbS, and ApS conceived and designed the study, drafted the manuscript, and provided overall supervision. AA, AbS, TT, and AD performed the data acquisition, analysis, or interpretation. AA, AbS, TT, AD, and ApS critically revised important intellectual content in the manuscript and approved the final version of the manuscript.

FUNDING

This work was supported by Ministry of Education and Science of the Kyrgyz Republic (Grant No. 0005823).

REFERENCES

Bauters, F., Rietzschel, E. R., Hertegonne, K. B., and Chirinos, J. A. (2016). The link between obstructive sleep apnea and cardiovascular disease. *Curr. Atheroscler. Rep.* 18:1. doi: 10.1007/s11883-015-0556-z

Beall, C. M. (2006). Andean, Tibetan, and Ethiopian patterns of adaptation to high-altitude hypoxia. *Integr. Comp. Biol.* 46, 18–24. doi: 10.1093/icb/icj004

Beall, C. M., Brittenham, G. M., Strohl, K. P., Blangero, J., Williams-Blangero, S., Goldstein, M. C., et al. (1998). Hemoglobin concentration of high-altitude Tibetans and Bolivian Aymara. *Am. J. Phys. Anthropol.* 106, 385–400. doi: 10.1002/(SICI)1096-8644(199807)106:3<385::AID-AJPA10>3.0.CO;2-X

Brito, J., Siques, P., Leon-Velarde, F., De La Cruz, J. J., Lopez, V., and Herruzo, R. (2007). Chronic intermittent hypoxia at high altitude exposure for over 12 years: assessment of hematological, cardiovascular, and renal effects. *High Alt. Med. Biol.* 8, 236–244. doi: 10.1089/ham.2007.8310

Brito, J., Siques, P., López, R., Romero, R., León-Velarde, F., Flores, K., et al. (2018). Long-Term intermittent work at high altitude: right heart functional and morphological status and associated cardiometabolic factors. *Front. Physiol.* 9:248. doi: 10.3389/fphys.2018.00248

Brown, D. W., Giles, W. H., and Croft, J. B. (2001). Hematocrit and the risk of coronary heart disease mortality. *Am. Heart J.* 142, 657–663. doi: 10.1067/mhj.2001.118467

Burtscher, M. (2014). Effects of living at higher altitudes on mortality: a narrative review. *Aging Dis.* 5, 274–280. doi: 10.14336/ad.2014.0500274

Burtscher, M., Gatterer, H., Burtscher, J., and Mairbaurl, H. (2018). Extreme terrestrial environments: life in thermal stress and hypoxia. a narrative review. *Front. Physiol.* 9:572. doi: 10.3389/fphys.2018.00572

Carallo, C., Irace, C., De Franceschi, M. S., Coppoletta, F., Tiriolo, R., Scicchitano, C., et al. (2011). The effect of aging on blood and plasma viscosity. An 11.6 years follow-up study. *Clin. Hemorheol. Microcirc.* 47, 67–74. doi: 10.3233/ch-2010-1367

Coppola, L., Caserta, F., De Lucia, D., Guastafierro, S., Grassia, A., Coppola, A., et al. (2000). Blood viscosity and aging. *Arch. Gerontol. Geriatr.* 31, 35–42. doi: 10.1016/S0167-4943(00)00063-7

Corante, N., Anza-Ramirez, C., Figueroa-Mujica, R., Macarlupu, J. L., Vizcardo-Galindo, G., Bilo, G., et al. (2018). Excessive erythrocytosis and cardiovascular risk in andean highlanders. *High Alt. Med. Biol.* 19, 221–231. doi: 10.1089/ham.2017.0123

de Lima, F. F., Mazzotti, D. R., Tufik, S., and Bittencourt, L. (2016). The role inflammatory response genes in obstructive sleep apnea syndrome: a review. *Sleep Breath* 20, 331–338. doi: 10.1007/s11325-015-1226-7

D'Hulst, G., and Deldicque, L. (2017). Human skeletal muscle wasting in hypoxia: a matter of hypoxic dose? *J. Appl. Physiol.* 122, 406–408. doi: 10.1152/japplphysiol.00264.2016

D'Hulst, G., Ferri, A., Naslain, D., Bertrand, L., Horman, S., Francaux, M., et al. (2016). Fifteen days of 3,200 m simulated hypoxia marginally regulates markers for protein synthesis and degradation in human skeletal muscle. *Hypoxia* 4, 1–14. doi: 10.2147/hp.s101133

Drager, L. F., Polotsky, V. Y., O'Donnell, C. P., Cravo, S. L., Lorenzi-Filho, G., and Machado, B. H. (2015). Translational approaches to understanding metabolic dysfunction and cardiovascular consequences of obstructive sleep apnea. *Am. J. Physiol. Heart Circ. Physiol.* 309, H1101–H1111. doi: 10.1152/ajpheart.00094.2015

Farias, J. G., Jimenez, D., Osorio, J., Zepeda, A. B., Figueroa, C. A., and Pulgar, V. M. (2013). Acclimatization to chronic intermittent hypoxia in mine workers: a challenge to mountain medicine in Chile. *Biol. Res.* 46, 59–67. doi: 10.4067/s0716-97602013000100009

Frackiewicz, J., Wlodarek, D., Brzozowska, A., Wierzbicka, E., Slowinska, M. A., Wadolowska, L., et al. (2018). Hematological parameters and all-cause mortality: a prospective study of older people. *Aging Clin. Exp. Res.* 30, 517–526. doi: 10.1007/s40520-017-0791-y

Garvican-Lewis, L. A., Sharpe, K., and Gore, C. J. (2016a). Last word on viewpoint: time for a new metric for hypoxic dose? *J. Appl. Physiol.* 121:359. doi: 10.1152/japplphysiol.00457.2016

Garvican-Lewis, L. A., Sharpe, K., and Gore, C. J. (2016b). Time for a new metric for hypoxic dose? *J. Appl. Physiol.* 121, 352–355. doi: 10.1152/japplphysiol.00579.2015

Ghadiri-Anari, A., Nazemian, N., and Vahedian-Ardakani, H.-A. (2014). Association of body mass index with hemoglobin concentration and iron parameters in Iranian population. *ISRN Hematol.* 2014:525312. doi: 10.1155/2014/525312

Gunga, H. C., Rocker, L., Behn, C., Hildebrandt, W., Koralewski, E., Rich, I., et al. (1996). Shift working in the Chilean Andes (> 3,600 m) and its influence on erythropoietin and the low-pressure system. *J. Appl. Physiol.* 81, 846–852. doi: 10.1152/jappl.1996.81.2.846

Heinicke, K., Prommer, N., Cajigal, J., Viola, T., Behn, C., and Schmidt, W. (2003). Long-term exposure to intermittent hypoxia results in increased hemoglobin mass, reduced plasma volume, and elevated erythropoietin plasma levels in man. *Eur. J. Appl. Physiol.* 88, 535–543. doi: 10.1007/s00421-002-0732-z

Hoppeler, H., Kleinert, E., Schlegel, C., Claassen, H., Howald, H., Kayar, S. R., et al. (1990). Morphological adaptations of human skeletal muscle to chronic hypoxia. *Int. J. Sports Med.* 11(Suppl. 1), S3–S9. doi: 10.1055/s-2007-1024846

Jacobs, R. A., Lundby, A. K., Fenk, S., Gehrig, S., Siebenmann, C., Fluck, D., et al. (2016). Twenty-eight days of exposure to 3454 m increases mitochondrial volume density in human skeletal muscle. *J. Physiol.* 594, 1151–1166. doi: 10.1113/jp271118

Kendzerska, T., Gershon, A. S., Hawker, G., Leung, R. S., and Tomlinson, G. (2014). Obstructive sleep apnea and risk of cardiovascular events and all-cause mortality: a decade-long historical cohort study. *PLoS Med.* 11:e1001599. doi: 10.1371/journal.pmed.1001599

Kunnas, T., Solakivi, T., Huuskonen, K., Kalela, A., Renko, J., and Nikkari, S. T. (2009). Hematocrit and the risk of coronary heart disease mortality in the TAMRISK study, a 28-year follow-up. *Prev. Med.* 49, 45–47. doi: 10.1016/j.ypmed.2009.04.015

Leon-Velarde, F., Gamboa, A., Chuquiza, J. A., Esteba, W. A., Rivera-Chira, M., and Monge, C. C. (2000). Hematological parameters in high altitude residents living at 4,355, 4,660, and 5,500 meters above sea level. *High Alt. Med. Biol.* 1, 97–104. doi: 10.1089/15270290050074233

Lundby, C., Pilegaard, H., Andersen, J. L., van Hall, G., Sander, M., and Calbet, J. A. (2004). Acclimatization to 4100 m does not change capillary density or mRNA expression of potential angiogenesis regulatory factors in human skeletal muscle. *J. Exp. Biol.* 207(Pt 22), 3865–3871. doi: 10.1242/jeb.01225

MacDougall, J. D., Green, H. J., Sutton, J. R., Coates, G., Cymerman, A., Young, P., et al. (1991). Operation Everest II: structural adaptations in skeletal muscle in response to extreme simulated altitude. *Acta Physiol. Scand.* 142, 421–427. doi: 10.1111/j.1748-1716.1991.tb09176.x

Mansukhani, M. P., Kara, T., Caples, S. M., and Somers, V. K. (2014). Chemoreflexes, sleep apnea, and sympathetic dysregulation. *Curr. Hypertens. Rep.* 16:476. doi: 10.1007/s11906-014-0476-2

Mejia, C. R., Quinones-Laveriano, D. M., Gomero, R., and Perez-Perez, L. (2017). [Hemoglobin changes (Hb) in miners exposed to high altitude and associated factors]. *Gac. Med. Mex.* 153, 166–172.

Micozzi, M. S., Albanes, D., and Stevens, R. G. (1989). Relation of body size and composition to clinical biochemical and hematologic indices in US men and women. *Am. J. Clin. Nutr.* 50, 1276–1281. doi: 10.1093/ajcn/50.6.1276

Miele, C. H., Schwartz, A. R., Gilman, R. H., Pham, L., Wise, R. A., Davila-Roman, V. G., et al. (2016). Increased cardiometabolic risk and worsening hypoxemia at high altitude. *High Alt. Med. Biol.* 17, 93–100. doi: 10.1089/ham.2015.0084

Mizuno, M., Savard, G. K., Areskog, N. H., Lundby, C., and Saltin, B. (2008). Skeletal muscle adaptations to prolonged exposure to extreme altitude: a role of physical activity? *High Alt. Med. Biol.* 9, 311–317. doi: 10.1089/ham.2008.1009

Neubauer, J. A. (2001). Invited review: Physiological and pathophysiological responses to intermittent hypoxia. *J. Appl. Physiol.* 90, 1593–1599. doi: 10.1152/jappl.2001.90.4.1593

Passali, D., Corallo, G., Yaremchuk, S., Longini, M., Proietti, F., Passali, G. C., et al. (2015). Oxidative stress in patients with obstructive sleep apnoea syndrome. *Acta Otorhinolaryngol. Ital.* 35, 420–425. doi: 10.14639/0392-100x-895

Peng, Q. Q., Basang, Z., Cui, C. Y., Li, L., Qian, J., Gesang, Q., et al. (2013). Physiological responses and evaluation of effects of BMI, smoking and drinking in high altitude acclimatization: a cohort study in Chinese Han young males. *PLoS One* 8:e79346. doi: 10.1371/journal.pone.0079346

Pereira-Victorio, C. J., Huamanquispe-Quintana, J., and Castelo-Tamayo, L. E. (2014). [Arterial blood gases in clinically healthy adults living at 3,350 meters of altitude]. *Rev. Peru. Med. Exp. Salud. Pub.* 31, 473–479.

Powell, F. L., and Garcia, N. (2000). Physiological effects of intermittent hypoxia. *High Alt. Med. Biol.* 1, 125–136. doi: 10.1089/15270290050074279

Rasmussen, P., Siebenmann, C., Diaz, V., and Lundby, C. (2013). Red cell volume expansion at altitude: a meta-analysis and Monte Carlo simulation. *Med. Sci. Sports Exerc.* 45, 1767–1772. doi: 10.1249/MSS.0b013e31829047e5

Richalet, J. P., Donoso, M. V., Jimenez, D., Antezana, A. M., Hudson, C., Cortes, G., et al. (2002). Chilean miners commuting from sea level to 4500 m: a prospective study. *High Alt. Med. Biol.* 3, 159–166. doi: 10.1089/15270290260131894

Sarybaev, A. S., Palasiewicz, G., Usupbaeva, D. A., Plywaczewski, R., Maripov, A. M., Sydykov, A. S., et al. (2003). Effects of intermittent exposure to high altitude on pulmonary hemodynamics: a prospective study. *High Alt. Med. Biol.* 4, 455–463. doi: 10.1089/152702903322616209

Serebrovskaya, T. V., and Xi, L. (2016). Intermittent hypoxia training as non-pharmacologic therapy for cardiovascular diseases: Practical analysis on methods and equipment. *Exp. Biol. Med.* 241, 1708–1723. doi: 10.1177/1535370216657614

Siques, P., Brito, J., Leon-Velarde, F., Barrios, L., De La Cruz, J. J., Lopez, V., et al. (2007). Hematological and lipid profile changes in sea-level natives after exposure to 3550-m altitude for 8 months. *High Alt. Med. Biol.* 8, 286–295. doi: 10.1089/ham.2007.8405

Skjelbakken, T., Dahl, I. M. S., and Lochen, M.-L. (2010). Changes in body mass index and smoking habits have a different impact on hemoglobin concentration in men and women: a longitudinal follow-up of the Tromso Study, 1994-2002. *Gender Med.* 7, 230–239. doi: 10.1016/j.genm.2010.06.006

Vinnikov, D., Brimkulov, N., and Redding-Jones, R. (2011). Four-year prospective study of lung function in workers in a high altitude (4000 m) mine. *High Alt. Med. Biol.* 12, 65–69. doi: 10.1089/ham.2010.1033

Wachsmuth, N. B., Volzke, C., Prommer, N., Schmidt-Trucksass, A., Frese, F., Spahl, O., et al. (2013). The effects of classic altitude training on hemoglobin mass in swimmers. *Eur. J. Appl. Physiol.* 113, 1199–1211. doi: 10.1007/s00421-012-2536-0

West, J. B. (2002). Intermittent exposure to high altitude. *High Alt. Med. Biol.* 3, 141–143. doi: 10.1089/15270290260131858

West, J. B. (2004). The physiologic basis of high-altitude diseases. *Ann. Intern. Med.* 141, 789–800. doi: 10.7326/0003-4819-141-10-200411160-00010

West, J. B. (2012). High-altitude medicine. *Am. J. Respir. Crit. Care Med.* 186, 1229–1237. doi: 10.1164/rccm.201207-1323CI

14

Imbalance in Renal Vasoactive Enzymes Induced by Mild Hypoxia: Angiotensin-Converting Enzyme Increases While Neutral Endopeptidase Decreases

Carlos P. Vio[1,2], Daniela Salas[1], Carlos Cespedes[1], Jessica Diaz-Elizondo[1], Natalia Mendez[1,3], Julio Alcayaga[4] and Rodrigo Iturriaga[5]*

[1] Department of Physiology, Center for Aging and Regeneration CARE UC, Facultad de Ciencias Biológicas, Pontificia Universidad Católica de Chile, Santiago, Chile, [2] Facultad de Medicina y Ciencia, Universidad San Sebastián, Santiago, Chile, [3] Institute of Anatomy, Histology, and Pathology, Facultad de Medicina, Universidad Austral de Chile, Valdivia, Chile, [4] Laboratorio de Fisiología Celular, Departamento de Biología, Facultad de Ciencias, Universidad de Chile, Santiago, Chile, [5] Laboratorio de Neurobiología, Department of Physiology, Facultad de Ciencias Biológicas, Pontificia Universidad Católica de Chile, Santiago, Chile

***Correspondence:**
Carlos P. Vio
cvio@uc.cl

Chronic hypoxia has been postulated as one of the mechanisms involved in salt-sensitive hypertension and chronic kidney disease (CKD). Kidneys have a critical role in the regulation of arterial blood pressure through vasoactive systems, such as the renin-angiotensin and the kallikrein–kinin systems, with the angiotensin-converting enzyme (ACE) and kallikrein being two of the main enzymes that produce angiotensin II and bradykinin, respectively. Neutral endopeptidase 24.11 or neprilysin is another enzyme that among its functions degrade vasoactive peptides including angiotensin II and bradykinin, and generate angiotensin 1–7. On the other hand, the kidneys are vulnerable to hypoxic injury due to the active electrolyte transportation that requires a high oxygen consumption; however, the oxygen supply is limited in the medullary regions for anatomical reasons. With the hypothesis that the chronic reduction of oxygen under normobaric conditions would impact renal vasoactive enzyme components and, therefore; alter the normal balance of the vasoactive systems, we exposed male Sprague-Dawley rats to normobaric hypoxia (10% O_2) for 2 weeks. We then processed renal tissue to identify the expression and distribution of kallikrein, ACE and neutral endopeptidase 24.11 as well as markers of kidney damage. We found that chronic hypoxia produced focal damage in the kidney, mainly in the cortico-medullary region, and increased the expression of osteopontin. Moreover, we observed an increase of ACE protein in the brush border of proximal tubules at the outer medullary region, with increased mRNA levels. Kallikrein abundance did not change significantly with hypoxia, but a tendency toward reduction was observed at protein and mRNA levels. Neutral endopeptidase 24.11 was localized in proximal tubules, and was abundantly expressed under normoxic conditions, which markedly decreased both at protein and mRNA levels with chronic hypoxia. Taken together, our results suggest that chronic hypoxia produces focal kidney damage along with an imbalance of key components of the renal vasoactive system, which could be the initial steps for a long-term contribution to salt-sensitive hypertension and CKD.

Keywords: renal hypoxia, kallikrein, angiotensin-converting enzyme, neprilysin, neutral endopeptidase, subtle renal injury

INTRODUCTION

Hypertension and chronic kidney disease (CKD) are major public health problems worldwide, with chronic hypoxia being one of the suggested mechanisms involved in the genesis of salt-sensitive hypertension and to the progression of CKD (Suga et al., 2001; Nangaku and Fujita, 2008). Several factors, such as angiotensin II, cyclosporine A, phenylephrine, and hypokalemia have been postulated to induce local vasoconstriction and renal hypoxia, which subsequently may lead to CKD (Johnson et al., 2002; Vio and Jeanneret, 2003).

Renal function and arterial blood pressure regulation are under physiological control by renal vasoactive substances, through the activation of different systems such as the following: nitric oxide synthases, the endothelin system, the renin-angiotensin system (RAS), the kallikrein–kinin system (KKS), and renal eicosanoids produced by cyclooxygenases 1 and 2. Among nitric oxide synthases, neuronal nitric oxide synthase (nNOS, NOS-1) plays an important role in the kidneys by regulating renal hemodynamics in the immature kidney during pre and postnatal stages (Rodebaugh et al., 2012). Additionally, NOS-1 and NOS-3 are upregulated by acute hypoxia (Gess et al., 1997). On the other hand, endothelin-1, which is a multifunctional peptide, has potent vasoconstrictor and profibrotic effects on the systemic vasculature and kidneys. The endothelin system seems to play a fundamental role in diabetes, proteinuric renal disease, hypertension, and renovascular disease (Hargrove et al., 2000; Kelsen et al., 2011; Meyers and Sethna, 2013). Our laboratory mainly studied the following two systems: the RAS, the KKS, and renal eicosanoids, which are related to both systems. We have focused on enzymes in both systems, since they are currently known as important targets of inhibitors in antihypertensive treatment, and are used in CKD. The RAS leads to vasoconstriction and sodium retention, and its main active peptide is angiotensin II. The latter is produced by the angiotensin-converting enzyme (ACE), and is metabolized by aminopeptidase A to angiotensin III (Mizutani et al., 2008) and by neutral endopeptidase 24.11 (NEP) or neprilysin to inactive metabolites (Rice et al., 2004; Campbell, 2017). The KKS produces vasorelaxation and sodium excretion through bradykinin produced by kallikrein, which is the key enzyme of the system. The renal KKS participates in renal and extrarenal events such as regulation of blood pressure and control of sodium and water excretion. Kallikrein originates in the connecting tubule (CNT) and generates bradykinin, which is the effector hormone in the kidney regulating sodium excretion and glomerular hemodynamics, among other effects (Jaffa et al., 1992; Vio et al., 1992; Madeddu et al., 2007; Zhang et al., 2018). Bradykinin levels are regulated by ACE and NEP. There is another family of natriuretic peptides that participates in the regulation of arterial blood pressure, with atrial natriuretic peptide being the main one that involves renal action (Chen, 2005). Furthermore, the availability of vasoactive hormones is regulated by peptidases that degrade them. In kidneys, NEP has the critical function of degrading bradykinin, angiotensin II and natriuretic peptides, and transforming angiotensin I into angiotensin 1–7 (Rice et al., 2004; Judge et al., 2015; Campbell, 2017).

Renal vasoactive systems are involved in a delicate balance of opposite effects that lead to the production of either vasoconstrictor or vasodilator hormones, which activate sodium-retaining or excretory mechanisms, and have profibrotic or antifibrotic consequences (Bader and Ganten, 2008). For example, ACE and NEP have opposite actions in the regulation of vasoactive peptides: ACE transforms angiotensin I into angiotensin II (with hypertensive effects) and NEP transforms angiotensin I into angiotensin 1–7 (with antihypertensive effects). Angiotensin 1–7 can be further degraded by ACE into angiotensin 1–5 (Rice et al., 2004; Campbell, 2017).

Alterations of vasoactive enzymes have been described during the progression of CKD and hypertension. In fact, most drugs used to treat hypertension have been designed to inhibit members of the RAS family. Furthermore, new studies suggest that the use of the angiotensin II receptor antagonist in addition to the NEP inhibitor is a promising strategy to treat heart failure associated to hypertension (Volpe et al., 2016).

It is known that the kidney is very sensitive to changes in oxygen supply. Partial pressure of oxygen (PO_2) is carefully balanced between the cortex and the outer medulla, where under normoxia, the PO_2 gradient within the kidney has been found to reach about 70 mmHg in the cortex and outer medulla, and up to 10 mmHg in the inner medulla and papilla (Leichtweiss et al., 1969; Baumgärtl et al., 1972; Günther et al., 1974; Lübbers and Baumgärtl, 1997; O'Neill et al., 2015). Adequate kidney oxygenation is crucial to fuel active transportation processes of electrolytes and water in the nephron. Although kidneys receive a very high blood flow, oxygen extraction is relatively low. Consequently, kidneys are particularly susceptible to hypoxic injury because small changes in flow, which can be generated by vasoconstriction for example, are translated into local hypoxia (Epstein, 1997). This can then generate focal lesions, and lead to manifestations of kidney damage when the condition becomes chronic.

Based on the current knowledge exposed above, the present study was guided by the hypothesis that chronic reduction of oxygen, under normobaric conditions, affects renal vasoactive enzyme components, altering the normal balance of vasoactive systems, and favoring the vasoconstrictor profibrotic RAS.

MATERIALS AND METHODS

Animals and Experimental Procedures

Experiments were performed in 12 adult male Sprague-Dawley rats (180–200 g, n = 6 for each group, normoxia and hypoxia). This study was carried out in accordance with recommendations in the "Manual de Normas de Bioseguridad" (*Biosafety Norms Manual*, 2nd Ed., 2008, FONDECYT-CONICYT). The experimental protocol for animals was approved by the Bio-Ethics Committee of the School of Science at Universidad de Chile. Animals were housed in a 12 h light/dark cycle with free access to food (Prolab RMH 3000, Purina LabDiet) and water, and were randomly assigned to either a control group (normoxia) or to chronic normobaric hypoxia for 2 weeks.

TABLE 1 | Body weight and hematocrit values in normoxic and hypoxic animals.

	Normoxia	Hypoxia
Body weight (g)	337.8 ± 7.7	219.3 ± 5.2*
Hematocrit (%)	44.3 ± 0.3	74.2 ± 1.2*

*$P < 0.001$.

Chronic Normobaric Hypoxia Exposure

Animals (n = 12) were exposed to normoxia (n = 6), serving as controls for normobaric hypoxia (n = 6) for 2 weeks as previously described (Icekson et al., 2013). Briefly, three rats were allocated to a cage (D × W × H; 48 cm × 26 cm × 15 cm) and two cages were placed in a 300 L (60 cm × 50 cm × 100 cm) acrylic chamber with a hermetic lid. The oxygen content (FiO_2) in the chamber was continuously monitored through an oxygen sensor (AX300, Teledyne Analytical Instruments, CA, United States), whose output was fed to an automatic programmable controller (Zelio SR2B121BD, Schneider Electric, France) that controlled two solenoid valves (2026BV172, Jefferson Solenoid Valves, FL, United States). A relief output valve opened simultaneously with the admission valves, and remained opened for 40 s after the closure of the latter ones, while two mechanic relief valves opened whenever the pressure inside the chamber exceeded approximately 17 mmHg. Thus, the mean pressure in the chamber was slightly larger (ΔP = 1.3 ± 0.1 mmHg) than the atmospheric one (717.2 ± 0.3 mmHg). The atmosphere within

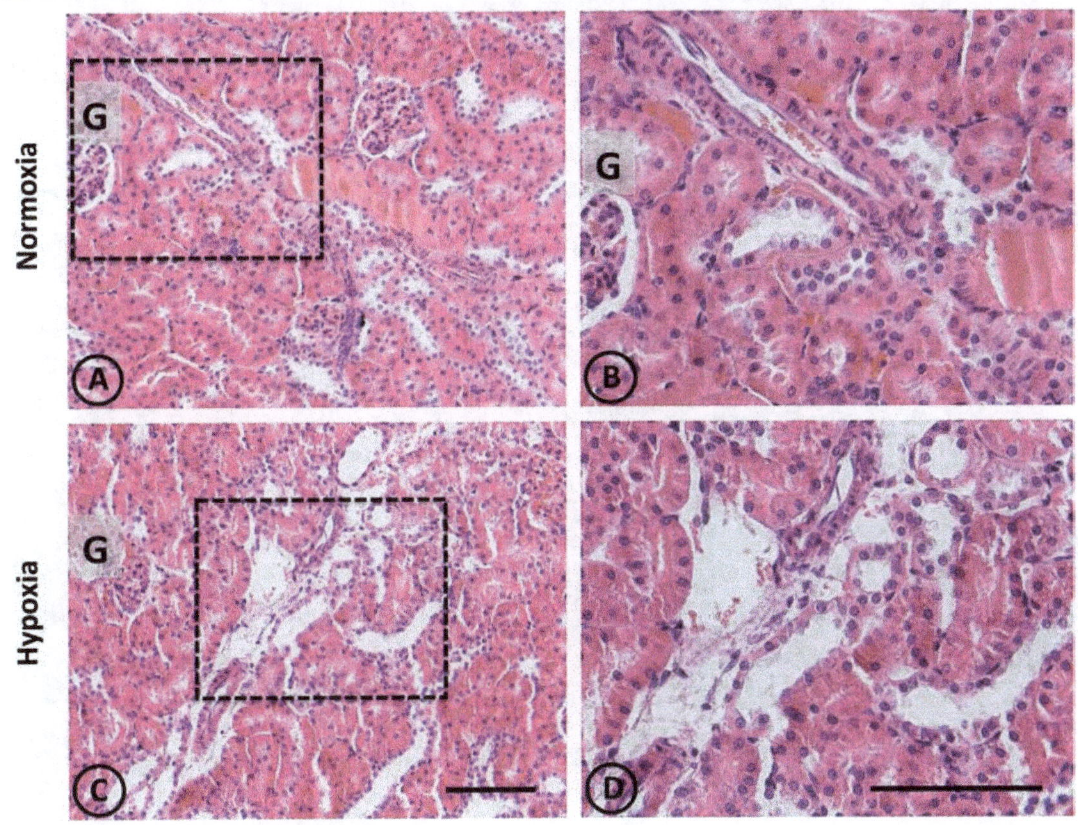

FIGURE 1 | Conventional staining with H-E in renal tissue from normoxic and hypoxic animals. Representative images of kidneys from animals in control **(A,B)** and hypoxic **(C,D)** conditions. **(A,B)** Normoxic tissue has tubules and tubulointerstitial space of normal aspect, both in the medullary zone and in the cortex. Blood vessels present usual appearance. **(C,D)** In hypoxic kidneys, it is possible to observe tubular dilation in some areas of the field, affecting certain blood vessels that irrigate such areas. Dotted areas correspond to higher magnification images on the right column. G = Glomerulus. Scale bar = 100 μm.

the chamber was continuously homogenized by four internal fans. After closure, chamber air was purged for approximately 5 min with pure N_2, until attaining approximately 9.5% of FiO_2. From then on, the system automatically regulated FiO_2 levels in the chamber by admitting N_2 or compressed air into the chamber if FiO_2 values were over 9.8% or below 8.7%, respectively. Mean FiO_2 within the chamber was $9.33 \pm 0.12\%$ (mean $\pm$ SD). CO_2 produced by animal ventilation was trapped by using $CaCO_3$ (250 g), and urinary NH_3 with H_3BO_3 (60 g). The chamber remained open for about 5 min every other day to clean the internal cages and replenish the water containers, whereas CO_2 and NH_3 traps were changed every four days. The cages were rotated within the chamber to maximize homogeneity. The pressure inside the chamber was continuously measured with a gauge transducer (Statham P20), and the FiO_2 signal was recorded at 1 Hz with a computerized analog to digital acquisition system (DI-158U, DATAQ Instruments Inc., OH, United States). The temperature in the chamber was recorded at 5 min intervals throughout the 14 days of hypoxia with a data logger (EL-USB-2, Lascar Electronics Inc., PA, United States).

At the end of the treatment, rats were deeply anesthetized with isoflurane (isoflurane in O_2, induction 4–5%) and euthanized by exsanguination. Blood was obtained from Vena Cava in heparin-tubes, and both kidneys were removed. Then, isoflurane was increased until breathing stopped and death of the animals was confirmed. Pneumothorax was performed as a secondary physical method of euthanasia.

Kidneys were rapidly decapsulated and approximately 100 mg slices were cut with a transverse cross section in the middle of the kidney (discarding both poles) to obtain samples for quantitative polymerase chain reaction (qRT-PCR). Samples for qRT-PCR were stored at −80°C until they were processed.

The hematocrit was determined by microcentrifugation using two uncoated hematocrit glass tubes (length 75 mm) per sample, filled and centrifuged for 5 min in a micro-hematocrit centrifuge (Hermle Z200). The hematocrit was established using a micro-hematocrit tube reader, and the mean value was calculated.

Source of Antisera and Chemicals

ACE antiserum (SC-12187) was purchased from Santa Cruz Biotechnology, United States. Osteopontin (OPN) monoclonal antibody (MPIIIB10) was obtained from Developmental Studies Hybridoma Bank, IA, United States, and NEP antiserum (AB-5458) from EMD Millipore. Kallikrein antibody was used

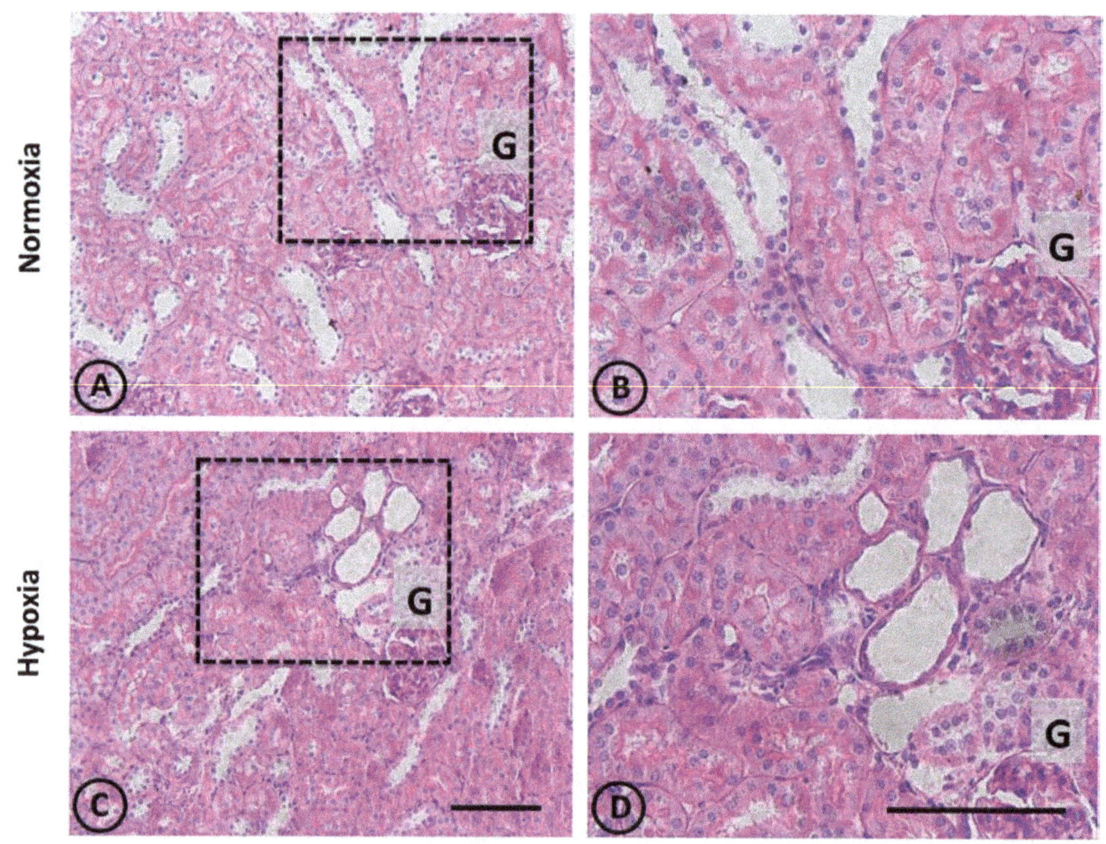

FIGURE 2 | Conventional staining with PAS in renal tissue from normoxic and hypoxic animals. **(A,C)** show a general view of cortical and medullary zones for each group. **(A,B)** correspond to the normoxia group. The color fuchsia is present mainly in the basal membrane and the brush border of proximal tubules. No signs of injury are observed in this group. **(C,D)** correspond to the hypoxia group, showing an area that presents focal damage. Only a few tubules present dilation, while the area that surrounds it presents normal appearance. Dotted areas indicate higher magnification images presented in the right column. G = Glomerulus. Scale bar = 100 μm.

as reported previously (Salas et al., 2007). Random primer dNTPs and FAST SYBR Green Master Mix were acquired from Thermo Fisher Scientific. Secondary antibody and corresponding peroxidase-anti-peroxidase (PAP) complex were purchased from MP Biomedicals, Inc., Germany.

Tissue Processing and Immunohistochemical Analysis

Renal tissue samples (3 mm thick) were fixed by immersion in Bouin's solution for 24 h at room temperature. Tissue was then dehydrated, embedded in Paraplast Plus, serially sectioned at 5 μm thick with a Leica rotatory microtome, mounted on glass slides, and stored.

Conventional staining of tissue sections was performed with Hematoxylin-Eosin (H-E), Periodic Acid-Schiff (PAS) for histological analysis, and Picrosirius red for collagen staining (Villanueva et al., 2006, 2014).

Immunostaining was carried out using an indirect immunoperoxidase technique to localize kallikrein, ACE, OPN, and NEP in rat kidneys. Briefly, tissue sections were dewaxed, rehydrated, rinsed in 0.05 M Tris-phosphate-saline (TPS) buffer, pH 7.6, and incubated overnight at 22°C with a primary antiserum raised against kallikrein, ACE, OPN, or NEP. The secondary antibody and corresponding PAP complex were applied for 30 min each at 22°C. The immunoperoxidase reaction was visualized after incubation of sections in 0.1% (wt/vol) diaminobenzidine and 0.03% hydrogen peroxide. Sections were rinsed with TPS buffer between incubations, counterstained with hematoxylin, dehydrated, cleared with xylene and then coverslipped. Controls for the immunostaining procedure were prepared by omission of the first antibody. Images were examined with conventional light microscopy and acquired using a Nikon Eclipse E600 microscope and Nikon DS-Ri1 digital camera.

Quantitative RT-PCR

Total RNA was extracted from whole kidney tissue using TRIzol, according to the manufacturer's instructions. RNA integrity was determined by 1% agarose gel electrophoresis and its concentration, by absorbance at 260/280 nm using a 2.5 μg aliquot of total RNA to cDNA synthesis. Samples were treated with DNAse I using MMLV, dNTPs and random primers to obtain cDNA. The housekeeping gene used was glyceraldehyde-3-phosphate dehydrogenase (GAPDH)

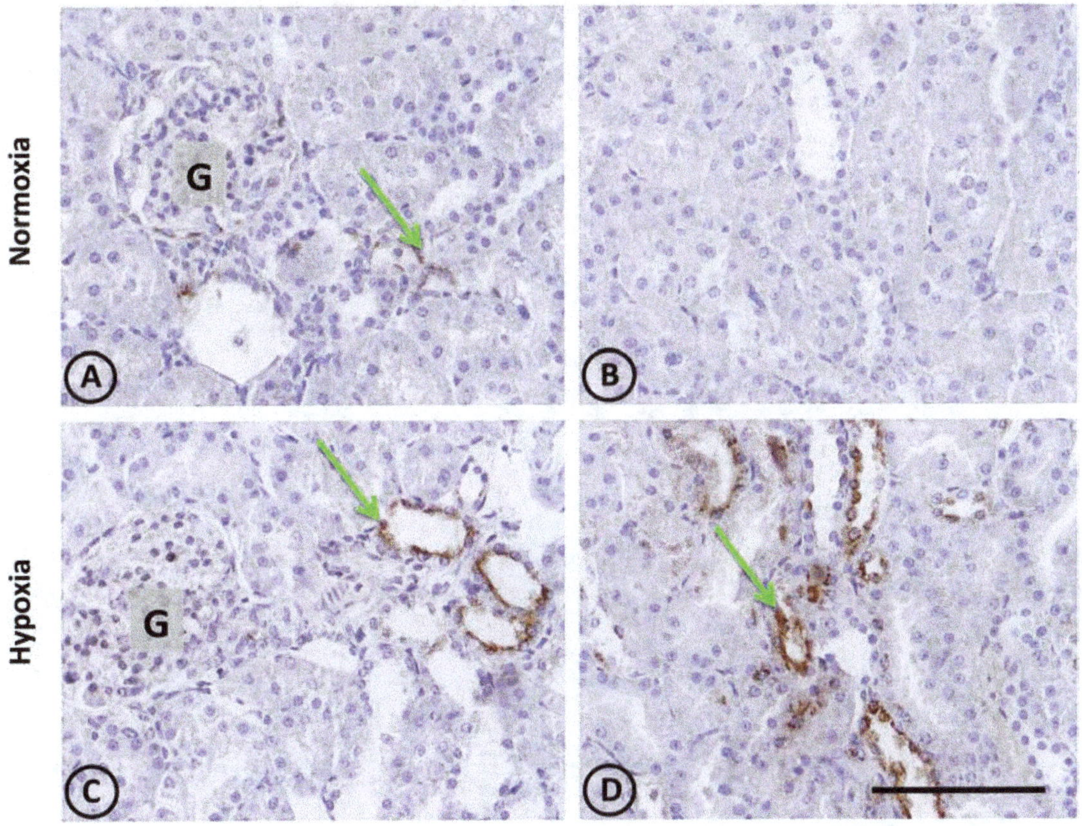

FIGURE 3 | Osteopontin in renal tissue from normoxic and hypoxic animals. The arrows indicate the localization of OPN that appears stained in brown. **(A,B)** correspond to the normoxia group. In **(A)** it is possible to observe a little OPN stain that indicates low expression levels of this protein. Brown stains are totally absent in **(B)**, and the same happens in others fields of the same renal section, representing normal conditions. **(C,D)** correspond to the hypoxia group. It is possible to observe an increase of OPN staining, expressed mainly in tubular cells. The left panel shows a cortical area where a glomerulus is observed (G). The right panel corresponds to the outer stripe of the outer medulla. All images have the same magnification. Scale bar = 100 μm.

(forward primer: 5′-CACGGCAAGTTCAACGGC-3′, reverse primer 5′-GGTGGTGAAGACGCCAGTA-3′). The primer sequences used were the following: kallikrein, forward primer: 5′-GCATCACACCTGACGGATTG-3′, reverse primer: 5′-GGCCTCCTGAGTCACCCTTG -3′; ACE, forward primer: 5′-AACACGGCTCGTGCAGAAG-3′, reverse primer: 5′-CCTGCTGTGGTTCCAGGTACA-3′; and NEP, forward primer: 5′-TCAGCCTTTCTGTGCTCGTC-3′, reverse primer: 5′-ATTGCGTTTCAACCAGCCTC-3′. Quantitative PCR was performed in duplicate in a StepOnePlus Real-Time PCR System (Applied Biosystems) using FAST SYBR Green Master Mix for amplification. Results were normalized by GAPDH. Mathematical quantification was made using the $2^{-\Delta\Delta CT}$ method (Livak and Schmittgen, 2001).

Statistics

All data are presented as mean ± SEM. Statistical analyses were performed using an unpaired Student's *t*-test and GraphPad Prism software (version 5.0c for Windows, GraphPad Software, CA, United States). Differences with $P < 0.05$ were considered statistically significant.

RESULTS

General Features and Morphological Traits

An increase in hematocrit and a decrease in body weight were observed in hypoxic animals compared to controls, over the 2-week period of hypoxia, which is characteristic of this experimental condition (**Table 1**).

For the morphological study we selected conventional stains with different properties to address tissue structure at the light microscopy level. They were H-E, PAS and Picrosirius Red. They provide information about general structure (H-E), more detailed information of structural shapes of tubules, glomeruli and vessels, provided by the glycoprotein and basement membrane staining (PAS), and collagen staining as an index of tissue damage (Picrosirius red).

The immunohistochemistry technique was used to evaluate *de novo* expression of tubular OPN, which is a key macrophage chemokine that is not normally expressed in adult kidneys, and is induced by tubular damage of different origins (Lombardi et al., 2001).

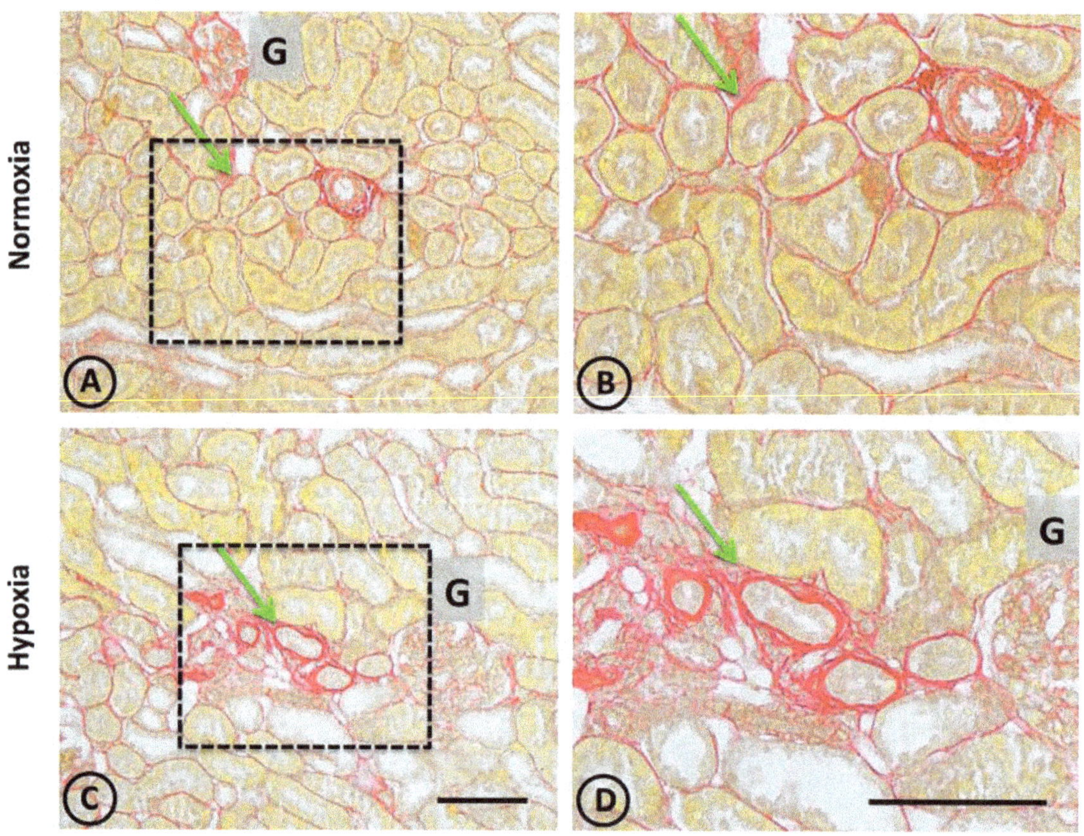

FIGURE 4 | Collagen staining with Picrosirius red stain in renal tissue from normoxic and hypoxic animals. **(A,B)** correspond to the normoxia group. **(C,D)** correspond to the hypoxia group. The left panel shows a panoramic view of the cortical and medullary zones of both groups. The dotted area indicates images with higher magnification on the right column. The arrows indicate the location of collagen stained in red. Note that peritubular collagen is scarce in all images. However, in the hypoxia group it is possible to observe small areas of fibrosis, characterized by an increase in local collagen. In **(A,B)** an arterial blood vessel is observed with perivascular collagen, which does not constitute fibrosis. All structures other than collagen are stained in yellow. G corresponds to the glomerulus. Scale bar = 100 μm.

Also, immunohistochemistry was used to characterize the protein expression at tissue level and the distribution in the kidney of the vasoactive enzymes kallikrein, ACE, and NEP.

Renal tissue specimens were examined in coded samples by two of the researchers (C.Cespedes and C.Vio), and systematic analysis of kidney tissue samples was done focusing on the overall morphological aspect, and on cortical and medullary tubules, glomeruli, blood vessels, interstitial space, and intratubular spaces.

An overall and detailed examination of renal tissue with conventional PAS and H-E staining of kidneys from normoxic animals showed no signs of pathological alterations in the cortex or the medulla. No vascular changes were observed, tubules were shaped normally in terms of diameter and cell size, and no signs of cell infiltration and inflammation were observed in the tubulointerstitial space. Glomeruli from cortical or juxtamedullary nephrons had normal aspect (**Figures 1A,B, 2A,B**).

A panoramic examination of kidney tissue from hypoxic animals over the cortex and medulla revealed a mild and focalized morphological alteration, characterized by focal lesions in the outer medullary and inner cortical zone, as evidenced with H-E staining (**Figure 1**). More detailed information was obtained with PAS staining, showing the focal alteration at this outer medullary region (**Figure 2**).

Focal areas with signs of alterations consisted of "spotty" areas mainly located in the outer medulla and inner cortical zone, close to juxtamedullary nephrons (**Figures 1, 2**). They contained dilated tubules with atrophic tubular epithelia, and basophilic aspect. Such atrophic and dilated tubules had a mild cellular infiltration in the corresponding tubulointerstitial space (**Figures 2C,D**).

In control animals, the presence of renal OPN was observed with a very scarce distribution in tubular cells of the cortex, as expected for normal tissue (**Figures 3A,B**). In contrast to normal tissue, kidneys from hypoxic animals showed an increased expression of OPN in cortical tubules with a focal distribution, as shown in **Figures 3C,D**, which corresponds to the typical pattern of *de novo* expression of OPN in renal injury.

In normal tissue, staining with Picrosirius red revealed typical collagen staining around arteries, and very faint staining in peritubular locations (**Figures 4A,B**). On the other hand, focal staining was observed in tissue from hypoxic animals in discrete areas corresponding to focal areas of local injury, as presented in

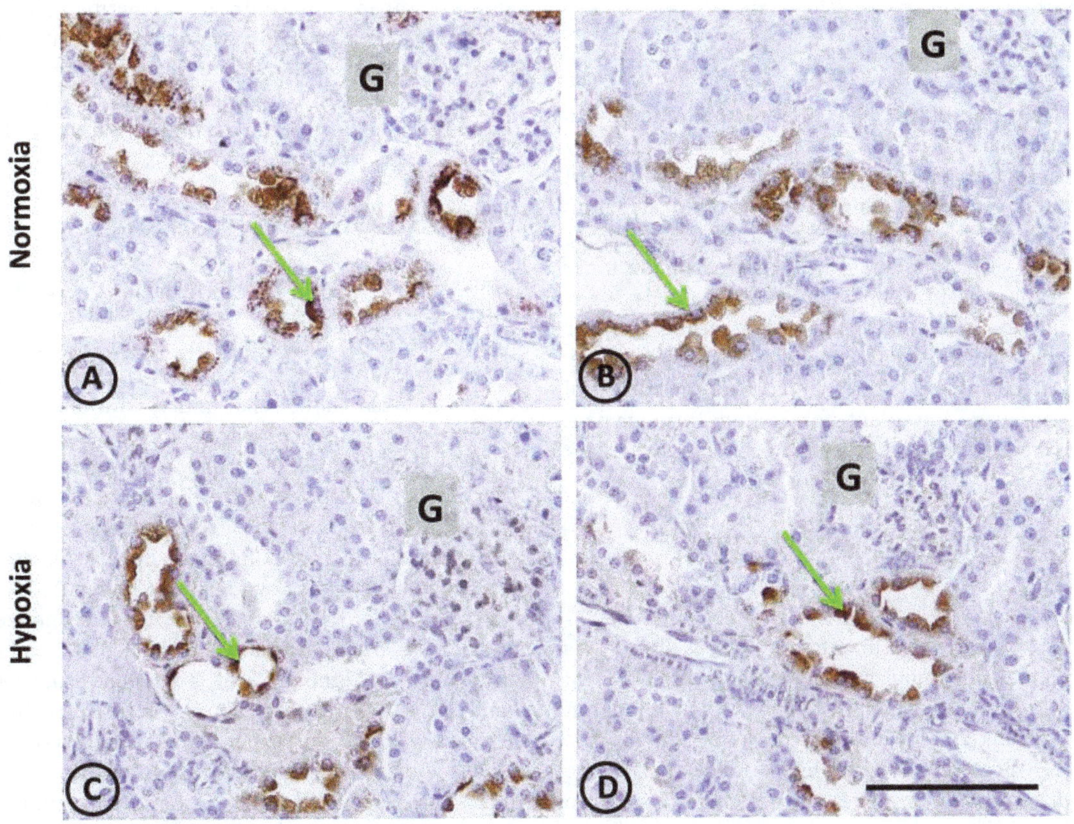

FIGURE 5 | Kallikrein immunostaining in renal tissue from normoxic and hypoxic animals. Green arrows indicate the localization of kallikrein (brown immunostaining) in both groups. It is expressed only in the cortical zone, specifically in the apical pole and perinuclear area of connecting tubule cells. **(A,B)** correspond to the normoxia group. Greater expression of kallikrein stains are observed in this group compared to the hypoxia group **(C,D)**, which presents less staining in the same cell type. The immunostained mark is not present in the collecting duct or another tubule type, in the glomerulus (G), or in blood vessels. All images of the cortical zone have the same magnification. Scale bar = 100 μm.

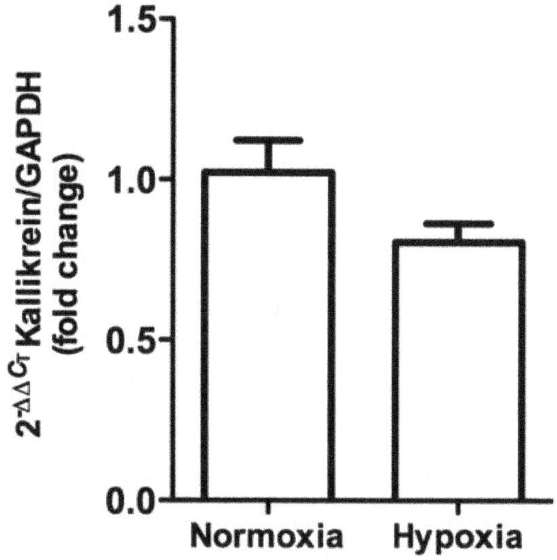

FIGURE 6 | Kallikrein gene expression in whole kidney tissue samples from normoxic and hypoxic animals. The graph represents the standardized average of kallikrein gene expression in both conditions, expressed as fold change between control versus hypoxic group. Results were averaged and mean values were compiled for statistical analysis. A slight decrease is observed, which does not constitute a statistically significant difference between the normoxia and hypoxia groups. GAPDH was used as a housekeeping gene.

Figures 4C,D, where peritubular signs of fibrosis around dilated and injured tubules were observed.

Thus, the histological evidence presented above is consistent with mild manifestations of lesions, with focal distribution patterns located in the outer medulla and inner cortical zone of the kidneys. No similar lesions were observed in the inner medulla or in the outer cortical zone of normoxic animals.

It is relevant to note that this outer medullary/inner cortical area is the zone where juxtamedullary nephrons reside. Juxtamedullary nephrons are fewer than cortical or superficial nephrons, but are very important for sodium management and blood pressure regulation because they generate medullary circulation.

Vasoactive Enzyme Expression and Distribution

Kallikrein

In normal and hypoxic experimental groups, kallikrein is restricted to connecting tubular cells (CNTc) of CNT of distal nephrons. In normal tissue, CNTc display abundant immunoreactive kallikrein in the apical pole and in the perinuclear area, where the Golgi complex resides. CNTc are intermingled with kallikrein negative cells, which correspond to intercalated cells. CNT are always in close anatomical relation with afferent arterioles close to glomeruli (**Figures 5A,B**). Kallikrein distribution in renal tissue from hypoxic animals was similar to control animals in the CNTc. However, decreased immunostaining intensity and stained focal areas were observed, and there was faint staining in focal tubules (**Figures 5C,D**).

Kallikrein gene expression measured by qRT-PCR was not significantly modified ($P > 0.05$), although it tended to decrease (**Figure 6**).

Angiotensin-Converting Enzyme

In normal animals, ACE was located exclusively in the S3 segment of proximal tubules, and was more concentrated in the inner cortical zone and outer medulla. The enzyme was present in the brush border of the apical cellular pole. No ACE was observed in other tubular cells or in the tubulointerstitial space (**Figures 7A,B**). In hypoxic animals, the same pattern of localization was observed over the proximal tubules, although with more intensity. Furthermore, strong staining in more disarranged proximal tubules was observed in focal areas, and focal ACE staining on the peritubular side (**Figures 7C,D**).

ACE gene expression, as measured by qRT-PCR, was significantly higher ($P < 0.001$) in hypoxic animals compared to controls (**Figure 8**).

Neutral Endopeptidase 24.11 or Neprylisin

This was observed in control animals in the brush border of proximal tubules, and more concentrated in the outer medulla than in the cortex. Heavy staining was observed in control renal tissue (**Figures 9A,B**), whereas less area was stained in hypoxic kidneys compared to controls. Furthermore, the presence of NEP in focal areas was observed in rather dilated and atrophied tubules (**Figures 9C,D**). Moreover, NEP gene expression, as measured by qRT-PCR, significantly decreased ($P < 0.001$) by almost 50% in hypoxic animals compared to controls (**Figure 10**).

DISCUSSION

Hypoxia due to renal vasoconstriction has been proposed to contribute to early stages of CKD and salt-sensitive hypertension (Suga et al., 2001; Johnson et al., 2002). The main findings of the present study are that normobaric hypoxia (10% O_2) for 2 weeks induced subtle renal injury, with discrete focal lesions, and local changes in components of renal vasoactive systems, such as increases in kallikrein and ACE, and less NEP expression.

Normobaric hypoxia may be induced by a variety of conditions that reduce the supply of oxygen to organs, such as chronic obstructive pulmonary disease (Kent et al., 2011), obstructive sleep apnea syndrome (Chiang, 2006), CKD (Shoji et al., 2014), and certain conditions that induce local renal hypoxia like cyclosporine A, hypokalemia, angiotensin II or contrast media (Lombardi et al., 2001; Suga et al., 2001; Zhou and Duan, 2014; Fähling et al., 2017). Normobaric hypoxia studies have an advantage over experiments using hypobaric conditions in that hypoxia effects are not mixed with those of low pressure. In fact, arterial blood pressure has been reported to remain unchanged in chronic hypobaric hypoxia (Rabinovitch et al., 1979; Hsieh et al., 2015), but to increase in chronic normobaric hypoxia (Schwenke et al., 2008; Moraes et al., 2014; Flor et al., 2018). The latter highlights the importance of choosing the right type of hypoxia depending on the pathological conditions to be studied, since both conditions may evoke distinct physiological responses (Savourey et al., 2003; Richard and Koehle, 2012). Hence, we used the normobaric hypoxia model in order to mimic the low oxygen supply that kidneys face under pathological conditions, and to distinguish the effects of hypoxia from hypobaria.

Morphological Alterations

Hypoxia is a key pathogenic event that can activate a vicious cycle of destructive processes. In our model, we observed a discrete focal lesion of tubular damage with conventional H-E, and Picrosirius red staining without glomerular damage, indicating the mild and patchy nature of the lesion. The expression of tubular OPN, which is a key macrophage chemokine, without infiltrative cells was somehow unexpected. However, it suggests that longer periods or more severe hypoxia are required to induce infiltration. When compared to other models of mild damage (angiotensin II, hypokalemia, phenylephrine and cyclosporine A) (Johnson et al., 2002), the present model displays a similar damage pattern, but with less intensity. A possible explanation for the low intensity of the damage is that this degree of hypoxia is counteracted in kidneys by regulatory mechanisms that supply oxygen to kidneys as the increased hematocrit (**Table 1**). Similar results have been shown in proximal and distal tubular cells in renal ischemia, tubulointerstitial nephritis, glomerulonephritis, and acute hypoxia (Hampel et al., 2003; Mazzali et al., 2003). These effects are in agreement with upregulation of inflammatory and profibrotic genes in response to hypoxia (Fu et al., 2016; Ow et al., 2018). Fibrosis and subsequent tubular damage exacerbate hypoxia, and induce the activation of genes that favor the expression of vasoconstrictor mediators such as endothelin-1, which could reduce oxygen delivery even more (Hampel et al., 2003). Considering that the outer medulla of the kidney is particularly vulnerable to reduced oxygen supply due to an imbalance between oxygen requirements and medullary blood flow (Fine et al., 2000; Zhou and Duan, 2014), we and others have proposed that a common pathway is perhaps local hypoxia, which creates a vicious circle that initiates and maintains focal renal injury (Vio and Jeanneret, 2003).

A larger inflammatory response was described in rats subjected to chronic hypoxia (81.9 mmHg) (Mazzali et al., 2003). The latter study achieved low PO_2 by reducing barometric pressure to an equivalent altitude of 5550 m, although PO_2 reduction was more severe in the present study (67.1 mmHg). This reduction in barometric pressure, however, may induce

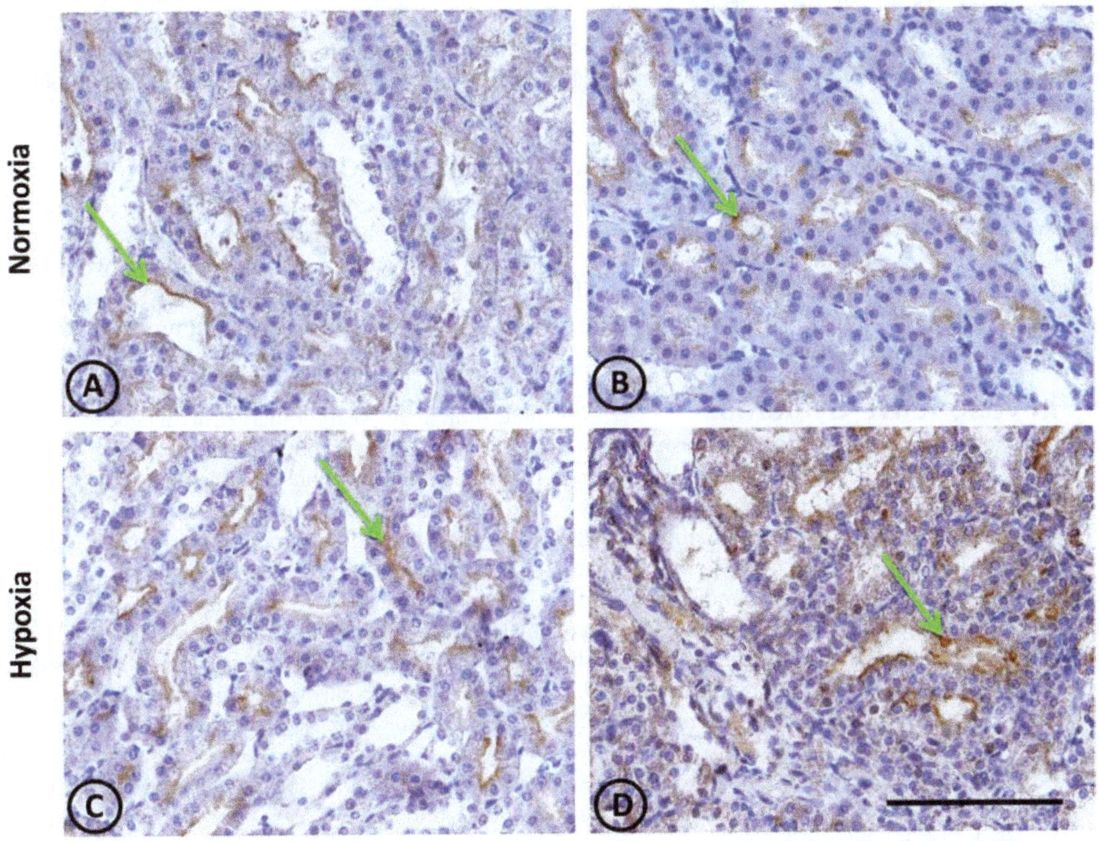

FIGURE 7 | Angiotensin-converting enzyme (ACE) immunostaining in renal tissue from normoxic and hypoxic animals. ACE localization (immunostained in brown) is indicated with green arrows. It is mainly expressed in the medullary zone, at the brush border of the proximal tubule; more specifically in segment S3. **(A,B)** correspond to the normoxia group. The ACE stain is less in the control group compared to the hypoxia group **(C,D)**. Additionally, in image **(D)**, the immunostained mark appears in the tubulointerstitial space, where there is also a higher number of infiltrative cells. All images correspond to the medullary zone with the same magnification. Scale bar = 100 μm.

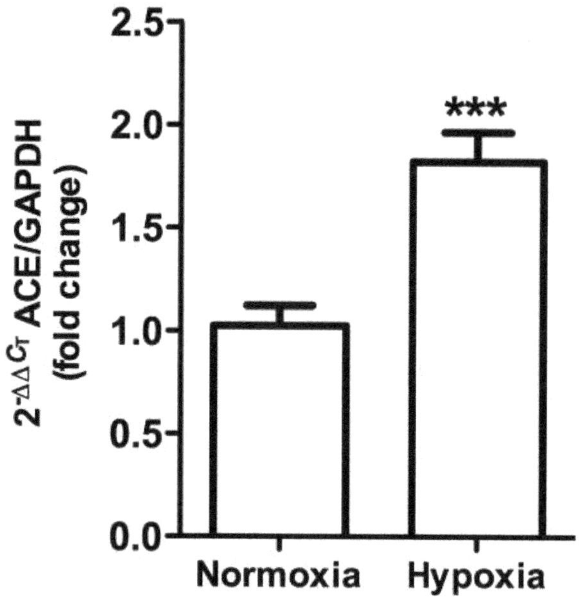

FIGURE 8 | Angiotensin-converting enzyme gene expression in whole kidney tissue samples from normoxic and hypoxic animals. The graph exhibits the average of ACE gene expression. Units were defined as fold change between control versus hypoxic group. Results were averaged and mean values were compiled for statistical analysis. There is a significant increase (***$P < 0.001$) in ACE gene expression in the hypoxia group when compared to the normoxia group. GAPDH was used as a housekeeping gene.

physiological responses that are independent from PO_2 reduction (Savourey et al., 2003, 2007; Richard and Koehle, 2012). Moreover, the exposure period was 10 days shorter in the experiments reported here. In chronic intermittent hypoxic experiments, changes in arterial pressure did not develop until 3 weeks of exposure (Del Rio et al., 2010). Thus, differences may arise from the different exposure period and barometric pressure.

Alterations in Vasoactive Systems

Changes in renal vasoactive components have been proposed to contribute to early stages of CKD and salt-sensitive hypertension. In fact, Johnson et al. (2002) proposed that changes in vasoactive systems constitute a common base for a variety of stimuli (e.g., hypokalemia, angiotensin II, phenylephrine, cyclosporine A) that induce vasoconstriction, leading to ischemia and subsequent subtle renal injury. In such conditions, rats are more sensitive to high-salt induced hypertension, even though arterial blood pressure augmentation is reversed after removing the stimuli. This suggests that renal damage is at the base of this mechanism.

Decreased Kallikrein Levels

Kallikrein is a serine protease with a key function for kidneys, since it produces bradykinin, which is one of the main vasorelaxing peptides that also inhibits sodium reabsorption through the activation of bradykinin receptor type 2 (Mukai et al., 1996; Sivritas et al., 2008). Our histology and immunohistochemistry data showed a local decrease of kallikrein in CNTc. It is worth noting that kallikrein-containing cells are always in close contact with arterioles underlying the anatomical link between KKS and RAS (Vio et al., 1988). Even though changes in kallikrein gene expression were not significant, there was a tendency to decrease. We have previously reported that hypokalemia, ischemia and phenylephrine (stimuli that produce renal hypoxia and kidney damage) also reduced kallikrein expression, which could contribute to the imbalance of vasoactive enzymes that favor vasoconstriction and sodium retention. The latter may, in turn, lead to the onset of renal injury and hypertension (Martinez et al., 1990; Suga et al., 2001; Johnson et al., 2002; Basile et al., 2005). Further studies are required to determine whether kallikrein reduction is a cause or a consequence of hypoxia. Thongboonkerd et al. (2002) reported a dual role of kallikrein, where episodic hypoxia (which mimics obstructive sleep apnea syndrome) reduced its activity associated with hypertension, while sustained hypoxia increased kallikrein levels. The difference in kallikrein expression observed under the experimental conditions reported here may have been due to the reoxygenation produced between the end of hypoxia and the extraction of renal tissue. This could be explained by the oxidative stress generated during reoxygenation, which may activate different pathways, and could influence kallikrein expression (Milano et al., 2004; Bianciardi et al., 2006). Reduced kallikrein expression favors vasoconstriction, which may worsen hypoxia and lead to kidney damage, since overexpression of human kallikrein in kidneys has been observed to protect rats from hypoxia-induced hypertension (Thongboonkerd et al., 2002).

Increased ACE Levels

ACE plays a critical role in RAS signaling: It produces angiotensin II (the main vasoconstrictor peptide), which activates pathways leading to hypertension and fibrosis, while also degrading bradykinin. Results from immunohistochemistry in this study showed a local increase of ACE in proximal tubules at the outer medullary region. The observed change in protein expression is consistent with greater gene expression, as measured by qRT-PCR. For many years, much effort has been placed on creating drugs to inhibit ACE, but very little is known about its regulation. It has been reported that phenylephrine, angiotensin II infusion and hypokalemia induce the ACE expression, which has been associated with kidney hypoxia and damage (Johnson et al., 1999; Lombardi et al., 2001; Suga et al., 2001; Vio and Jeanneret, 2003).

It seems that ACE regulation differs depending on the tissue analyzed (Jackson et al., 1986; Oparil et al., 1988; King et al., 1989). For instance, Oparil et al. (1988) reported that hypoxia reduced ACE activity in lungs (associated to angiotensin II reduction), but increased its activity in renal tissue, which was reversed to normal levels when rats were returned to normoxia. Reasons behind organ-specific regulation of ACE are not known, but lungs and kidneys seem to present opposite ACE regulations. Vascular endothelial growth factor (VEGF) is postulated to be the major growth factor modified in response to hypoxia, which increases local production of ACE (Enholm et al., 1997; Saijonmaa et al., 2001), and generates synergy between the RAS and VEGF, hence contributing to angiogenesis and vascular remodeling in response to hypoxia.

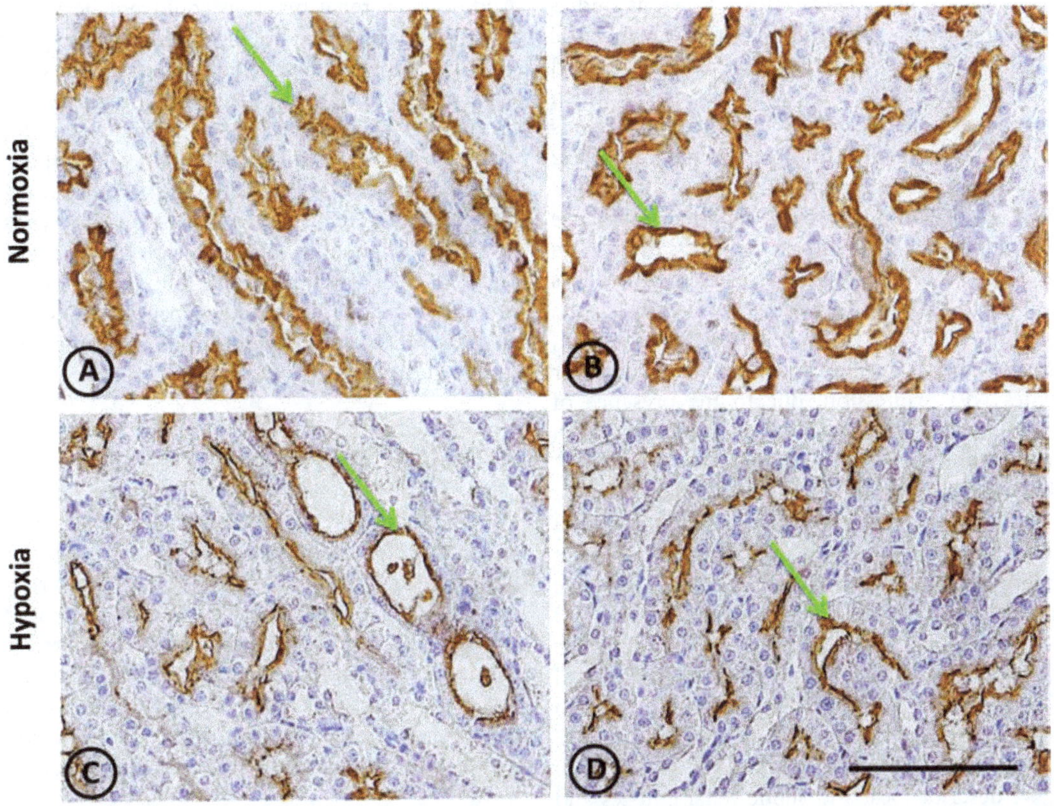

FIGURE 9 | Neutral endopeptidase immunostaining in renal tissue from normoxic and hypoxic animals. The NEP protein is indicated with green arrows, and it appears immunostained in brown. Its expression was located in proximal tubules, being more concentrated in the S3 segment (both in superficial and juxtamedullary nephrons) at the medullary ray and outer strip of the medulla, respectively. **(A,B)** correspond to the normoxia group. NEP expression is higher in the control group compared to the hypoxia group **(C,D)**. All images correspond to the medullary zone, and they have the same magnification. Scale bar = 100 μm.

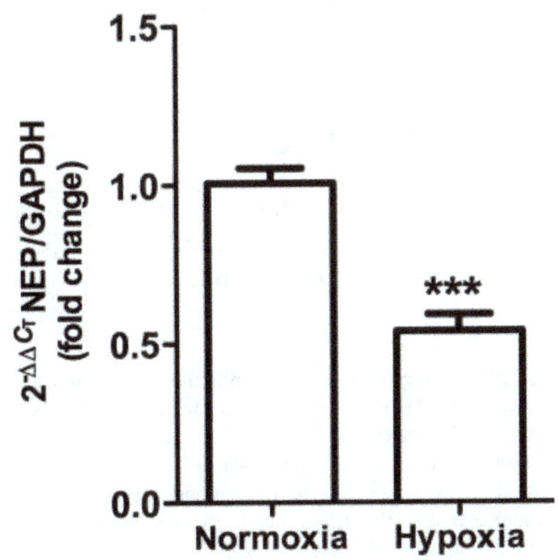

FIGURE 10 | Neutral endopeptidase gene expression in whole kidney tissue samples from normoxic and hypoxic animals. The graph shows the average of NEP gene expression. Arbitrary units were defined as fold change between control versus hypoxic group. Results were averaged and mean values were compiled for statistical analysis. There is a significant decrease in NEP gene expression in the hypoxia group compared to the normoxia group (***$P < 0.001$). GAPDH was used as a housekeeping gene.

Increases in ACE may be acting in the following two ways: (1) to increase the amount of angiotensin II that leads to greater vascular resistance and fibrosis, and (2) to decrease the amount of kallikrein by degradation, contributing to an imbalance of vasoactive enzymes and thus to the onset of renal injury observed during hypoxia.

Decreased NEP Levels

Together with ACE, NEP is the most important kinin-degrading enzyme in the cardiovascular system. Renal NEP is responsible for processing a range of substrates as vasoactive peptides, including bradykinin, endothelins, angiotensin I and angiotensin II, among others (Rice et al., 2004; Judge et al., 2015; Campbell, 2017). In our model, we observed that hypoxia decreased NEP expression both at protein and gene expression levels. Immunohistochemical staining showed that NEP is abundantly expressed in proximal tubules at the outer medullary region under normoxic conditions, but hypoxia reduced its expression. One of the consequences of NEP reduction is a lower generation of angiotensin 1-7, an antihypertensive peptide that counteracts the effects of angiotensin II, which is consistent with a hypertensive phenotype.

There are few studies that report on NEP localization, although the enzyme exhibits vast tissue distribution, with greater abundance in kidneys and lungs (Li et al., 1995). Previous studies by Carpenter and Stenmark (2001) showed that normobaric hypoxia, although for a much shorter time (72 h), caused a decline in NEP expression at the pulmonary level, which caused increases in vascular permeability. The latter corresponds to a phenotype that is reversed through recombinant NEP administration or a bradykinin receptor antagonist. Down-regulation of NEP by hypoxia has been reported in mouse primary cortical and hippocampal neurons as well as in prostate cancer cell lines, where NEP decrease is associated with a loss of beneficial effects mediated by the specific degradation of the substrate (Wang et al., 2011; Nalivaeva et al., 2012; Mitra et al., 2013). It has been shown that the hypoxia inducible factor negatively regulates NEP expression, due to the presence of hypoxia-responsive elements in its promoter (Mitra et al., 2013), which could be responsible for NEP reduction.

Taken together, the changes in the enzymes that regulate the production/degradation of the vasoactive peptides observed in our experimental conditions suggest that hypoxia induces a hypertensive phenotype due to an imbalance of the vasoactive peptides, leading to an increase in the vasoconstrictors and a decrease in vasodilators, such as: decreased bradykinin (antihypertensive peptide) due to decreased kallikrein and increased ACE; increased angiotensin II (hypertensive peptide) due to increased ACE; and reduction of angiotensin 1-7 (antihypertensive peptides) due to decreased NEP.

In summary, we describe local and subtle renal injuries and changes in renal vasoactive components that could damage the kidney, making it more sensitive to high-salt induced hypertension under conditions such as high salt load. Future experiments could involve challenging renal function with high sodium diets to increase oxygen consumption and induce salt-sensitive hypertension.

STUDY LIMITATIONS

Although this study attempted to limit oxygenation time before collecting the samples (2 h maximum) and during feeding/cleaning the animals (5 min every 48 h), changes occurring during reoxygenation (e.g., changes in redox status) could not be ruled out, and may have altered our results. Additionally, renal function could not be measured, since the metabolic cages could not be placed under hypoxic conditions.

Due to space limitations in the hypoxic chambers, the experiments were performed using only male rats. Considering the important differences between males and females in terms of cardiovascular and renal function, it is important to perform these experiments on females in the future to evaluate the possible differences that may exist in the response to hypoxia.

Finally, changes in the expression of key enzymes of the RAS and the KKS were measured, but it cannot be assumed that this will translate into changes in peptide levels. Local levels of angiotensin II and bradykinin will be measured and evaluated in future studies.

AUTHOR CONTRIBUTIONS

CV, JA, RI, and CC conceived and designed the study, analyzed and interpreted the data, drafted the manuscript, critically revised important intellectual content in the manuscript, and provided overall supervision. DS, CC, JA, and JD-E performed the experiments and analyzed the data and drafted the manuscript, and contributed to intellectual content in the manuscript. NM analyzed and interpreted the data and contributed to intellectual content in the manuscript. All authors approved the final manuscripts and agreed to be accountable for all aspects of the work.

FUNDING

This work was supported by a grant from CONICYT awarded to the CARE UC Center, grant AFB 170005, FONDECYT grant 11170245 to NM, FONDECYT grant 1090157 to JA, and FONDECYT grant 1150040 to RI.

ACKNOWLEDGMENTS

The authors are grateful to Maria Alcoholado for technical assistance in tissue sections. DS, JD-E, and NM are postdoctoral fellows from the CARE UC Center and CONICYT.

REFERENCES

Bader, M., and Ganten, D. (2008). Update on tissue renin-angiotensin systems. *J. Mol. Med.* 86, 615–621. doi: 10.1007/s00109-008-0336-0

Basile, D. P., Fredrich, K., Alausa, M., Vio, C. P., Liang, M., Rieder, M. R., et al. (2005). Identification of persistently altered gene expression in the kidney after functional recovery from ischemic acute renal failure. *Am. J. Physiol. Renal Physiol.* 288, F953–F963. doi: 10.1152/ajprenal.00329.2004

Baumgärtl, H., Leichtweiss, H. P., Lübbers, D. W., Weiss, C., and Hurland, H. (1972). The oxygen supply of the dog kidney: measurements of intrarenal pO2. *Microvasc. Res.* 4, 247–257. doi: 10.1016/0026-2862(72)90036-2

Bianciardi, P., Fantacci, M., Caretti, A., Ronchi, R., Milano, G., Morel, S., et al. (2006). Chronic in vivo hypoxia in various organs: hypoxia-inducible factor-1alpha and apoptosis. *Biochem. Biophys. Res. Commun.* 342, 875–880. doi: 10.1016/j.bbrc.2006.02.042

Campbell, D. J. (2017). Long-term neprilysin inhibition - implications for ARNIs. *Nat. Rev. Cardiol.* 14, 171–186. doi: 10.1038/nrcardio.2016.200

Carpenter, T. C., and Stenmark, K. R. (2001). Hypoxia decreases lung neprilysin expression and increases pulmonary vascular leak. *Am. J. Physiol. Lung Cell. Mol. Physiol.* 281, L941–L948. doi: 10.1152/ajplung.2001.281.4.L941

Chen, Y. F. (2005). Atrial natriuretic peptide in hypoxia. *Peptides* 26, 1068–1077. doi: 10.1016/j.peptides.2004.08.030

Chiang, A. A. (2006). Obstructive sleep apnea and chronic intermittent hypoxia: a review. *Chin. J. Physiol.* 249, 234–243.

Del Rio, R., Moya, E. A., and Iturriaga, R. (2010). Carotid body and cardiorespiratory alterations in intermittent hypoxia: the oxidative link. *Eur. Respir. J.* 36, 136–142. doi: 10.1183/09031936.0015 8109

Enholm, B., Paavonen, K., Ristimäki, A., Kumar, V., Gunji, Y., Klefstrom, J., et al. (1997). Comparison of VEGF, VEGF-B, VEGF-C and Ang-1 mRNA regulation by serum, growth factors, oncoproteins and hypoxia. *Oncogene* 14, 2475–2483. doi: 10.1038/sj.onc.1201090

Epstein, F. H. (1997). Oxygen and renal metabolism. *Kidney Int.* 51, 381–385. doi: 10.1038/ki.1997.50

Fähling, M., Mathia, S., Scheidl, J., Abramovitch, R., Milman, Z., Paliege, A., et al. (2017). Cyclosporin a induces renal episodic hypoxia. *Acta Physiol.* 219, 625–639. doi: 10.1111/apha.12811

Fine, L. G., Bandyopadhay, D., and Norman, J. T. (2000). Is there a common mechanism for the progression of different types of renal diseases other than proteinuria? Towards the unifying theme of chronic hypoxia. *Kidney Int. Suppl.* 75, S22–S26. doi: 10.1046/j.1523-1755.2000.07512.x

Flor, K. C., Silva, E. F., Menezes, M. F., Pedrino, G. R., Colombari, E., and Zoccal, D. B. (2018). Short-term sustained hypoxia elevates basal and hypoxia-induced ventilation but not the carotid body chemoreceptor activity in rats. *Front. Physiol.* 9:134. doi: 10.3389/fphys.2018.00134

Fu, Q., Colgan, S. P., and Shelley, C. S. (2016). Hypoxia: the force that drives chronic kidney disease. *Clin. Med. Res.* 14, 15–39. doi: 10.3121/cmr.2015.1282

Gess, B., Schricker, K., Pfeifer, M., and Kurtz, A. (1997). Acute hypoxia upregulates NOS gene expression in rats. *Am. J. Physiol. Regul. Integr. Comp. Physiol.* 273, R905–R910. doi: 10.1152/ajpregu.1997.273.3.R905

Günther, H., Aumüller, G., Kunke, S., Vaupel, P., and Thews, G. (1974). Verteilung der O2-drucke in der rattenniere unter normbedingungen. *Res. Exp. Med.* 163, 251–264. doi: 10.1007/BF01851672

Hampel, D. J., Sansome, C., Romanov, V. I., Kowalski, A. J., Denhardt, D. T., and Goligorsky, M. S. (2003). Osteopontin traffic in hypoxic renal epithelial cells. *Nephron Exp. Nephrol.* 94, e66–e76. doi: 10.1159/000071285

Hargrove, G. M., Dufresne, J., Whiteside, C., Muruve, D. A., and Wong, N. C. (2000). Diabetes mellitus increases endothelin-1 gene transcription in rat kidney. *Kidney Int.* 58, 1534–1545. doi: 10.1046/j.1523-1755.2000.00315.x

Hsieh, Y. H., Jacono, F. J., Siegel, R. E., and Dick, T. E. (2015). Respiratory modulation of sympathetic activity is attenuated in adult rats conditioned with chronic hypobaric hypoxia. *Respir. Physiol. Neurobiol.* 206, 53–60. doi: 10.1016/j.resp.2014.11.011

Icekson, G., Dominguez, C. V., Dedios, V. P., Arroyo, J., and Alcayaga, J. (2013). Petrosal ganglion responses to acetylcholine and ATP are enhanced by chronic normobaric hypoxia in the rabbit. *Respir. Physiol. Neurobiol.* 189, 624–631. doi: 10.1016/j.resp.2013.07.023

Jackson, R. M., Narkates, A. J., and Oparil, S. (1986). Impaired pulmonary conversion of angiotensin I to angiotensin II in rats exposed to chronic hypoxia. *J. Appl. Physiol.* 60, 1121–1127. doi: 10.1152/jappl.1986.60.4.1121

Jaffa, A. A., Vio, C. P., Silva, R. H., Vavrek, R. J., Stewart, J. M., Rust, P. F., et al. (1992). Evidence for renal kinins as mediators of amino acid-induced hyperperfusion and hyperfiltration in the rat. *J. Clin. Invest* 89, 1460–1468. doi: 10.1172/JCI115736

Johnson, R. J., Gordon, K. L., Suga, S., Duijvestijn, A. M., Griffin, K., and Bidani, A. (1999). Renal injury and salt-sensitive hypertension after exposure to catecholamines. *Hypertension* 34, 151–159. doi: 10.1161/01.HYP.34.1.151

Johnson, R. J., Herrera-Acosta, J., Schreiner, G. F., and Rodriguez-Iturbe, B. (2002). Subtle acquired renal injury as a mechanism of salt-sensitive hypertension. *N. Engl. J. Med.* 346, 913–923. doi: 10.1056/NEJMra011078

Judge, P., Haynes, R., Landray, M. J., and Baigent, C. (2015). Neprilysin inhibition in chronic kidney disease. *Nephrol. Dial. Transplant.* 30, 738–743. doi: 10.1093/ndt/gfu269

Kelsen, S., Hall, J. E., and Chade, A. R. (2011). Endothelin-A receptor blockade slows the progression of renal injury in experimental renovascular disease. *Am. J. Physiol. Renal Physiol.* 301, F218–F225. doi: 10.1152/ajprenal.00089.2011

Kent, B. D., Mitchell, P. D., and McNicholas, W. T. (2011). Hypoxemia in patients with COPD: cause, effects, and disease progression. *Int. J. Chron. Obstruct. Pulmon. Dis.* 6, 199–208. doi: 10.2147/COPD.S10611

King, S. J., Booyse, F. M., Lin, P. H., Traylor, M., Narkates, A. J., and Oparil, S. (1989). Hypoxia stimulates endothelial cell angiotensin-converting enzyme antigen synthesis. *Am. J. Physiol. Cell Physiol.* 256, C1231–C1238. doi: 10.1152/ajpcell.1989.256.6.C1231

Leichtweiss, H. P., Lübbers, D. W., Weiss, C., Baumgärtl, H., and Reschke, W. (1969). The oxygen supply of the rat kidneys: measurements of intrarenal pO2. *Pflügers Arch.* 309, 328–349. doi: 10.1007/BF00587756

Li, C., Booze, R. M., and Hersh, L. B. (1995). Tissue-specific expression of rat neutral endopeptidase (neprilysin) mRNAs. *J. Biol. Chem.* 270, 5723–5728. doi: 10.1074/jbc.270.11.5723

Livak, K. J., and Schmittgen, T. D. (2001). Analysis of relative gene expression data using real-time quantitative PCR and the $2^{-\Delta\Delta CT}$ method. *Methods* 25, 402–408. doi: 10.1006/meth.2001.1262

Lombardi, D. M., Viswanathan, M., Vio, C. P., Saavedra, J. M., Schwartz, S. M., and Johnson, R. J. (2001). Renal and vascular injury induced by exogenous angiotensin II is AT1 receptor-dependent. *Nephron* 87, 66–74. doi: 10.1159/000045886

Lübbers, D. W., and Baumgärtl, H. (1997). Heterogeneities and profiles of oxygen pressure in brain and kidney examples of pO2 distribution in the living tissue. *Kidney Int.* 51, 372–380. doi: 10.1038/ki.1997.49

Madeddu, P., Emanueli, C., and El-Dahr, S. (2007). Mechanisms of disease: the tissue kallikrein-kinin system in hypertension and vascular remodeling. *Nat. Clin. Pract. Nephrol.* 3, 208–221. doi: 10.1038/ncpneph0444

Martinez, L., Vio, C. P., Valdés, G., Kychenthal, W., and Mendoza, S. (1990). Decreased kallikrein excretion in renal transplant treated with cyclosporine A. *Transplant. Proc.* 22, 294–296.

Mazzali, M., Jefferson, J. A., Ni, Z., Vaziri, N. D., and Johnson, R. J. (2003). Microvascular and tubulointerstitial injury associated with chronic hypoxia-induced hypertension. *Kidney Int.* 63, 2088–2093. doi: 10.1046/j.1523-1755.2003.00011.x

Meyers, K. E., and Sethna, C. (2013). Endothelin antagonists in hypertension and kidney disease. *Pediatr. Nephrol.* 28, 711–720. doi: 10.1007/s00467-012-2316-4

Milano, G., Bianciardi, P., Corno, A. F., Raddatz, E., Morel, S., von Segesser, L. K., et al. (2004). Myocardial impairment in chronic hypoxia is abolished by short aeration episodes: involvement of K+ATP channels. *Exp. Biol. Med.* 229, 1196–1205. doi: 10.1177/153537020422901115

Mitra, R., Chao, O. S., Nanus, D. M., and Goodman, O. B. Jr. (2013). Negative regulation of NEP expression by hypoxia. *Prostate* 73, 706–714. doi: 10.1002/pros.22613

Mizutani, S., Ishii, M., Hattori, A., Nomura, S., Numaguchi, Y., Tsujimoto, M., et al. (2008). New insights into the importance of aminopeptidase A in hypertension. *Heart Fail. Rev.* 13, 273–284. doi: 10.1007/s10741-007-9065-7

Moraes, D. J. A., Bonagamba, L. G. A., Costa, K. M., Costa-Silva, J. H., Zoccal, D. B., and Machado, B. H. (2014). Short-term sustained hypoxia induces changes in the coupling of sympathetic and respiratory activities in rats. *J. Physiol.* 592, 2013–2033. doi: 10.1113/jphysiol.2013.262212

Mukai, H., Fitzgibbon, W. R., Bozeman, G., Margolius, H. S., and Ploth, D. W. (1996). Bradykinin B2 receptor antagonist increases chloride and water absorption in rat medullary collecting duct. *Am. J. Physiol. Regul. Integr. Comp. Physiol.* 271, R352–R360. doi: 10.1152/ajpregu.1996.271.2.R352

Nalivaeva, N. N., Belyaev, N. D., Zhuravin, I. A., and Turner, A. J. (2012). The Alzheimer's amyloid-degrading peptidase, neprilysin: can we control it? *Int. J. Alzheimers Dis.* 2012:383796. doi: 10.1155/2012/383796

Nangaku, M., and Fujita, T. (2008). Activation of the renin-angiotensin system and chronic hypoxia of the kidney. *Hypertens. Res.* 31, 175–184. doi: 10.1291/hypres.31.175

O'Neill, J., Fasching, A., Pihl, L., Patinha, D., Franzén, S., and Palm, F. (2015). Acute SGLT inhibition normalizes O2 tension in the renal cortex but causes hypoxia in the renal medulla in anaesthetized control and diabetic rats. *Am. J. Physiol. Renal Physiol.* 309, F227–F234. doi: 10.1152/ajprenal.00689.2014

Oparil, S., Narkates, A. J., Jackson, R. M., and Ann, H. S. (1988). Altered-angiotensin converting enzyme in lung and extrapulmonary tissues of hypoxia-adapted rats. *J. Appl. Physiol.* 65, 218–227. doi: 10.1152/jappl.1988.65.1.218

Ow, C. P. C., Ngo, J. P., Ullah, M. M., Hilliard, L. M., and Evans, R. G. (2018). Renal hypoxia in kidney disease: cause or consequence? *Acta Physiol.* 222:e12999. doi: 10.1111/apha.12999

Rabinovitch, M., Gamble, W., Nadas, A. S., Miettinen, O. S., and Reid, L. (1979). Rat pulmonary circulation after chronic hypoxia: hemodynamic and structural features. *Am. J. Physiol. Heart Circ. Physiol.* 236, H818–H827. doi: 10.1152/ajpheart.1979.236.6.H818

Rice, G. I., Thomas, D. A., Grant, P. J., Turner, A. J., and Hooper, N. M. (2004). Evaluation of angiotensin-converting enzyme (ACE), its homologue ACE2 and neprilysin in angiotensin peptide metabolism. *Biochem. J.* 383, 45–51. doi: 10.1042/BJ20040634

Richard, N. A., and Koehle, M. S. (2012). Differences in cardio-ventilatory responses to hypobaric and normobaric hypoxia: a review. *Aviat. Space Environ. Med.* 83, 677–684. doi: 10.3357/ASEM.3182.2012

Rodebaugh, J., Sekulic, M., Davies, W., Montgomery, S., Khraibi, A., Solhaug, M. J., et al. (2012). Neuronal nitric oxide synthase, nNOS, regulates renal hemodynamics in the postnatal developing piglet. *Pediatr. Res.* 71, 144–149. doi: 10.1038/pr.2011.23

Saijonmaa, O., Nyman, T., Kosonen, R., and Fyhrquist, F. (2001). Upregulation of angiotensin-converting enzyme by vascular endothelial growth factor. *Am. J. Physiol. Heart Circ. Physiol.* 280, H885–H891. doi: 10.1152/ajpheart.2001.280.2.H885

Salas, S. P., Giacaman, A., Romero, W., Downey, P., Aranda, E., Mezzano, D., et al. (2007). Pregnant rats treated with a serotonin precursor have reduced fetal weight and lower plasma volume and kallikrein levels. *Hypertension* 50, 773–779. doi: 10.1161/HYPERTENSIONAHA.107.094540

Savourey, G., Launay, J. C., Besnard, Y., Guinet, A., and Travers, S. (2003). Normo- and hypobaric hypoxia: are there any physiological differences? *Eur. J. Appl. Physiol.* 89, 122–126. doi: 10.1007/s00421-002-0789-8

Savourey, G., Launay, J. C., Besnard, Y., Guinet-Lebreton, A., Alonso, A., Sauvet, F., et al. (2007). Normo or hypobaric hypoxia tests: propositions for the determination of the individual susceptibility to altitude illnesses. *Eur. J. Appl. Physiol.* 100, 193–205. doi: 10.1007/s00421-007-0417-8

Schwenke, D. O., Tokudome, T., Shirai, M., Hosoda, H., Horio, T., Kishimoto, I., et al. (2008). Exogenous ghrelin attenuates the progression of chronic hypoxia-induced pulmonary hypertension in conscious rats. *Endocrinology* 149, 237–244. doi: 10.1210/en.2007-0833

Shoji, K., Tanaka, T., and Nangaku, M. (2014). Role of hypoxia in progressive chronic kidney disease and implications for therapy. *Curr. Opin. Nephrol. Hypertens.* 23, 161–168. doi: 10.1097/01.mnh.0000441049.98664.6c

Sivritas, S. H., Ploth, D. W., and Fitzgibbon, W. R. (2008). Blockade of renal medullary bradykinin B2 receptors increases tubular sodium reabsorption in rats fed a normal-salt diet. *Am. J. Physiol. Renal Physiol.* 295, F811–F817. doi: 10.1152/ajprenal.90225.2008

Suga, I., Phillips, I., Ray, P. E., Raleigh, J. A., Vio, C. P., Kim, Y. G., et al. (2001). Hypokalemia induces renal injury and alterations in vasoactive mediators that favor salt sensitivity. *Am. J. Physiol. Renal Physiol.* 281, F620–F629. doi: 10.1152/ajprenal.2001.281.4.F620

Thongboonkerd, V., Gozal, E., Sachleben, L. R. Jr., Arthur, J. M., Pierce, W. M., Cai, J., et al. (2002). Proteomic analysis reveals alterations in the renal kallikrein pathway during hypoxia-induced hypertension. *J. Biol. Chem.* 277, 34708–34716. doi: 10.1074/jbc.M203799200

Villanueva, S., Cespedes, C., and Vio, C. P. (2006). Ischemic acute renal failure induces the expression of a wide range of nephrogenic proteins. *Am. J. Physiol. Regul. Integ. Comp. Phys.* 290, R861–R870. doi: 10.1152/ajpregu.00384.2005

Villanueva, S., Contreras, F., Tapia, A., Carreño, J. E., Vergara, C., Ewertz, E., et al. (2014). Basic fibroblast growth factor reduces functional and structural damage in chronic kidney disease. *Am. J. Physiol. Renal Physiol.* 306, F430–F441. doi: 10.1152/ajprenal.00720.2012

Vio, C. P., Figueroa, C. D., and Caorsi, I. (1988). Anatomical relationship between kallikrein containing tubules and the juxtaglomerular apparatus in the human kidney. *Am. J. Hypertens.* 1, 269–271. doi: 10.1093/ajh/1.3.269

Vio, C. P., and Jeanneret, V. A. (2003). Local induction of angiotensin-converting enzyme in the kidney as a mechanism of progressive renal diseases. *Kidney Int. Suppl.* 86, S57–S63. doi: 10.1046/j.1523-1755.64.s86.11.x

Vio, C. P., Loyola, S., and Velarde, V. (1992). Localization of components of the kallikrein-kinin system in the kidney: relation to renal function State of the art lecture. *Hypertension* 19, 10–16. doi: 10.1161/01.HYP.19.2_Suppl.II10

Volpe, M., Carnovali, M., and Mastromarino, V. (2016). The natriuretic peptides system in the pathophysiology of heart failure: from molecular basis to treatment. *Clin. Sci.* 130, 57–77. doi: 10.1042/CS20150469

Wang, Z., Yang, D., Zhang, X., Li, T., Li, J., Tang, Y., et al. (2011). Hypoxia-induced down-regulation of neprilysin by histone modification in mouse primary cortical and hippocampal neurons. *PLoS One* 6:e19229. doi: 10.1371/journal.pone.0019229

Zhang, D. D., Gao, Z. X., Vio, C. P., Xiao, Y., Wu, P., Zhang, H., et al. (2018). Bradykinin stimulates renal Na+ and K+ excretion by inhibiting the K+ channel (Kir4.1) in the distal convoluted tubule. *Hypertension* 72, 361–369. doi: 10.1161/HYPERTENSIONAHA.118.11070

Zhou, L., and Duan, S. (2014). Effects of angiotensin converting enzyme inhibitors and angiotensin receptor blockers in contrast-induced nephropathy. *Kidney Blood Press. Res.* 38, 165–171. doi: 10.1159/00035576

15

Circulating Apoptotic Signals During Acute and Chronic Exposure to High Altitude in Kyrgyz Population

*Djuro Kosanovic[1,2], Simon Maximilian Platzek[1], Aleksandar Petrovic[1], Akylbek Sydykov[1], Abdirashit Maripov[3], Argen Mamazhakypov[1], Meerim Sartmyrzaeva[3], Kubatbek Muratali Uulu[3], Meerim Cholponbaeva[3], Aidana Toktosunova[3], Nazgul Omurzakova[3], Melis Duishobaev[3], Christina Vroom[1], Oleg Pak[1], Norbert Weissmann[1], Hossein Ardeschir Ghofrani[1], Akpay Sarybaev[3] and Ralph Theo Schermuly[1]**

[1] Chair for Pulmonary Pharmacotherapy, Member of the German Center for Lung Research, Universities of Giessen and Marburg Lung Center, Giessen, Germany, [2] Sechenov First Moscow State Medical University (Sechenov University), Moscow, Russia, [3] Kyrgyz National Centre for Cardiology and Internal Medicine, named after Academician Mirsaid Mirrakhimov, Bishkek, Kyrgyzstan

***Correspondence:**
Ralph Theo Schermuly
ralph.schermuly@innere.med.uni-giessen.de

Background: Circulating apoptotic signals (CASs) have been described in the pathologies associated with dysregulated apoptosis, such as cancer, heart diseases, and pulmonary hypertension (PH). However, nothing is known about the expression profiles of these markers in the circulation of humans exposed to acute and chronic effects of high altitude (HA).

Methods: Gene expression levels of different apoptotic signals (ASs) were analyzed in human pulmonary artery smooth muscle cells (PASMCs) upon hypoxia incubation. In addition, we measured the plasma values of relevant CAS in Kyrgyz volunteers during acute and chronic exposure to HA. Finally, we analyzed the effects of pro-apoptotic mediator Fas ligand (FasL) on apoptosis and proliferation of human PASMCs.

Results: Several cellular AS were increased in PASMCs exposed to hypoxia, in comparison to normoxia condition. Among analyzed CAS, there was a prominent reduction of FasL in lowlanders exposed to HA environment. Furthermore, decreased circulatory levels of FasL were found in highlanders with HA-induced PH (HAPH), as compared to the lowland controls. Furthermore, FasL concentration in plasma negatively correlated with tricuspid regurgitant gradient values. Finally, FasL exerted pro-apoptotic and anti-proliferative effects on PASMCs.

Conclusion: Our data demonstrated that circulating levels of FasL are reduced during acute and chronic exposure to HA environment. In addition, dysregulated FasL may play a role in the context of HAPH due to its relevant functions on apoptosis and proliferation of PASMCs.

Keywords: high altitude, circulating apoptotic markers, Fas ligand, hypoxic pulmonary hypertension, pulmonary artery smooth muscle cells

INTRODUCTION

High altitude is a well-known extreme environment characterized by hypoxia, among other abiotic factors, and may exert prominent acute and chronic effects on respiratory and cardiovascular systems (Maggiorini and Leon-Velarde, 2003; West, 2012; Mirrakhimov and Strohl, 2016). An important part of the human population inhabits high altitudes of our planet and a large number of people visit these elevations periodically due to several reasons (Mirrakhimov and Strohl, 2016; Azad et al., 2017). Short-term exposure of non-acclimatized people to high altitude may provoke the appearance of several acute mountain disorders, including acute mountain sickness and high-altitude pulmonary edema (West, 2012). Long-term exposure to this challenging external surrounding may lead to development of high altitude-induced pulmonary hypertension (HAPH), which is a pathological condition currently classified in the group 3 of pulmonary hypertension (PH) (Maggiorini and Leon-Velarde, 2003; Simonneau et al., 2013; Mirrakhimov and Strohl, 2016).

In general, pulmonary vascular remodeling as the main attribute of PH pathology appears due to significant dysregulation of normal processes in the pulmonary vascular cells, such as proliferation and apoptosis (Schermuly et al., 2011; Malczyk et al., 2016; Stenmark et al., 2018; Thenappan et al., 2018). Abnormal regulation of apoptosis and occurrence of "apoptotic-resistant" phenotype in pulmonary vascular cells, such as pulmonary artery smooth muscle cells (PASMCs), are important hallmarks of hypoxia-induced PH pathogenesis (Yang et al., 2001; Chen et al., 2014; Li et al., 2017; You et al., 2018). Due to the existence of these cellular abnormalities, e.g., increased proliferation and resistance to apoptosis, PH is often described as a "tumor-like disease" in recent years (Chan and Rubin, 2017; Marshall et al., 2018). However, despite clear advancement in understanding of the role of apoptosis in hypoxia-associated PH and PH in general, many questions remain unresolved and insufficiently investigated.

A disbalance between pro- and anti-apoptotic molecular pathways has been described as an important phenomenon in the cancer field (Holdenrieder and Stieber, 2004). In addition to the general pathobiology of cellular apoptosis, several circulating apoptotic signals (CASs) have been evaluated as promising biomarkers relevant to the tumor pathologies (Holdenrieder and Stieber, 2010). In the field of cardiovascular diseases, some of the apoptotic markers have been also identified in the blood circulation (Parissis et al., 2004; Niessner et al., 2009). With regard to the pulmonary vascular disease, it has been demonstrated that the levels of CASs, namely Fas ligand (FasL) and tumor necrosis factor (TNF)-related apoptosis-inducing ligand (TRAIL), are changed in response to therapy or altered in patients with PH, respectively (Akagi et al., 2013; Liu et al., 2015). However, almost nothing is known about the profiles of circulating apoptotic markers in the context of human individuals exposed to high altitude hypoxic condition.

Therefore, we investigated for the first time the potential changes in the plasma levels of different apoptotic signals, including FasL, TRAIL and apolipoprotein C1 (ApoC1), in human individuals who live permanently in high altitude regions and lowland subjects who spent a short period of time in such environment. Finally, the potential alteration in gene expression profile of various apoptotic players, for example caspase (Casp) 1 and 3, survivin, Fas-associated death domain protein (FADD)-like ICE inhibitory protein (FLIP), ApoC1, TRAIL and FasL, was analyzed in human PASMCs exposed to hypoxia for different time durations.

MATERIALS AND METHODS

Study Design

In order to analyze the circulating profiles of various apoptotic markers during acute and chronic exposure to high altitude hypoxia, we have performed two studies among the Kyrgyz population.

First, for the purpose of investigating the people permanently living at high altitude environment, we have selected the human community of Sary-Mogol and Achyk-Suu villages, which are located in Alay and Chon-Alay districts of the province of Osh in the southern part of Kyrgyzstan. These villages are settled at altitudes of 3000–3100 m, but the most of the residents usually spend 3–4 months per year at even higher elevations (3200–3600 m). Importantly, we ensured that all subjects enrolled in the study were ethnic Kyrgyz and were born and permanently living at high altitudes. As the lowland control, we have included the volunteers from Bishkek, Kyrgyzstan (approximately 760 m above the sea level). All participants of the study underwent the general anthropometric and echocardiographic measurements (please see below), followed by collection of the peripheral blood and separation of the citrated platelet free plasma (PFP).

Secondly, for the purpose of investigating the people acutely exposed to high altitude hypoxia, we had a group of healthy Kyrgyz males. Initially, the subjects underwent examination in Bishkek (low altitude (LA 1) at 760 m, with the outside temperature ranging from 28 to 35°C during the study execution). After that, the participants were transported by road to an altitude of 3200 m (Tuya-Ashuu pass, Kyrgyzstan) (**Figure 1**), where the outside temperature was in the range 5–20°C, while inside the rooms in the research station the temperature was maintained at 22 ± 2°C. The first 2 days after arrival to high altitude environment the subjects took

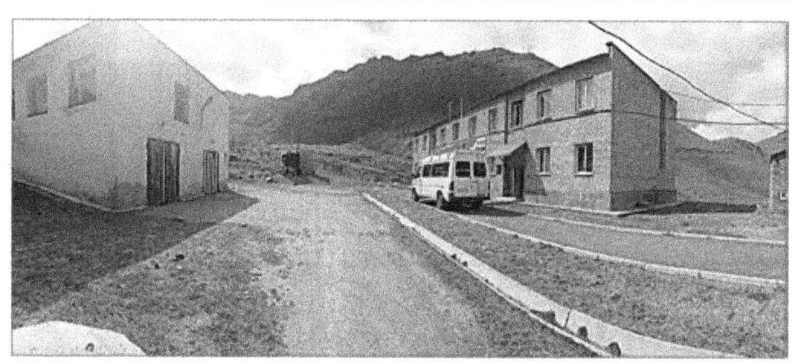

FIGURE 1 | High altitude research station near to the Tuya-Ashuu pass (3200 m), Kyrgyzstan. The photograph is original work of one of the authors.

complete rest. During the next 2 days they were allowed to walk at plains and downhill. Thereafter, the participants were involved in common activities, such as indoor games, watching TV, playing table tennis or billiard, along with morning drill, walking and other galley duties. Importantly, all subjects were free of cardiac or neurological problems and were not consuming any kind of medications. In addition to the basal examination in Bishkek (LA 1) at low altitude, all individuals underwent echocardiographic measurements, followed by the collection of the peripheral blood and separation of the EDTA plasma on days 2 (HA 2), 7 (HA 7), and 20 (HA 20) of high altitude exposure, and on the second day after descent to Bishkek at low altitude again (LA 2). In addition, anthropometry was performed in all participants.

Both studies protocols were approved by the Ethics Committees of the National Centre for Cardiology and Internal Medicine, Bishkek, Kyrgyzstan (01-1/08 and 01-1/07) and the faculty of Medicine at Justus-Liebig University, Giessen, Germany (AZ: 236/16). The study was performed in agreement to the principles outlined in the Declaration of Helsinki of the World Medical Association. Finally, written informed consent was obtained from all participants.

Anthropometric and Echocardiographic Measurements

Several general parameters were obtained, such as age, gender ratio, body mass index (BMI), and body surface area (BSA). BMI (kg/m^2) was calculated using the formula: BMI = weight (kg)/(height $(m)^2$). BSA (m^2) was calculated using the Du Bois formula as follows: BSA = $0.007184 \times [(\text{height (m)} \times 100)^{0.725}] \times (\text{weight (kg)})^{0.425}$). The right ventricular to right atrial pressure gradient was used as a surrogate of the estimated systolic pulmonary artery pressure. Continuous-wave Doppler echocardiography was employed to estimate the tricuspid regurgitant gradient (TRG, in mmHg) from the peak flow tricuspid regurgitation velocity by means of the simplified Bernoulli equation measured using continuous-wave Doppler, as previously described (Yock and Popp, 1984). All the above mentioned parameters are presented in the **Table 1** (acute high altitude exposure) and **Table 2** (chronic exposure to high altitude). In the case of acute high altitude study, all general parameters, including age, gender, BMI, and BSA were comparable among all participants (**Table 1**). TRG values were initially increased on the second day (HA 2) of high altitude exposure in comparison to the lowlands (LA 1), and later gradually decreased until return to the low altitude (LA 2) (**Table 1**). There were statistically significant elevations of TRG on the days 2 and 7 at high altitude, as compared to the lowland conditions (LA 1) (**Table 1**). Also, there was a significant increase of TRG values on the day 2 of high altitude exposure, in comparison to the low altitude upon return (LA 2) (**Table 1**).

In the case of chronic exposure to high altitude (**Table 2**), BMI and BSA were comparable among all 3 groups: lowland control subjects (LA), highlanders without (HA; TRG $\leq$ 23 mmHg) and with PH (HA-PH; TRG $\geq$ 40 mmHg). However, there were noticeable differences in gender ratio and age (lowland control group consisted only of younger males). This fact is a potential limitation of our study. TRG values were significantly increased in highlanders with PH, as compared to the lowland controls and highlanders without PH (**Table 2**).

TABLE 2 | Chronic exposure to high altitude – human subjects' anthropometric and echocardiographic data.

	Age (years)	Gender ratio m/f (%)	BMI (kg/m^2)	BSA (m^2)	TRG (mmHg)
LA	20.6 ± 2.9	100/0	23.1 ± 1.6	1.9 ± 0.1	20.9 ± 1.6
HA	50.5 ± 11.3	60/40	23.9 ± 4.0	1.7 ± 0.1	20.7 ± 0.4
HA-PH	53.1 ± 14.6	42/58	25.5 ± 5.3	1.7 ± 0.1	46.7 ± 6.0****$$$$

*Adult human subjects permanently living at lowland regions (LA) (n = 10) and high altitude (HA) locations were included for the study. Individuals settled at high altitude regions were separated into two groups: highlanders without pulmonary hypertension (PH) (HA) (n = 10) and highlanders with PH (HA-PH) (n = 12). Various anthropometric and echocardiographic parameters were presented. Results are shown as Mean ± SD (n = 10–12). ****p < 0.0001 LA compared to the HA-PH; $$$$ p < 0.0001 HA compared to the HA-PH. one-way ANOVA with Tukey's multiple comparisons test was performed for statistical analysis. m, male; f, female; BMI, body mass index (in kg/m²); BSA, body surface area (in m²); TRG, tricuspid regurgitant gradient (in mmHg).*

Cell Culture and RT-qPCR

Primary human PASMCs were purchased from Lonza and cultured in Smooth Muscle Growth Medium-2 containing supplement-mix. Human PASMCs passage 7 were incubated at 37°C in a humidified atmosphere of 5% CO_2 in either normoxic (21% O_2) or hypoxic conditions (1% O_2) for a period of 24, 48, and 72 h. Upon the end of the incubation period cells were lysed in RLT buffer (Qiagen) and total cell RNA was extracted using the RNeasy Mini Kit (Qiagen). Complementary DNA (cDNA)

TABLE 1 | Acute exposure to high altitude – human subjects' anthropometric and echocardiographic data.

Age (years)	Gender Ratio m/f(%)	BMI (kg/m^2)	BSA (m^2)	TRG (mmHg)				
				LA1	HA 2	HA 7	HA 20	LA 2
25.4 ± 4.2	100/0	23.0 ± 1.9	1.8 ± 0.1	18.5 ± 1.1	23.0 ± 2.2***$$	20.9 ± 0.8*	19.5 ± 1.6	18.4 ± 1.1

*Adult human subjects who initially came from the lowlands (LA 1) (n = 8) were exposed to high altitude (HA) for 2 (HA 2) (n = 8), 7 (HA 7) (n = 8), and 20 (HA 20) (n = 8) days. After 20 days, they returned to the lowlands again (LA 2) (n = 8). Various anthropometric and echocardiographic parameters at different time points were presented in the table. Results are shown as Mean ± SD (n = 8). *p < 0.05; ***p < 0.001 compared to the LA 1. $$ p < 0.01 compared to the LA 2. Friedman test with Dunn's multiple comparisons test was performed for statistical analysis. m, male, f, female; BMI, body mass index (in kg/m²); BSA, body surface area (in m²); TRG, tricuspid regurgitant gradient (in mmHg).*

TABLE 3 | Primer sequences are given from (5′ to 3′).

Target	FP	RP
Human ApoC1	AGC AAG GAT TCA GAG TGC CCC	CCT TCA GCT TAT CCA AGG CAC TG
Human Casp1	TGG GAC TCT CAG CAG ATC AAA CA	GGA TGT GGG CAT AGC TGG GT
Human Casp3	GTA GAA GAG TTT CGT GAG TGC TCG	GCA CAC CCA CCG AAA ACC AG
Human FasL	GGA GAA GCA AAT AGG CCA CCC	CCA GAG GCA TGG ACC TTG AGT
Human FLIP	CGG ACT ATA GAG TGC TGA TGG CA	TCC AAC TCA ACC ACA AGG TCC A
Human survivin	AAA GAG CCA AGA ACA AAA TTG C	GAG AGA GAA GCA GCC ACT GTT AC
Human TRAIL	TCC GTC AGC TCG TTA GAA AGA TGAT	GGT CCC AGT TAT GTG AGC TGC
Human porphobilinogen deaminase (PBGD)	CCC ACG CGA ATC ACT CTC AT	TGT CTG GTA ACG GCA ATG CG

FP, forward primer; RP, reverse primer.

was produced by reverse transcriptase polymerase chain reaction via iScript cDNA Synthesis Kit (Bio-Rad). Real-time PCR was performed in Mx3000P qPCR system (Stratagene) using the iTaq Universal SYBR Green Supermix (Bio-Rad). Primer sequences are given from (5′ to 3′) and presented in the **Table 3**. Human porphobilinogen deaminase (PBGD) served as a housekeeping gene. In order to confirm specific amplification of the expected PCR product, gel electrophoresis and melting curve analysis were performed.

Apoptosis and Proliferation Assays

For assessment of apoptosis, human PASMCs (3000 cells per well) were seeded in 96-well white-walled plate in Smooth Muscle Growth Medium-2. After 48 h of recovery time cells were stimulated with different concentrations of SuperFasLigand (Enzo Life Sciences) and incubated at 37°C in water saturated incubators for 24 h under normoxic conditions (21% O_2). The apoptosis Caspase-Glo 3/7 assay (Promega) was performed following the manufacturer's instructions. The luminescence of the caspase cleaved substrate reaction was measured after 30 min of incubation at room temperature.

Proliferation of human PASMCs exposed to normoxic (21% O_2) or hypoxic conditions (1% O_2) was assessed by Cell Proliferation ELISA, 5-bromo-2′-deoxyuridine (BrdU) assay (Sigma Aldrich). In more details, 7500 cells per well were seeded into 24-well plates and following the 24 h starvation period PASMCs were incubated for 24 or 48 h in Smooth Muscle Growth Medium-2. After that the cells were treated with different concentrations of SuperFasLigand or 500 ng/ml of neutralizing anti-Fas antibody ZB4 (Millipore). In addition, PASMCs were incubated for 48 h in Smooth Muscle Basal Medium and stimulated with 50 ng/ml of platelet-derived growth factor (PDGF) (R&D Systems) and/or 500 ng/ml of neutralizing anti-Fas antibody ZB4. The absorbance of the substrate reaction was measured at 370 nm (reference wavelength 492 nm).

Enzyme-Linked Immunosorbent Assay (ELISA)

Citrated platelet free plasma (PFP) or EDTA plasma samples were obtained from the peripheral blood from all participants of the study. In order to analyze the circulating levels of different markers, several ELISA measurements were performed for the following targets (ELISA kits): ApoC1 (Abnova), TRAIL (R&D Systems), FasL (LSBio/R&D Systems) and B-type natriuretic peptide (BNP) (Abnova). The concentrations of the markers were expressed as μg or pg per mL of plasma.

Data Analysis

Results are presented as Mean ± SD. Unpaired t-test with Welch's correction or ordinary one-way ANOVA with Dunnett's or Tukey's multiple comparisons test were used to compare data derived from the cell culture. Data based on ELISA and echocardiographic measurements were analyzed using Friedman test with Dunn's multiple comparisons test, RM one-way ANOVA with Tukey's multiple comparisons test or ordinary one-way ANOVA with Tukey's multiple comparisons test. Spearman or Pearson tests were used for the correlation analysis. Statistical significance was considered when p-value was < 0.05, < 0.01, < 0.001, and < 0.0001.

RESULTS

Alteration in the Gene Expression Levels of Various Apoptotic Markers in Human PASMCs After Hypoxic Incubation

As already described in Section "Materials and Methods," human PASMCs were exposed to hypoxia condition for different time durations (24, 48, and 72 h), followed by quantification of the gene expression levels of various apoptotic markers, such as Casp1 and 3, survivin, FLIP, ApoC1, TRAIL, and FasL (**Figures 2**, **3**). In general, all investigated apoptotic signals had increased their expression profiles upon hypoxic stimuli in human PASMCs (**Figures 2**, **3**), as compared to the normoxia condition. However, there were no clear and uniform time-dependent changes in the expression profiles of investigated apoptotic markers. The most prominent and statistically significant upregulation was noticed in the case of survivin and FasL, during all time points of hypoxia exposure, in comparison to the respective normoxic controls (**Figures 2C**, **3C**).

Circulating Profiles of Apoptotic Markers in Human Subjects Exposed to Acute High Altitude Conditions

We have already mentioned in the Section "Materials and Methods" that circulating levels of different apoptotic markers, such as ApoC1, TRAIL and FasL, were measured by ELISA in the plasma samples of human volunteers taken at different time points: in the lowland conditions (LA 1), on days 2 (HA 2), 7 (HA 7), and 20 (HA 20) of high altitude exposure, and

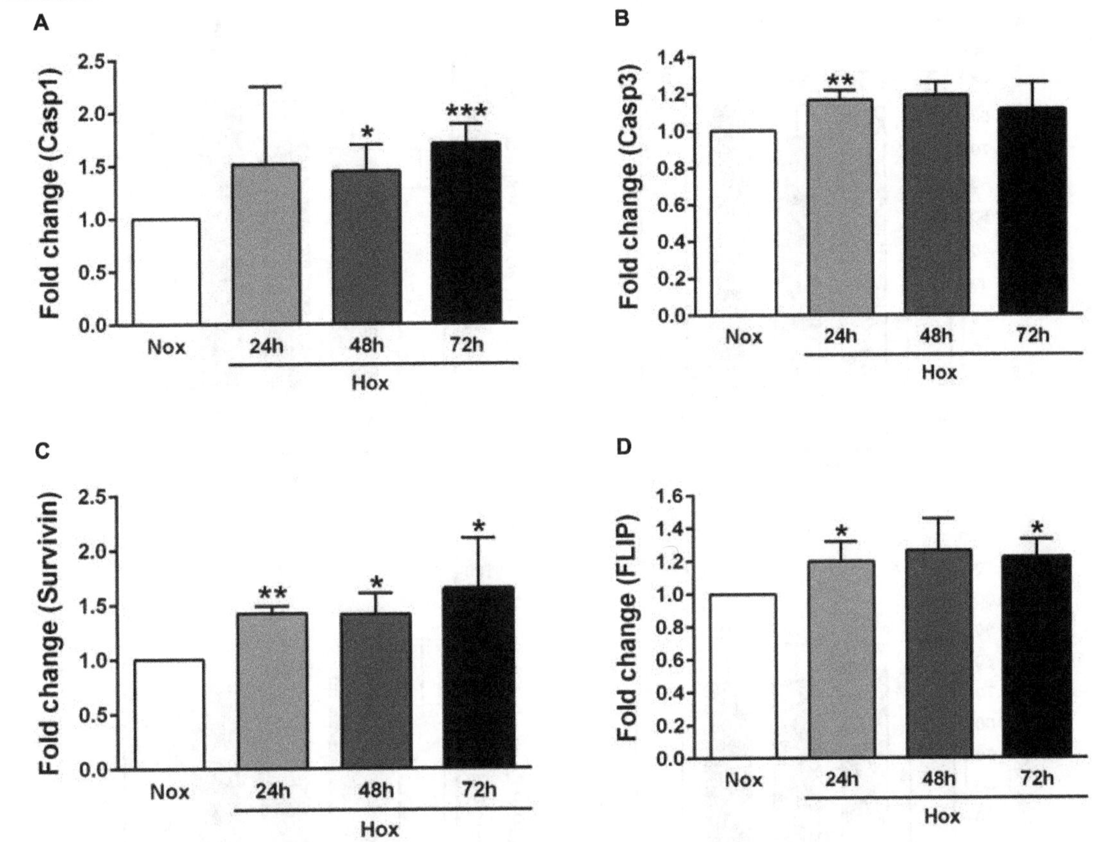

FIGURE 2 | Gene expression profiles of different apoptotic markers in human pulmonary arterial smooth muscle cells (PASMCs) exposed to hypoxia I. Human PASMCs were exposed to hypoxia (Hox) for different time durations (24, 48, and 72 h), followed by RT-qPCR for measurement of various apoptotic markers, such as: **(A)** caspase 1 (Casp1) and **(B)** 3 (Casp3), **(C)** survivin, and **(D)** Fas-associated death domain protein (FADD)-like ICE inhibitory protein (FLIP). Normoxia (Nox) exposure served as a control. Results are presented as a fold change normalized to the respective normoxic controls. Results are expressed as Mean ± SD (n = 4). *$p < 0.05$, **$p < 0.01$; ***$p < 0.001$ Nox versus Hox. Unpaired t-test with Welch's correction was performed for statistical analyses.

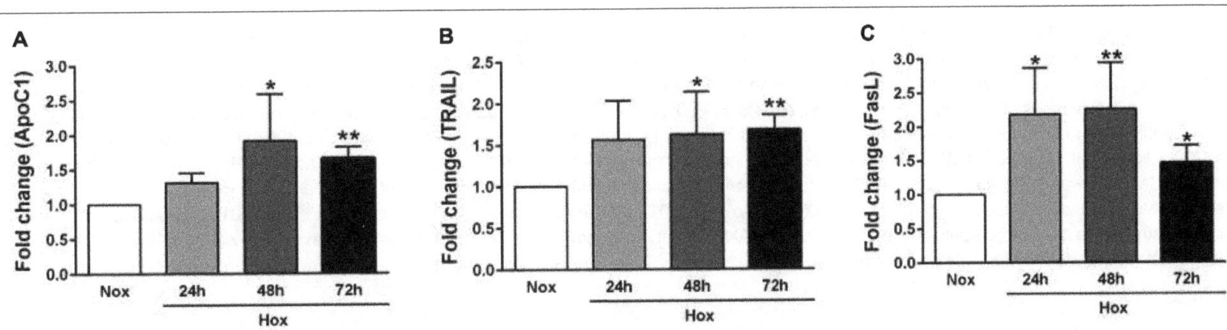

FIGURE 3 | Gene expression profiles of different apoptotic markers in human PASMCs exposed to hypoxia II. Human PASMCs were exposed to hypoxia (Hox) for different time durations (24, 48, and 72 h), followed by RT-qPCR for measurement of various apoptotic markers, such as: **(A)** apolipoprotein C1 (ApoC1), **(B)** tumor necrosis factor (TNF)-related apoptosis-inducing ligand (TRAIL), and **(C)** Fas ligand (FasL). Normoxia (Nox) exposure served as a control. Results are presented as a fold change normalized to the respective normoxic controls. Results are expressed as Mean ± SD (n = 4). *$p < 0.05$; **$p < 0.01$ Nox versus Hox. Unpaired t-test with Welch's correction was performed for statistical analyses.

after return to the low altitude (LA 2). In addition, ELISA was performed in the plasma samples during the same time points in order to analyze the level of circulating BNP. Investigated circulating apoptotic markers had different expression profiles and due to the technical reasons not all values for all enrolled subjects are available. Apo C1 circulating levels (in μg/mL) were comparable among different time points, except on day 7 (HA 7) of high altitude exposure, when the levels of this marker were significantly decreased in comparison to the low altitude upon descent from the high altitude (**Figure 4A**). Further, circulating

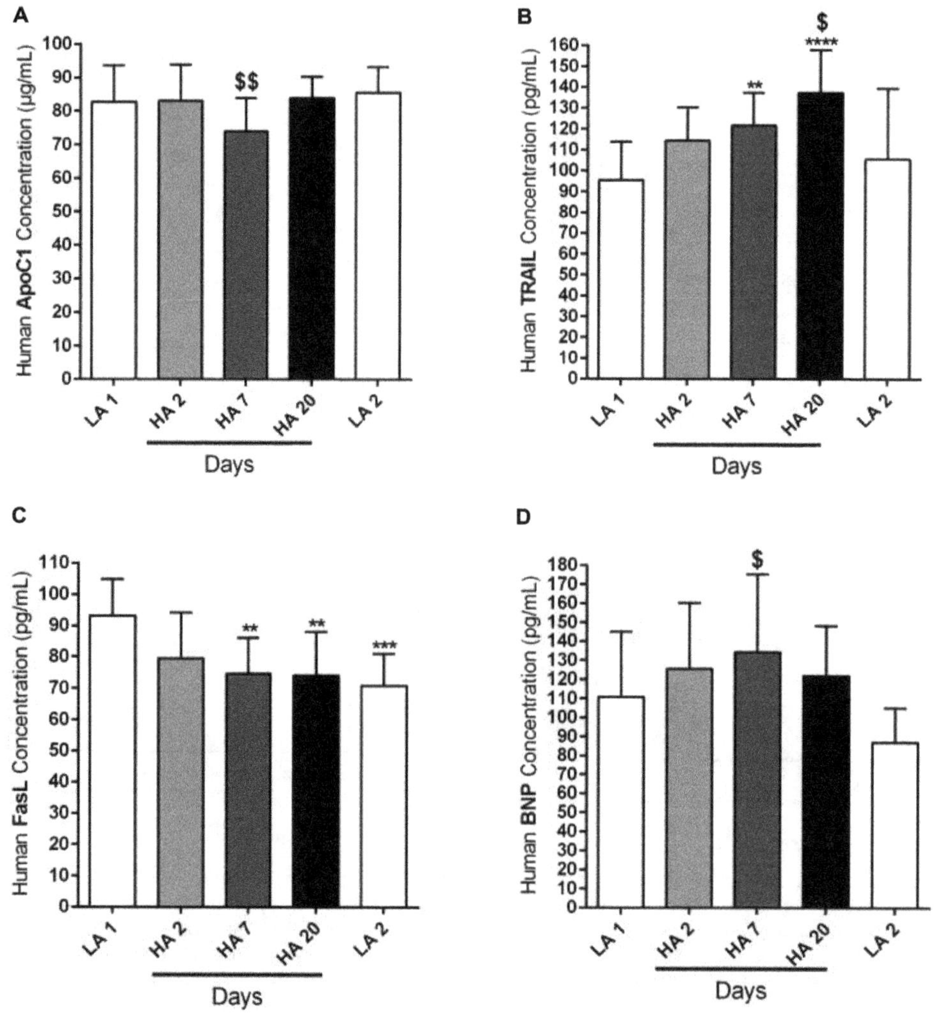

FIGURE 4 | Circulating apoptotic markers in human subjects during acute exposure to high altitude. Healthy volunteers living at lowland regions of Kyrgyzstan (LA 1) (n = 7–8) were exposed to high altitude (HA) environment (3200 m) in total duration of 20 days. After exposure to this extreme environment they returned to the lowlands again (LA 2) (n = 8). Echocardiographic measurements and collection of the peripheral blood were performed during the following time points: in low altitude location (LA 1), after 2 (HA 2) (n = 8), 7 (HA 7) (n = 8), and 20 (HA 20) (n = 8) days spending at high altitude, and after return to the lowlands again (LA 2). Plasma was separated and enzyme-linked immunosorbent assay (ELISA) was performed for the detection and quantification of the following circulating apoptotic markers: **(A)** apolipoprotein C1 (ApoC1), **(B)** TNF-related apoptosis-inducing ligand (TRAIL), and **(C)** Fas ligand (FasL). In addition, the circulating profile of B-type natriuretic peptide (BNP) was analyzed by ELISA. **(D)** Results are expressed as concentrations of the above mentioned markers (in µg or pg per mL of plasma) and presented as Mean ± SD (n = 7–8). $^{**}p < 0.01$; $^{***}p < 0.001$; $^{****}p < 0.0001$ compared to the LA 1 group. $^{\$}p < 0.05$; $^{\$\$}p < 0.01$ compared to the LA 2 group. Friedman test with Dunn's multiple comparisons test, RM one-way ANOVA with Tukey's multiple comparisons test or ordinary one-way ANOVA with Tukey's multiple comparisons test were performed for statistical analyses.

levels of TRAIL (in pg/mL) were gradually increasing due to high altitude exposure, with being significantly enhanced on days 7 (HA 7) and 20 (HA 20), in comparison to the lowland conditions (LA 1) (**Figure 4B**). After returning to the lowlands again, there was a significant decrease of circulating TRAIL levels (**Figure 4B**). In the case of FasL (in pg/mL), there was clear, but not time-dependent reduction of the circulating levels of this marker in high altitude conditions, as compared to the lowlands (LA 1) (**Figure 4C**). Surprisingly, decreased levels of circulating FasL were kept upon return to the low altitude (**Figure 4C**). Finally, there was a noticeable trend of increased levels of circulating BNP (in pg/mL) during different time points at high altitude, with prominent reduction upon return to the lowlands (**Figure 4D**). However, the significant difference was present only between the circulating levels of this marker on day 7 (HA 7) and the second low altitude condition (LA 2) (**Figure 4D**).

Circulating Profiles of Apoptotic Markers in Kyrgyz Highlanders and Lowlanders

As already indicated in the Section "Materials and Methods," circulating levels of different apoptotic markers, such as ApoC1, TRAIL and FasL, were measured by ELISA in the plasma samples of human subjects permanently living at high altitudes,

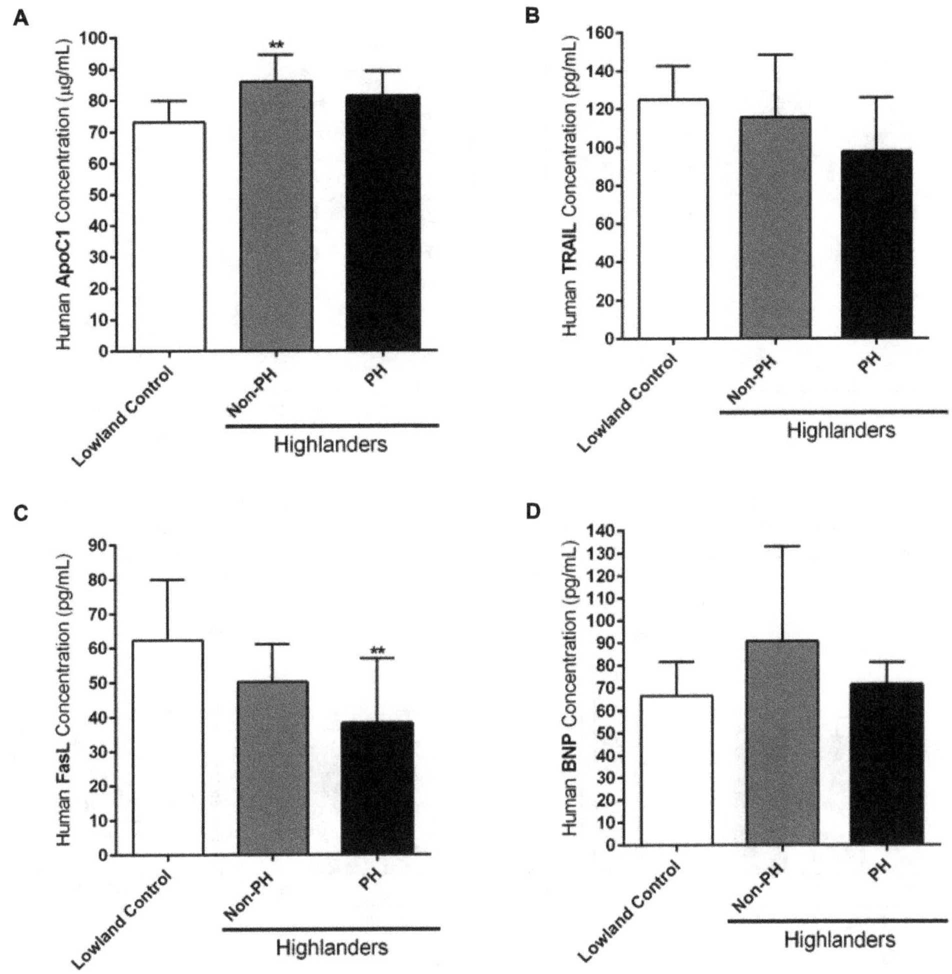

FIGURE 5 | Circulating apoptotic markers in human subjects permanently living at high altitude. Human subjects permanently living at high altitude regions of Kyrgyzstan (highlanders) were separated into two groups: individuals without developed pulmonary hypertension (Non-PH) (n = 9–10) and individuals with this pulmonary vascular disease (PH) (n = 10). People living at the low altitude served as a control (n = 9–10). Echocardiographic measurements and collection of the peripheral blood were performed for all volunteers. Plasma was separated and enzyme-linked immunosorbent assay (ELISA) was performed for the detection and quantification of the following circulating apoptotic markers: **(A)** apolipoprotein C1 (ApoC1), **(B)** TNF-related apoptosis-inducing ligand (TRAIL), and **(C)** Fas ligand (FasL). In addition, the circulating profile of B-type natriuretic peptide (BNP) was analyzed by ELISA. **(D)** Results are expressed as concentrations of the above mentioned markers (in µg or pg per mL of plasma) and presented as Mean ± SD (n = 9–10). $^{**}p < 0.01$ compared to the lowland control. One-way ANOVA with Tukey's multiple comparisons test was performed for statistical analysis.

in comparison to the people settled in the lowland locations (Lowland Control). Highlanders were further divided into two groups, those who developed PH (PH) and those who did not develop this pulmonary vascular disease (Non-PH). In addition, ELISA was performed in the plasma samples of these three groups, in order to analyze the level of circulating BNP. Due to the technical reasons not all values for all enrolled subjects are available. ApoC1 circulating levels (in µg/mL) were increased in both highlander groups, with being statistically significant in the case of highlanders without PH, in comparison to the lowland controls (**Figure 5A**). TRAIL circulating profile (in pg/mL) did not reveal significant changes among groups, however, there was a trend of reduction in the level of this marker in highlanders with PH, as compared to the people living at low altitude (**Figure 5B**). Further, there was a visible decrease in the circulating levels of FasL (in pg/mL) in both highlander groups, with statistically significant alteration in highlanders with PH, in comparison to the lowland control (**Figure 5C**). Finally, there were no significant changes in the context of BNP (in pg/mL) among different groups (**Figure 5D**). Surprisingly, there was a trend of elevated levels of circulating BNP in highlanders without PH, as compared to other two groups (**Figure 5D**).

Circulating FasL Levels Negatively Correlate With TRG Values in Kyrgyz Population

Furthermore, we have investigated the correlation between the circulating levels of FasL (pg/mL) in both acute and chronic exposure of Kyrgyz volunteers with TRG values (**Figure 6**).

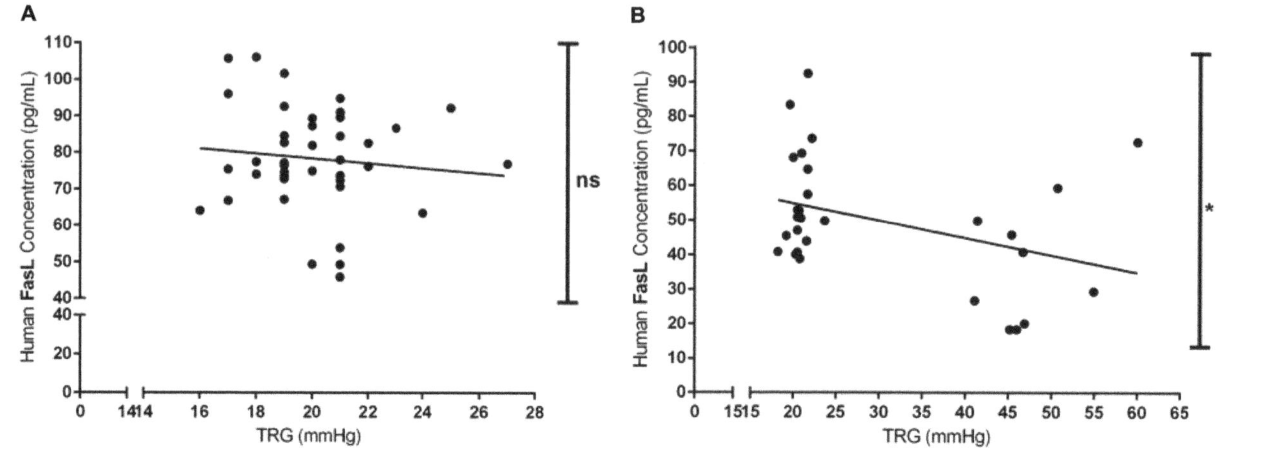

FIGURE 6 | Correlations between the circulating levels of Fas ligand and tricuspid regurgitant gradient (TRG) during acute and chronic exposure to high altitude. Correlations between the concentrations of circulating Fas ligand (FasL, in pg/mL) and TRG (in mmHg) values in human subjects exposed to acute **(A)** and chronic **(B)** effects of high altitude environment are shown. Spearman or Pearson tests were performed for statistical analyses. *$p < 0.05$; ns, not significant.

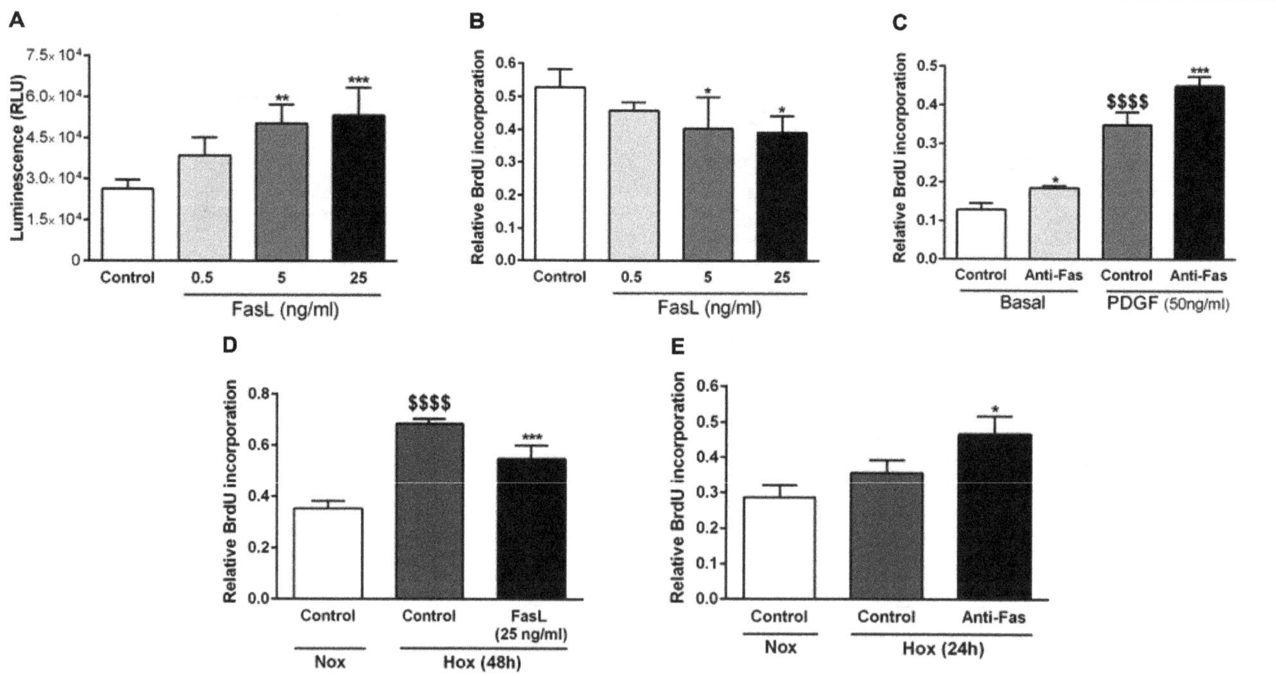

FIGURE 7 | Pro-apoptotic and anti-proliferative functions of Fas ligand in human PASMCs. Human PASMCs were exposed to normoxic (Nox) **(A–C)** or hypoxic (Hox) **(D,E)** conditions and treated with different concentrations (ng/ml) of Fas ligand (FasL) or anti-Fas, followed by measurements of cellular apoptosis and proliferation, using apoptosis assay **(A)** and 5-bromo-2′-deoxyuridine (BrdU) incorporation assays **(B–E)**, respectively. Results are presented as Mean ± SD ($n = 4$). *$p < 0.05$; **$p < 0.01$; ***$p < 0.001$ compared to the respective controls. $$$$$p < 0.0001$ basal/normoxic control compared to the PDGF/hypoxic control, respectively. Ordinary one-way ANOVA with Dunnett's or Tukey's multiple comparisons test was performed for statistical analysis. PDGF, platelet-derived growth factor.

Although there was a slight trend, there was no significant correlation between these two parameters in human subjects exposed acutely to high altitude environment (**Figure 6A**). However, there was a significant negative correlation between circulating levels of FasL and TRG in permanent residents of lowlands and highlands in investigated Kyrgyz population (**Figure 6B**).

FasL Exerts Pro-apoptotic and Anti-proliferative Effects in Human PASMCs

Finally, we have analyzed the relevant cellular functions of FasL in human PASMCs, such as apoptosis and proliferation (**Figure 7**). We have found that different concentrations

(5 and 25 ng/ml) of FasL significantly increased apoptosis of PASMCs (**Figure 7A**). Furthermore, the same concentrations of this ligand significantly reduced the proliferation of PASMCs under normoxic conditions (**Figure 7B**). In addition, anti-Fas enhanced the cellular proliferation under the basal conditions as well as during the stimulation with PDGF (**Figure 7C**). PASMCs were also exposed to hypoxic conditions (**Figures 7D,E**) and FasL (25 ng/ml) significantly decreased the proliferation of these cells (**Figure 7D**). Finally, anti-Fas resulted in augmentation of the PASMCs proliferation (**Figure 7E**). Clearly, FasL demonstrates pro-apoptotic and anti-proliferative properties in human PASMCs.

DISCUSSION

In general, the findings of our study revealed that:

(1) There was a prominent enhancement in gene expression of various apoptotic players in human PASMCs exposed to hypoxia condition,
(2) There were differential changes in investigated circulating apoptotic markers during acute and chronic exposure to high altitude in humans, with the most uniform alteration in FasL,
(3) FasL levels in plasma negatively correlated with TRG values in Kyrgyz population permanently settled in low and high altitudes, and,
(4) FasL exerted pro-apoptotic and anti-proliferative functions in human PASMCs.

Cellular apoptosis is an important, complicate and complex process (Sartorius et al., 2001). Under various stimuli, caspases' may activate and perform the apoptosis (Sartorius et al., 2001). Results of our study demonstrated an augmentation in gene expression of Casp 1 and 3 after the hypoxia incubation in PASMCs. Despite the fact that PH in general is characterized by "apoptosis-resistant" events, the increase in Casp3 expression was found in the lungs of monocrotaline model and the interpretation has to be taken with caution, since there are also some evidences that caspases may even exert anti-apoptotic features (Sartorius et al., 2001; Yang and Widmann, 2001; Le Goff et al., 2012; Hong et al., 2014).

With regard to other apoptotic players, our study indicated an increase in gene expression profiles of ApoC1, FLIP, and survivin in PASMCs exposed to hypoxia, in comparison to the respective normoxic controls. The literature suggested that ApoC1, FLIP, and survivin are generally considered as anti-apoptotic signals in different conditions (Sartorius et al., 2001; Takano et al., 2008; Portt et al., 2011; Fan et al., 2015; Zhang et al., 2015, 2016). Importantly, survivin is well-investigated in the context of hypoxia-induced PH and our data are in line with the literature sources (Fan et al., 2015; Zhang et al., 2015, 2016).

In the case of TRAIL and FasL, we have shown a noticeable increase in the gene expression for both targets during the hypoxic exposure of PASMCs, as compared to their respective normoxic controls. Limited evidences from the literature implicated these two signals in the context of pulmonary vascular disease (Hameed et al., 2012; Saito et al., 2015). Interestingly, although TRAIL is usually considered as pro-apoptotic mediator, its role in experimental PH pathogenesis has been described (Hameed et al., 2012). Taken together, it is clear that there is a complex play of different apoptotic mediators and this cellular process is indeed dysregulated in the pulmonary vascular cells exposed to hypoxia, however, it goes beyond the simplistic explanation based only on the expression patterns (increased/decreased) or historically known pro- or anti-apoptotic features of these signals.

In the cancer field, abnormally regulated apoptosis causes the release of apoptotic products into circulation, and they may represent potential biomarkers (Holdenrieder and Stieber, 2010). Up to date, there is no evidence about the expression profile of circulating apoptotic markers in humans exposed to acute and chronic effects of high altitude. In our study, we have investigated the concentration of ApoC1, TRAIL, and FasL in the plasma of Kyrgyz lowlanders who spent a short period of time in high altitude environment. The same signals were explored in the circulation of the permanent dwellers of high altitude who did or did not develop the HAPH, as well as in the blood of lowlanders. In addition, we have analyzed the circulating BNP, which is usually considered as an important cardiac biomarker, relevant to the PH field (Mellor et al., 2014; Anwar et al., 2016). Briefly, BNP has shown a trend to initially increase with days spent at high altitude in the circulation of Kyrgyz volunteers, as compared to the lowland conditions, and after day 7 there was a tendency to decrease, with a visible reduction upon descent to the lowlands again. Similarly, there was no clear change in the circulating profile of this cardiac marker in highlanders compared to the lowlanders, except non-significant augmentation in highlanders without PH.

ApoC1 circulatory levels were mostly comparable during the acute exposure of subjects to high altitude conditions, while there was some signal of increased values of this marker in the circulation of highlanders, in comparison to lowlanders. Yet, the data do not convincingly suggest the significant alteration of ApoC1 neither during acute nor chronic exposure to high altitude conditions.

Interestingly, the circulating concentrations of TRAIL showed the opposite manner in acute versus chronic exposure to high altitude in human volunteers. On one hand, there was a clear augmentation of this marker with days spent at high altitude in the blood of lowlanders, with significant reduction upon descent to low altitude again. On the other hand, there was noticeable, yet insignificant reduction of the circulating levels of TRAIL in highlanders (particularly those who developed HAPH) in comparison to the lowlanders. Furthermore, the literature suggested the elevated values of this marker in PH patients (Liu et al., 2015). Therefore, further studies are crucially needed to reveal the precise role of this apoptotic signal in both acute and chronic exposure to high altitude.

Finally, clearer and more informative results were obtained with focus on FasL in the circulation of humans in both acute and chronic exposure to high altitude geographic locations. There was a significant reduction of circulating FasL values in lowlanders exposed to high altitude environment for a short period of time. In addition, the circulating concentrations of this apoptotic marker were significantly decreased in highlanders with PH, as compared to the lowlanders. Interestingly, there were attenuated values of FasL in highlanders without PH also, in comparison to the lowland control, however, the change was not statistically significant. Lastly, there was a negative correlation between the circulatory levels of FasL and TRG, clearly indicated the potential biomarker properties of this apoptotic signal in the case of chronic effects of high altitude and HAPH. In accordance with our findings, FasL serum values were shown to be relevant to the field of pulmonary vascular diseases, as evident in the literature (Akagi et al., 2013; Saito et al., 2015). Importantly, FasL expression was increased in PASMCs derived from patients with idiopathic pulmonary arterial hypertension upon the treatment with prostaglandin I2, which was associated with induction of apoptosis (Akagi et al., 2013). Following this line of thinking, we have also demonstrated in this study that FasL enhanced the apoptotic process in PASMCs. Consistently, pro-apoptotic features of FasL in PASMCs were described in the literature (Zhang et al., 2003; Wang et al., 2010). Furthermore, we have shown that the same concentrations of FasL used for the assessment of apoptosis significantly reduced the proliferation of these pulmonary vascular cells under normoxic conditions. In addition, the blockage of FasL resulted in increased proliferation of PASMCs under the basal conditions as well as during the stimulation with PDGF. Of note, PDGF signaling is a very well-known player associated with hypoxia and pulmonary vascular remodeling (Schermuly et al., 2005; ten Freyhaus et al., 2011; Veith et al., 2014). Finally, we have demonstrated that FasL exerted anti-proliferative effects on PASMCs exposed to hypoxic conditions, and blockage of FasL resulted in enhancement of the proliferation process.

Overall, our study identified for the first time that circulating levels of apoptotic signal FasL are reduced during acute and chronic exposure to high altitude environment. In addition, due to its pro-apoptotic and anti-proliferative functions in the relevant cells of the pulmonary vasculature, dysregulated FasL signal may play an important role in the context of HAPH.

AUTHOR CONTRIBUTIONS

DK, HG, ASa, and RS conceived, designed, and created the study. DK, SP, AP, ASy, AbM, ArM, MS, KMU, MC, AT, NO, MD, and CV organized the expeditions and performed the field and laboratory measurements. DK, ASa, AbM, HG, ASy, and RS drafted and wrote the manuscript. OP and NW contributed with significant intellectual content. All authors read and approved the manuscript.

FUNDING

This study was supported by the Cardiovascular Medical Research and Education Fund (CMREF), Universities of Giessen and Marburg Lung Center (UGMLC), Excellence Cluster Cardio-Pulmonary System (ECCPS), and Ministry of Education and Science of the Kyrgyz Republic (Grant No. 0005823).

ACKNOWLEDGMENTS

We are eternally thankful to all Kyrgyz volunteers for participation in this study.

REFERENCES

Akagi, S., Nakamura, K., Matsubara, H., Kusano, K. F., Kataoka, N., Oto, T., et al. (2013). Prostaglandin I2 induces apoptosis via upregulation of Fas ligand in pulmonary artery smooth muscle cells from patients with idiopathic pulmonary arterial hypertension. *Int. J. Cardiol.* 165, 499–505. doi: 10.1016/j.ijcard.2011.09.004

Anwar, A., Ruffenach, G., Mahajan, A., Eghbali, M., and Umar, S. (2016). Novel biomarkers for pulmonary arterial hypertension. *Respir. Res.* 17:88. doi: 10.1186/s12931-016-0396-6

Azad, P., Stobdan, T., Zhou, D., Hartley, I., Akbari, A., Bafna, V., et al. (2017). High-altitude adaptation in humans: from genomics to integrative physiology. *J. Mol. Med.* 95, 1269–1282. doi: 10.1007/s00109-017-1584-7

Chan, S. Y., and Rubin, L. J. (2017). Metabolic dysfunction in pulmonary hypertension: from basic science to clinical practice. *Eur. Respir. Rev.* 26:170094. doi: 10.1183/16000617.0094-2017

Chen, M., Liu, Y., Yi, D., Wei, L., Li, Y., and Zhang, L. (2014). Tanshinone IIA promotes pulmonary artery smooth muscle cell apoptosis in vitro by inhibiting the JAK2/STAT3 signaling pathway. *Cell. Physiol. Biochem.* 33, 1130–1138. doi: 10.1159/000358682

Fan, Z., Liu, B., Zhang, S., Liu, H., Li, Y., Wang, D., et al. (2015). YM155, a selective survivin inhibitor, reverses chronic hypoxic pulmonary hypertension in rats via upregulating voltage-gated potassium channels. *Clin. Exp. Hypertens.* 37, 381–387. doi: 10.3109/10641963.2014.987390

Hameed, A. G., Arnold, N. D., Chamberlain, J., Pickworth, J. A., Paiva, C., Dawson, S., et al. (2012). Inhibition of tumor necrosis factor-related apoptosis-inducing ligand (TRAIL) reverses experimental pulmonary hypertension. *J. Exp. Med.* 209, 1919–1935. doi: 10.1084/jem.20112716

Holdenrieder, S., and Stieber, P. (2004). Apoptotic markers in cancer. *Clin. Biochem.* 37, 605–617. doi: 10.1016/j.clinbiochem.2004.05.003

Holdenrieder, S., and Stieber, P. (2010). Circulating apoptotic markers in the management of non-small cell lung cancer. *Cancer Biomark.* 6, 197–210. doi: 10.3233/CBM-2009-0130

Hong, Y. M., Kwon, J. H., Choi, S., and Kim, K. C. (2014). Apoptosis and inflammation associated gene expressions in monocrotaline-induced pulmonary hypertensive rats after bosentan treatment. *Korean Circ. J.* 44, 97–104. doi: 10.4070/kcj.2014.44.2.97

Le Goff, A., Ji, Z., Leclercq, B., Bourette, R. P., Mougel, A., Guerardel, C., et al. (2012). Anti-apoptotic role of caspase-cleaved GAB1 adaptor protein in hepatocyte growth factor/scatter factor-MET receptor protein signaling. *J. Biol. Chem.* 287, 35382–35396. doi: 10.1074/jbc.M112.409797

Li, Y. X., Run, L., Shi, T., and Zhang, Y. J. (2017). CTRP9 regulates hypoxia-mediated human pulmonary artery smooth muscle cell proliferation, apoptosis and migration via TGF-beta1/ERK1/2 signaling pathway. *Biochem. Biophys. Res. Commun.* 490, 1319–1325. doi: 10.1016/j.bbrc.2017.07.020

Liu, H., Yang, E., Lu, X., Zuo, C., He, Y., Jia, D., et al. (2015). Serum levels of tumor necrosis factor-related apoptosis-inducing ligand correlate with the severity of pulmonary hypertension. *Pulm. Pharmacol. Ther.* 33, 39–46. doi: 10.1016/j.pupt.2015.06.002

Maggiorini, M., and Leon-Velarde, F. (2003). High-altitude pulmonary hypertension: a pathophysiological entity to different diseases. *Eur. Respir. J.* 22, 1019–1025. doi: 10.1183/09031936.03.00052403

Malczyk, M., Veith, C., Schermuly, R. T., Gudermann, T., Dietrich, A., Sommer, N., et al. (2016). NADPH oxidases-do they play a role in TRPC regulation under hypoxia? *Pflugers Arch.* 468, 23–41. doi: 10.1007/s00424-015-1731-3

Marshall, J. D., Bazan, I., Zhang, Y., Fares, W. H., and Lee, P. J. (2018). Mitochondrial dysfunction and pulmonary hypertension: cause, effect or both. *Am. J. Physiol. Lung Cell. Mol. Physiol.* 314, L782–L796. doi: 10.1152/ajplung.00331.2017

Mellor, A., Boos, C., Holdsworth, D., Begley, J., Hall, D., Lumley, A., et al. (2014). Cardiac biomarkers at high altitude. *High Alt. Med. Biol.* 15, 452–458. doi: 10.1089/ham.2014.1035

Mirrakhimov, A. E., and Strohl, K. P. (2016). High-altitude pulmonary hypertension: an update on disease pathogenesis and management. *Open Cardiovasc. Med. J.* 10, 19–27. doi: 10.2174/1874192401610010019

Niessner, A., Hohensinner, P. J., Rychli, K., Neuhold, S., Zorn, G., Richter, B., et al. (2009). Prognostic value of apoptosis markers in advanced heart failure patients. *Eur. Heart J.* 30, 789–796. doi: 10.1093/eurheartj/ehp004

Parissis, J. T., Adamopoulos, S., Antoniades, C., Kostakis, G., Rigas, A., Kyrzopoulos, S., et al. (2004). Effects of levosimendan on circulating pro-inflammatory cytokines and soluble apoptosis mediators in patients with decompensated advanced heart failure. *Am. J. Cardiol.* 93, 1309–1312. doi: 10.1016/j.amjcard.2004.01.073

Portt, L., Norman, G., Clapp, C., Greenwood, M., and Greenwood, M. T. (2011). Anti-apoptosis and cell survival: a review. *Biochim. Biophys. Acta.* 1813, 238–259. doi: 10.1016/j.bbamcr.2010.10.010

Saito, Y., Nakamura, K., Akagi, S., Sarashina, T., Ejiri, K., Miura, A., et al. (2015). Epoprostenol sodium for treatment of pulmonary arterial hypertension. *Vasc. Health Risk Manag.* 11, 265–270. doi: 10.2147/VHRM.S50368

Sartorius, U., Schmitz, I., and Krammer, P. H. (2001). Molecular mechanisms of death-receptor-mediated apoptosis. *Chembiochem.* 2, 20–29. doi: 10.1002/1439-7633(20010105)2:1<20::AID-CBIC20>3.0.CO;2-X

Schermuly, R. T., Dony, E., Ghofrani, H. A., Pullamsetti, S., Savai, R., Roth, M., et al. (2005). Reversal of experimental pulmonary hypertension by PDGF inhibition. *J. Clin. Invest.* 115, 2811–2821. doi: 10.1172/JCI24838

Schermuly, R. T., Ghofrani, H. A., Wilkins, M. R., and Grimminger, F. (2011). Mechanisms of disease: pulmonary arterial hypertension. *Nat. Rev. Cardiol.* 8, 443–455. doi: 10.1038/nrcardio.2011.87

Simonneau, G., Gatzoulis, M. A., Adatia, I., Celermajer, D., Denton, C., Ghofrani, A., et al. (2013). Updated clinical classification of pulmonary hypertension. *J. Am. Coll. Cardiol.* 62, D34–D41. doi: 10.1016/j.jacc.2013.10.029

Stenmark, K. R., Frid, M. G., Graham, B. B., and Tuder, R. M. (2018). Dynamic and diverse changes in the functional properties of vascular smooth muscle cells in pulmonary hypertension. *Cardiovasc. Res.* 114, 551–564. doi: 10.1093/cvr/cvy004

Takano, S., Yoshitomi, H., Togawa, A., Sogawa, K., Shida, T., Kimura, F., et al. (2008). Apolipoprotein C-1 maintains cell survival by preventing from apoptosis in pancreatic cancer cells. *Oncogene* 27, 2810–2822. doi: 10.1038/sj.onc.1210951

ten Freyhaus, H., Dagnell, M., Leuchs, M., Vantler, M., Berghausen, E. M., Caglayan, E., et al. (2011). Hypoxia enhances platelet-derived growth factor signaling in the pulmonary vasculature by down-regulation of protein tyrosine phosphatases. *Am. J. Respir. Crit. Care Med.* 183, 1092–1102. doi: 10.1164/rccm.200911-1663OC

Thenappan, T., Ormiston, M. L., Ryan, J. J., and Archer, S. L. (2018). Pulmonary arterial hypertension: pathogenesis and clinical management. *BMJ* 360:j5492. doi: 10.1136/bmj.j5492

Veith, C., Zakrzewicz, D., Dahal, B. K., Balint, Z., Murmann, K., Wygrecka, M., et al. (2014). Hypoxia- or PDGF-BB-dependent paxillin tyrosine phosphorylation in pulmonary hypertension is reversed by HIF-1α depletion or imatinib treatment. *Thromb. Haemost.* 112, 1288–1303. doi: 10.1160/TH13-12-1031

Wang, S., Wang, Y., Jiang, J., Wang, R., Li, L., Qiu, Z., et al. (2010). 15-HETE protects rat pulmonary arterial smooth muscle cells from apoptosis via the PI3K/Akt pathway. *Prostaglandins Other Lipid Mediat.* 91, 51–60. doi: 10.1016/j.prostaglandins.2009.12.007

West, J. B. (2012). High-altitude medicine. *Am. J. Respir. Crit. Care. Med.* 186, 1229–1237. doi: 10.1164/rccm.201207-1323CI

Yang, C., Wang, S., Liang, T., Wang, J., Wang, K., and Wang, B. (2001). The roles of bcl-2 gene family in the pulmonary artery remodeling of hypoxia pulmonary hypertension in rats. *Chin. Med. Sci. J.* 16, 182–184.

Yang, J. Y., and Widmann, C. (2001). Antiapoptotic signaling generated by caspase-induced cleavage of RasGAP. *Mol. Cell. Biol.* 21, 5346–5358. doi: 10.1128/MCB.21.16.5346-5358.2001

Yock, P. G., and Popp, R. L. (1984). Noninvasive estimation of right ventricular systolic pressure by Doppler ultrasound in patients with tricuspid regurgitation. *Circulation* 70, 657–662. doi: 10.1161/01.CIR.70.4.657

You, B., Liu, Y., Chen, J., Huang, X., Peng, H., Liu, Z., et al. (2018). Vascular peroxidase 1 mediates hypoxia-induced pulmonary artery smooth muscle cell proliferation, apoptosis resistance and migration. *Cardiovasc. Res.* 114, 188–199. doi: 10.1093/cvr/cvx234

Zhang, S., Fantozzi, I., Tigno, D. D., Yi, E. S., Platoshyn, O., Thistlethwaite, P. A., et al. (2003). Bone morphogenetic proteins induce apoptosis in human pulmonary vascular smooth muscle cells. *Am. J. Physiol. Lung Cell. Mol. Physiol.* 285, L740–L754. doi: 10.1152/ajplung.00284.2002

Zhang, S., Liu, B., Fan, Z., Wang, D., Liu, Y., Li, J., et al. (2016). Targeted inhibition of survivin with YM155 promotes apoptosis of hypoxic human pulmonary arterial smooth muscle cells via the upregulation of voltage-dependent K(+) channels. *Mol. Med. Rep.* 13, 3415–3422. doi: 10.3892/mmr.2016.4977

Zhang, S., Liu, B., Zhang, B., and Fan, Z. (2015). [The effect of survivin expression on the apoptosis and proliferation of hypoxic human pulmonary arterial smooth muscle cells]. *Zhonghua jie he he hu xi za zhi* 38, 45–49.

16

Prediction of Critical Power and W′ in Hypoxia: Application to Work-Balance Modelling

Nathan E. Townsend[1], David S. Nichols[1], Philip F. Skiba[2], Sebastien Racinais[1] and Julien D. Périard[1]*

[1] *Athlete Health and Performance Centre, Aspetar Orthopaedic and Sports Medicine Hospital, Doha, Qatar,* [2] *Department of Sports Medicine, Advocate Lutheran General Hospital, Park Ridge, IL, USA*

Correspondence:
Nathan E. Townsend
nathan.townsend@aspetar.com

Purpose: Develop a prediction equation for critical power (CP) and work above CP (W′) in hypoxia for use in the work-balance (W'_{BAL}) model.

Methods : Nine trained male cyclists completed cycling time trials (TT; 12, 7, and 3 min) to determine CP and W′ at five altitudes (250, 1,250, 2,250, 3,250, and 4,250 m). Least squares regression was used to predict CP and W′ at altitude. A high-intensity intermittent test (HIIT) was performed at 250 and 2,250 m. Actual and predicted CP and W′ were used to compute W′ during HIIT using differential ($W'_{BALdiff}$) and integral (W'_{BALint}) forms of the W'_{BAL} model.

Results : CP decreased at altitude ($P < 0.001$) as described by 3rd order polynomial function ($R^2 = 0.99$). W′ decreased at 4,250 m only ($P < 0.001$). A double-linear function characterized the effect of altitude on W′ ($R^2 = 0.99$). There was no significant effect of parameter input (actual vs. predicted CP and W′) on modelled W'_{BAL} at 2,250 m ($P = 0.24$). $W'_{BALdiff}$ returned higher values than W'_{BALint} throughout HIIT ($P < 0.001$). During HIIT, $W'_{BALdiff}$ was not different to 0 kJ at completion, at 250 m (0.7 ± 2.0 kJ; $P = 0.33$) and 2,250 m (-1.3 ± 3.5 kJ; $P = 0.30$). However, W'_{BALint} was lower than 0 kJ at 250 m (-0.9 ± 1.3 kJ; $P = 0.058$) and 2,250 m (-2.8 ± 2.8 kJ; $P = 0.02$).

Conclusion: The altitude prediction equations for CP and W′ developed in this study are suitable for use with the W'_{BAL} model in acute hypoxia. This enables the application of W'_{BAL} modelling to training prescription and competition analysis at altitude.

Keywords: high-intensity intermittent exercise, cycling, altitude, hypoxia, fatigue

INTRODUCTION

The critical power (CP) concept was originally introduced by Monod and Scherrer (1965), and describes the relationship between sustainable power output and duration for severe-intensity exercise. A simple hyperbolic, two parameter model was proposed:

$$W' = t_{lim}/(P - CP) \tag{1}$$

where W′ = total work accumulated above CP until task failure, t_{lim} = duration until task failure, P = power output, and CP = critical power, defined as a rate limited sustainable power output below which no net expenditure of W′ occurs. Equation (1) can be conceptualized according to a hydraulic model (Margaria, 1976; Morton, 2006), whereby the value W′ progressively depletes during exercise whenever P > CP and reconstitutes when P < CP. Additionally, it can also be seen that if W′ depletes to zero, then t_{lim} also reaches zero and hence task failure is attained. A continuous integral function has been proposed, termed the "work-balance" (W'_{BAL}) model, which mathematically describes the depletion and reconstitution of W′ (Skiba et al., 2012, 2014a, 2015). A differential equation form of the W'_{BAL} has also been proposed (Skiba et al., 2015). As per the abovementioned hydraulic model, the W'_{BAL} models predict that task failure during an intermittent task is attained when W' depletes to 0 kJ. Both versions of the W'_{BAL} model require CP and W′ as input variables, hence accurate estimation of CP and W′ is a prerequisite for computing W'_{BAL}. However, studies have reported that moderate hypoxia decreases CP (Dekerle et al., 2012; Simpson et al., 2015; Shearman et al., 2016) and severe hypoxia decreases both CP and W′ (Valli et al., 2011). Since it is impractical to measure CP and W′ at all possible altitudes, a prediction model which corrects CP and W′ for the effect of hypoxia would permit W'_{BAL} computation at any given altitude.

The mechanistic basis of the two parameter CP model has been extensively studied (Jones et al., 2010). Numerous investigations have demonstrated that CP corresponds to the highest exercise intensity at which pulmonary $\dot{V}O_2$ (Poole et al., 1988; Jones et al., 2008; Vanhatalo et al., 2016), and intramuscular high energy phosphates (Jones et al., 2008; Chidnok et al., 2013), can achieve a steady state. The achievement of steady-state $\dot{V}O_2$ kinetics indicates the net energetic demand of the task can be met by oxidative metabolism (Poole et al., 2016). When the task requirement increases beyond CP the additional energetic demand is supplemented by substrate level phosphorylation (Vanhatalo et al., 2016) which induces non-steady state $\dot{V}O_2$ kinetics, accelerated degradation of high energy phosphates, and accumulation of metabolites involved in peripheral muscle fatigue (Jones et al., 2008; Poole et al., 2016). Since the total amount of work accumulated above CP is terminated at the moment of task failure, the mechanisms leading to task failure itself also determine the value of W′. Recent work examining the etiology of neuromuscular fatigue during high intensity exercise reveals that some combination of both central and peripheral fatigue mechanisms is always present at the moment of task failure, whilst the relative contribution of each depends on the task (Hureau et al., 2016). Observed values for [PCr], [P_i], and [H^+] at task failure have been shown to remain similar despite manipulations in pacing strategy during continuous exercise (Burnley et al., 2010), or recovery duration (Chidnok et al., 2012) and recovery power (Chidnok et al., 2013) during intermittent exercise. Also, following exhaustive high-intensity exercise the magnitude of peripheral fatigue, assessed via twitch interpolation, remains consistent in normoxia and moderate hypoxia (Amann et al., 2006b; Romer et al., 2007). Recently it was demonstrated that changes in peripheral fatigue (assessed via twitch potentiation) was significantly correlated to changes in both [P_i] and [H^+] during exercise when lower limb muscle afferent feedback was impaired using lumbar intrathecal fentanyl (Blain et al., 2016). Collectively, these findings have led to the theory that within a given task, peripheral muscle fatigue may be regulated via group III/IV afferent feedback, which limits central motor drive to the locomotor muscle (Hureau et al., 2016). The existence of such a feedback loop might explain why W′ appears to resemble a fixed capacity within a given task (Broxterman et al., 2015). From a mathematical perspective, a fixed value of W′ allows performance during high-intensity tasks to be predicted using the 2-parameter CP model.

During exercise in hypoxia, convective O_2 transport to the working muscle is reduced (Amann and Calbet, 2008), and multiple studies have reported a significant decrease in CP without a corresponding change in W′ (Dekerle et al., 2012; Simpson et al., 2015; Shearman et al., 2016). If CP is lower in hypoxia, then according to the CP model a given absolute exercise intensity in the severe domain will result in a faster rate of W′ depletion. Previously we reported a large error in modelled W'_{BAL} during intermittent exercise performed in hypoxia when the normoxic CP estimate is used (Shearman et al., 2016). Therefore, CP must either be tested in hypoxia, or estimated from measurements in normoxia. Various studies have examined the effect of increasing altitude on $\dot{V}O_{2max}$ reporting either a linear decrease (Wehrlin and Hallén, 2006; Clark et al., 2007), a curvilinear decrease (Péronnet et al., 1991; Bassett et al., 1999), or a curvilinear interaction between altitude and sea level $\dot{V}O_{2max}$ (MacInnis et al., 2015). To our knowledge, no studies have examined the dose-response effect of increasing altitude on CP and W′. Moreover, a large reduction in W′ was reported at high altitude (5,050 m) (Valli et al., 2011), whereas another study found no change at simulated altitude equivalent to 3,800 m (Simpson et al., 2015). Hence, the approximate threshold altitude where W′ begins to decline remains unclear. The purpose of this study was to examine the dose-response effect of increasing altitude on both CP and W′, and thereafter to develop a prediction equation enabling W'_{BAL} computation in hypoxia. A secondary aim was to compare the integral vs. the differential equation form of the W'_{BAL} model. We hypothesized that CP would decline in a curvilinear fashion commencing from the lowest altitude above sea level (1,250 m) tested, whereas W′ would only begin to decline at altitudes above ≈3,800 m.

Abbreviations: P, Power; W, Watt; CP, Critical power; asymptote of the power–duration relationship; W′, "W-prime" curvature constant of the power–duration relationship; t_{lim}, Time to exhaustion; W'_{BAL}, Work-balance: Amount or balance of W′ remaining; W'_{BALint}, Integral equation form of W'_{BAL} model; $W'_{BALdiff}$, Differential equation form of W'_{BAL} model; $\tau_{W'}$, Time constant for reconstitution of W′; PCr, Intramuscular phosphocreatine; P_i, Intramuscular inorganic phosphate; H^+, Intramuscular hydrogen ion; ADP_{free}, Intramuscular adenosine di-phosphate free; AMP_{free}, Intramuscular adenosine mono-phosphate free; O_2, Oxygen; $\dot{V}O_2$, Volume of oxygen consumption; HIIT, High-intensity intermittent test; 3TT, 3 min time trial; FiO_2, Fraction of inspired oxygen.

METHODS

Participants

Nine trained male cyclists (mean ± SD; age 34 ± 6 year, 78.1 ± 8.0 kg; $\dot{V}O_{2peak}$ 4.57 ± 0.47 $L.min^{-1}$) volunteered to participate in this study, which was approved by the Anti-Doping Lab Qatar Institutional Review Board. All procedures conformed to the standards of the Declaration of Helsinki. Participant inclusion was based on age (18–40 years), training history (2 year minimum cycling training history, 7 $h.wk^{-1}$ minimum average training), and health status (free from injury or illness). All participants were experienced at conducting cycling time trials. Written informed consent was obtained following explanation of the experimental procedures, associated risks, and potential benefits.

Experimental Overview

Participants completed a total of eight testing sessions over a period of 2 months. A minimum of 2, and a maximum of 14 days was specified between any two consecutive lab visits, however, two participants completed one lab visit each outside of this window due to unavoidable personal commitments. The first visit to laboratory involved an $\dot{V}O_{2peak}$ ramp incremental test (30 $W.min^{-1}$) for subject characteristics, followed by a 30 min recovery period and then a 7 min familiarization time trial (TT). Thereafter, on five separate lab visits, participants completed TT's to determine CP and W′ at the following target FiO_2: 0.203, 0.18, 0.159, 0.14, and 0.123, which corresponds to simulated altitudes of 250, 1,250, 2,250, 3,250, and 4,250 m, respectively. The order of condition was counterbalanced according to a latin square design, with participants blinded to the experimental condition. On the remaining two visits, a HIIT at 250 m and 2,250 m was completed. These sessions were not performed after completion of all five TT testing sessions, but rather on the next lab visit immediately following the TT testing at the same altitude. We chose this experimental protocol to minimize the effect of either training or altitude acclimation, on performance during the HIIT. Participants were instructed to avoid strenuous exercise for 24 h prior to each testing session, and to abstain from caffeine and alcohol on the day of testing.

Equipment and Measures

All exercise tests were performed on an electronically braked cycle ergometer (Schoberer Rad Messtechnik, Jülich, Germany) with power was measured at 1 Hz. All simulated altitude conditions were conducted inside a temperature controlled (20°C) altitude chamber (LoxyMed, Berlin, Germany) with stability of target altitude within ±100 m.

Critical Power Testing

The CP test was equivalent to that described and validated by Karsten et al. (2014, 2016). This protocol consists of three TT efforts lasting 12, 7, and 3 min in descending order, interspersed with 30 min of active recovery. We chose to use TTs rather than time to exhaustion (TTe) tests on the grounds that TTs exhibit lower typical error than TTe tests (Paton and Hopkins, 2001) and secondly, recent evidence suggests that CP and W′ parameters estimated from self-paced TTs lead to better prediction of actual TT performance duration then parameters estimated from constant load trials (Black et al., 2015). Participants were blinded to power output, but not duration. Upon completion of the 12 and 7 min TTs, participants exited the altitude chamber within 1-2 min so the first 20 min of the recovery period was always conducted in normoxia. The last 10 min of recovery was conducted inside the chamber at the simulated altitude as specified by the experimental condition.

CP and W′ were initially modelled using three versions of the 2-parameter CP model (1) linear 1/time model, (2) linear work-time model, and (3) nonlinear hyperbolic model (Jones et al., 2008). In each case the standard error of the estimate (SEE) was determined for CP and W′. The lowest SEE for the majority of tests occurred for the linear 1/time model. Therefore, all data analysis used estimates from this model.

High-Intensity Intermittent Test (HIIT)

The HIIT consisted of nine discreet work intervals performed at a target power output predicted to produce task failure during constant load exercise in 5 min according to the 2-parameter CP model:

$$P_5 = (W'/t_{desired}) + CP \tag{2}$$

Where P_5 is power output and $t_{desired}$ is the desired time to task failure (300 s). Interval duration ranged from 40 to 60 s and recovery duration from 30 to 60 s. Immediately following every 3rd work interval a maximal sprint effort (3–5 s) was performed in isokinetic mode at 100 $rev.min^{-1}$. After the 9th work interval, there was a 2.5 min recovery period followed by a self-paced, maximal effort 3 min TT (3TT). Power during all recovery periods was 60 W.

Altitude Prediction and W'_{BAL} Modelling

Mean CP and W′ estimates from each altitude were expressed as a percentage of the values obtained during testing at 250 m. These values were fitted to a 3rd order polynomial using ordinary least squares regression (GraphPad PRISM, USA). Change in W′ with increasing altitude was described using a two-segment linear regression approach since it was expected that no change would occur in W′ until the highest altitude tested (Valli et al., 2011; Dekerle et al., 2012; Simpson et al., 2015; Shearman et al., 2016). Slope one was constrained to 0 ($\%.km^{-1}$) and intercept one was constrained to 100% of baseline level (250 m). Breakpoint, slope and intercept two were left unconstrained. Only measured values for CP and W′ were used to model W'_{BAL} during the intermittent task at 250 m, whereas both the actual measures of CP and W′, and corrected values based on the prediction models, were used to compute W'_{BAL} at 2,250 m.

Modelling of W'_{BAL} during HIIT was conducted using two different equations referred to as the "integral" (W'_{BALint}) model (Skiba et al., 2012) and the "differential" ($W'_{BALdiff}$) model (Skiba et al., 2015). A detailed mathematical derivation from $W'_{BALdiff}$ to W'_{BALint} can be found in the appendix section of Skiba et al. (Skiba et al., 2015). Briefly, the W'_{BALint} model deducts cumulative work expended (or recovered) from the initial W′ to determine W'_{BAL} remaining during an intermittent task. The discharge and reconstitution rate of W'_{BAL} occurs exponentially as shown in Equation (3):

$$W'_{BALint} = W' - \int_0^t W'_{exp} \cdot e^{\frac{-(t-u)}{\tau_{W'}}} \cdot du \tag{3}$$

Where W'_{exp} is the amount of W′ presently expended, and (t-u) is equal to the time in seconds where the athlete is recovering below CP. The time constant for the reconstitution of W′ ($\tau_{W'}$) is a function of the difference between the recovery power and the individual's CP (D_{CP}) according to the following equation (Skiba et al., 2012):

$$\tau_{W'} = 546 \cdot e^{(-0.01 D_{CP})} + 316 \quad (4)$$

The $W'_{BALdiff}$ model treats W′ as a chemical reactant. As per the integral form, W′ reconstitution follows an exponential time course, whilst discharge is strictly linear. However, the time constant is calculated by dividing the starting W′ by D_{CP} rather than fitting data as per equation 4. The discharge of W′ when P>CP using the differential form of the W'_{BAL} is given by:

$$W'_{BALdiff} = W'_0 - \left(W'_0 - W'(u)\right) e^{-\frac{D_{CP}}{W'_0}(t-u)} \quad (5)$$

Where W'_0 is the initial starting value of W′ prior to a work segment where P>CP, and as above (t-u) is equal to the segment of time where P>CP. Recovery of $W'_{BALdiff}$ occurs during a segment of time when P<CP according to Equation (6):

$$W'_{BALdiff} = W'_0 - W'_{exp}\, e^{-D_{CP}t/W'_0} \quad (6)$$

Where W'_{exp} is the W′ expended during the prior segment in which P>CP. The time course for the entire HIIT is computed by sequentially determining depletion and recovery for each successive segment, where P>CP and P<CP, respectively.

Modelled W'_{BAL} for both the integral and differential equations was computed at 1 Hz throughout the HIIT, but only values at completion of each interval (1 through 9), and the final 3TT, are reported.

Statistical Analysis

Statistical analysis was completed on all data using the Statistical Package for Social Sciences (SPSS) Version 22.0 (SPSS Inc., Champaign, IL). Normality of the data was checked using the Shapiro-Wilk test with ($P < 0.05$) indicating non-normality. Linear mixed modelling was used to examine the fixed effect of altitude on CP and W′, and also to examine fixed effects of model (W'_{BALint} vs. $W'_{BALdiff}$), parameter input (actual vs. altitude corrected CP), altitude (250 vs. 2,250 m), and interval (1 to 9 + 3TT), on modelled W'_{BAL}. Random effects were designated as participant slope and intercept. *Post-hoc* pairwise comparisons were conducted using Sidak's correction and effect sizes were calculated using Hedges' *g*. All pairwise comparisons are reported as mean difference (95% confidence interval: lower, upper; hedges' *g*; *P*-value).

RESULTS

Effect of Altitude on CP and W′

Individual and group mean changes at altitude in CP and W′ are presented in **Figures 1A,B**. At 250 m, mean CP was 269.9 W (95% CI: 250.6, 289.1 W). There was a significant effect of altitude on both CP ($P < 0.001$) and W′ ($P < 0.001$). Compared with 250 m, *post-hoc* comparison showed that CP decreased significantly at 1250 m by 13.0 W (95% CI: 5.6, 20.3; $g = 0.41$; $P < 0.001$), at 2,250 m by 34.9 W (95% CI: 24.8, 44.9; $g = 1.22$; $P < 0.001$), at 3,250 m by 52.3 W (95% CI: 39.9, 64.8; $g = 1.64$; $P < 0.001$), and at 4,250 m by 74.0 W (95% CI: 59.7, 90.1; $g = 2.87$; $P < 0.001$). Mean W′ at 250 m was 17.2 kJ (95% CI: 14.3, 20.1 kJ). Compared with 250 m, no significant differences were found at 1,250 m (−0.5 kJ; 95% CI: −1.6, 2.7; $g = 0.11$; $P = 0.99$), 2,250 m (−0.5 kJ; 95% CI: −2.8, 1.7; $g = 0.12$; $P = 0.99$), or 3,250 m (−1.7 kJ; 95% CI: −4.0, 0.7; $g = 0.39$; $P = 0.3$). At 4,250 m W′ was significantly lower than 250 m (−4.7 kJ; 95% CI: −7.1, −2.3; $g = 1.18$; $P < 0.001$).

Modelling CP and W′ at Altitude

Baseline CP at 250 m was correlated with the magnitude of decline in CP at altitude (expressed as ΔW/km altitude. $r = 0.89$; $P = 0.001$). However, when the decline in CP at altitude was expressed as percent changes, this relationship was not significant ($r = 0.47$; $P = 0.21$). Therefore, to simplify the CP prediction equation, we chose to fit the data as percent changes. Using least squares regression, the decrease in CP with increasing altitude (**Figure 1C**) was best fit to a 3rd order polynomial function ($r^2 = 0.99$) as follows:

$$y = 0.0016x^3 - 0.0157x^2 - 0.027x + 1.0025 \quad (7)$$

Where y = the percent decline in CP from sea level values, and x = altitude in km.

The effect of altitude on W′ was described using a two segment linear model, whereby the intercept and gradient of line one were constrained to 100 and 0%, respectively. The gradient for line 2 was −18.3% (per km) and the breakpoint was 2.76 km. Assuming a mean 95% confidence interval range for W′ measures at all altitudes, this two-segment model predicts W′ measured at sea level, to decline significantly beyond ≈3,500 m (**Figure 1D**).

W'_{BAL} Modelling during Intermittent Task

Figure 2 shows modelled W'_{BAL} during the HIIT for an individual subject. **Table 1** presents group mean data for all W'_{BAL} computations. There was no significant effect of parameter input (actual vs. corrected CP and W′) on modelled W'_{BAL} at 2,250 m ($P = 0.24$). A significant main effect of model (W'_{BALint} vs. $W'_{BALdiff}$) was observed ($P < 0.001$), and also altitude (250 vs. 2,250 m. $P < 0.01$). The altitude by model interaction was significant ($P = 0.02$), where *post-hoc* comparison revealed a significant effect of altitude for the $W'_{BALdiff}$ model only (−0.6 kJ; 95% CI: −0.8, −0.4; $g = 0.86$; $P < 0.001$).

Figure 3 displays computed W'_{BAL} at completion of the 3TT (which concludes the HIIT) for all model variants. $W'_{BALdiff}$ was not different to a value of 0 kJ, which theoretically represents the limit of tolerance during high intensity exercise, at either 250 m (0.7 kJ; 95% CI: −0.9, 2.2 kJ; $g = 0.34$; $P = 0.33$), or 2,250 m for actual model inputs (−1.3 kJ; 95% CI: −3.9, 1.4 kJ; $g = 0.37$; $P = 0.30$), and altitude corrected inputs (−1.1 kJ; 95% CI: −3.6, 1.4 kJ; $g = 0.33$; $P = 0.35$). W'_{BALint} was different to 0 kJ at 2,250 m for both actual (−2.8 kJ; 95% CI: −4.9, −0.7 kJ; $g = 1.03$; $P = 0.02$)

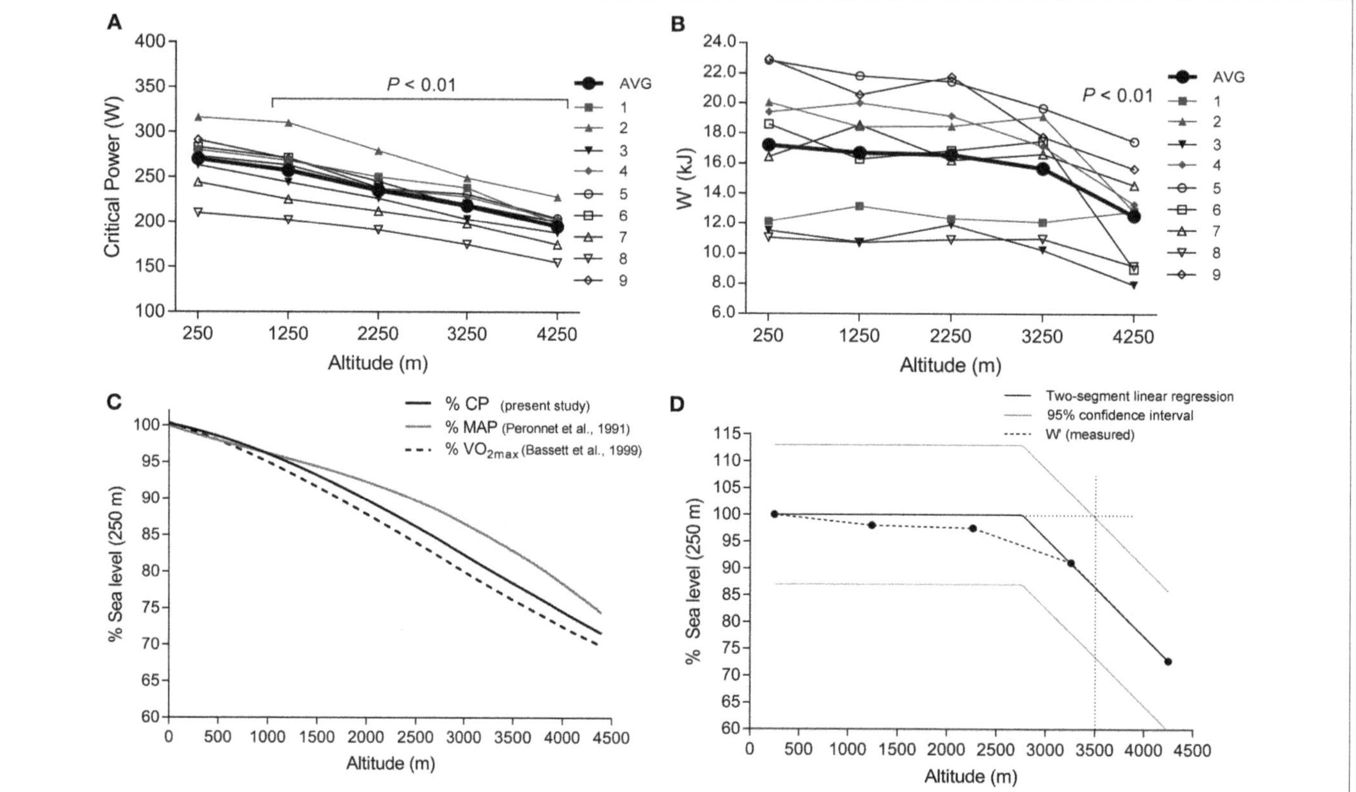

FIGURE 1 | Effect of increasing altitude on group mean and individual subject critical power (A) and W′ **(B)**. Model predicted critical power also showing comparison to maximal aerobic power (MAP) and $\dot{V}O_{2max}$ **(C)**, and W′ **(D)**, expressed as percent of sea level measured values. In **(D)** light gray solid lines represent 95% CI. Intersection of the dotted lines indicates predicted altitude where a statistically significant decline in W′ would occur. $P < 0.05$ indicates significant difference compared to 250 m.

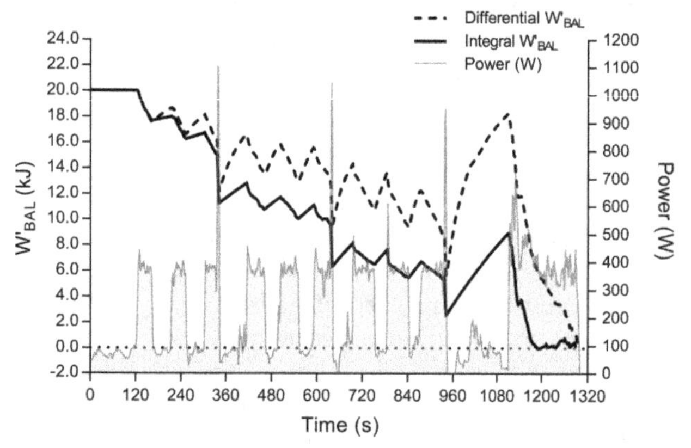

FIGURE 2 | W'_{BAL} responses, showing both integral (solid black line) and differential (dotted line) model computations, during the high intensity intermittent test. Light gray shaded area shows actual power output.

and altitude corrected inputs (−2.6 kJ; 95% CI: −4.5, −0.6 kJ; $g = 1.02$; $P = 0.02$), whilst the difference approached significance at 250 m (−0.9 kJ; 95% CI: −1.9, 0.04 kJ; $g = 0.74$; $P = 0.058$). An example of a field based practical application of the altitude correction to $W'_{BALdiff}$ is shown in **Figure 4**, which was computed from field data during the 2015 Giro d'Italia.

DISCUSSION

Previous studies have quantified the decrease in $\dot{V}O_{2max}$ that occurs at altitude (Bassett et al., 1999; Wehrlin and Hallén, 2006; Clark et al., 2007; MacInnis et al., 2015), however this is the first to examine the effect of altitude on CP and W′. Consistent with data on the dose-response effect of hypoxia on $\dot{V}O_{2max}$ (Bassett et al., 1999; MacInnis et al., 2015), we observed a curvilinear decrease in CP. Secondly, the effect of hypoxia on W′ appears to display threshold type characteristics since there were no significant changes at lower altitudes, whereas a decrease occurred at the highest altitude only (4,250 m). Lastly, we have demonstrated for the first time that a prediction equation can be used in place of actual measurements of CP + W′ at simulated altitude of 2,250 m, to characterize intermittent high-intensity exercise using the W'_{BAL} model.

With increasing altitude, $\dot{V}O_{2max}$ has been shown to decrease linearly (Wehrlin and Hallén, 2006; Clark et al., 2007), or curvilinearly (Bassett et al., 1999; MacInnis et al., 2015). The curvilinear decrease in CP observed in this study (see **Figures 1A,C**) was similar to that for $\dot{V}O_{2max}$ reported by

TABLE 1 | Mean ± SD modelled W'_{BAL} responses at the completion of each interval during the HIIT.

		Intermittent task interval number										
		Initial W′	**1**	**2**	**3**	**4**	**5**	**6**	**7**	**8**	**9**	**3TT**
250 M												
$W'_{BALdiff}$	Actual	17.2 ± 4.7	15.0 ± 4.1	13.7 ± 3.5	13.4 ± 3.3	11.1 ± 2.7	10.6 ± 2.4	10.8 ± 2.3	8.7 ± 2.1	8.0 ± 1.5	7.4 ± 1.3	0.7 ± 2.0
W'_{BALint}	Actual	17.2 ± 4.7	15.1 ± 4.2	13.5 ± 3.6	12.5 ± 3.3	8.6 ± 2.9**	7.8 ± 2.7**	7.6 ± 2.6**	4.7 ± 2.5**	4.4 ± 2.2**	4.1 ± 2.0**	−0.9 ± 1.3*
2,250 M												
$W'_{BALdiff}$	Actual	16.9 ± 4.0	14.8 ± 3.4	13.6 ± 3.1	13.2 ± 2.9	10.7 ± 2.4	10.2 ± 2.3	10.3 ± 2.2	7.7 ± 2.0†	7.0 ± 1.9†	6.4 ± 1.8†	−1.3 ± 3.5††
	Corrected	16.9 ± 4.0	14.8 ± 3.7	13.6 ± 3.4	13.3 ± 3.2	10.7 ± 2.6	10.3 ± 2.6	10.4 ± 2.6	7.9 ± 2.3	7.2 ± 2.1	6.6 ± 2.0	−1.1 ± 3.3
W'_{BALint}	Actual	16.9 ± 4.0	14.9 ± 3.5	13.4 ± 3.1	12.5 ± 3.0	8.6 ± 2.6**	8.0 ± 2.6**	7.7 ± 2.6**	4.5 ± 2.4**	4.1 ± 2.4**	3.9 ± 2.3**	−2.8 ± 2.8*††
	Corrected	16.9 ± 4.0	14.9 ± 3.5	13.4 ± 3.2	12.6 ± 3.1	8.7 ± 2.8**	8.1 ± 2.9**	7.8 ± 3.0**	4.6 ± 2.8**	4.3 ± 2.7**	4.1 ± 2.7**	−2.6 ± 2.6*

$P < 0.05$ Integral vs. differential.
**$P < 0.01$ Integral vs. differential.*
†$P < 0.05$ 2,250 m vs. 250 m.*
††$P < 0.01$ 2,250 m vs. 250 m.*

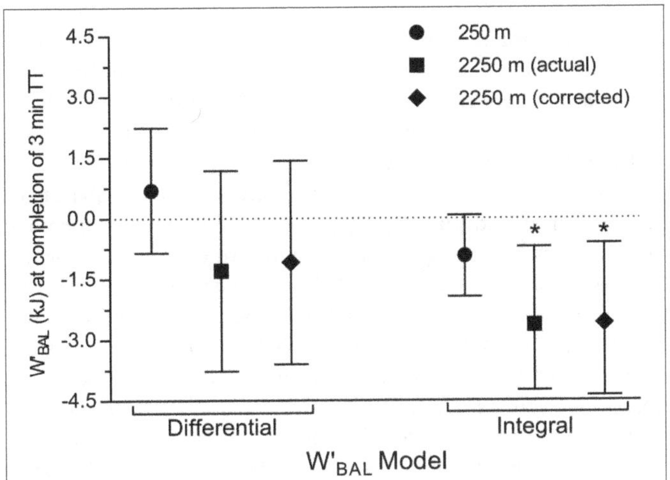

FIGURE 3 | Modelled W'_{BAL} at completion of the 3TT which concludes the HIIT expressed as mean ± 95% CI. Dotted line at $W'_{BAL} = 0$ kJ indicates the theoretical point of exhaustion. *$P < 0.05$ difference compared with 0 kJ.

Bassett et al. (1999). Whilst the effect of hypoxia on the factors that determine $\dot{V}O_{2max}$ are well understood (Wagner, 1996), less is known about the determinants of CP in hypoxia. Traditionally, CP has been considered to reflect a rate limited aerobic energetic supply (Jones et al., 2010). However, it is important to note that $\dot{V}O_2$ at CP is below $\dot{V}O_{2max}$ (Poole et al., 1988; Vanhatalo et al., 2016), and therefore oxidative metabolism at CP cannot be "rate limited." Rather, CP is associated with the highest exercise intensity where a $\dot{V}O_2$ steady state, and muscle "metabolic stability" can be achieved (Poole et al., 1988; Jones et al., 2008; Vanhatalo et al., 2016). Metabolic stability is characterized by minimal disturbance to intramuscular [PCr], [P_i], [H^+], [ADP_{free}], [AMP_{free}] and Gibbs free energy of ATP hydrolysis (Grassi et al., 2011). In hypoxia, a decrease in convective O_2 transport to working muscle occurs (Amann and Calbet, 2008), and the $\dot{V}O_2$ primary component decelerates (Hughson and Kowalchuk, 1995). Since the $\dot{V}O_2$ primary component is considered an "epiphenomenon" of metabolic stability (Grassi et al., 2011), and has been shown to correlate with CP (Murgatroyd et al., 2011), then an O_2 supply limitation on $\dot{V}O_2$ kinetics may impair metabolic stability, and thus explain why CP is reduced in hypoxia (Dekerle et al., 2012; Simpson et al., 2015; Shearman et al., 2016).

In the present study we found no significant differences in W′ at moderate altitudes up to 3,250 m, however a marked reduction (≈27%) occurred at 4,250 m (see **Figure 1B**). These results broadly align with several other investigations examining the effect of differing magnitudes of hypoxia on W′ (Valli et al., 2011; Dekerle et al., 2012; Simpson et al., 2015; Shearman et al., 2016). In recent years improved understanding of the mechanistic basis of W′ has developed. When the exercise intensity increases beyond CP, there is progressive recruitment of type IIx muscle fibers (Copp et al., 2010) and a slowing of $\dot{V}O_2$ uptake kinetics (Brittain et al., 2001). Slower $\dot{V}O_2$ uptake kinetics allows progressive deterioration of muscle metabolic stability to occur which has been demonstrated for both constant load (Jones et al., 2008), and intermittent exercise (Chidnok et al., 2013). The cellular changes associated with failure of metabolic stability are believed to be linked to the emergence of the $\dot{V}O_2$ slow component, and to underlie mechanisms of peripheral muscle fatigue (Grassi et al., 2015). Murgatroyd et al. (Murgatroyd et al., 2011) reported a significant correlation between the $\dot{V}O_2$ slow component magnitude and W′, which suggests the capacity to complete work above CP until the point of exhaustion is ultimately determined by the mechanisms of fatigue contributing to task failure. In moderate hypoxia (FiO_2: ≈0.15), the absolute magnitude of peripheral muscle fatigue, assessed via twitch interpolation, remains similar to normoxia following either constant load work to task failure (Amann et al., 2007), or self-paced TT exercise (Amann et al., 2006a). Additionally, Romer et al. (Romer et al., 2007) found the rate of peripheral fatigue development to increase in hypoxia (FiO_2: ≈0.13) compared with normoxia, but the absolute magnitude remained similar. These findings support the notion that the apparent fixed nature of W′ may be linked to the existence of a peripheral muscle fatigue limit which cannot be surpassed despite

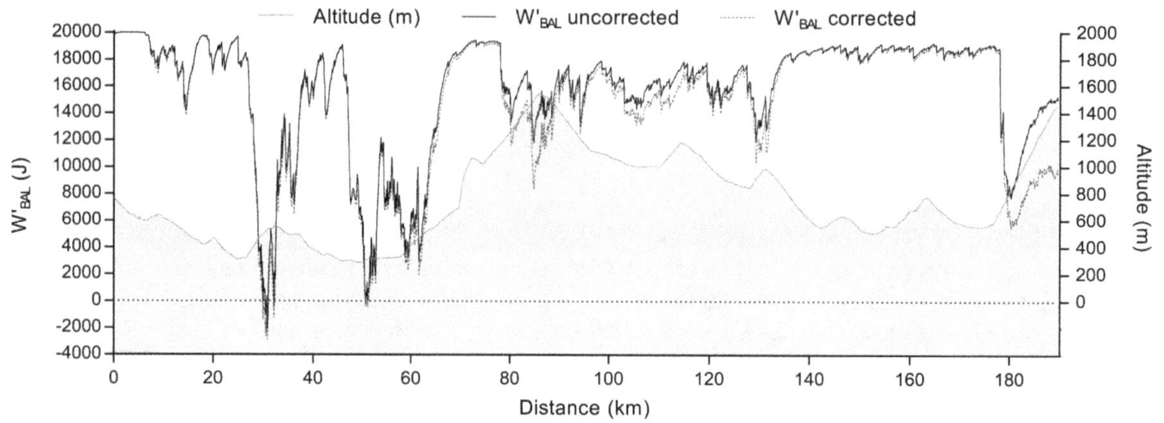

FIGURE 4 | Field data collected during the 2015 Giro d'Italia showing the effect of altitude correction of CP and W′ on modelled $W'_{BALdiff}$ response.

varying experimental conditions, including hypoxia (Amann et al., 2006b; Romer et al., 2007; Poole et al., 2016). However, since hypoxia reduces CP, a given absolute workrate in the severe domain corresponds to a higher intensity *relative* to CP, compared with normoxic conditions. Therefore, according to the CP model, W′ should deplete faster and time to exhaustion would decline. This would be associated with an exacerbated rate of fatigue development in hypoxia, as shown by Romer et al. (Romer et al., 2007). Hence, rather than conceptualizing hypoxia *per se* as the mechanism which exacerbates fatigue, it is the effect of hypoxia on decreasing CP that indirectly leads to a more rapid onset of fatigue, coincident with depletion of W′, at a given absolute workrate.

This study is the first to examine the effect of increasing altitude on W′. Our finding that W′ was markedly reduced only in severe hypoxia (≈27% at 4,250 m) led to the construction of a two-segment linear model (see **Figure 1D**). Using an average confidence interval across all trials, we estimated that a significant decrease in W′ would occur at altitudes beyond ≈3,500 m. Simpson et al. (2015) reported a small decrease in W′ at 3,800 m, but this did not reach statistical significance, whilst Valli et al. (2011) found a large decrease (≈55%) in W′ at 5,050 m. Thus, it appears likely that severe hypoxia reduces W′, yet some uncertainty remains regarding the lowest altitude at which this occurs. Measurement of W′ shows high within-subject variability (Karsten et al., 2014) though, which may confound attempts to accurately determine such a threshold altitude. Valli et al. (2011) suggested the decrease in W′ was consistent with reduced muscle-venous O_2 storage. More recent evidence reveals a decrease in central motor drive in severe hypoxia (≈5,250 m), but no change in moderate hypoxia (≈2,500 m), compared with sea level (Amann et al., 2007). Group III/IV afferent feedback from the locomotor muscles has been suggested to regulate central motor drive (Amann et al., 2006a, 2007), although evidence also suggests that a direct effect of cerebral hypoxia, independent of afferent feedback, may contribute to reduced performance and altered central motor drive in severe hypoxia (Millet et al., 2012). A direct inhibitory effect of cerebral hypoxia on central motor drive might explain the reduction in W′ found in this study and that of Valli et al. (2011), and also the finding that peripheral fatigue is significantly reduced at task failure only in severe hypoxia, but not moderate hypoxia (Amann et al., 2007).

In order to extend the applicability of the constant load CP model to intermittent high-intensity exercise, Skiba et al. (2012) introduced the W'_{BALint} model. This model includes the following assumptions, (1) expenditure of W′ occurs when the power output exceeds CP, (2) reconstitution of the W′ occurs when the power output falls below CP, and (3) the reconstitution of W′ follows a predictable monoexponential time course. The W'_{BALint} model has been validated empirically in normoxia (Skiba et al., 2012, 2014b), whilst a receiver-operator characteristic analysis found subjective rating of exhaustion to occur when the modelled W'_{BAL} fell below 1.5 kJ (Skiba et al., 2014a). Previously, we demonstrated the W'_{BALint} model to be applicable during intermittent high intensity exercise at ≈2,450 m (Shearman et al., 2016). However, this model was only valid when CP and W′ were also measured at the same FiO_2 (Shearman et al., 2016). In the present study, we have shown that a predictable decline in CP occurs with increasing altitude up to 4,250 m (**Figures 1A,C**), and therefore, W'_{BAL} can be calculated in hypoxia using measurements of CP and W′ in normoxia. We found no difference in computed W'_{BALint} or $W'_{BALdiff}$ during intermittent high-intensity cycling at 2,250 m, when either actual measurements of CP and W′ at 2,250 m were used, or predicted values based on measures at 250 m (see **Table 1**).

A modified version of the W'_{BALint} model (Skiba et al., 2012) was recently published (Skiba et al., 2015). This newer model adopted principles of chemical reaction kinetics and takes the form of a differential equation, hence it was referred to as the W'_{BAL} "differential" model. The advantage of a differential equation is that the time constant of W′ recovery does not require prior fitting to empirical data (Skiba et al., 2015), or estimation from Equation 4. The present study though, is the first to directly compare the W'_{BALint} model (Skiba et al., 2012) vs. the $W'_{BALdiff}$ model (Skiba et al., 2015), within a single subject sample (see **Table 1**). We found significantly higher values for computed $W'_{BALdiff}$ from the fourth interval onwards during the HIIT, at which point W'_{BALint} had declined by ≈50% from initial W′. This difference can largely be explained by the smaller time constant (hence faster recovery kinetics) observed for $W'_{BALdiff}$ vs. the W'_{BALint} model (Skiba et al., 2015). Upon completion of the 3TT at both 250 or 2250 m, $W'_{BALdiff}$ values displayed only small effect sizes and non-significant differences compared with a theoretical criterion of 0 kJ. However, the difference in W'_{BALint} values was moderate at 250 m and large at 2,250 m. This finding contrasts our previous work (Shearman et al., 2016), in which the W'_{BALint} model showed good agreement with a criterion range of $W'_{BAL} = 0 \pm 1.5$ kJ at task failure. In the present study however, we included all-out sprint efforts in addition to self-paced TT exercise during the HIIT. Whilst the $W'_{BALdiff}$ model appeared better suited to the HIIT in this study, the short recovery time constant led to faster W′ reconstitution than reported by Ferguson et al. (2010) for longer recovery durations. Further research is required to understand the limitations of the current mathematical approaches and to develop a more robust model of intermittent exercise.

Since interval training and road cycling competition is highly stochastic in nature, there are limitless permutations of intensity and work to rest ratios. The application of W'_{BAL} approach though, enables analysis of all such permutations within a single unifying mathematical framework. A key justification for the present study was to extend the practical application of W'_{BAL} during dynamic environmental conditions such as a mountain climb in cycling. **Figure 4** presents competition field data from the 2015 Giro d'Italia, during a stage which ascends beyond 1,400 m. The effect of increasing altitude can be seen by comparing the uncorrected CP vs. corrected (for altitude) parameter input into W'_{BAL} model. Interestingly, despite a maximum reported effort on the final hill climb, it appears as though W'_{BAL} is reconstituting since the power is below CP. The failure to deplete W'_{BAL} in this instance likely reflects prolonged accumulation of fatigue mechanisms such as glycogen depletion and/or increasing central fatigue (Thomas et al., 2015), which are not taken into account within the framework of the current models. Glycogen depletion has been shown to decrease the value of W′ (Miura et al., 2000), and fatigue induced inefficiency might decrease CP (Grassi et al., 2015). Accordingly, further research is warranted to develop a robust W'_{BAL} model for a variety of different task requirements. Prolonged endurance exercise would be one such example.

It is well known that endurance exercise performance is reduced upon ascent to altitude (Amann and Calbet, 2008). Secondly, recent progress has been made in the field of mathematical modelling intermittent high-intensity performance, which has practical applications in training load prescription and monitoring (Skiba et al., 2014a, 2015; Shearman et al., 2016). In the present investigation, we report a curvilinear decrease in CP with increasing altitude as well as a significant reduction in W′ occurring only at 4,250 m. The predictable decline in CP, combined with lack of change in W′ up to 3,250 m, enables modelling of W'_{BAL} in hypoxic environments without the requirement for testing at all altitudes. This enables the prescription of equivalent relative intensity interval training workouts in hypoxic conditions compared with normoxia. Whilst we validated use of the altitude correction factor within the W'_{BAL} at 2,250 m, since it is known that W′ contains relatively high typical error (Karsten et al., 2014, 2016), and there may be changes in W′ at higher altitudes, caution is required when interpreting modelled intermittent performance in severe hypoxia above ≈3,500 m.

AUTHOR CONTRIBUTIONS

NT, DN, PS, and JP contributed to experimental concept and design. NT, DN, SR, and JP contributed to data collection and analysis. NT, PS, SR, and JP contributed to manuscript preparation. The authors declare that the results of the study are presented clearly, honestly, and without fabrication, falsification, or inappropriate data manipulation.

ACKNOWLEDGMENTS

NT, DN, PS, SR, and JP would like to acknowledge the contribution of Scott Cocking and Mathew Wilson who assisted with data collection, and also Mark Liversedge and Damien Grauser for Golden Cheetah cycling analytics software development. The authors thank the cyclists for their effort.

REFERENCES

Amann, M., and Calbet, J. A. (2008). Convective oxygen transport and fatigue. *J. Appl. Physiol.* 104, 861–870. doi: 10.1152/japplphysiol.01008.2007

Amann, M., Eldridge, M. W., Lovering, A. T., Stickland, M. K., Pegelow, D. F., and Dempsey, J. A. (2006a). Arterial oxygenation influences central motor output and exercise performance via effects on peripheral locomotor muscle fatigue in humans. *J. Physiol.* 575(Pt 3), 937–952. doi: 10.1113/jphysiol.2006.113936

Amann, M., Romer, L. M., Pegelow, D. F., Jacques, A. J., Hess, C. J., and Dempsey, J. A. (2006b). Effects of arterial oxygen content on peripheral locomotor muscle fatigue. *J. Appl. Physiol.* 101, 119–127. doi: 10.1152/japplphysiol.01596.2005

Amann, M., Romer, L. M., Subudhi, A. W., Pegelow, D. F., and Dempsey, J. A. (2007). Severity of arterial hypoxaemia affects the relative contributions of peripheral muscle fatigue to exercise performance in healthy humans. *J. Physiol.* 581(Pt 1), 389–403. doi: 10.1113/jphysiol.2007.129700

Bassett, D. R. Jr., Kyle, C. R., Passfield, L., Broker, J. P., and Burke, E. R. (1999). Comparing cycling world hour records, -1967-1996: modeling with empirical data. *Med. Sci. Sports Exerc.* 31, 1665–1676. doi: 10.1097/00005768-199911000-00025

Black, M. I., Jones, A. M., Bailey, S. J., and Vanhatalo, A. (2015). Self-pacing increases critical power and improves performance during severe-intensity exercise. *Appl. Physiol. Nutr. Metab.* 40, 662–670. doi: 10.1139/apnm-2014-0442

Blain, G. M., Mangum, T. S., Sidhu, S. K., Weavil, J. C., Hureau, T. J., Jessop, J. E., et al. (2016). Group III/IV muscle afferents limit the intramuscular metabolic perturbation during whole body exercise in humans. *J. Physiol.* 594, 5303–5315. doi: 10.1113/JP272283

Brittain, C. J., Rossiter, H. B., Kowalchuk, J. M., and Whipp, B. J. (2001). Effect of prior metabolic rate on the kinetics of oxygen uptake during moderate-intensity exercise. *Eur. J. Appl. Physiol.* 86, 125–134. doi: 10.1007/s004210100514

Broxterman, R. M., Craig, J. C., Ade, C. J., Wilcox, S. L., and Barstow, T. J. (2015). The effect of resting blood flow occlusion on exercise tolerance and W′. *Am. J. Physiol. Regul. Integr. Comp. Physiol.* 309, R684–R691. doi: 10.1152/ajpregu.00283.2015

Burnley, M., Vanhatalo, A., Fulford, J., and Jones, A. M. (2010). Similar metabolic perturbations during all-out and constant force exhaustive exercise in humans: a (31)P magnetic resonance spectroscopy study. *Exp. Physiol.* 95, 798–807. doi: 10.1113/expphysiol.2010.052688

Chidnok, W., Dimenna, F. J., Bailey, S. J., Vanhatalo, A., Morton, R. H., Wilkerson, D. P., et al. (2012). Exercise tolerance in intermittent cycling: application of the critical power concept. *Med. Sci. Sports Exerc.* 44, 966–976. doi: 10.1249/MSS.0b013e31823ea28a

Chidnok, W., Fulford, J., Bailey, S. J., DiMenna, F. J., Skiba, P. F., Vanhatalo, A., et al. (2013). Muscle metabolic determinants of exercise tolerance following exhaustion: relationship to the "critical power." *J. Appl. Physiol.* 115, 243–250. doi: 10.1152/japplphysiol.00334.2013

Clark, S. A., Bourdon, P. C., Schmidt, W., Singh, B., Cable, G., Onus, K. J., et al. (2007). The effect of acute simulated moderate altitude on power, performance and pacing strategies in well-trained cyclists. *Eur. J. Appl. Physiol.* 102, 45–55. doi: 10.1007/s00421-007-0554-0

Copp, S. W., Hirai, D. M., Musch, T. I., and Poole, D. C. (2010). Critical speed in the rat: implications for hindlimb muscle blood flow distribution and fibre recruitment. *J. Physiol.* 588, 5077–5087. doi: 10.1113/jphysiol.2010. 198382

Dekerle, J., Mucci, P., and Carter, H. (2012). Influence of moderate hypoxia on tolerance to high-intensity exercise. *Eur. J. Appl. Physiol.* 112, 327–335. doi: 10.1007/s00421-011-1979-z

Ferguson, C., Rossiter, H. B., Whipp, B. J., Cathcart, A. J., Murgatroyd, S. R., and Ward, S. A. (2010). Effect of recovery duration from prior exhaustive exercise on the parameters of the power-duration relationship. *J. Appl. Physiol.* 108, 866–874. doi: 10.1152/japplphysiol.91425.2008

Grassi, B., Porcelli, S., Salvadego, D., and Zoladz, J. A. (2011). Slow $\dot{V}O_2$ kinetics during moderate-intensity exercise as markers of lower metabolic stability and lower exercise tolerance. *Eur. J. Appl. Physiol.* 111, 345–55. doi: 10.1007/s00421-010-1609-1

Grassi, B., Rossiter, H. B., and Zoladz, J. A. (2015). Skeletal muscle fatigue and decreased efficiency: two sides of the same coin? *Exerc. Sport Sci. Rev.* 43, 75–83. doi: 10.1249/JES.0000000000000043

Hughson, R. L., and Kowalchuk, J. M. (1995). Kinetics of oxygen uptake for submaximal exercise in hyperoxia, normoxia, and hypoxia. *Can. J. Appl. Physiol.* 20, 198–210. doi: 10.1139/h95-014

Hureau, T. J., Romer, L. M., and Amann, M. (2016). The "sensory tolerance limit": a hypothetical construct determining exercise performance? *Eur. J. Sport Sci.* doi: 10.1080/17461391.2016.1252428. [Epub ahead of print].

Jones, A. M., Vanhatalo, A., Burnley, M., Morton, R. H., and Poole, D. C. (2010). Critical power: implications for determination of $\dot{V}O_2$ max and exercise tolerance. *Med. Sci. Sports Exerc.* 42, 1876–1890. doi: 10.1249/MSS.0b013e3181d9cf7f

Jones, A. M., Wilkerson, D. P., DiMenna, F., Fulford, J., and Poole, D. C. (2008). Muscle metabolic responses to exercise above and below the "critical power" assessed using 31P-MRS. *Am. J. Physiol. Regul. Integr. Comp. Physiol.* 294, R585–R593. doi: 10.1152/ajpregu.00731.2007

Karsten, B., Hopker, J., Jobson, S. A., Baker, J., Petrigna, L., Klose, A., et al. (2016). Comparison of inter-trial recovery times for the determination of critical power and W′ in cycling. *J. Sports Sci.* 1–6. doi: 10.1080/02640414.2016.1215500

Karsten, B., Jobson, S. A., Hopker, J., Jimenez, A., and Beedie, C. (2014). High agreement between laboratory and field estimates of critical power in cycling. *Int. J. Sports Med.* 35, 298–303. doi: 10.1055/s-0033-1349844

MacInnis, M. J., Nugent, S. F., MacLeod, K. E., and Lohse, K. R. (2015). Methods to estimate $\dot{V}O_2$ max upon acute hypoxia exposure. *Med. Sci. Sports Exerc.* 47, 1869–1876. doi: 10.1249/MSS.0000000000000628

Margaria, R. (1976). *Biomechanics and Energetics of Muscular Exercise*. Oxford: Clarendon Press.

Millet, G. Y., Muthalib, M., Jubeau, M., Laursen, P. B., and Nosaka, K. (2012). Severe hypoxia affects exercise performance independently of afferent feedback and peripheral fatigue. *J. Appl. Physiol.* 112, 1335–1344. doi: 10.1152/japplphysiol.00804.2011

Miura, A., Sato, H., Sato, H., Whipp, B. J., and Fukuba, Y. (2000). The effect of glycogen depletion on the curvature constant parameter of the power-duration curve for cycle ergometry. *Ergonomics* 43, 133–141. doi: 10.1080/001401300184693

Monod, H., and Scherrer, J. (1965). The work capacity of a synergic muscular group. *Ergonomics* 8, 329–38. doi: 10.1080/00140136508930810

Morton, R. H. (2006). The critical power and related whole-body bioenergetic models. *Eur. J. Appl. Physiol.* 96, 339–354. doi: 10.1007/s00421-005-0088-2

Murgatroyd, S. R., Ferguson, C., Ward, S. A., Whipp, B. J., and Rossiter, H. B. (2011). Pulmonary O_2 uptake kinetics as a determinant of high-intensity exercise tolerance in humans. *J. Appl. Physiol.* 110, 1598–1606. doi: 10.1152/japplphysiol.01092.2010

Paton, C. D., and Hopkins, W. G. (2001). Tests of cycling performance. *Sports Med.* 31, 489–496. doi: 10.2165/00007256-200131070-00004

Péronnet, F., Thibault, G., and Cousineau, D. L. (1991). A theoretical analysis of the effect of altitude on running performance. *J. Appl. Physiol.* 70, 399–404.

Poole, D. C., Burnley, M., Vanhatalo, A., Rossiter, H. B., and Jones, A. M. (2016). Critical power: an important fatigue threshold in exercise physiology. *Med. Sci. Sports Exerc.* 48, 2320–2334. doi: 10.1249/MSS.0000000000000939

Poole, D. C., Ward, S. A., Gardner, G. W., and Whipp, B. J. (1988). Metabolic and respiratory profile of the upper limit for prolonged exercise in man. *Ergonomics* 31, 1265–1279. doi: 10.1080/00140138808966766

Romer, L. M., Haverkamp, H. C., Amann, M., Lovering, A. T., Pegelow, D. F., and Dempsey, J. A. (2007). Effect of acute severe hypoxia on peripheral fatigue and endurance capacity in healthy humans. *Am. J. Physiol. Regul. Integr. Comp. Physiol.* 292, R598–R606. doi: 10.1152/ajpregu.00269.2006

Shearman, S., Dwyer, D., Skiba, P., and Townsend, N. (2016). Modeling intermittent cycling performance in hypoxia using the critical power concept. *Med. Sci. Sports Exerc.* 48, 527–535. doi: 10.1249/MSS.0000000000000794

Simpson, L. P., Jones, A. M., Skiba, P. F., Vanhatalo, A., and Wilkerson, D. (2015). Influence of Hypoxia on the power-duration relationship during high-intensity exercise. *Int. J. Sports Med.* 36, 113–119. doi: 10.1055/s-0034-1389943

Skiba, P. F., Chidnok, W., Vanhatalo, A., and Jones, A. M. (2012). Modeling the expenditure and reconstitution of work capacity above critical power. *Med. Sci. Sports Exerc.* 44, 1526–1532. doi: 10.1249/MSS.0b013e3182517a80

Skiba, P. F., Clarke, D., Vanhatalo, A., and Jones, A. M. (2014a). Validation of a novel intermittent W′ model for cycling using field data. *Int. J. Sports Physiol. Perform.* 9, 900–904. doi: 10.1123/ijspp.2013-0471

Skiba, P. F., Fulford, J., Clarke, D. C., Vanhatalo, A., and Jones, A. M. (2015). Intramuscular determinants of the ability to recover work capacity above critical power. *Eur. J. Appl. Physiol.* 115, 703–713. doi: 10.1007/s00421-014-3050-3

Skiba, P. F., Jackman, S., Clarke, D., Vanhatalo, A., and Jones, A. M. (2014b). Effect of work and recovery durations on W′ reconstitution during intermittent exercise. *Med. Sci. Sports Exerc.* 46, 1433–1440. doi: 10.1249/MSS.0000000000000226

Thomas, K., Goodall, S., Stone, M., Howatson, G., St Clair Gibson ,A., and Ansley, L. (2015). Central and peripheral fatigue in male cyclists after 4-, 20-, and 40-km time trials. *Med. Sci. Sports Exerc.* 47, 537–546. doi: 10.1249/MSS.0000000000000448

Valli, G., Cogo, A., Passino, C., Bonardi, D., Morici, G., Fasano, V., et al. (2011). Exercise intolerance at high altitude (5050 m): critical power and W′. *Respir. Physiol. Neurobiol.* 177, 333–341. doi: 10.1016/j.resp.2011.05.014

Vanhatalo, A., Black, M. I., DiMenna, F. J., Blackwell, J. R., Schmidt, J. F., Thompson, C., et al. (2016). The mechanistic bases of the power–time relationship: muscle metabolic responses and relationships to muscle fibre type. *J. Physiol.* 594, 4407–4423. doi: 10.1113/JP271879

Wagner, P. D. (1996). A theoretical analysis of factors determining $\dot{V}O_2$ MAX at sea level and altitude. *Respir. Physiol.* 106, 329–343. doi: 10.1016/S0034-5687(96)00086-2

Wehrlin, J. P., and Hallén, J. (2006). Linear decrease in. VO_{2max} and performance with increasing altitude in endurance athletes. *Eur. J. Appl. Physiol.* 96, 404–12. doi: 10.1007/s00421-005-0081-9

17

Task Failure During Exercise to Exhaustion in Normoxia and Hypoxia is Due to Reduced Muscle Activation Caused by Central Mechanisms While Muscle Metaboreflex does not Limit Performance

*Rafael Torres-Peralta[1,2], David Morales-Alamo[1,2], Miriam González-Izal[3], José Losa-Reyna[1,2], Ismael Pérez-Suárez[1,2], Mikel Izquierdo[3] and José A. L. Calbet[1,2]**

[1] Department of Physical Education, University of Las Palmas de Gran Canaria, Las Palmas de Gran Canaria, Spain, [2] Research Institute of Biomedical and Health Sciences (IUIBS), Las Palmas de Gran Canaria, Spain, [3] Department of Health Sciences, Public University of Navarra, Tudela, Spain

***Correspondence:**
José A. L. Calbet
lopezcalbet@gmail.com

To determine whether task failure during incremental exercise to exhaustion (IE) is principally due to reduced neural drive and increased metaboreflex activation eleven men (22 ± 2 years) performed a 10 s control isokinetic sprint (IS; 80 rpm) after a short warm-up. This was immediately followed by an IE in normoxia (Nx, P_IO_2:143 mmHg) and hypoxia (Hyp, P_IO_2:73 mmHg) in random order, separated by a 120 min resting period. At exhaustion, the circulation of both legs was occluded instantaneously (300 mmHg) during 10 or 60 s to impede recovery and increase metaboreflex activation. This was immediately followed by an IS with open circulation. Electromyographic recordings were obtained from the *vastus medialis* and *lateralis*. Muscle biopsies and blood gases were obtained in separate experiments. During the last 10 s of the IE, pulmonary ventilation, VO_2, power output and muscle activation were lower in hypoxia than in normoxia, while pedaling rate was similar. Compared to the control sprint, performance (IS-Wpeak) was reduced to a greater extent after the IE-Nx (11% lower $P < 0.05$) than IE-Hyp. The root mean square (EMG_{RMS}) was reduced by 38 and 27% during IS performed after IE-Nx and IE-Hyp, respectively (Nx vs. Hyp: $P < 0.05$). Post-ischemia IS-EMG_{RMS} values were higher than during the last 10 s of IE. Sprint exercise mean (IS-MPF) and median (IS-MdPF) power frequencies, and burst duration, were more reduced after IE-Nx than IE-Hyp ($P < 0.05$). Despite increased muscle lactate accumulation, acidification, and metaboreflex activation from 10 to 60 s of ischemia, IS-Wmean (+23%) and burst duration (+10%) increased, while IS-EMG_{RMS} decreased (−24%, $P < 0.05$), with IS-MPF and IS-MdPF remaining unchanged. In conclusion, close to task failure, muscle activation is lower in hypoxia than in normoxia. Task failure is predominantly caused by central mechanisms, which recover to great extent within 1 min even when the legs remain ischemic. There is dissociation between the recovery of EMG_{RMS} and performance. The reduction of surface electromyogram MPF, MdPF and burst duration due to fatigue is associated but not caused by muscle acidification and lactate accumulation. Despite metaboreflex stimulation, muscle activation and power output recovers partly in ischemia indicating that metaboreflex activation has a minor impact on sprint performance.

Keywords: electromyography, EMG, exhaustion, fatigue, high-intensity, hypoxia, lactate, performance

INTRODUCTION

Muscle fatigue has been defined as "any exercise-induced reduction in the ability to exert muscle force or power, regardless of whether the task can be sustained (Bigland-Ritchie and Woods, 1984), that can be reversed by rest" (Gandevia, 2001). The mechanisms leading to task failure may involve physiological processes at neural (central fatigue) or muscular levels (peripheral fatigue), with failure distal to the neuromuscular junction included in the "peripheral" component. It has been suggested that the rate of muscle fatigue development is regulated by the central nervous system (CNS) with feedback from the type III and IV muscle afferents (Amann and Dempsey, 2008), which sense metabolite accumulation, particularly H^+, lactate, and ATP (Light et al., 2008). Type III/IV muscle afferents have been reported to inhibit corticospinal drive (Amann and Dempsey, 2008; Rossman et al., 2012; Kennedy et al., 2015), with greater inhibitory effect on extensor than flexor muscles (Martin et al., 2006). However, whether metabolite accumulation and the expected metaboreflex stimulation impair muscle activation and limit peak power during whole-body sprint exercise remains unknown.

During whole-body exercise in severe acute hypoxia ($F_IO_2 <$ 0.115, or altitude above 4500 m) the level of peripheral fatigue at exhaustion seems lower, indicating that central mechanisms, likely linked to reduced brain oxygenation (Rasmussen et al., 2010), predominate over local mechanisms in determining the cessation of exercise (Amann et al., 2007). In agreement with this hypothesis, an instantaneous increase of the inspired O_2 fraction (F_IO_2) from 0.21 to 1.00 does not eliminate muscle fatigue at the end of an incremental exercise test performed at sea level (Calbet et al., 2003a). In contrast, during constant-intensity or incremental exercise to exhaustion in severe hypoxia ($P_IO_2 \approx 75$ mmHg), muscle fatigue is swiftly relieved by mild hyperoxic gas or room air (Kayser et al., 1994; Calbet et al., 2003a,b; Amann et al., 2007). These findings led to the concept that during incremental exercise to exhaustion in normoxia, task failure is most likely caused by peripheral mechanisms while central mechanisms prevail in severe hypoxia (Calbet et al., 2003a; Amann et al., 2007). In support, peripheral fatigue, as assessed via decreases in potentiated quadriceps twitch force 2 min after constant-intensity exercise to exhaustion, was lower when the exercise was performed in severe hypoxia than in normoxia (Amann et al., 2007). Nevertheless, this observation was not accompanied by an assessment of muscle metabolites and obviates the fact that reduced potentiated quadriceps twitch force may occur without reduction of peak power output (Fernandez-del-Olmo et al., 2013; Hureau et al., 2014). Moreover, the recovery process starts as early as muscle contraction ceases, and given the fast kinetics of phosphocreatine re-synthesis at the end of exercise (Bogdanis et al., 1996; Dawson et al., 1997; Yoshida et al., 2013), most of the recovery has already occurred within the first 2 min post-exercise (Sargeant and Dolan, 1987; Froyd et al., 2013). Also, muscle fatigue is task-specific (Gandevia, 2001), implying that a procedure using a similar pattern of movement, and hence recruitment of neural pathways, is expected to be more sensitive to detect fatigue.

In this context, every possible combination of effects and interpretation of results has been reported in regard to the contribution of central and peripheral mechanisms to muscle fatigue after dynamic contractions in normoxia (Sidhu et al., 2009, 2012; Marcora and Staiano, 2010; Fernandez-del-Olmo et al., 2013) and hypoxia (Amann et al., 2007; Goodall et al., 2010; Millet et al., 2012). Some of these discrepancies can be attributed to the fact that neural mechanisms of muscle fatigue are task-specific (Sidhu et al., 2012), to different levels of input from type III and IV muscle afferents (Sidhu et al., 2012), and to methodological limitations (Rodriguez-Falces et al., 2013; Héroux et al., 2015; Bachasson et al., 2016). Although the inhibition of type III and IV muscle afferents has been shown to attenuate muscle fatigue in certain exercise models (Sidhu et al., 2014), whether type III and IV muscle afferent input contributes to reduce exercise performance by a central mechanism remains controversial (Millet et al., 2009, 2012; Marcora, 2010; Amann et al., 2013a; Kennedy et al., 2015). Part of the discrepancies may be due to the fact that type III and IV muscle afferent discharge cannot be directly measured during whole-body exercise in humans, combined with the difficulty in interpreting the effects of intrathecal fentanyl when this drug differently alters ventilation, arterial O_2 content, arterial $PaCO_2$, heart rate and mean arterial blood pressure, depending on the exercise intensity, exercise duration, and the study population (Dempsey et al., 2014; Olson et al., 2014; Poon and Song, 2015). Thus, we decided to explore the role of III/IV muscle afferents on exercise performance (peak power output) using a completely different experimental approach.

Abbreviations: ADP, Adenosine diphosphate; ATP, Adenosine triphosphate; CNS, Central nervous system; d.w., Dry weight; DEXA, Dual-energy x-ray absorptiometry; EMG, Surface electromyogram; EMG_{RMS}, Root mean square of the EMG; F_IO_2, Inspired oxygen fraction; HR, Heart rate; HRmax, Maximal heart rate; Hyp, Hypoxia; Hypb, session in hypoxia with biopsies taken; IE, Incremental exercise to exhaustion; IS, Isokinetic sprint; MPF, Mean power frequency; MdPF, Median power frequency; MVC, Maximal voluntary contraction; Nx, Normoxia; Nxb, Session in normoxia with biopsies taken; PaO_2, Arterial oxygen pressure; PCr, Phosphocreatine; P_IO_2, Inspired O_2 pressure; RMS, root mean square; RMSNz, Normalized root mean square; V_E, Minute ventilation; VO_2, Oxygen consumption; VO_2max, Maximal oxygen uptake; VO_2peak, Peak oxygen uptake; Wpeak-i, Instantaneous peak power output; Wmax, Peak power output at exhaustion during the incremental exercise test; Wmean, mean power output during the 10 s sprints; w.w., wet weight; TAI, Total activation index.

The main aim of this investigation was to determine whether task failure during an incremental exercise to exhaustion is principally due to central mechanisms that cause a reduction in neural activation, modulated by the level of oxygenation. This hypothesis has been previously examined but with different procedures (Kayser et al., 1994; Amann et al., 2007, 2013b) which did not include measurements of muscle metabolites or performance immediately after exhaustion. Another aim was to determine if increased afferent feedback from metabolite accumulation in an exhausted muscle has a negative influence on sprint performance by reducing neural activation, as assessed through electromyogram (EMG) recordings.

We aimed to test these two hypotheses: (i) task failure during incremental exercise to exhaustion in hypoxia occurs with lower levels of muscle activation compared to normoxia, and (ii) increased afferent feedback from III and IV muscle afferents impairs sprint performance.

METHODS

Subjects

Eleven healthy men (age: 21.5 ± 2.0 years, height: 174 ± 8 cm, body mass: 72.3 ± 9.3 kg, body fat: 16.1 ± 4.9%, VO_2max: 51 ± 5 mL.kg^{-1}.min^{-1}) agreed to participate in this investigation. Before volunteering, subjects received full oral and written information about the experiments and possible risks associated with participation. Written consent was obtained from each subject. The study was performed by the Helsinki Declaration and was approved by the Ethical Committee of the University of Las Palmas de Gran Canaria (CEIH-2010-01 and CEIH-2009-01).

General Overview

This study was a part of a larger project that included several experiments designed to address the mechanisms limiting whole-body exercise performance in humans. The results focusing on O_2 transport and muscle metabolism have been published (Calbet et al., 2015; Morales-Alamo et al., 2015). Body composition was determined by dual-energy x-ray absorptiometry (DEXA) (Hologic QDR-1500, Hologic Corp., software version 7.10, Waltham, MA) (Calbet et al., 1997), during the familiarization sessions. The leg muscle mass was calculated from the DEXA scans using Wang's et al. model (Wang et al., 1999).

The experimental protocol is summarized in **Figure 1**, and an example of the electromyographic recordings from one subject is given in **Figure 2**. On the experimental days, subjects reported to the laboratory at 08.00 h. after an overnight fast from 22.00 h. The subjects performed an incremental exercise test to exhaustion in normoxia (P_IO_2: ~143 mmHg) or acute hypoxia (P_IO_2: ~73 mmHg, Altitrainer200, SMTEC, Switzerland), in random order and separated by a 120 min rest. Before the exercise test, bilateral cuffs were placed around the thighs and connected to a rapid cuff inflator (SCD10, Hokanson E20 AG101, Bellevue, USA). The test started with a warm-up (2 min at 50 W + 2 min 100 W + 1 min at 160 W) followed by 4.5 min of slow unloaded pedaling. This was followed by a 30 s rest period while the subjects became ready to sprint at the 5th minute after the end of the warm-up. The volunteers were requested to sprint as hard and fast as possible during 10 s with the ergometer set in isokinetic mode and at 80 rpm (Excalibur Sport 925900, Lode, Groningen, The Netherlands). This sprint was used as a control sprint and was always performed in normoxia. Five minutes later, the incremental exercise began. For the test in normoxia, the load was increased by 30 W every 2 min until exhaustion, starting from an initial load of 80 W. In hypoxia, the incremental test started from 60 W, and the load was increased by 20 W every 2 min until exhaustion. Exhaustion during the incremental exercise tests was defined by the subject stopping pedaling or dropping pedaling rate below 50 rpm during 5 s, despite strong verbal encouragement. At exhaustion, the cuffs were inflated at maximal speed and pressure (i.e., 300 mmHg) to completely and instantaneously occlude the circulation (ischemia). This prevented any increase of oxygenation during the recovery and caused anoxia within 3–5 s of the application of the occlusion as reported elsewhere (Morales-Alamo et al., 2015). A limitation of previous studies was that the impact of the early recovery could not be accounted for (Marcora and Staiano, 2010; Coelho et al., 2015), and certainly some recovery occurs during the time elapsed between the end of the exercise and the start of the sprint. To circumvent this limitation we applied complete ischemia during the recovery and we used short (10 s) and long (60 s) ischemia periods. We surmised that peripheral fatigue would be exacerbated by the prolonged ischemia at the end of an incremental exercise to exhaustion.

The incremental exercise test in normoxia and hypoxia ended with two different periods of ischemia of 10 or 60 s, during which the subjects breathed normoxic gas. Following a countdown, the subject performed a 10 s isokinetic sprint as hard and fast as possible while the ergometer was set at 80 rpm. The cuffs were always instantaneously deflated at the beginning of the post-ischemia sprints. In the unfatigued state, peak power increases with pedaling rate, but peak power is less affected by pedaling rate in the fatigued state (Beelen and Sargeant, 1991). Importantly, the difference in peak power between the fatigued and unfatigued state increases the higher the pedaling rate used in the control sprint (unfatigued) (Beelen and Sargeant, 1991). Thus, to avoid the limitations associated with varying pedaling rates sprints were performed in isokinetic mode at 80 rpm, a pedaling rate that allows maximal power output in the fatigued state (Beelen and Sargeant, 1991).

A few weeks later, the IEs were repeated in two additional experimental sessions; 1 day in normoxia (Nxb, P_IO_2: ~143 mmHg) and the other in hypoxia (Hypb, P_IO_2: ~73 mmHg; "b" indicates biopsy session). In the Nxb session, after 10 min rest in the supine position, a muscle biopsy was obtained from the m. *vastus lateralis* with local anesthesia (lidocaine 2%, 2 ml), using the Bergstrom technique with suction (Bergstrom, 1962). This biopsy was obtained with the needle pointing distally with 45° inclination (Guerra et al., 2011). An additional incision was performed before the beginning of the exercise in the contralateral leg. Afterward, the incisions were covered with a transient plaster, and a cuff was placed around the left leg. The subjects then sat on the cycle ergometer and resting

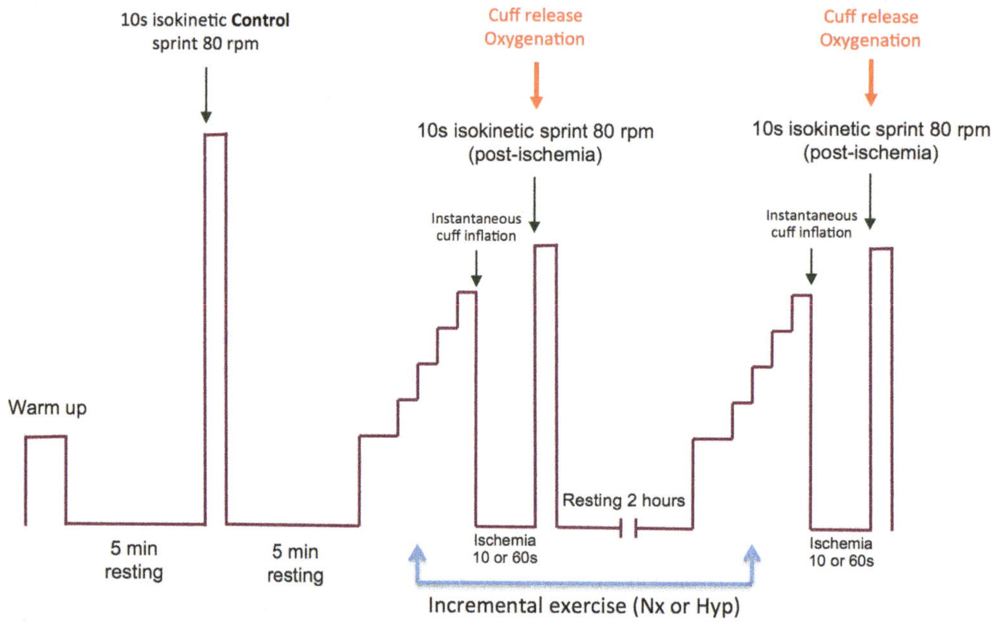

FIGURE 1 | Experimental protocol. The experimental day started with a warm-up followed by 4.5 min of slow unloaded pedaling and a 30 s resting phase, while the subjects became ready to perform the first sprint (isokinetic, 10 s at 80 rpm) at the 5th minute after the end of the warm-up. This sprint was used as a control sprint and was always performed in normoxia. Five minutes later, an incremental exercise to exhaustion began in normoxia (P_IO_2: ~143 mmHg) or acute hypoxia (P_IO_2: ~73 mmHg). The order of the incremental exercise test was randomized. Between the two incremental exercise tests, the subjects were allowed to rest during 120 min. At the end of the incremental exercise test, bilateral cuffs were inflated at maximal speed and pressure (i.e., 300 mmHg) to occlude completely and instantaneously the circulation (ischemia) of the legs. The incremental exercise test in normoxia and hypoxia ended with an ischemia period of 10 s on one experimental day and 60 s on another day. The order of the duration of the ischemia period was randomized. At the end of the ischemia period, the subjects performed a 10 s isokinetic sprint as hard and fast as possible (80 rpm) while the cuffs were always instantaneously deflated at the beginning of the post-ischemia sprints.

measurements were performed. Two minutes later, the IE was begun as described above. At exhaustion, the cuff was inflated instantaneously at 300 mmHg, and a biopsy was taken exactly 10 s after the end of the incremental exercise test. The biopsy needle was introduced perpendicular to the thigh. This biopsy was followed by a final biopsy at 60 s with the needle pointing proximally (45° inclination). In the Hypb session, essentially the same procedures were applied. All biopsies were immediately frozen in liquid nitrogen and stored at −80°C. Hypb and Nxb sessions were performed in random order.

Power Output, Oxygen Uptake and Hemoglobin Oxygen Saturation

Power output during the sprint was reported as instantaneous peak power output (Wpeak-i) and mean power output (Wmean) during the 10 s duration of the sprint. Oxygen uptake was measured with a metabolic cart (Vmax N29; Sensormedics, Yorba Linda, California, USA), calibrated before each test according to the manufacturer instructions, with high-grade calibration gasses (Carburos Metálicos, Las Palmas de Gran Canaria, Spain). Respiratory variables were analyzed breath-by-breath and averaged every 20 s during the incremental exercise tests. The highest 20-s averaged VO_2 recorded in normoxia was taken as the VO_2max. The same criterion was applied to determine the VO_2peak in hypoxia. Hemoglobin oxygen saturation (SpO_2) was determined with a finger pulse oximeter (OEM III module, 4549-000, Plymouth, MN).

Muscle Metabolites

From each muscle biopsy, 30 mg of wet tissue were freeze-dried, cleaned and powdered with a manual mortar on ice. Subsequently, the samples were suspended in 0.5 M $HClO_4$ and centrifuged at 15,000 g at 4°C for 15 min. The supernatant was neutralized with $KHCO_3$ 2.1M. ATP, phosphocreatine (PCr), creatine, pyruvate and lactate concentrations were enzymatically determined in neutralized extracts by fluorometric analysis (Lowry and Passonneau, 1972; Morales-Alamo et al., 2013).

Electromyography

Electrical muscle activation was monitored using surface electromyography (EMG). EMG signals were continuously recorded from the *vastus medialis* and *vastus lateralis*. Before the application of the EMG electrodes the skin surface was carefully shaved and wiped with alcohol to reduce skin impedance. Bipolar single differential electrodes were placed longitudinally on the muscles following the SENIAM recommendations (Merletti and Hermens, 2000) and taped to the skin to minimize movement artifacts. The reference electrode was placed on the skin over the acromion. The position of the electrodes was marked on the skin with indelible ink, and these references were used for precise electrode placement on repeated experiments.

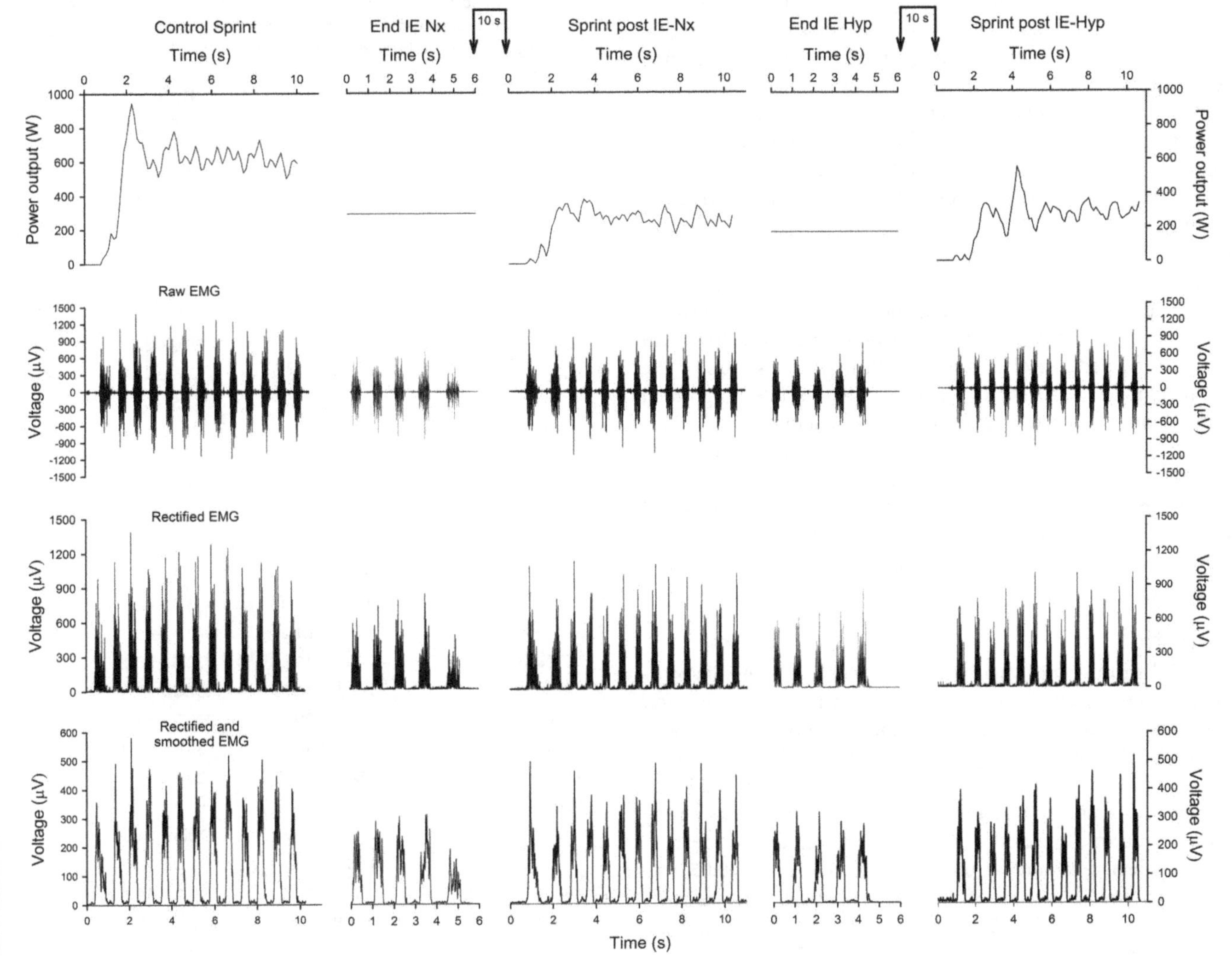

FIGURE 2 | Power output and EMG of a representative subject. Schematic representation of the power output (upper panels), raw EMG (2nd row), rectified EMG (3rd row) and rectified and smoothed EMG (lower panels), during the control sprint, last 6 s of the incremental exercise (IE) in normoxia (Nx), subsequent 10-s isokinetic sprint at 80 rpm (normoxia), IE in hypoxia (Hyp) and subsequent 10-s isokinetic sprint at 80 rpm (normoxia). The connected vertical arrows indicate the duration of the ischemia period, which in this example was 10 s.

The EMG signals were acquired using a 16-channel recording system (Myomonitor IV, Delsys Inc., Boston, MA) at a sampling rate of 1000 Hz using rectangular shaped (19.8 mm wide and 35 mm long) bipolar surface electrodes with 1 × 10 mm 99.9% Ag conductors, and with an inter-conductor distance of 10 mm (DE-2.3 Delsys Inc.). The EMG data were filtered with a high-pass filter of 20 Hz and a low-pass filter of 450 Hz using a fifth-order Butterworth filter. The system has an input impedance of > $10^{15}\Omega$ per 0.2pF of input capacitance, a common mode rejection ratio of >80 dB, signal-to-noise ratio <1.2 μV, and a pre-amplifier gain 1000 V/V ±1%. Each pedal revolution was detected using an electrogoniometer (Goniometer Biosignal Sensor S700 Joint Angle Shape Sensor; Delsys Inc. Boston) fixed on the left knee and sampled at 500 Hz. EMG and joint movement were simultaneously recorded by a portable device (Myomonitor IV, Delsys Inc. Boston) and wirelessly transmitted to a computer (EMGWorks Wireless application and EMGWorks Acquisition 3.7.1.3; Delsys, Inc. Boston).

The EMG signal corresponding to each muscle contraction was analyzed using code developed "in house" (Matlab R2012b, MathWorks, Natick, MA, USA). The EMG recordings were full-wave rectified and to provide an index of muscle activation, the amplitude characteristics were analyzed via average RMS of a 25-ms moving window for the duration of the burst. Burst onset and offset detection were determined using 20% of the maximal EMG_{RMS} activity of each burst as a reference (Baum and Li, 2003; Hug and Dorel, 2009; Torres-Peralta et al., 2014), rather than a mean threshold value from 15 consecutive bursts (Ozgünen et al., 2010). This approach yielded the same result as direct simple visual discrimination with 100% detection of all bursts. The EMG_{RMS} recorded during the last minute of a 2 min 80 W load (in normoxia) was used to normalize the remaining EMG_{RMS} data. Besides, we defined a total activity index during the sprint (TAI) as TAI = EMG_{RMS} × burst duration (ms) × number of pedal strokes during the sprint. The total activity index is similar to the integrated EMG signal, but was computed separately for each burst and excluded the baseline EMG between burst (Torres-Peralta et al., 2014). The TAI recorded during the last minute of a 2 min 80 W load (in normoxia) was used to normalize the rest of the TAI values.

The mean (MPF) and median (MdPF) power spectrum frequencies were calculated using the Fast Fourier Transform (Solomonow et al., 1990). All variables were reported as the mean values of the pedal strokes recorded during the last 10 s of the incremental exercise or the 10 s sprints. EMG variables responded similarly during the four control sprints. Therefore, to reduce EMG variability the four control sprints were averaged. EMG data are reported separately for *vastus medialis* and *lateralis*, and also as the average of the two muscles. Since the incremental exercise tests in normoxia and hypoxia were repeated, the mean of each pair was used in further analysis to represent either normoxia or hypoxia.

Statistics

Normal distribution of variables was checked with the Shapiro-Wilks test. A repeated-measures ANOVA with F_IO_2 condition (normoxia vs. hypoxia) and occlusion duration (10 vs. 60 s) was used to analyze the responses observed during the sprints. Pairwise comparisons at specific time points were performed with Student t-tests, and adjusted for multiple comparisons using the Holm–Bonferroni method. Values are reported as the mean ± standard deviation (unless otherwise stated). $P \leq 0.05$ was considered statistically significant. All statistical analyses were performed using SPSS v.15.0 for Windows (SPSS Inc., Chicago, IL) and Excel 2011 (Microsoft, Redmond, WA, USA).

RESULTS

Incremental Exercise

Compared to normoxia, Wmax, pulmonary ventilation, respiratory rate, heart rate and VO_2peak were reduced during the last 10 s of exercise in hypoxia. Additional information regarding the respiratory and cardiovascular responses to the IE can be found elsewhere (Calbet et al., 2015; Morales-Alamo et al., 2015). The ergospirometric variables corresponding to the last 10 s of incremental exercise are reported in **Table 1**, together with the corresponding electromyographic responses.

Muscle Fatigue

Compared to the control sprints, post-IE sprint performance was reduced (32–46%, $P < 0.05$; **Figure 3**) as previously reported (Morales-Alamo et al., 2015). Sprint Wpeak-i was 11% lower following post-IE in normoxia than hypoxia. Similar effects were observed in Wmean. Sprint performance was improved after ischemic recovery. Wpeak-i and Wmean were 11 and 23% higher, respectively, following 60 than 10 s of occlusion ($P < 0.05$), as previously reported (Morales-Alamo et al., 2015).

TABLE 1 | Ergospirometric and electromyographic responses during the last 10 s of the incremental exercise to exhaustion in normoxia ($P_IO_2 \approx$ 143 mmHg) and severe hypoxia ($P_IO_2 \approx$ 73 mmHg).

	Normoxia	Hypoxia	P
F_IO_2 (%)	20.8 ± 0.1	10.8 ± 0.1	<0.001
SpO_2 (%)	93.1 ± 4.4	64.6 ± 4.6	<0.001
Wmax (W)	259.2 ± 32.0	170.1 ± 21.0	<0.001
VO_2peak (l.min^{-1})	3.62 ± 0.37	2.41 ± 0.29	<0.001
V_E (l.min^{-1})	143.5 ± 19.5	123.8 ± 22.5	<0.001
RR (breaths.min^{-1})	60.2 ± 7.6	53.8 ± 7.0	<0.001
HR (beats.min^{-1})	185.4 ± 6.0	175.1 ± 9.0	<0.001
$P_{ET}O_2$(mmHg)	113.2 ± 2.3	58.6 ± 2.8	<0.001
$P_{ET}CO_2$(mmHg)	32.1 ± 2.6	27.5 ± 2.1	<0.001
RER	1.15 ± 0.03	1.35 ± 0.11	<0.001
VCO_2(l.min^{-1})	4.12 ± 0.49	3.23 ± 0.41	<0.001
Pedaling rate (rpm)	56.7 ± 7.4	55.4 ± 5.9	0.5
VM RMSraw (μV)	134.2 ± 60.1	113.3 ± 48.9	<0.05
VL RMSraw (μV)	103.0 ± 30.9	88.9 ± 30.9	0.12
Average RMSraw (μV)	121.0 ± 37.7	101.1 ± 33.7	<0.01
VM RMSNz (A.U.)	219.1 ± 77.6	182.3 ± 45.5	<0.05
VL RMSNz (A.U.)	193.7 ± 76.4	165.0 ± 62.4	0.07
Average RMSNz (A.U.)	206.4 ± 61.2	173.7 ± 41.8	<0.05
VM TAINz (A.U.)	289.5 ± 109.6	222.6 ± 88.1	<0.001
VL TAINz (A.U.)	246.5 ± 102.2	187.5 ± 73.1	<0.05
Average TAINz (A.U.)	268.0 ± 80.1	205.0 ± 68.2	<0.001
VM MPF (Hz)	84.2 ± 18.4	89.6 ± 18.0	0.13
VL MPF (Hz)	84.1 ± 18.6	89.6 ± 17.8	0.13
Average MPF (Hz)	84.2 ± 18.5	89.6 ± 17.9	0.13
VM MdPF (Hz)	68.6 ± 12.3	73.3 ± 14.8	<0.05
VL MdPF (Hz)	68.5 ± 12.5	73.0 ± 14.6	<0.05
Average MdPF (Hz)	68.6 ± 12.4	73.1 ± 14.7	<0.05
VM Burst (ms)	401.9 ± 51.7	362.5 ± 55.9	0.12
VL Burst (ms)	401.4 ± 55.2	368.3 ± 55.7	0.10
Average Burst (ms)	401.7 ± 49.4	365.4 ± 52.8	0.10

F_IO_2, inspiratory oxygen fraction; SpO_2, hemoglobin saturation in capillary blood measured by pulse oximetry; Wmax, power output at exhaustion; VO_2, oxygen consumption; V_E, pulmonary ventilation; RR, respiratory rate; HR, heart rate; $P_{ET}O_2$, end-tidal O_2 pressure; $P_{ET}CO_2$, end-tidal CO_2 pressure; RER, respiratory exchange ratio; VCO_2, CO_2 production; rpm, revolutions per minute; VL, vastus lateralis; VM, vastus medialis; RMSraw, raw root mean square; RMSNz, normalized root mean square; TAINz, Normalized total activation index (arbitrary units, A.U.); MPF, mean power frequency; MdPF, median power frequency; Burst, burst duration; Average, mean of VM and VL.

EMG responses

Vastus Lateralis EMGs

Figure 2 depicts an example of the EMG recordings during one experimental day. During the last 10 s of the incremental exercise to exhaustion the raw (average of the two muscles) and normalized RMS were 16% lower in hypoxia than in normoxia ($P < 0.05$) (**Table 1**). The average normalized TAI was also lower (23%) in hypoxia than in normoxia ($P < 0.001$). The median frequency was 6% lower in normoxia than hypoxia ($P <$ 0.05). The mean and median frequencies during the last 10 s of the IE remained at the same level during the subsequent sprints.

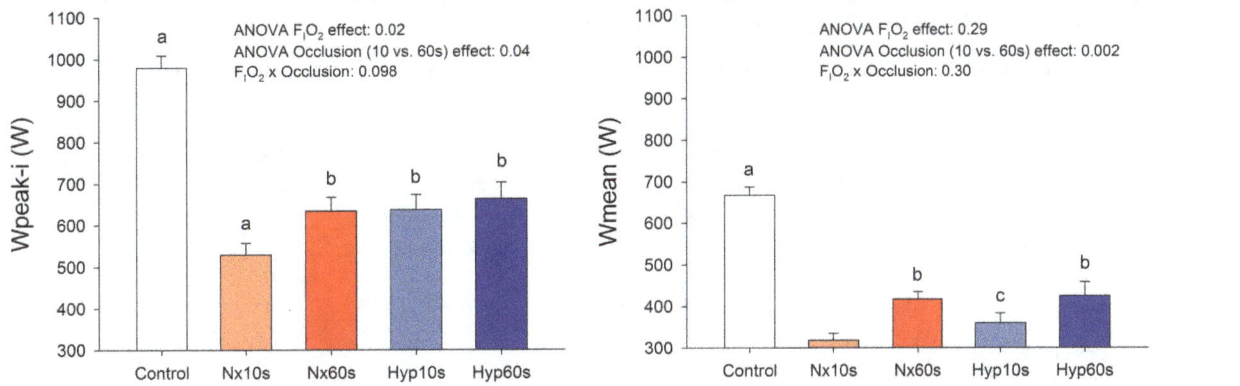

FIGURE 3 | Power output. Peak (Wpeak-i) and mean (Wmean) power output during sprint exercise performed at the end of an incremental exercise to exhaustion in normoxia ($P_IO_2 \approx 143$ mmHg) and severe hypoxia ($P_IO_2 \approx 73$ mmHg), after 10 or 60 s of occlusion of the circulation. [a]$P < 0.05$ compared with the other conditions; [b]$P < 0.05$ compared with Nx10s; [c]$P < 0.05$ compared with Nx60s.

TABLE 2 | *Vastus lateralis* electromyographic variables in response to sprint exercise performed at the end of an incremental exercise to exhaustion in normoxia ($P_IO_2 \approx 143$ mmHg) and severe hypoxia ($P_IO_2 \approx 73$ mmHg), after 10 or 60 s of occlusion of the circulation.

	Control sprint	Nx10s	Nx60s	Hyp10s	Hyp60s	Main Oxy (*P*)	Main Occ (*P*)	Interaction Oxy x Occ (*P*)
RMSraw (μV)	238.1 ± 82.0[a]	153.2 ± 64.7	137.1 ± 53.2	160.2 ± 68.7	161.8 ± 61.8	0.220	0.706	0.429
RMSNz (A.U.)	475.1 ± 155.2[a]	317.3 ± 95.1	254.6 ± 110.0	344.2 ± 126.4[c]	317.0 ± 172.4	0.112	0.059	0.436
Burst (ms)	331.9 ± 24.6[b,d]	299.7 ± 22.7[c]	324.6 ± 27.7	305.5 ± 23.8[c]	337.3 ± 34.4[b,d]	0.026	0.001	0.381
TAINz (A.U.)	1023.1 ± 340.6[a]	600.8 ± 268.8	581.5 ± 244.2	642.9 ± 297.0	715.8 ± 288.2	0.12	0.729	0.326
MPF (Hz)	93.9 ± 9.7[b,c]	81.9 ± 14.2	79.5 ± 16.4	86.3 ± 20.3	89.5 ± 17.2	0.006	0.837	0.212
MdPF (Hz)	80.2 ± 6.0[b,c,d]	66.4 ± 9.4[e]	67.0 ± 13.6	71.4 ± 16.6	74.7 ± 13.9[c]	0.011	0.255	0.500

[a]$P < 0.05$ compared with the other conditions.
[b]$P < 0.05$ compared with Nx10s.
[c]$P < 0.05$ compared with Nx60s.
[d]$P < 0.05$ compared with Hyp10s.
[e]$P < 0.05$ compared with Hyp60s.
RM ANOVA (2 × 2) Main Oxy: main oxygenation effect due to the conditions in which was performed the incremental exercise test (Nx, Normoxia; Hyp, hypoxia); RM ANOVA (2 × 2) Main Occ, Main Occlusion effect due to the duration of the occlusion (10 vs. 60 s); Wpeak-i, instantaneous peak power in the sprint; Wmean, mean power in the 10 s sprint; RMSraw, raw root mean square; RMSNz, Normalized root mean square; Burst, burst duration; TAINz, Normalized total activation index (arbitrary units, A.U.); MPF, mean power frequency; MdPF, median power frequency.

The average RMS, RMSNz, and TAINz were 1.6-, 1.7-, and 2.9-fold higher during the sprints post-IE than during the last 10 s of the IE (all, $P < 0.05$). Compared to the control sprints, the RMSraw and the normalized RMSNz were reduced by 36 and 35%, respectively, in the sprints performed after the IE (**Table 2**). Although the 60 s occlusion caused a 14% lower RMSNz compared to the 10 s occlusion, this difference did not reach statistical significance (Main effect $P = 0.059$). Compared to the control sprints the TAINz was reduced by 42 and 34% during the sprints performed after the incremental test in normoxia and hypoxia, respectively ($P < 0.05$).

Compared to the control sprint, the median frequency was reduced by 18 and 9% in the sprints that followed the IEs in normoxia and hypoxia, respectively (both, $P < 0.05$) (**Table 3**). Thus, the median frequency was 9% lower in the sprints that followed IE in normoxia than in hypoxia (Main effect $P = 0.011$). MPF changes were essentially similar to MdPF (**Tables 1–4**).

Compared to the control sprints, the duration of the bursts was reduced by 9% in the sprints performed after 10 s occlusions. Nevertheless, after 60 s of occlusion, the duration of burst in the following sprints achieved the same value as in the control sprints (331.9 ± 24.6 and 331.0 ± 29.7 ms, control and 60 s after IE, respectively, $P = 0.91$). The duration of the bursts was 3% longer in the sprints that followed an IE in hypoxia than normoxia ($P = 0.03$). The average contraction time (i.e., burst duration x pedaling rate) was 15% lower during the last 10 s of IE than during the post-IE sprints ($P < 0.001$).

Vastus Medialis EMGs

The *vastus medialis* EMG responses to incremental (**Table 1**) and sprint exercise (**Table 3**) were similar to those described for the *vastus lateralis*. Therefore, we combined both *vastus* EMGs responses to reduce variability (**Table 4**). The combined response was similar to that reported for *vastus lateralis* and *medialis*, but with lower variability, confirming some of the effects that did not reach statistical significance when only analyzed using a single muscle EMG recordings.

TABLE 3 | *Vastus medialis* electromyographic variables in response to sprint exercise performed at the end of an incremental exercise to exhaustion in normoxia and severe hypoxia ($P_IO_2 \approx 73$ mmHg), after 10 or 60 s of occlusion of the circulation.

	Control sprint	Nx10s	Nx60s	Hyp10s	Hyp60s	Main Oxy (*P*)	Main Occ (*P*)	Interaction Oxy × Occ (*P*)
RMSraw (μV)	263.5 ± 115.7[b,c,e]	177.4 ± 95.0[d]	193.9 ± 121.3	204.2 ± 103.1	183.9 ± 81.1	0.333	0.943	0.038
RMSNz (A.U.)	410.4 ± 163.3[a]	284.0 ± 97.1[d]	276.4 ± 126.1	333.0 ± 143.1	279.7 ± 104.8[d]	0.078	0.137	0.098
Burst (ms)	342.2 ± 27.7[b]	309.4 ± 42.5[c]	355.2 ± 49.4[d]	322.0 ± 53.1	347.8 ± 37.9[b]	0.743	0.017	0.154
TAINz (A.U.)	1152.1 ± 463.3[a]	701.1 ± 359.9[d]	809.0 ± 498.6	829.7 ± 397.9	820.7 ± 335.6	0.118	0.638	0.119
MPF (Hz)	94.3 ± 9.9[b,c,d]	81.9 ± 14.0	79.8 ± 15.8	85.8 ± 19.2	89.4 ± 17.4	0.008	0.703	0.241
MdPF (Hz)	80.8 ± 6.7[a]	66.2 ± 9.2	67.1 ± 13.4	71.3 ± 16.6	74.6 ± 14.1[b,c]	0.011	0.218	0.587

[a]$P < 0.05$ compared with the other conditions.
[b]$P < 0.05$ compared with Nx10s.
[c]$P < 0.05$ compared with Nx60s.
[d]$P < 0.05$ compared with Hyp10s.
[e]$P < 0.05$ compared with Hyp60s.
RM ANOVA (2 × 2) Main Oxy, main oxygenation effect due to the conditions in which was performed the incremental exercise test (Nx, Normoxia; Hyp, hypoxia); RM ANOVA (2 × 2) Main Occ, Main Occlusion effect due to the duration of the occlusion (10 vs. 60 s); RMSraw, raw root mean square; RMSNz, Normalized root mean square; Burst, burst duration; TAINz, Normalized total activation index (arbitrary units, A.U.); MPF, mean power frequency; MdPF, median power frequency.

TABLE 4 | Electromyographic variables (average of *vastus medialis* and *lateralis*) in response to sprint exercise performed at the end of an incremental exercise to exhaustion in normoxia ($P_IO_2 \approx 143$ mmHg) and severe hypoxia ($P_IO_2 \approx 73$ mmHg), after 10 or 60 s of occlusion of the circulation.

	Control	Nx10s	Nx60s	Hyp10s	Hyp60s	Main Oxy (*P*)	Main Occ (*P*)	Interaction Oxy × Occ (*P*)
RMSraw (μV)	250.8 ± 89.1[a]	165.3 ± 69.6[d]	165.5 ± 76.5	182.2 ± 79.8	172.9 ± 50.7	0.164	0.793	0.536
RMSNz (A.U.)	442.7 ± 141.9[a]	300.6 ± 88.9[d]	265.5 ± 93.9[d]	338.6 ± 122.7	298.3 ± 117.7[d]	0.042	0.043	0.835
Burst (ms)	337.1 ± 23.9[b,d]	304.5 ± 29.8[c]	339.9 ± 36.0[d]	313.7 ± 36.0	342.6 ± 35.3[b,d]	0.305	0.005	0.754
TAINz (A.U.)	1089.7 ± 355.0	653.1 ± 274.8[d]	720.1 ± 323.5	739.6 ± 331.4	769.7 ± 238.9	0.082	0.510	0.575
MPF (Hz)	94.1 ± 9.8[b,c,d]	81.9 ± 14.1	79.6 ± 16.1	86.0 ± 19.7	89.5 ± 17.3[b,c]	0.007	0.769	0.221
MdPF (Hz)	80.5 ± 6.3[b,c,d]	66.3 ± 9.2	67.0 ± 13.5	71.3 ± 16.6	74.6 ± 14.0[b,c]	0.011	0.234	0.543

[a]$P < 0.05$ compared with the other conditions.
[b]$P < 0.05$ compared with Nx10s.
[c]$P < 0.05$ compared with Nx60s.
[d]$P < 0.05$ compared with Hyp10s.
RM ANOVA (2 × 2) Main Oxy, main oxygenation effect due to the conditions in which was performed the incremental exercise test (Nx, Normoxia; Hyp, hypoxia); RM ANOVA (2 × 2) Main Occ, Main Occlusion effect due to the duration of the occlusion (10 vs. 60 s); RMSraw, raw root mean square; RMSNz, Normalized root mean square; Burst, burst duration; TAINz, Normalized total activation index (arbitrary units, A.U.); MPF, mean power frequency; MdPF, median power frequency.

Muscle Metabolites

Muscle metabolites and the aerobic and anaerobic energy yield during the sprints have been reported elsewhere (Morales-Alamo et al., 2015). Briefly, ATP and PCr concentrations were reduced to a similar extent both in normoxia and hypoxia (ANOVA time effect: $P < 0.05$). From the 10th to 60th s of ischemic recovery ATP concentration remained unchanged while PCr declined an additional ~5% (ANOVA time effect: $P < 0.05$ compared to Post and $P < 0.001$, compared to PRE). Muscle lactate concentration was increased to similar values 10 s after both incremental exercise tests (93.5 ± 24.3 and 88.3 ± 26.6 mmol kg d.w.$^{-1}$, in normoxia and hypoxia, respectively (ANOVA time effect: $P < 0.001$). From the 10th to 60th s of ischemia muscle lactate was increased by 24.0 ± 20.7 and 21.6 ± 24.5 mmol kg d.w.$^{-1}$, and muscle pH reduced by 0.102 ± 0.040 and 0.109 ± 0.041 units, after the IE in normoxia and hypoxia, respectively (ANOVA time effect: $P < 0.01$).

DISCUSSION

This investigation confirms, in agreement with previous studies using constant intensity (Marcora and Staiano, 2010) and incremental exercise to exhaustion in normoxia (Coelho et al., 2015), that task failure during incremental exercise in normoxia is not caused by muscle fatigue. The present study extends these findings to whole-body incremental exercise in severe hypoxia. We have also shown that muscle activation during the last 10 s of an incremental exercise to exhaustion is lower in severe hypoxia than in normoxia. This reduction in muscle activation cannot be explained by differences in metabolite accumulation between hypoxia and normoxia, and likely reflects central mechanisms of fatigue, which recovered, at least partly, during the next 10 or 60 s of ischemia, as reflected by the greater activation of the muscles during the subsequent sprint. The latter occurred despite the lower energy availability and the greater accumulation of metabolites after the ischemic recoveries. We have shown that neuromuscular performance, as assessed by a sprint test, at the end of an incremental exercise to exhaustion, is greater when the incremental exercise has been performed in severe acute hypoxia than in normoxia despite similar muscle metabolite accumulation. This is also compatible with the incremental exercise in hypoxia ending by central mechanism/s acting earlier, i.e., with a lower amount of peripheral fatigue in hypoxia than in normoxia. This reduction in sprint performance is accompanied by a greater reduction in muscle activation (as reflected by the EMG_{RMS} changes) in the sprints carried out after IE in normoxia than hypoxia. This could also be interpreted as indicative of slower recovery of central mechanisms of fatigue during the 10 s of ischemic recovery that followed the IE performed in normoxia compared to the sprint performed after the IE in hypoxia.

Strikingly, following 60 s of recovery with complete occlusion of the circulation sprint performance was higher than that observed immediately following 10 s of occlusion, as previously reported (Morales-Alamo et al., 2015). This improvement in performance was achieved with lower EMG_{RMS} compared to the sprints executed after 10 s of ischemia. Thus, this investigation demonstrates dissociation between the recovery of the EMG_{RMS} and the recovery of power output. Since occlusion resulted in an increase of muscle lactate and H^+ accumulation from 10 to 60 s of occlusion (Morales-Alamo et al., 2015), the present experiments support the concept that muscle acidification contributes to reduce EMG_{RMS}. In addition, we have demonstrated that despite similar muscle concentrations of lactate and H^+ at the beginning of the respective sprints, the MPF and MdPF during sprint exercise are reduced by muscle fatigue when the sprint is performed after an incremental exercise in normoxia, but not in hypoxia. MPF and MdPF did not recover from the end of the incremental exercise to the start of the sprints, or from the 10th to the 60th second of ischemia, despite cessation of neural activation and appropriate oxygenation of the brain. These results point to peripheral mechanisms being primarily responsible for the reduction of MPF and MdPF during the sprints post-IE (Juel, 1988; Brody et al., 1991). Moreover, despite greater lactate and H^+ accumulation after 60 s of ischemic recovery, sprint exercise MPF and MdPF were not further reduced; therefore these two metabolites do not seem to account for the observed reduction of MPF and MdPF with muscle fatigue (Vestergaard-Poulsen et al., 1995). We have also shown that the duration of the bursts is reduced in fatigued muscles contracting under isokinetic conditions, recovering to non-fatigued levels within 60 s, regardless of the muscular concentrations of lactate and H^+. We lastly provided evidence for a minor impact, if any, of increased group III/IV afferent feedback on sprint exercise performance.

Surface EMG Changes are More Sensitive to Central than Peripheral Fatigue

To demonstrate the existence of central fatigue it is necessary to show that during a maximal voluntary contraction, direct stimulation of motor neural pathways or cortical motoneurons results in greater levels of force than elicited voluntarily (Merton, 1954; Gandevia et al., 1996). These procedures have several constraints limiting their application to complex tasks, such as pedaling. To circumvent these problems, a commonly used approach has been to carry out potentiated and interpolated twitch assessments at exhaustion as fast as possible, i.e., 1–2 min after the task failure, when most of the reduction in power output has already been recovered (Sargeant and Dolan, 1987; Fernandez-del-Olmo et al., 2013; Froyd et al., 2013; Coelho et al., 2015). Another limitation of stimulation techniques is that muscle fatigue is task-specific (Gandevia, 2001). Stimulation techniques cannot reproduce the complexity of motor orders involving thousands of motor units from different muscles firing at different rates, which are recruited with specific timings to achieve a coordinated movement. Also, in fatigued muscles, the increase in force elicited by an interpolated twitch may be due in part to intracellular mechanisms (i.e., a peripheral mechanism that is likely related to the force/$[Ca^{2+}]_i$ relationship) (Gandevia et al., 2013), not necessarily reflecting increased central fatigue.

An alternative approach for assessing muscle fatigue is to measure the maximal power that can be generated during the task that elicits muscle fatigue (Cairns et al., 2005; Marcora and Staiano, 2010; Coelho et al., 2015). However, during whole-body exercise on the cycle ergometer, pedaling frequency slows down close to task failure (Torres-Peralta et al., 2014). Given the dependency of power on muscle contraction velocity, fatigue should ideally be tested under similar muscle contraction velocities as during isokinetic pedaling (Sargeant and Dolan, 1987).

In the present experiments, the sprints were performed in isokinetic conditions, i.e., the duration of each pedaling cycle was always the same, regardless of the state of muscle fatigue (**Figure 2**). This isokinetic approach was possible because the cycle ergometer servo-control instantaneously varied the resistance applied to the pedals depending on the force exerted resulting in a constant pedaling rate of 80 rpm. These conditions allowed us to examine the impact of fatigue on certain components of the EMG signal without the variability induced by the speed of movement.

At a given pedaling rate, the duration of contraction bursts increases with the intensity of exercise, reaching maximal values at intensities close to Wmax (Torres-Peralta et al., 2014). In all conditions and every subject, the mean intensity achieved during the 10 s sprints was above the intensity reached at exhaustion during the IEs. This result implies that concerning intensity, burst duration should have been maximal during all sprints. However, burst duration during the sprints performed after 10 s of ischemic recovery was reduced, meaning that muscles were activated during a shorter fraction of the pedaling cycle compared to the control sprints. This effect might have been caused by reduced sarcolemmal excitability as a consequence of fatigue (Sejersted and Sjogaard, 2000; Sidhu et al., 2012). Reduced sarcolemmal excitability during hand grip exercise has been associated with lactic acidosis in blood (Hilbert et al., 2012). However, if present at exhaustion, sarcolemmal excitability appears to recover in less than 60 s after a fatiguing sprint exercise (Fernandez-del-Olmo et al., 2013). In agreement, burst duration recovered within the 60 s of ischemic rest after both IEs. Despite the observed recovery of burst duration, the EMG_{RMS} was further reduced following 60 s of ischemia. Since the reduction in EMG_{RMS}

was accompanied by increased power output and normal burst duration, it seems unlikely that the lower sprint EMG_{RMS} after 60 s of ischemia originates from a failure of the muscle cells to respond to neural activation.

During high-intensity contractions, the myosin ATPase and ion pumps account for most of the energy expenditure in muscles because no energy can be diverted to biosynthetic processes as the required enzymes are blocked (Morales-Alamo and Calbet, 2014). In our experimental conditions, upon cessation of incremental exercise the ion pumps are expected to be maximally activated, particularly the Na^+-K^+ pump, which has a critical role in restoring sarcolemmal excitability (Pedersen et al., 2003; Hostrup et al., 2014). During ischemia, the energy needed to maintain the activity of the ion pumps was provided by the glycolysis and to a lesser extent by the minute amount of remaining PCr (Morales-Alamo et al., 2015). The O_2 that still remained bound to myoglobin at the end of incremental exercise was rapidly used upon occlusion due to the strong activation of mitochondrial respiration by the increased ADP concentration at task failure (Morales-Alamo et al., 2015). Femoral vein and mean capillary PO_2 were lower at exhaustion after the incremental exercise test in severe hypoxia than in normoxia (Calbet et al., 2015). Therefore, the potential contribution of the small amount of O_2 trapped in the occluded leg (or remaining bound to myoglobin) to ATP re-synthesis should have been lower in hypoxia than in normoxia. However, although more O_2 was available at exhaustion for the initial recovery in normoxia, i.e., within the first 10 s of occlusion, performance was more impaired in the sprint performed after 10 s of ischemic recovery that followed the normoxic rather than the hypoxic IEs. This result concurs with task failure occurring with a lower level of peripheral fatigue during IE in hypoxia than normoxia, as our results indicate.

Studies in cats (Hill et al., 1992; Lagier-Tessonnier et al., 1993) and rabbits (Arbogast et al., 2000) have shown increased baseline discharge frequency of group III and IV muscle afferents by PO_2 close to the values observed in the femoral vein in the present investigation (Calbet et al., 2015). Thus, lower interstitial PO_2 values in hypoxia than normoxia could have enhanced III/IV afferent feedback to cause increased inhibition of the corticospinal drive during exercise in severe acute hypoxia, as previously suggested (Calbet et al., 2015). Muscle III and IV afferent, and perhaps other sensory endings in joints and tendons, have been postulated to contribute to central fatigue (Reid, 1927; Bigland-Ritchie et al., 1986; Garland, 1991; Amann et al., 2008, 2013a). Animal studies have shown that when motoneurons are stimulated repetitively many neurons reduce their discharge frequency or stop firing (Kernell and Monster, 1982a,b; Spielmann et al., 1993). This phenomenon is likely accentuated by hypoxia. Consequently, reduced responsiveness of some motoneurons pools (central fatigue) combined with increased III/IV muscle afferent feedback and increased ventilatory demand at any given absolute intensity might have increased the perception of effort (Marcora, 2009), leading to task failure at the end of IE in hypoxia with a lower level of peripheral fatigue than in normoxia (Pierrefiche et al., 1997). Oxygenation upon exhaustion might have restored faster central fatigue at the end of the IE in hypoxia than normoxia, by reinstating within seconds normoxic interstitial PO_2 levels in the CNS. In agreement, with altitude acclimatization, oxygen delivery at VO_2max is almost restored to sea level values (Calbet and Lundby, 2009), improving brain oxygenation compared to acute hypoxia and reducing supraspinal fatigue (Goodall et al., 2014a,b).

The absolute exercise intensity at task failure was lower in hypoxia than normoxia. However, metabolite accumulation was similar regardless of F_IO_2 and, hence, differences in absolute exercise intensity do not seem to account for the differences in peripheral fatigue.

Group III and IV Muscle Afferent Stimulation does not Limit Peak Power Output during Whole-Body Sprint Exercise in Healthy Humans

Group III/IV muscle afferent neurons include a complex family of afferent endings some of which act as nociceptors while others respond to thermal, mechanical or chemical stimulation (Light et al., 2008; McCord and Kaufman, 2010; Jankowski et al., 2013). Metabolic products of muscle contraction like H^+ (Rotto and Kaufman, 1988; Light et al., 2008), lactate (Light et al., 2008), adenosine (Middlekauff et al., 1997), ATP (Light et al., 2008), nitric oxide (Arbogast et al., 2001), and inflammation mediators may also increase III/IV muscle afferent discharge (Light et al., 2008; McCord and Kaufman, 2010). It is particularly important that the response to the isolated increase of H^+, ATP and lactate is much lower than observed to the combination of the three (Light et al., 2008). Some metaboreceptive III and IV muscle afferents seem specialized in detecting innocuous levels of metabolites, while others respond to noxious levels and contribute to muscle pain (Kniffki et al., 1978; Mense, 1996). It is thought that both low and high concentration responding-endings could contribute to sympathetic reflexes and to increase the perception of effort (Light et al., 2008).

Using lumbar intrathecal fentanyl administration before exercise to block μ-opioid receptor-sensitive group, Amann and co-workers (Amann et al., 2009, 2011) studied the influence of group III and IV afferents on voluntary activation (assessed by the twitch-interpolation technique) after constant-intensity bicycling exercise. After 3 min of recovery, voluntary activation was reduced by 1.2% during the placebo trial (non-significant) and 1.7% during the fentanyl trial (Amann et al., 2011). Moreover, 3 min after a time trial that caused fatigue in 7.5 min, voluntary activation was reduced by 1.6% (compared to 0.8% in the placebo trial) (Amann et al., 2009). These results further emphasize that any potentially negative influence of III and IV muscle afferents on voluntary activation is likely small after whole-body exercise or that voluntary activation capacity recovers rather quickly (Bigland-Ritchie et al., 1986; Kennedy et al., 2015; Pageaux et al., 2015).

Amann et al. (2011) reported that despite the inhibition of III and IV muscle afferents, fentanyl markedly reduced performance (from 8.7 to 6.8 min) during a constant-intensity trial to exhaustion. In another study by the same group

(Amann et al., 2009), where the subjects performed a time trial, performance was similar in the fentanyl and placebo experiments. The reason for these discrepant effects of III/IV muscle afferents inhibition on performance is not clear (Marcora, 2010). In the case of the constant-intensity trial, there was a substantial impairment in O_2 transport in the fentanyl trial, an effect caused by reduced ventilation, leading to lower hemoglobin saturation and VO_2 with fentanyl than placebo. A slightly lower impairment of O_2 transport was reported in the time trial experiments, which could have been compensated for by increased involvement of the anaerobic metabolism (Amann et al., 2009). Marcora (2010) have suggested that during the time trial, the "belief effect" induced by reducing leg muscle pain with fentanyl-induced a fast start, which compensated for the negative effect of fentanyl on cardiorespiratory responses. As a result, exercise performance was unchanged during the time trial. During the constant-intensity trial, the "belief effect" could not induce a fast start and consequently exercise performance was reduced.

Interestingly, in both experiments with fentanyl the reduction of quadriceps potentiated twitch forces elicited by magnetic neural stimulation were greater than in the control trials (Amann et al., 2009, 2011). Assuming that a reduction in the force elicited by potentiated twitches indicates a greater level of peripheral fatigue and that the subjects exercised to their limits in all trials, Amann and co-workers studies give support to the concept that III/IV afferent feedback is used to set the limit of peripheral fatigue that is permitted. However, these experiments, combined with the present findings, show that task failure at the end of an IE to exhaustion (current study), or at the end of constant-intensity (Marcora and Staiano, 2010; Bosio et al., 2012) or a simulated time-trial competition (Amann and co-workers studies) is not due to a peripheral failure. Both types of experiments show that greater levels of peripheral fatigue are possible, but not reached because the exercise ends due to central mechanisms of fatigue (Kayser, 2003). The critical question is whether peripheral fatigue causes central fatigue and task failure through a central mechanism by activating the metaboreflex. If the latter is the main mechanism causing central fatigue and task failure a reduction in sprint performance under conditions with increased metaboreflex activation will be expected. However, our results show that this is not the case.

Metabolite accumulation at task failure and during ischemia should have promoted a sustained discharge of III/IV muscle afferents (Darques and Jammes, 1997; Darques et al., 1998; Light et al., 2008; McCord and Kaufman, 2010), an effect that would be expected to be greater after 60 than 10 s occlusions in the present investigation. Nevertheless, sprint exercise power output was higher after 60 than 10 s of ischemia. Increased metaboreflex activation should exacerbate the ventilatory response to exercise (Amann et al., 2010), as observed during the sprints performed following 60 s of ischemia in the present investigation (Morales-Alamo et al., 2015). Thus, despite increased metaboreflex activation during the sprints after 60 s of ischemia, and a theoretically worsened metabolic situation, peak and mean power output was higher during the sprints after 60 than 10 s of ischemia. Our findings appear to be at odds with the recent study by Kennedy et al. (2015), in which the occlusion of the circulation during 2 min after a 2-min sustained MVC of the knee extensors resulted in a progressive reduction of the maximal voluntary contraction (MVC) (see Figure 3A of Kennedy et al., 2015). This effect was accompanied by a progressive reduction of maximal voluntary activation indicative of increasing central fatigue (see Figure 3B of Kennedy et al., 2015). In agreement with our results, Kennedy et al. (2015) observed a fast recovery of voluntary activation upon release of the cuff, indicating that the negative influence of III/IV afferent discharge on voluntary activation was also relieved very rapidly. This quick response could be due to (i) the release of the direct compression on the femoral nerve, (ii) the washout of metabolites combined with oxygenation due to reactive hyperemia, or (iii) the combination of these effects. In our experimental conditions, the hyperemic response to the release of the cuff was likely much greater than in Kennedy et al. (2015) as reflected by the rapid increase of pulmonary VO_2 and the elevated heart rate at the beginning of the sprint (Morales-Alamo et al., 2015). Another interesting aspect of the study by Kennedy et al. (2015) is that the level of peripheral fatigue as assessed by potentiated twitches remained at the same level during the 2 min of ischemia, despite 5 × 2-s long MVC maneuvers (i.e., 10 s of maximal contractile activity with occlusion of the circulation). Thus, the 2 min of post-exercise ischemia did not worsen peripheral fatigue (Kennedy et al., 2015). Although Kennedy et al. (2015) did not measure muscle metabolites, 10 s of maximal contractile activity during the 2 min of ischemia, in combination with increased metabolic demand due to the preceding MVC (sustained during 2 min), should have increased peripheral fatigue according to the prevailing paradigm.

The present investigation strongly suggests that the inhibitory role of muscle afferent discharge on the corticospinal motor drive during maximal intensity whole-body exercise is either small or counteracted by a strong corticospinal drive (central command). Otherwise, the III/IV muscle afferent feedback due to ischemia (PO_2 close to 0 mmHg in our experimental conditions) and the metabolites accumulated during the IEs should have decreased Wpeak and Wmean during the 10 or 60 s post-ischemia sprints below the Wmax achieved at task failure in the IEs. This finding contrasts with experiments using single joint (Gandevia et al., 1996; Kennedy et al., 2015) or handgrip dynamic contractions (Broxterman et al., 2015), where a clear inhibition of voluntary activation is consistently shown.

In the present investigation, increased III/IV muscle afferent feedback could explain why the observed EMG_{RMS} were lower in the sprints performed after 60 s than after 10 s of ischemia. Likewise, that MPF and MdPF remained at task failure levels during the post-IE sprints is also consistent with an on-going negative feedback reducing motoneurons firing frequencies (Broxterman et al., 2015). However, the power output achieved during the sprints after 60 s of ischemia is close to the maximal power attainable by our subjects without phosphagens (Morales-Alamo et al., 2015), leaving little room for central mechanisms to limit sprint performance after 60 s of ischemia. Thus, it seems that 60 s of ischemic recovery allows for restoration of the central mechanisms of fatigue, despite the discharge from the III/IV muscle afferents. The latter was likely counteracted by a strong central command and a rapid reperfusion of the muscle upon the release of the cuff during the post-IE sprints. In agreement with this interpretation, Amann et al. (2009) reported no effect of intrathecal fentanyl on time trial performance, although the power output profile was dramatically changed.

Reduced Sprint EMG_{RMS} But Increased Power Output after 60 than 10 s Post-Exercise Ischemia

In vitro experiments have shown that lactate and H^+ accumulation may facilitate peripheral recovery by increasing chloride conductance (Nielsen et al., 2001; Pedersen et al., 2003; Karelis et al., 2004). Thus, an elevated glycolytic rate combined with a progressive rise of muscle temperature due to flow arrest during ischemic recovery could have exerted two opposing actions. Positively, increased glycolysis may have facilitated peripheral recovery by enhancing sarcolemmal excitability (Pedersen et al., 2003), which was likely depressed immediately after the IEs. Negatively, increased glycolysis and the subsequent metabolite accumulation may have increased III/IV muscle afferent discharge, interfering with muscle activation. The combination of both mechanisms could explain the lower EMG_{RMS} values observed during the sprints performed 60 s compared to 10 s after the IEs. If we assume that the normalized EMG_{RMS} is a valid index of corticospinal motor output, only reduced when the corticospinal motor drive is lower, a greater reduction in sprint EMG_{RMS} after prolonged (60 s) compared to shorter (10 s) ischemia would lead to the untenable conclusion that all of the improvement in Wpeak and Wmean observed from 10 to 60 s of ischemic recovery is due to peripheral mechanisms. Moreover, this peripheral-based improvement would have to be sufficient to counteract the reduced motor command. A more plausible explanation is that for a given level of neural activation, EMG_{RMS} is reduced by metabolite accumulation; i.e., EMG_{RMS} does not faithfully reflect the level of neural activation (Vestergaard-Poulsen et al., 1995). In agreement with this interpretation, it has been shown that central fatigue recovers rapidly upon cessation of contractile activity, even when peripheral fatigue remains at the same level (Bigland-Ritchie et al., 1986; Gandevia et al., 1996). Therefore, the observed reduction in sprint EMG_{RMS} after 60 s compared to 10 s of ischemic recovery is unlikely to be caused only by increased central mechanisms of fatigue.

Fatigue Reduces the Duration of the Burst during Isokinetic Sprints

The duration of the burst was similarly decreased in the sprints performed 10 s after the incremental exercise in hypoxia and normoxia. However, sprint power output was greater after the incremental exercise in hypoxia. To generate greater power, more mechanical impulse must be produced. As the duration of the bursts (a surrogate of contraction time) was similar in the sprints performed 10 s after both IEs, the subjects must have applied a greater force on the pedals after the hypoxic IE. Therefore, greater motor cortical drive was required in the sprint that occurred after hypoxia. In agreement, with this conclusion, the MPF and MdPF were higher in the sprints preceded by IE in hypoxia than normoxia, suggesting greater firing rates (Solomonow et al., 1990; Gerdle and Fugl-Meyer, 1992; Sbriccoli et al., 2003) and a lower degree of central fatigue during the sprint 10 s after the IE in hypoxia. Alternatively, central fatigue could have recovered more rapidly after the IE in hypoxia, likely due to a direct effect of oxygenation on the CNS, as previously postulated (Kayser et al., 1994; Calbet et al., 2003a,b; Amann et al., 2007; Goodall et al., 2014a).

Limitations

At the end of the incremental exercise muscle activation was much lower than during the subsequent sprints, despite the fact muscles remained ischemic and that metabolite accumulation reduces EMG_{RMS}. This finding indicates that task failure was not due to muscle fatigue; it was caused by reduced muscle activation. However, this conclusion is not based on genuine assessments of central fatigue and peripheral fatigue with stimulation techniques. Nonetheless, there is not an ideal method to quantify the extent of change in neuromuscular function (Cairns et al., 2005). Current methods based on stimulation techniques have also limitations. For example, the response of fatigued muscles to potentiated twitches depends on the method of stimulation (Froyd et al., 2013). Moreover, methods based on electrical or magnetic stimulation may give results different from those obtained using voluntary dynamic contractions. Few minutes after a 30 s all out sprint exercise (Wingate test) potentiated quadriceps twitches indicate substantial peripheral fatigue, when at the same time peak power output has completely recovered (Fernandez-del-Olmo et al., 2013).

In summary, task failure at the end of an incremental exercise to exhaustion depends more on central than peripheral mechanisms, as indicated by the fact that the level of muscle activation observed during the last 10 s of the incremental exercise was much lower than that reached 10 s later during a 10 s sprint, despite the fact that muscle remained ischemic from the end of exercise to the start of the sprint. The central components of fatigue appear to recover to a greater extent, during the first 10 s following an incremental exercise to exhaustion in hypoxia than in normoxia, concomitant with a rapid change to normoxic breathing during the recovery. We have also shown that ischemic recovery after incremental exercise to exhaustion allows for a partial restoration of power output despite increased acidification and reduced EMG_{RMS}. Moreover, this study demonstrates that MPF, MdPF and the duration of the bursts during isokinetic sprints are reduced with fatigue. Lastly, this investigation indicates that increased group III/IV muscle afferent discharge has a minor, if any, negative impact on sprint exercise performance in healthy humans.

AUTHOR CONTRIBUTIONS

Conception and design of the experiments: JC; pre-testing, experimental preparation, data collection and analysis: RT, DM, JL, IP, and JC; EMG analysis: RT, MG, and MI. The first version of the manuscript was written by RT and JC. All co-authors read, contributed comments and approved the final version of the manuscript.

ACKNOWLEDGMENTS

This study was supported by a grant from the Ministerio de Educación y Ciencia of Spain (DEP2009-11638 and FEDER) and VII Convocatoria de Ayudas a la Investigación Cátedra Real Madrid-Universidad Europea de Madrid (2015/04RM). Especially thanks are given to José Navarro de Tuero for his excellent technical assistance.

REFERENCES

Amann, M., Blain, G. M., Proctor, L. T., Sebranek, J. J., Pegelow, D. F., and Dempsey, J. A. (2010). Group III and IV muscle afferents contribute to ventilatory and cardiovascular response to rhythmic exercise in humans. *J. Appl. Physiol.* 109, 966–976. doi: 10.1152/japplphysiol.00462.2010

Amann, M., Blain, G. M., Proctor, L. T., Sebranek, J. J., Pegelow, D. F., and Dempsey, J. A. (2011). Implications of group III and IV muscle afferents for high-intensity endurance exercise performance in humans. *J. Physiol.* 589, 5299–5309. doi: 10.1113/jphysiol.2011.213769

Amann, M., and Dempsey, J. A. (2008). Locomotor muscle fatigue modifies central motor drive in healthy humans and imposes a limitation to exercise performance. *J. Physiol.* 586, 161–173. doi: 10.1113/jphysiol.2007.141838

Amann, M., Goodall, S., Twomey, R., Subudhi, A. W., Lovering, A. T., and Roach, R. C. (2013b). AltitudeOmics: on the consequences of high-altitude acclimatization for the development of fatigue during locomotor exercise in humans. *J. Appl. Physiol. (1985)* 115, 634–642. doi: 10.1152/japplphysiol.00606.2013

Amann, M., Proctor, L. T., Sebranek, J. J., Eldridge, M. W., Pegelow, D. F., and Dempsey, J. A. (2008). Somatosensory feedback from the limbs exerts inhibitory influences on central neural drive during whole body endurance exercise. *J. Appl. Physiol.* 105, 1714–1724. doi: 10.1152/japplphysiol.90456.2008

Amann, M., Proctor, L. T., Sebranek, J. J., Pegelow, D. F., and Dempsey, J. A. (2009). Opioid-mediated muscle afferents inhibit central motor drive and limit peripheral muscle fatigue development in humans. *J. Physiol.* 587, 271–283. doi: 10.1113/jphysiol.2008.163303

Amann, M., Romer, L. M., Subudhi, A. W., Pegelow, D. F., and Dempsey, J. A. (2007). Severity of arterial hypoxaemia affects the relative contributions of peripheral muscle fatigue to exercise performance in healthy humans. *J. Physiol.* 581, 389–403. doi: 10.1113/jphysiol.2007.129700

Amann, M., Venturelli, M., Ives, S. J., McDaniel, J., Layec, G., Rossman, M. J., et al. (2013a). Peripheral fatigue limits endurance exercise via a sensory feedback-mediated reduction in spinal motoneuronal output. *J. Appl. Physiol.* 115, 355–364. doi: 10.1152/japplphysiol.00049.2013

Arbogast, S., Darques, J. L., Bregeon, F., and Jammes, Y. (2001). Effects of endogenous nitric oxide in activation of group IV muscle afferents. *Muscle Nerve* 24, 247–253. doi: 10.1002/1097-4598(200102)24:2<247::AID-MUS100>3.0.CO;2-T

Arbogast, S., Vassilakopoulos, T., Darques, J. L., Duvauchelle, J. B., and Jammes, Y. (2000). Influence of oxygen supply on activation of group IV muscle afferents after low-frequency muscle stimulation. *Muscle Nerve* 23, 1187–1193. doi: 10.1002/1097-4598(200008)23:8<1187::AID-MUS5>3.0.CO;2-9

Bachasson, D., Temesi, J., Gruet, M., Yokoyama, K., Rupp, T., Millet, G. Y., et al. (2016). Transcranial magnetic stimulation intensity affects exercise-induced changes in corticomotoneuronal excitability and inhibition and voluntary activation. *Neuroscience* 314, 125–133. doi: 10.1016/j.neuroscience.2015.11.056

Baum, B. S., and Li, L. (2003). Lower extremity muscle activities during cycling are influenced by load and frequency. *J. Electromyogr. Kinesiol.* 13, 181–190. doi: 10.1016/S1050-6411(02)00110-4

Beelen, A., and Sargeant, A. J. (1991). Effect of fatigue on maximal power output at different contraction velocities in humans. *J. Appl. Physiol.* 71, 2332–2337.

Bergstrom, J. (1962). Muscle electrolytes in man. *Scand. J. Clin. Lab. Invest. Suppl.* 68, 1–110.

Bigland-Ritchie, B., and Woods, J. J. (1984). Changes in muscle contractile properties and neural control during human muscular fatigue. *Muscle Nerve* 7, 691–699. doi: 10.1002/mus.880070902

Bigland-Ritchie, B. R., Dawson, N. J., Johansson, R. S., and Lippold, O. C. (1986). Reflex origin for the slowing of motoneurone firing rates in fatigue of human voluntary contractions. *J. Physiol.* 379, 451–459. doi: 10.1113/jphysiol.1986.sp016263

Bogdanis, G. C., Nevill, M. E., Boobis, L. H., and Lakomy, H. K. (1996). Contribution of phosphocreatine and aerobic metabolism to energy supply during repeated sprint exercise. *J. Appl. Physiol.* 80, 876–884.

Bosio, A., de Morree, H. M., Rampinini, E., and Marcora, S. M. (2012). "Is exercise tolerance limited by muscle fatigue in humans?" in *The Biomedical Basis of Elite Performance* (London: The Physiological Society), PC98.

Brody, L. R., Pollock, M. T., Roy, S. H., De Luca, C. J., and Celli, B. (1991). pH-induced effects on median frequency and conduction velocity of the myoelectric signal. *J. Appl. Physiol.* 71, 1878–1885.

Broxterman, R. M., Ade, C. J., Craig, J. C., Wilcox, S. L., Schlup, S. J., and Barstow, T. J. (2015). Influence of blood flow occlusion on muscle oxygenation characteristics and the parameters of the power-duration relationship. *J. Appl. Physiol.* 118, 880–889. doi: 10.1152/japplphysiol.00875.2014

Cairns, S. P., Knicker, A. J., Thompson, M. W., and Sjøgaard, G. (2005). Evaluation of models used to study neuromuscular fatigue. *Exerc. Sport. Sci. Rev.* 33, 9–16.

Calbet, J. A., Boushel, R., Rådegran, G., Søndergaard, H., Wagner, P. D., and Saltin, B. (2003a). Determinants of maximal oxygen uptake in severe acute hypoxia. *Am. J. Physiol. Regul.* 284, R291–R303. doi: 10.1152/ajpregu.00155.2002

Calbet, J. A., Boushel, R., Radegran, G., Sondergaard, H., Wagner, P. D., and Saltin, B. (2003b). Why is VO_2max after altitude acclimatization still reduced despite normalization of arterial O_2 content? *Am. J. Physiol. Regul.* 284, R304–R316. doi: 10.1152/ajpregu.00156.2002

Calbet, J. A., Chavarren, J., and Dorado, C. (1997). Fractional use of anaerobic capacity during a 30- and a 45-s Wingate test. *Eur. J. Appl.* 76, 308–313. doi: 10.1007/s004210050253

Calbet, J. A., Losa-Reyna, J., Torres-Peralta, R., Rasmussen, P., Ponce-González, J. G., Sheel, A. W., et al. (2015). Limitations to oxygen transport and utilization during sprint exercise in humans: evidence for a functional reserve in muscle O_2 diffusing capacity. *J. Physiol.* 593, 4649–4664. doi: 10.1113/JP270408

Calbet, J. A., and Lundby, C. (2009). Air to muscle O_2 delivery during exercise at altitude. *High. Alt. Med. Biol.* 10, 123–134. doi: 10.1089/ham.2008.1099

Coelho, A. C., Cannon, D. T., Cao, R., Porszasz, J., Casaburi, R., Knorst, M. M., et al. (2015). Instantaneous quantification of skeletal muscle activation, power production, and fatigue during cycle ergometry. *J. Appl. Physiol.* 118, 646–654. doi: 10.1152/japplphysiol.00948.2014

Darques, J. L., Decherchi, P., and Jammes, Y. (1998). Mechanisms of fatigue-induced activation of group IV muscle afferents: the roles played by lactic acid and inflammatory mediators. *Neurosci. Lett.* 257, 109–112. doi: 10.1016/S0304-3940(98)00816-7

Darques, J. L., and Jammes, Y. (1997). Fatigue-induced changes in group IV muscle afferent activity: differences between high- and low-frequency electrically induced fatigues. *Brain Res.* 750, 147–154. doi: 10.1016/S0006-8993(96)01341-8

Dawson, B., Goodman, C., Lawrence, S., Preen, D., Polglaze, T., Fitzsimons, M., et al. (1997). Muscle phosphocreatine repletion following single and repeated short sprint efforts. *Scand. J. Med. Sci. Sports* 7, 206–213. doi: 10.1111/j.1600-0838.1997.tb00141.x

Dempsey, J. A., Blain, G. M., and Amann, M. (2014). Are type III-IV muscle afferents required for a normal steady-state exercise hyperpnoea in humans? *J. Physiol.* 592, 463–474. doi: 10.1113/jphysiol.2013.261925

Fernandez-del-Olmo, M., Rodriguez, F. A., Marquez, G., Iglesias, X., Marina, M., Benitez, A., et al. (2013). Isometric knee extensor fatigue following a Wingate test: peripheral and central mechanisms. *Scand. J. Med. Sci. Sports* 23, 57–65. doi: 10.1111/j.1600-0838.2011.01355.x

Froyd, C., Millet, G. Y., and Noakes, T. D. (2013). The development of peripheral fatigue and short-term recovery during self-paced high-intensity exercise. *J. Physiol.* 591, 1339–1346. doi: 10.1113/jphysiol.2012.245316

Gandevia, S. C. (2001). Spinal and supraspinal factors in human muscle fatigue. *Physiol. Rev.* 81, 1725–1789.

Gandevia, S. C., Allen, G. M., Butler, J. E., and Taylor, J. L. (1996). Supraspinal factors in human muscle fatigue: evidence for suboptimal output from the motor cortex. *J. Physiol.* 490(Pt 2), 529–536. doi: 10.1113/jphysiol.1996.sp021164

Gandevia, S. C., McNeil, C. J., Carroll, T. J., and Taylor, J. L. (2013). Twitch interpolation: superimposed twitches decline progressively during a tetanic contraction of human adductor pollicis. *J. Physiol.* 591, 1373–1383. doi: 10.1113/jphysiol.2012.248989

Garland, S. J. (1991). Role of small diameter afferents in reflex inhibition during human muscle fatigue. *J. Physiol.* 435, 547–558. doi: 10.1113/jphysiol.1991.sp018524

Gerdle, B., and Fugl-Meyer, A. R. (1992). Is the mean power frequency shift of the EMG a selective indicator of fatigue of the fast twitch motor units? *Acta Physiol. Scand.* 145, 129–138.

Goodall, S., Ross, E. Z., and Romer, L. M. (2010). Effect of graded hypoxia on supraspinal contributions to fatigue with unilateral knee-extensor contractions. *J. Appl. Physiol.* 109, 1842–1851. doi: 10.1152/japplphysiol.00458.2010

Goodall, S., Twomey, R., and Amann, M. (2014a). Acute and chronic hypoxia: implications for cerebral function and exercise tolerance. *Fatigue Biomed. Health Behav.* 2, 73–92. doi: 10.1080/21641846.2014.909963

Goodall, S., Twomey, R., Amann, M., Ross, E. Z., Lovering, A. T., Romer, L. M., et al. (2014b). AltitudeOmics: exercise-induced supraspinal fatigue is attenuated in healthy humans after acclimatization to high altitude. *Acta Physiol. (Oxf.)* 210, 875–888. doi: 10.1111/apha.12241

Guerra, B., Gomez-Cabrera, M. C., Ponce-Gonzalez, J. G., Martinez-Bello, V. E., Guadalupe-Grau, A., Santana, A., et al. (2011). Repeated muscle biopsies through a single skin incision do not elicit muscle signaling, but IL-6 mRNA and STAT3 phosphorylation increase in injured muscle. *J. Appl. Physiol.* 110, 1708–1715. doi: 10.1152/japplphysiol.00091.2011

Héroux, M. E., Taylor, J. L., and Gandevia, S. C. (2015). The use and abuse of transcranial magnetic stimulation to modulate corticospinal excitability in humans. *PLoS ONE* 10:e0144151. doi: 10.1371/journal.pone.0144151

Hilbert, M., Shushakov, V., and Maassen, N. (2012). The influence of respiratory acid-base changes on muscle performance and excitability of the sarcolemma during strenuous intermittent hand grip exercise. *J. Appl. Physiol. (1985)* 112, 571–579. doi: 10.1152/japplphysiol.00869.2010

Hill, J. M., Pickar, J. G., Parrish, M. D., and Kaufman, M. P. (1992). Effects of hypoxia on the discharge of group III and IV muscle afferents in cats. *J. Appl. Physiol.* 73, 2524–2529.

Hostrup, M., Kalsen, A., Ortenblad, N., Juel, C., Mørch, K., Rzeppa, S., et al. (2014). beta2-adrenergic stimulation enhances Ca^{2+} release and contractile properties of skeletal muscles, and counteracts exercise-induced reductions in Na^+-K^+-ATPase Vmax in trained men. *J. Physiol.* 592, 5445–5459. doi: 10.1113/jphysiol.2014.277095

Hug, F., and Dorel, S. (2009). Electromyographic analysis of pedaling: a review. *J. Electromyogr. Kinesiol.* 19, 182–198. doi: 10.1016/j.jelekin.2007.10.010

Hureau, T. J., Olivier, N., Millet, G. Y., Meste, O., and Blain, G. M. (2014). Exercise performance is regulated during repeated sprints to limit the development of peripheral fatigue beyond a critical threshold. *Exp. Physiol.* 99, 951–963. doi: 10.1113/expphysiol.2014.077974

Jankowski, M. P., Rau, K. K., Ekmann, K. M., Anderson, C. E., and Koerber, H. R. (2013). Comprehensive phenotyping of group III and IV muscle afferents in mouse. *J. Neurophysiol.* 109, 2374–2381. doi: 10.1152/jn.01067.2012

Juel, C. (1988). Muscle action potential propagation velocity changes during activity. *Muscle Nerve* 11, 714–719. doi: 10.1002/mus.880110707

Karelis, A. D., Marcil, M., Péronnet, F., and Gardiner, P. F. (2004). Effect of lactate infusion on M-wave characteristics and force in the rat plantaris muscle during repeated stimulation *in situ*. *J. Appl. Physiol.* 96, 2133–2138. doi: 10.1152/japplphysiol.00037.2004

Kayser, B. (2003). Exercise starts and ends in the brain. *Eur. J. Appl.* 90, 411–419. doi: 10.1007/s00421-003-0902-7

Kayser, B., Narici, M., Binzoni, T., Grassi, B., and Cerretelli, P. (1994). Fatigue and exhaustion in chronic hypobaric hypoxia: influence of exercising muscle mass. *J. Appl. Physiol.* 76, 634–640.

Kennedy, D. S., Fitzpatrick, S. C., Gandevia, S. C., and Taylor, J. L. (2015). Fatigue-related firing of muscle nociceptors reduces voluntary activation of ipsilateral but not contralateral lower limb muscles. *J. Appl. Physiol.* 118, 408–418. doi: 10.1152/japplphysiol.00375.2014

Kernell, D., and Monster, A. W. (1982a). Motoneurone properties and motor fatigue. An intracellular study of gastrocnemius motoneurones of the cat. *Exp. Brain Res.* 46, 197–204.

Kernell, D., and Monster, A. W. (1982b). Time course and properties of late adaptation in spinal motoneurones of the cat. *Exp. Brain Res.* 46, 191–196.

Kniffki, K. D., Mense, S., and Schmidt, R. F. (1978). Responses of group IV afferent units from skeletal muscle to stretch, contraction and chemical stimulation. *Exp. Brain Res.* 31, 511–522. doi: 10.1007/BF00239809

Lagier-Tessonnier, F., Balzamo, E., and Jammes, Y. (1993). Comparative effects of ischemia and acute hypoxemia on muscle afferents from tibialis anterior in cats. *Muscle Nerve* 16, 135–141. doi: 10.1002/mus.880160203

Light, A. R., Hughen, R. W., Zhang, J., Rainier, J., Liu, Z., and Lee, J. (2008). Dorsal root ganglion neurons innervating skeletal muscle respond to physiological combinations of protons, ATP, and lactate mediated by ASIC, P2X, and TRPV1. *J. Neurophysiol.* 100, 1184–1201. doi: 10.1152/jn.01344.2007

Lowry, O. H., and Passonneau, J. V. (1972). *A Flexible System of Enzymatic Analysis.* New York, NY: Academic Press.

Marcora, S. (2009). Perception of effort during exercise is independent of afferent feedback from skeletal muscles, heart, and lungs. *J. Appl. Physiol.* 106, 2060–2062. doi: 10.1152/japplphysiol.90378.2008

Marcora, S. (2010). Counterpoint: afferent feedback from fatigued locomotor muscles is not an important determinant of endurance exercise performance. *J. Appl. Physiol.* 108, 454–456. discussion: 456–457. doi: 10.1152/japplphysiol.00976.2009a

Marcora, S. M., and Staiano, W. (2010). The limit to exercise tolerance in humans: mind over muscle? *Eur. J. Appl.* 109, 763–770. doi: 10.1007/s00421-010-1418-6

Martin, P. G., Smith, J. L., Butler, J. E., Gandevia, S. C., and Taylor, J. L. (2006). Fatigue-sensitive afferents inhibit extensor but not flexor motoneurons in humans. *J. Neurosci.* 26, 4796–4802. doi: 10.1523/JNEUROSCI.5487-05.2006

McCord, J. L., and Kaufman, M. P. (2010). "Reflex autonomic responses evoked by group III and IV muscle afferents," in *Translational Pain Research: From Mouse to Man*, eds L. Kruger and A. R. Light (Light Boca Raton, FL: CRC Press; Taylor and Francis Group), 283–298.

Mense, S. (1996). Group III and IV receptors in skeletal muscle: are they specific or polymodal? *Prog. Brain Res.* 113, 83–100. doi: 10.1016/S0079-6123(08)61082-1

Merletti, R., and Hermens, H. (2000). Introduction to the special issue on the SENIAM European Concerted Action. *J. Electromyogr. Kinesiol.* 10, 283–286. doi: 10.1016/S1050-6411(00)00019-5

Merton, P. A. (1954). Voluntary strength and fatigue. *J. Physiol.* 123, 553–564. doi: 10.1113/jphysiol.1954.sp005070

Middlekauff, H. R., Nitzsche, E. U., Nguyen, A. H., Hoh, C. K., and Gibbs, G. G. (1997). Modulation of renal cortical blood flow during static exercise in humans. *Circ. Res.* 80, 62–68. doi: 10.1161/01.RES.80.1.62

Millet, G. Y., Aubert, D., Favier, F. B., Busso, T., and Benoît, H. (2009). Effect of acute hypoxia on central fatigue during repeated isometric leg contractions. *Scand. J. Med. Sci. Sports* 19, 695–702. doi: 10.1111/j.1600-0838.2008.00823.x

Millet, G. Y., Muthalib, M., Jubeau, M., Laursen, P. B., and Nosaka, K. (2012). Severe hypoxia affects exercise performance independently of afferent feedback and peripheral fatigue. *J. Appl. Physiol.* 112, 1335–1344. doi: 10.1152/japplphysiol.00804.2011

Morales-Alamo, D., and Calbet, J. A. (2014). Free radicals and sprint exercise in humans. *Free Radic. Res.* 48, 30–42. doi: 10.3109/10715762.2013.825043

Morales-Alamo, D., Losa-Reyna, J., Torres-Peralta, R., Martin-Rincon, M., Perez-Valera, M., Curtelin, D., et al. (2015). What limits performance during whole-body incremental exercise to exhaustion in humans? *J. Physiol.* 593, 4631–4648. doi: 10.1113/JP270487

Morales-Alamo, D., Ponce-Gonzalez, J. G., Guadalupe-Grau, A., Rodriguez-Garcia, L., Santana, A., Cusso, R., et al. (2013). Critical role for free radicals on sprint exercise-induced CaMKII and AMPKalpha phosphorylation in human skeletal muscle. *J. Appl. Physiol.* 114, 566–577. doi: 10.1152/japplphysiol.01246.2012

Nielsen, O. B., de Paoli, F., and Overgaard, K. (2001). Protective effects of lactic acid on force production in rat skeletal muscle. *J. Physiol.* 536, 161–166. doi: 10.1111/j.1469-7793.2001.t01-1-00161.x

Olson, T. P., Joyner, M. J., Eisenach, J. H., Curry, T. B., and Johnson, B. D. (2014). Influence of locomotor muscle afferent inhibition on the ventilatory response to exercise in heart failure. *Exp. Physiol.* 99, 414–426. doi: 10.1113/expphysiol.2013.075937

Ozgünen, K. T., Celik, U., and Kurdak, S. S. (2010). Determination of an optimal threshold value for muscle activity detection in EMG analysis. *J. Sports Sci. Med.* 9, 620–628.

Pageaux, B., Angius, L., Hopker, J. G., Lepers, R., and Marcora, S. M. (2015). Central alterations of neuromuscular function and feedback from group III-IV muscle afferents following exhaustive high-intensity one-leg dynamic exercise. *Am. J. Physiol. Regul.* 308, R1008–R1020. doi: 10.1152/ajpregu.00280.2014

Pedersen, T. H., Clausen, T., and Nielsen, O. B. (2003). Loss of force induced by high extracellular [K+] in rat muscle: effect of temperature, lactic acid and beta2-agonist. *J. Physiol.* 551, 277–286. doi: 10.1113/jphysiol.2003.041418

Pierrefiche, O., Bischoff, A. M., Richter, D. W., and Spyer, K. M. (1997). Hypoxic response of hypoglossal motoneurones in the *in vivo* cat. *J. Physiol.* 505(Pt 3), 785–795.

Poon, C. S., and Song, G. (2015). Type III-IV muscle afferents are not required for steady-state exercise hyperpnea in healthy subjects and patients with COPD or heart failure. *Respir. Physiol. Neurobiol.* 216, 78–85. doi: 10.1016/j.resp.2015.04.007

Rasmussen, P., Nielsen, J., Overgaard, M., Krogh-Madsen, R., Gjedde, A., Secher, N. H., et al. (2010). Reduced muscle activation during exercise related to brain oxygenation and metabolism in humans. *J. Physiol.* 588, 1985–1995. doi: 10.1113/jphysiol.2009.186767

Reid, C. (1927). The mechanism of voluntary muscular fatigue. *Br. Med. J.* 2, 545–546. doi: 10.1136/bmj.2.3481.545

Rodriguez-Falces, J., Maffiuletti, N. A., and Place, N. (2013). Twitch and M-wave potentiation induced by intermittent maximal voluntary quadriceps contractions: differences between direct quadriceps and femoral nerve stimulation. *Muscle Nerve* 48, 920–929. doi: 10.1002/mus.23856

Rossman, M. J., Venturelli, M., McDaniel, J., Amann, M., and Richardson, R. S. (2012). Muscle mass and peripheral fatigue: a potential role for afferent feedback? *Acta Physiol. (Oxf.)* 206, 242–250. doi: 10.1111/j.1748-1716.2012.02471.x

Rotto, D. M., and Kaufman, M. P. (1988). Effect of metabolic products of muscular contraction on discharge of group III and IV afferents. *J. Appl. Physiol.* 64, 2306–2313.

Sargeant, A. J., and Dolan, P. (1987). Effect of prior exercise on maximal short-term power output in humans. *J. Appl. Physiol.* 63, 1475–1480.

Sbriccoli, P., Bazzucchi, I., Rosponi, A., Bernardi, M., De Vito, G., and Felici, F. (2003). Amplitude and spectral characteristics of biceps Brachii sEMG depend upon speed of isometric force generation. *J. Electromyogr. Kinesiol.* 13, 139–147. doi: 10.1016/S1050-6411(02)00098-6

Sejersted, O. M., and Sjøgaard, G. (2000). Dynamics and consequences of potassium shifts in skeletal muscle and heart during exercise. *Physiol. Rev.* 80, 1411–1481.

Sidhu, S. K., Bentley, D. J., and Carroll, T. J. (2009). Locomotor exercise induces long-lasting impairments in the capacity of the human motor cortex to voluntarily activate knee extensor muscles. *J. Appl. Physiol.* 106, 556–565. doi: 10.1152/japplphysiol.90911.2008

Sidhu, S. K., Cresswell, A. G., and Carroll, T. J. (2012). Motor cortex excitability does not increase during sustained cycling exercise to volitional exhaustion. *J. Appl. Physiol.* 113, 401–409. doi: 10.1152/japplphysiol.00486.2012

Sidhu, S. K., Weavil, J. C., Venturelli, M., Garten, R. S., Rossman, M. J., Richardson, R. S., et al. (2014). Spinal mu-opioid receptor-sensitive lower limb muscle afferents determine corticospinal responsiveness and promote central fatigue in upper limb muscle. *J. Physiol.* 592, 5011–5024. doi: 10.1113/jphysiol.2014.275438

Solomonow, M., Baten, C., Smit, J., Baratta, R., Hermens, H., D'Ambrosia, R., et al. (1990). Electromyogram power spectra frequencies associated with motor unit recruitment strategies. *J. Appl. Physiol.* 68, 1177–1185.

Spielmann, J. M., Laouris, Y., Nordstrom, M. A., Robinson, G. A., Reinking, R. M., and Stuart, D. G. (1993). Adaptation of cat motoneurons to sustained and intermittent extracellular activation. *J. Physiol.* 464, 75–120. doi: 10.1113/jphysiol.1993.sp019625

Torres-Peralta, R., Losa-Reyna, J., González-Izal, M., Perez-Suarez, I., Calle-Herrero, J., Izquierdo, M., et al. (2014). Muscle activation during exercise in severe acute hypoxia: role of absolute and relative intensity. *High. Alt. Med. Biol.* 15, 472–482. doi: 10.1089/ham.2014.1027

Vestergaard-Poulsen, P., Thomsen, C., Sinkjaer, T., and Henriksen, O. (1995). Simultaneous 31P-NMR spectroscopy and EMG in exercising and recovering human skeletal muscle: a correlation study. *J. Appl. Physiol.* 79, 1469–1478.

Wang, W., Wang, Z., Faith, M. S., Kotler, D., Shih, R., and Heymsfield, S. B. (1999). Regional skeletal muscle measurement: evaluation of new dual-energy X-ray absorptiometry model. *J. Appl. Physiol.* 87, 1163–1171.

Yoshida, T., Abe, D., and Fukuoka, Y. (2013). Phosphocreatine resynthesis during recovery in different muscles of the exercising leg by 31P-MRS. *Scand. J. Med. Sci. Sports* 23, e313–e319. doi: 10.1111/sms.12081

18

High-Intensity Exercise in Hypoxia: Is Increased Reliance on Anaerobic Metabolism Important?

Brendan R. Scott[1]*, Paul S. R. Goods[2] and Katie M. Slattery[3]

[1] School of Psychology and Exercise Science, Murdoch University, Perth, WA, Australia, [2] Western Australian Institute of Sport, Perth, WA, Australia, [3] New South Wales Institute of Sport, Sydney Olympic Park, NSW, Australia

Keywords: metabolic stress, muscle, hypertrophy, sprints, training adaptation

***Correspondence:**
Brendan R. Scott
Brendan.Scott@murdoch.edu.au

INTRODUCTION

Hypoxic training strategies to optimize physiological exercise responses have been extensively investigated, although often with limited performance benefits over the equivalent normoxic training (Roels et al., 2007). Recently, novel methods including intermittent hypoxic resistance training (IHRT) and repeat sprint training in hypoxia (RSH) have begun to receive research attention. Early results indicate that IHRT can augment muscle hypertrophy and strength compared to normoxic training (Nishimura et al., 2010; Manimmanakorn et al., 2013a,b), while RSH improves fatigue resistance, resulting in an increased capacity for repeated maximal efforts (Galvin et al., 2013; Faiss et al., 2013b). Although performing these high-intensity activities in hypoxia appears to provide some benefits for training adaptations, the mechanisms underpinning these responses are not fully understood. The beneficial responses to high-intensity exercise in hypoxia may result from a greater reliance on anaerobic metabolism, suggesting that increased metabolic stress may drive (or at least contribute to) these adaptations (Faiss et al., 2013b; Scott et al., 2015a). Considering the likely importance of metabolic stress on adaptation to IHRT and RSH strategies, the purpose of this paper is to briefly discuss the potential benefits of high-intensity training in hypoxia with reference to the role of anaerobic processes.

IMPACTS OF HYPOXIA ON METABOLIC PROCESSES

Both resistance exercise and repeated sprints are characterized by multiple, maximal or near-maximal efforts separated by incomplete recovery periods. Performance during such activities is largely reliant on phosphocreatine (PCr) resynthesis rate (Girard et al., 2011). These high-energy phosphates provide a fuel source during brief high-intensity efforts (Girard et al., 2011), and are therefore necessary to mitigate a decline in performance across repeated efforts. Oxygen availability is an important moderator for PCr resynthesis kinetics, with slower PCr recovery under hypoxic (fraction of inspired oxygen [F_IO_2] = 10%) compared with normoxic conditions, and accelerated PCr recovery rates when breathing hyperoxic air (F_IO_2 = 100%) (Haseler et al., 1999). During IHRT and RSH, participants recover between efforts in hypoxia, likely impairing PCr resynthesis. Therefore, subsequent efforts are performed under progressively more challenging circumstances, with less energy contribution from PCr stores. This also rationalizes why performing a single set of repeat sprint exercise is relatively unaffected by hypoxic conditions (Goods et al., 2014), whereas impaired performance is observed across multiple sets (Balsom et al., 1994; Billaut et al., 2013; Kon et al., 2015; Morrison et al., 2015).

Exacerbated deoxygenation of skeletal muscle tissue in hypoxia has also been shown to increase reliance on glycolytic rather than aerobic energy production (Bowtell et al., 2014). Although it is not clear regarding the actual contributions of different systems to energy production during IHRT or RSH, research has demonstrated that short duration running performance can be maintained in hypoxia due to a shift toward anaerobic metabolism (Weyand et al., 1999). Corroborating these findings, research investigating both IHRT (Kon et al., 2010, 2012) and RSH (Goods et al., 2014; Morrison et al., 2015) has observed increased concentrations of blood lactate (a by-product of glycolysis) when exercising in hypoxia compared with normoxia. These data suggest that a decrease in oxygen availability during IHRT and RSH increases the contribution of anaerobic metabolism to total energy production, and may result in performance impairment, as first demonstrated by Balsom et al. (1994) over 20 years ago.

Nevertheless, it should be acknowledged that some research has not observed hypoxia to increase markers of metabolic stress during resistance exercise (Kurobe et al., 2015; Yan et al., 2016) or repeat sprint training (Billaut et al., 2013; Gatterer et al., 2014; Goods et al., 2015). In IHRT research, these contrasting findings may result from differences in the structure of exercise. If sufficient repetition volume during sets is not performed, the contraction time during which metabolites accumulate is decreased, and if inter-set rest periods are too long there is a greater chance for intramuscular metabolites to be removed into circulation and PCr resynthesis to occur (Scott et al., 2014, 2015a). Likewise, if adequate recovery is given between efforts during RSH training protocols, the replenishment of PCr stores may occur despite the hypoxic conditions (Girard et al., 2011). Considering that metabolic stress is a likely moderator of adaptation to hypoxic training, optimal training responses may require that exercise and work:rest ratios are structured to exaggerate anaerobic energy production and limit recovery between repeated sets.

ROLES OF METABOLIC STRESS IN ADAPTATIONS TO EXERCISE

Increased metabolic stress is proposed to stimulate various physiological processes associated with muscle hypertrophy (Schoenfeld, 2013). Nevertheless, the exact mechanisms by which this occurs are not fully understood. One possible explanation is an increase in motor unit recruitment. It is possible that metabolic acidosis causes premature fatigue in the fibers initially recruited during exercise, resulting in the activation of additional motor units to maintain the same level of force generation (Manini and Clark, 2009; Manimmanakorn et al., 2013b). This is supported by recent research that has demonstrated heightened integrated electromyography response during moderate-load IHRT compared to the same exercise in normoxia (Scott et al., 2016). If more motor units are recruited during training, a larger portion of the muscle will be stimulated to adapt (Scott et al., 2015a). Cell swelling is another potential mediator for muscle hypertrophy, resulting from metabolite accumulation within the cells and a resultant inflow of water to equilibrate the osmotic gradient (Loenneke et al., 2012). Cellular swelling can increase protein synthesis and decrease protein degradation in a range of cell types (Lang et al., 1998), and it is possible that similar responses occur in muscle cells (Loenneke et al., 2012). Finally, increased growth hormone concentrations have been reported following IHRT protocols (Kon et al., 2010, 2012, 2014), which may be caused by increased lactate build-up and/or metabolic acidosis (Loenneke et al., 2010). However, the role of exercise-induced endocrine responses may not have anabolic effects in healthy individuals as once thought (West and Phillips, 2010), and further research is required to clarify this and other potential mechanisms for hypertrophy during IHRT.

The additional stress associated with hypoxia during repeat sprint training has been demonstrated to improve glycolytic activity in muscle (Girard et al., 2011). This adaptation may be linked to an increased expression of glycolytic enzymes, such as phosphofructokinase (Puype et al., 2013), lactate dehydrogenase (Faiss et al., 2013b) and enzymes involved in pH regulation, such as carbonic anhydrase (Faiss et al., 2013b). Increased metabolic stress can also trigger adaptations that improve pH regulation and enhance blood buffering capacity following repeat sprint training (Girard et al., 2011; Faiss et al., 2013b). Likewise, the creation of a metabolically stressful environment signals adaptive processes that enhance oxygen utilization (via improved blood perfusion) (Casey and Joyner, 2012; Montero and Lundby, 2015) and delivery within the skeletal muscle to facilitate PCr resynthesis during recovery periods (Haseler et al., 1999; Faiss et al., 2013b). Finally, improved fast twitch fiber recruitment similar to that postulated for IHRT is also thought to play a role in enhanced exercise performance following RSH (Faiss et al., 2013a). It is therefore not surprising that the addition of hypoxia to place a further metabolic strain during repeat sprint training has been investigated with promising results regarding performance outcomes. While further research is needed to fully understand how metabolic stress may improve sea-level repeat sprint ability following RSH, the greater metabolic load imposed by hypoxia suggests that it does play an important part in the development of fatigue resistance within skeletal muscle during intense exercise.

RECOMMENDATIONS AND CONSIDERATIONS

Considering the apparent importance of metabolic stress on adaptations to IHRT and RSH, the actual exercise performed should be structured with this in mind. For IHRT, substantial repetition volume is likely required during sets to provide sufficient time-under-tension during which metabolic stress can accumulate. Researchers have shown that IHRT causes significant decreases in minimal oxygenation levels in working muscles (Kon et al., 2010), which indicates a more hypoxic intramuscular environment. This would theoretically place more emphasis on anaerobic energy production, increasing the concentration of metabolic by-products (Kon et al., 2010, 2012). If brief inter-set rest periods are implemented, it may be possible to attenuate the clearance of these metabolites, meaning that the next set would begin with already elevated metabolite concentrations within the muscles. Furthermore, brief rest periods would also not allow for PCr stores to be resynthesized to the same levels in hypoxia as in normoxia, whereas extended recovery periods may allow for similar PCr recover, irrespective of hypoxia (Scott et al., 2015a). Current evidence suggests that IHRT should be structured using light to moderate loads (20–70% 1-repetition maximum), which allow for substantial repetitions in each set (10–30 repetitions) and short recovery periods (30–60 s) (Scott et al., 2015a). However, the optimal level of hypoxia to use during IHRT has not yet been determined, and this could obviously have a large impact on training adaptations.

For RSH, an important consideration appears to be the level of hypoxia used, with extreme hypoxic conditions (i.e., $F_IO_2 \leq 13\%$) drastically compromising performance capacity (Goods et al., 2014). From a practical point of view, Gatterer et al. (2014) demonstrated that completing shuttle runs in the confined space of a hypoxic chamber is a viable option to gain the benefits of RSH while maintaining movement specificity. Brocherie et al. (2015) recently used this strategy with success, demonstrating that elite hockey players completing over-ground running RSH in an inflatable hypoxic marquee were able to improve and maintain repeated sprint ability for at least 3 weeks after a RSH intervention. This is critical, as previous researchers have identified limited crossover effects of RSH between cycling and running modalities (Goods et al., 2015). Regarding the actual exercise prescription for RSH, it seems that multiple sets of repeated sprints are required to observe increases in metabolic by-products (Morrison et al., 2015) and longer efforts (>6 s) are likely to have a larger impact on anaerobic metabolism (Faiss et al., 2013b; Puype et al., 2013). Additionally, as proposed for IHRT, short incomplete recoveries via exaggerated work:rest ratios (1:2–1:3) may be more successful for increasing glycolytic stress and therefore performance outcomes (Faiss et al., 2013b) than protocols employing work:rest ratios more commonly used for repeated sprint ability tests (1:5+) (Goods et al., 2015). Nevertheless, it must be acknowledged that some studies have reported varied effects of RSH on metabolic adaptation and performance improvements (Galvin et al., 2013; Brocherie et al., 2015; Goods et al., 2015). Further research is therefore needed to provide conclusive recommendations regarding RSH implementation.

It would also be remiss not to highlight that there are some potential limitations associated with IHRT and RSH strategies. It is possible that the additional stress of hypoxia may result in large performance decrements during training, which could mitigate any hypoxia-mediated benefits from such training. Decreases in concentric velocity during resistance exercise sets has been very strongly related to blood lactate concentration (a marker of anaerobic metabolism; $r = 0.93–0.97$) (Sánchez-Medina and González-Badillo, 2011), and it would therefore be expected that hypoxia-mediated increases in metabolic stress might cause a decline in resistance exercise performance. Nevertheless, our group has not observed hypoxia to impact negatively on performance during high-load resistance exercise (Scott et al., 2015b). Furthermore, several studies have reported an inability to match peak speeds, mean power output or mechanical work performed during RSH compared to normoxic repeat sprint training across an entire session (Billaut et al., 2013; Goods et al., 2014; Morrison et al., 2015). It has also been highlighted that central nervous system fatigue may play a role in decreased performance during hypoxic repeat-sprint exercise, indicating anticipatory central regulation of exercise performance (Billaut et al., 2013). This reduction in performance may attenuate the neuromuscular load of the sprint exercise, and should be considered in the planning and periodization of RSH training. The specific work:rest ratios and accumulated volume to achieve metabolic overload will also be dependent on the prior training status of each individual, which could result in different training adaptations between athletes. Similarly, it is possible that physiological responses to repeat sprint exercise may differ between males and females (Billaut and Bishop, 2009), which could result in altered training adaptations during RSH and should be examined further.

CONCLUSIONS

Adding the physiological stress of hypoxia during exercise essentially makes training more reliant on anaerobic pathways. Recent advances in scientific understanding of IHRT and RSH suggest that this metabolic stress may be an important moderator of adaptations to these novel training strategies, albeit via different mechanisms. It is likely that increased metabolic stress during IHRT causes increased motor unit recruitment and cellular swelling, which may drive (at least partially) hypertrophy of skeletal muscle (Schoenfeld, 2013). During RSH, higher intramuscular concentrations of metabolites may improve glycolytic activity, PCr resynthesis rate, oxygen utilization, and fast twitch muscle fiber behavior, effectively promoting peripheral fatigue resistance (Girard et al., 2011; Casey and Joyner, 2012; Faiss et al., 2013b).

AUTHOR CONTRIBUTIONS

BS, KS, and PG were involved in manuscript conceptualization, writing, and editing.

REFERENCES

Balsom, P., Gaitanos, G., Ekblom, B., and Sjödin, B. (1994). Reduced oxygen availability during high intensity intermittent exercise impairs performance. *Acta Physiol. Scand.* 152, 279–285. doi: 10.1111/j.1748-1716.1994.tb09807.x

Billaut, F., and Bishop, D. (2009). Muscle fatigue in males and females during multiple-sprint exercise. *Sports Med.* 39, 257–278. doi: 10.2165/00007256-200939040-00001

Billaut, F., Kerris, J. P., Rodriguez, R. F., Martin, D. T., Gore, C. J., and Bishop, D. J. (2013). Interaction of central and peripheral factors during repeated sprints at different levels of arterial O_2 saturation. *PLoS ONE* 8:e77297. doi: 10.1371/journal.pone.0077297

Bowtell, J. L., Cooke, K., Turner, R., Mileva, K. N., and Sumners, D. P. (2014). Acute physiological and performance responses to repeated sprints in varying degrees of hypoxia. *J. Sci. Med. Sport* 17, 399–403. doi: 10.1016/j.jsams.2013.05.016

Brocherie, F., Millet, G. P., Hauser, A., Steiner, T., Rysman, J., Wehrlin, J. P., et al. (2015). "Live high-train low and high" hypoxic training improves team-sport performance. *Med. Sci. Sports Exerc.* 47, 2140–2149. doi: 10.1249/MSS.0000000000000630

Casey, D. P., and Joyner, M. J. (2012). Compensatory vasodilatation during hypoxic exercise: mechanisms responsible for matching oxygen supply to demand. *J. Physiol.* 590, 6321–6326. doi: 10.1113/jphysiol.2012.242396

Faiss, R., Girard, O., and Millet, G. P. (2013a). Advancing hypoxic training in team sports: from intermittent hypoxic training to repeated sprint training in hypoxia. *Br. J. Sports Med.* 47, i45–50. doi: 10.1136/bjsports-2013-092741

Faiss, R., Leger, B., Vesin, J. M., Fournier, P. E., Eggel, Y., Deriaz, O., et al. (2013b). Significant molecular and systemic adaptations after repeated sprint training in hypoxia. *PLoS ONE* 8:e56522. doi: 10.1371/journal.pone.0056522

Galvin, H. M., Cooke, K., Sumners, D. P., Mileva, K. N., and Bowtell, J. L. (2013). Repeated sprint training in normobaric hypoxia. *Br. J. Sports Med.* 47, i74–i79. doi: 10.1136/bjsports-2013-092826

Gatterer, H., Philippe, M., Menz, V., Mosbach, F., Faulhaber, M., and Burtscher, M. (2014). Shuttle-run sprint training in hypoxia for youth elite soccer players: a pilot study. *J. Sport Sci. Med.* 13, 731–735.

Girard, O., Mendez-Villanueva, A., and Bishop, D. (2011). Repeated-sprint ability - part I: factors contributing to fatigue. *Sports Med.* 41, 673–694. doi: 10.2165/11590550-000000000-00000

Goods, P. S., Dawson, B., Landers, G. J., Gore, C. J., and Peeling, P. (2015). No additional benefit of repeat-sprint training in hypoxia than in normoxia on sea-level repeat-sprint ability. *J. Sport Sci. Med.* 14, 681–688.

Goods, P. S., Dawson, B. T., Landers, G. J., Gore, C. J., and Peeling, P. (2014). Effect of different simulated altitudes on repeat-sprint performance in team-sport athletes. *Int. J. Sports Physiol. Perform.* 9, 857–862. doi: 10.1123/ijspp.2013-0423

Haseler, L. J., Hogan, M. C., and Richardson, R. S. (1999). Skeletal muscle phosphocreatine recovery in exercise-trained humans is dependent on O_2 availability. *J. Appl. Physiol.* 86, 2013–2018.

Kon, M., Ikeda, T., Homma, T., Akimoto, T., Suzuki, Y., and Kawahara, T. (2010). Effects of acute hypoxia on metabolic and hormonal responses to resistance exercise. *Med. Sci. Sports Exerc.* 42, 1279–1785. doi: 10.1249/MSS.0b013e3181ce61a5

Kon, M., Ikeda, T., Homma, T., and Suzuki, Y. (2012). Effects of low-intensity resistance exercise under acute systemic hypoxia on hormonal responses. *J. Strength Cond. Res.* 26, 611–617. doi: 10.1519/JSC.0b013e3182281c69

Kon, M., Nakagaki, K., Ebi, Y., Nishiyama, T., and Russell, A. P. (2015). Hormonal and metabolic responses to repeated cycling sprints under different hypoxic conditions. *Growth Horm. IGF Res.* 25, 121–126. doi: 10.1016/j.ghir.2015.03.002

Kon, M., Ohiwa, N., Honda, A., Matsubayashi, T., Ikeda, T., Akimoto, T., et al. (2014). Effects of systemic hypoxia on human muscular adaptations to resistance exercise training. *Physiol. Rep.* 2:e12033. doi: 10.14814/phy2.12033

Kurobe, K., Huang, Z., Nishiwaki, M., Yamamoto, M., Kanehisa, H., and Ogita, F. (2015). Effects of resistance training under hypoxic conditions on muscle hypertrophy and strength. *Clin. Physiol. Funct. Imaging* 35, 197–202. doi: 10.1111/cpf.12147

Lang, F., Busch, G. L., Ritter, M., Volkl, H., Waldegger, S., Gulbins, E., et al. (1998). Functional significance of cell volume regulatory mechanisms. *Physiol. Rev.* 78, 247–306.

Loenneke, J. P., Fahs, C. A., Rossow, L. M., Abe, T., and Bemben, M. G. (2012). The anabolic benefits of venous blood flow restriction training may be induced by muscle cell swelling. *Med. Hypotheses* 78, 151–154. doi: 10.1016/j.mehy.2011.10.014

Loenneke, J. P., Wilson, G. J., and Wilson, J. M. (2010). A mechanistic approach to blood flow occlusion. *Int. J. Sports Med.* 31, 1–4. doi: 10.1055/s-0029-1239499

Manimmanakorn, A., Hamlin, M. J., Ross, J. J., Taylor, R., and Manimmanakorn, N. (2013a). Effects of low-load resistance training combined with blood flow restriction or hypoxia on muscle function and performance in netball athletes. *J. Sci. Med. Sport* 16, 337–342. doi: 10.1016/j.jsams.2012.08.009

Manimmanakorn, A., Manimmanakorn, N., Taylor, R., Draper, N., Billaut, F., Shearman, J. P., et al. (2013b). Effects of resistance training combined with vascular occlusion or hypoxia on neuromuscular function in athletes. *Eur. J. Appl. Physiol.* 113, 1767–1774. doi: 10.1007/s00421-013-2605-z

Manini, T. M., and Clark, B. C. (2009). Blood flow restricted exercise and skeletal muscle health. *Exerc. Sport Sci. Rev.* 37, 78–85. doi: 10.1097/JES.0b013e31819c2e5c

Montero, D., and Lundby, C. (2015). Enhanced performance after repeated sprint training in hypoxia: false or reality? *Med. Sci. Sports Exerc.* 47, 2483. doi: 10.1249/MSS.0000000000000711

Morrison, J., McLellan, C., and Minahan, C. (2015). A clustered repeated-sprint running protocol for team-sport athletes performed in normobaric hypoxia. *J. Sport Sci. Med.* 14, 857–863.

Nishimura, A., Sugita, M., Kato, K., Fukuda, A., Sudo, A., and Uchida, A. (2010). Hypoxia increases muscle hypertrophy induced by resistance training. *Int. J. Sports Physiol. Perform.* 5, 497–508. doi: 10.1123/ijspp.5.4.497

Puype, J., Van Proeyen, K., Raymackers, J. M., Deldicque, L., and Hespel, P. (2013). Sprint interval training in hypoxia stimulates glycolytic enzyme activity. *Med. Sci. Sports Exerc.* 45, 2166–2174. doi: 10.1249/MSS.0b013e31829734ae

Roels, B., Bentley, D. J., Coste, O., Mercier, J., and Millet, G. P. (2007). Effects of intermittent hypoxic training on cycling performance in well-trained athletes. *Eur. J. Appl. Physiol.* 101, 359–368. doi: 10.1007/s00421-007-0506-8

Sánchez-Medina, L., and González-Badillo, J. J. (2011). Velocity loss as an indicator of neuromuscular fatigue during resistance training. *Med. Sci. Sports Exerc.* 43, 1725–1734. doi: 10.1249/MSS.0b013e318213f880

Schoenfeld, B. J. (2013). Potential mechanisms for a role of metabolic stress in hypertrophic adaptations to resistance training. *Sports Med.* 43, 179–194. doi: 10.1007/s40279-013-0017-1

Scott, B. R., Slattery, K. M., and Dascombe, B. J. (2014). Intermittent hypoxic resistance training: does it provide added benefit? *Front. Physiol.* 5:397. doi: 10.3389/fphys.2014.00397

Scott, B. R., Slattery, K. M., and Dascombe, B. J. (2015a). Intermittent hypoxic resistance training: is metabolic stress the key moderator? *Med. Hypotheses* 84, 145–149. doi: 10.1016/j.mehy.2014.12.001

Scott, B. R., Slattery, K. M., Sculley, D. V., Hodson, J. A., and Dascombe, B. J. (2015b). Physical performance during high-intensity resistance exercise in normoxic and hypoxic conditions. *J. Strength Cond. Res.* 29, 807–815. doi: 10.1519/JSC.0000000000000680

Scott, B. R., Slattery, K. M., Sculley, D. V., Lockhart, C., and Dascombe, B. J. (2016). Acute physiological responses to moderate-load resistance exercise In hypoxia. *J. Strength Cond. Res.* doi: 10.1519/jsc.0000000000001649. [Epub ahead of print].

West, D. W., and Phillips, S. M. (2010). Anabolic processes in human skeletal muscle: restoring the identities of growth hormone and testosterone. *Phys. Sportsmed.* 38, 97–104. doi: 10.3810/psm.2010.10.1814

Weyand, P. G., Lee, C. S., Martinez-Ruiz, R., Bundle, M. W., Bellizzi, M. J., and Wright, S. (1999). High-speed running performance is largely unaffected by hypoxic reductions in aerobic power. *J. Appl. Physiol.* 86, 2059–2064.

Yan, B., Lai, X., Yi, L., Wang, Y., and Hu, Y. (2016). Effects of five-week resistance training in hypoxia on hormones and muscle strength. *J. Strength Cond. Res.* 30, 184–193. doi: 10.1519/JSC.0000000000001056

19

Variations in Hypoxia Impairs Muscle Oxygenation and Performance During Simulated Team-Sport Running

*Alice J. Sweeting[1], François Billaut[1, 2], Matthew C. Varley[1], Ramón F. Rodriguez[1], William G. Hopkins[1] and Robert J. Aughey[1]**

[1] Institute of Sport, Exercise and Active Living, Victoria University, Melbourne, VIC, Australia, [2] Département de Kinesiology, Université Laval, Québec, QC, Canada

Correspondence:
Robert J. Aughey
Robert.Aughey@vu.edu.au

Purpose: To quantify the effect of acute hypoxia on muscle oxygenation and power during simulated team-sport running.

Methods: Seven individuals performed repeated and single sprint efforts, embedded in a simulated team-sport running protocol, on a non-motorized treadmill in normoxia (sea-level), and acute normobaric hypoxia (simulated altitudes of 2,000 and 3,000 m). Mean and peak power was quantified during all sprints and repeated sprints. Mean total work, heart rate, blood oxygen saturation, and quadriceps muscle deoxyhaemoglobin concentration (assessed via near-infrared spectroscopy) were measured over the entire protocol. A linear mixed model was used to estimate performance and physiological effects across each half of the protocol. Changes were expressed in standardized units for assessment of magnitude. Uncertainty in the changes was expressed as a 90% confidence interval and interpreted via non-clinical magnitude-based inference.

Results: Mean total work was reduced at 2,000 m (−10%, 90% confidence limits ±6%) and 3,000 m (−15%, ±5%) compared with sea-level. Mean heart rate was reduced at 3,000 m compared with 2,000 m (−3, ±3 min^{-1}) and sea-level (−3, ±3 min^{-1}). Blood oxygen saturation was lower at 2,000 m (−8, ±3%) and 3,000 m (−15, ±2%) compared with sea-level. Sprint mean power across the entire protocol was reduced at 3,000 m compared with 2,000 m (−12%, ±3%) and sea-level (−14%, ±4%). In the second half of the protocol, sprint mean power was reduced at 3,000 m compared to 2,000 m (−6%, ±4%). Sprint mean peak power across the entire protocol was lowered at 2,000 m (−10%, ±6%) and 3,000 m (−16%, ±6%) compared with sea-level. During repeated sprints, mean peak power was lower at 2,000 m (−8%, ±7%) and 3,000 m (−8%, ±7%) compared with sea-level. In the second half of the protocol, repeated sprint mean power was reduced at 3,000 m compared to 2,000 m (−7%, ±5%) and sea-level (−9%, ±5%). Quadriceps muscle deoxyhaemoglobin concentration was lowered at 3,000 m compared to 2,000 m (−10, ±12%) and sea-level (−11, ±12%).

Conclusions: Simulated team-sport running is impaired at 3,000 m compared to 2,000 m and sea-level, likely due to a higher muscle deoxygenation.

Keywords: altitude, non-motorized treadmill, near-infrared spectroscopy, repeated sprints

INTRODUCTION

Athletic performance is reduced at altitude, including elevations of 580 m (Gore et al., 1997). Team-sport matches are contested at a range of terrestrial altitudes including 1,600 m (Johannesburg, South Africa) and 3,600 m (La Paz, Bolivia). The impact of moderate to high altitude on junior-elite soccer performance has recently been investigated (Aughey et al., 2013; Garvican et al., 2013; Buchheit et al., 2015). At 1,600 m, total distance and high-speed running were reduced by 9 and 15%, respectively (Garvican et al., 2013). At 3,600 m, the 5-min peak period of high-speed running and total distance covered was lowered by 20.8 and 9.1%, respectively (Aughey et al., 2013). Acclimatization to, and native residence at, 3,600 m does not protect against the detrimental effects of altitude on team-sport athlete match running (Aughey et al., 2013). Altitude therefore has a substantial impact on running performance during junior-elite soccer matches. Understanding the magnitude and impact of altitude exposure on team-sport match running may assist in optimizing athlete physical preparation for playing at altitude.

The influence of altitude on team-sport athlete match running is typically investigated through repeated sprint laboratory studies. The capacity to perform sprint efforts is considered important for scoring during team-sport matches (Faude et al., 2012). Laboratory repeated sprint tests, performed on a non-motorized treadmill, are generally designed to replicate periods of match running and allow measurement of an athlete's capacity to resist fatigue. In team-sport athletes, peak power during three sets of nine repeated sprints, of 4-s in duration, was maintained at a simulated altitude of 3,000 m but not 4,000 m (Goods et al., 2014). The peak speed performed by untrained individuals is reduced during 10 6-s repeated-sprints in varying hypoxic conditions compared to normoxia (Bowtell et al., 2014). The distance covered by amateur team-sport athletes during the final two sets of four 4-s repeated sprints was also reduced in normobaric hypoxia compared to normoxia (Morrison et al., 2015). Simulated altitude therefore has a detrimental effect on laboratory repeated sprint performance. However, assessing the impact of titrated altitude during controlled laboratory studies does not replicate the chaotic and complex nature of team-sport matches (Sirotic and Coutts, 2007). During repeated sprint laboratory studies, with known exercise and rest periods, participants may plan their physical output. In matches, team-sport athletes perform low-speed activity interspersed with high-intensity movement. Exercise intensity may be regulated dependent upon an individual's ability to perform high-intensity activity (Castagna and Abt, 2003). Under conditions of environmental stress, athletes may moderate this low-speed activity to preserve the capacity to perform hard efforts, including repeated sprints (Aughey et al., 2013, 2014). Laboratory studies designed to mimic environmental stress, such as simulating altitude, should therefore include periods of lower-intensity work interspersed with repeated sprint efforts to simulate the running performed by team-sport athletes during matches.

The impact of altitude on physical performance during a simulated team-sport movement protocol was recently examined (Aldous et al., 2015). Total and high-speed distance covered by team-sport athletes during a 90-min protocol was reduced by 4% at 1,000 m simulated altitude compared to sea-level. The distance covered in each of the two 45-min halves was 10% lower at altitude compared to sea-level, with total sprint distance also reduced in the final 15 min of the protocol. Perceived exertion across the entire protocol was also 7% lower at sea-level compared to altitude. Since team-sport matches are contested at a range of altitudes around the world, the dose-response relationship of varying altitudes on simulated match running should be explored. The subsequent impact of these altitudes on the physiological determinants of team-sport running should also be examined.

Physiological determinants including neural, ionic and metabolic factors underpin the capacity to perform repeated sprint efforts (Billaut et al., 2012). Moderately trained individuals with a high maximal oxygen uptake ($\dot{V}O_{2max}$) may have an increased resynthesis rate of phosphocreatine (PCr), a vital substrate during intermittent high-intensity exercise (Harris et al., 1976). Attained exclusively via aerobic sources, the resynthesis of PCr is dependent upon O_2 and can be completely suppressed via limb blood flow occlusion (Harris et al., 1976). Muscle O_2 kinetics and PCr resynthesis are also tightly linked (Kime et al., 2003). A high perfusion and reoxygenation rate of the active musculature during recovery periods, assessed via near-infrared spectroscopy (NIRS), is paramount to reproduce a high performance in a subsequent bout (Ufland et al., 2012). The delivery of O_2 is also highly sensitive to manipulations of environmental O_2 and compromised at altitude, which may contribute to impairment during repeated-sprint exercise (Billaut and Buchheit, 2013). The capacity of skeletal muscle to be reoxygenated during 30 s of passive rest between repeated sprint running efforts is reduced by up to 33% in hypoxia (Bowtell et al., 2014), although NIRS has not been utilized to assess muscle reoxygenation during simulated team-sport running at varying altitudes. Since PCr resynthesis is a main factor of performance during repeated sprint efforts, the slower repletion of this substrate at altitude may be detrimental to team-sport running performance. Therefore, the aim of the present study was to quantify the effect of acute, titrated hypoxia on physical output and physiological responses during simulated team-sport running.

METHODS

Participants

Seven (six males and one female) individuals (age 27.0 ± 6.6 years; height 179.7 ± 6.1 cm; $\dot{V}O_{2max}$ 59.5 ± 5.1 mL.kg^{-1}.min^{-1}; body mass 75.1 ± 10.2 kg at commencement of study, [mean ± Standard Deviation (SD)] provided written informed consent to participate in the study. Participants were from team-sport plus endurance backgrounds and trained at least twice per week. The study was approved by the university Human Research Ethics Committee and conformed to the declaration of Helsinki. Participants were sea-level natives and had not visited >2,000 m altitude for more than 24 h in the 4 months prior to participating in the study.

Study Design

A single-blind randomized design, with altitude counter-balanced, was employed. All testing was conducted within a 23.92 m^2 environmental exercise laboratory. During their first visit, participants completed a $\dot{V}O_{2max}$ test to assess maximal aerobic power. The test consisted of 3 × 4 min periods of incremental running before speed was maintained and gradient increased by 1% each minute until volitional exhaustion (Robertson et al., 2010). Participants then returned for a separate familiarization session, involving a 5 min warm-up at 100 W on a cycle ergometer (Velotron, Seattle, USA) followed by four maximal 4 s sprints, each separated by 14 s of passive recovery, on the non-motorized treadmill (Woodway Force, Waukesha, WI, USA). Individual speed ranges for the simulated team-sport movement protocol, described below, were established from the maximal speed attained during six sprint efforts on the non-motorized treadmill (Sirotic and Coutts, 2008). Participants then completed a modified (condensed to 13 min) version of the team-sport running protocol. The familiarization session, 1 week after the preliminary visit, involved completion of the entire simulated team-sport movement protocol and NIRS measurements. Participants then completed a testing session at sea-level followed by two randomized, counter-balanced sessions under titrated hypoxic conditions. Each session involved a standardized 5 min cycling warm-up at 100 W and completion of the simulated team-sport running protocol. Normobaric hypoxia was created through nitrogen injection into the environmental exercise laboratory. The F_iO_2 was ~0.163 and ~0.143, simulating altitudes of 2,000 m and 3,000 m, respectively. Simulated altitudes were based on the definition of low to moderate altitude (Bartsch et al., 2008). Each session was conducted at similar times of the day for each participant to limit influence of the circadian rhythm on sprint-induced neuromuscular fatigue (Giacomoni et al., 2006). All sessions were separated by 1 week. Participants were encouraged to refrain from physical activity and caffeine in the 24 h prior to each session.

Simulated Team-Sport Running Protocol

Participants were secured onto the non-motorized treadmill using a manufacturer provided belt. The belt connected to a horizontal force transducer, adjusted for each participant by measuring and reproducing the displacement between the anterior superior illiac spine and the belt, as per Serpiello et al. (2011). Participants were encouraged to keep this consistent throughout all sessions. The force transducers were calibrated, before each participant's session, according to the manufacturer's guidelines.

The 26.4 min protocol (Zois et al., 2013) required participants to move through six individually-established speed zones, displayed in **Figure 1**. The total percentage of each activity was; standing (33%), walking (23%), jogging (23%), running (13%), fast running (4%), and sprinting (4%). The protocol included three repeated-sprint tests (set 1 and 3; four 4 s sprints and set 2; two 4 s sprints, all interspersed with 14 s passive recovery) and 10 single sprint efforts, all 4 s in duration. Visual (screen above the non-motorized treadmill) and verbal (strong 3-2-1 countdown to the upcoming change in activity) instructions on the target speed were given. Visual instructions included a red line on the screen, or each participant's individual target speed, and a green line indicating their actual speed. Participants were required to match their current speed with the target speed as closely as possible for all of the six speed zones. Verbal cues were given by the same operator to reduce variability. Data was sampled at 50 Hz and exported to customized software to analyze the mean total work completed across each half of the protocol. The first half was activity performed with the first 12-min of the protocol and the second half was activity post the 13-min mark. Minute 12 to 13 was a passive resting period and consequently removed from analysis. The average mean and peak power was calculated for all sprints in each half. The average mean and peak power was also calculated for each of the first and third set of repeated sprints. All sprints were defined as the first occurrence of speed at 1 $m \cdot s^{-1}$ and from this point, a 4 s period was subsequently calculated (Serpiello et al., 2011). Peak power was determined as the highest single value recorded during a sprint. The coefficient of variation (CV) for mean power and mean peak power was 3.3 and 4.8%, respectively.

Physiological Measures

Blood oxygen saturation (S_pO_2) was continuously measured at the earlobe by pulse oximetry (SPO Medical equipment, Israel) and collected for each minute across the entire protocol. Average S_pO_2 data was analyzed for the first and second half of the protocol. Heart rate (HR) was recorded each minute of the protocol and averaged for the first plus second half. Rating of perceived exertion (RPE) was collected each minute, across both halves, via the Borg 6–20 scale. The mean RPE for each half of the protocol was analyzed.

Oxygenation of the vastus lateralis was monitored during all trials using a NIRS device (Oxymon MkIII, Artinis, The Netherlands). The emitter and detector probe pair, with an optode distance of 4 cm, were attached using black plastic spacers. Probes were placed on the muscle belly (~15 cm above the proximal border of the patella and 5 cm lateral to the midline of the thigh) of the dominant lower limb and protected from external light using black bandages. A modified form of the Beer–Lambert Law calculated micromolar changes in tissue oxyhaemoglobin [O_2Hb] and deoxyhaemoglobin [HHb] across time using received optical densities from two continuous wavelengths of NIR light (763 and 855 nM). The differential optical path-length factor was 4.95 (Billaut and Buchheit, 2013). Skinfold thickness (5.7 ± 1.4 mm) was less than half of the emitter-detector distance in each participant.

Analysis concentrated on Δ[HHb], as it is primarily independent of total hemoglobin (De Blasi et al., 1993). Maximal [HHb] was obtained post-exercise via pressure cuff inflation (~300 mmHg), at the base of the thigh until the increased Δ[HHb] plateaued. The leg ischemia was performed whilst standing to mimic the sprint position. All Δ[HHb] values presented are expressed as a percentage of the amplitude of change between baseline and maximal [HHb] values. Data was acquired at 10 Hz throughout the entire protocol and averaged for each minute of the protocol. Data was also obtained during

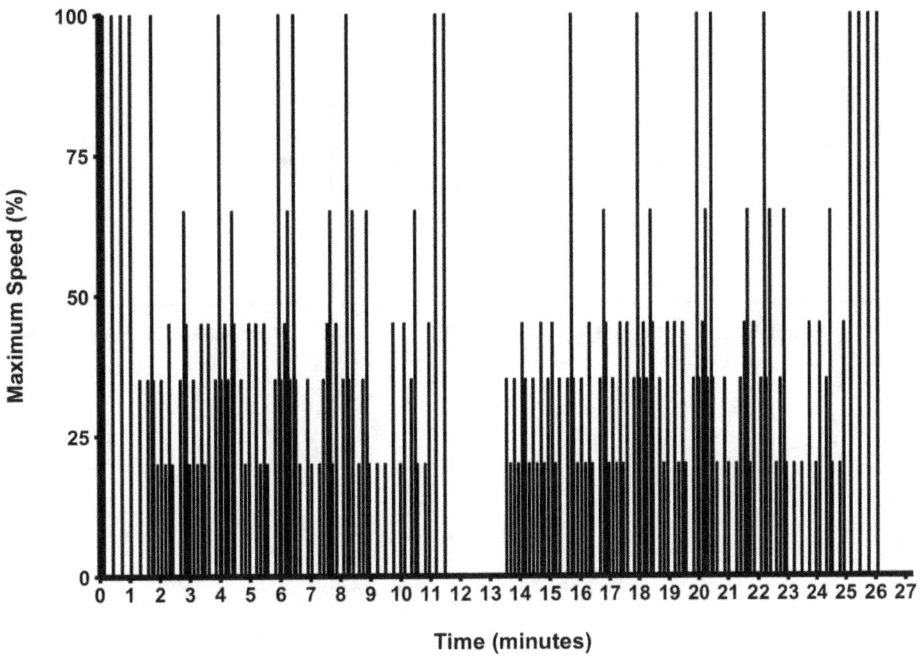

FIGURE 1 | The simulated team-sport running protocol.

the recovery periods from repeated sprint efforts, within the first and third set of repeated sprints.

Statistical Analysis

Separate analyses were performed for each of the measures derived from the non-motorized and physiological variables. Each analysis was performed with the same mixed model using the general linear mixed-model procedure (Proc Mixed) in the Statistical Analysis System (version 9.4, SAS Institute, Cary NC). The fixed effects in the model were altitude (three levels: sea-level, 2,000, 3,000 m), the interaction of altitude with a dummy variable representing the second half of the testing session (to estimate mean change between the first and second half, representing mean fatigue in the second half), and a dummy variable representing the second trial at altitude (to adjust the altitude effects to the first trial at altitude). The following random effects were specified: participant identity (to allow for repeated measurement on participants) and its interaction with the second-half dummy variable (with unstructured covariance, to allow for individual second-half means, representing individual differences in fatigue); participant identity interacted with trial identity (to allow for the repeated measurement on participants within trials); participant identity interacted with a dummy variable representing non-sea level (to estimate individual responses to altitude); and the residual (representing error of measurement from half to half). There were insufficient observations to allow successful specification of different but correlated individual responses to the two altitudes.

All measures, except for the physiological measures, were log-transformed before analysis then back-transformed to express the changes in percent units. The changes were also expressed in standardized units for assessment of magnitude. Standardization was performed by dividing the change score of the log-transformed measure by the between-participant standard deviation derived from the random effects for participant and its interaction with trial identity; this between-participant standard deviation represents the differences between participant free of residual (measurement) error. Uncertainty in the changes was expressed as 90% confidence intervals and interpreted via the non-clinical magnitude-based inference approach (Hopkins et al., 2009). Standardized changes of 0.20, 0.60, 1.20, 2.0, and 4.0 were thresholds for small, moderate, large, very large, and extremely large effects, respectively (Hopkins et al., 2009). When the confidence interval for a change included small positive and negative effects, the change was deemed unclear. For clear effects, the likelihood that the true effect was substantial was indicated with the following scale: *possibly* (25–75%), *likely* (75 to <95%), *very likely* (95–99.5%), and *most likely* (>99.5%).

RESULTS

The mean and ± standard deviation of mean heart rate, vastus lateralis deoxyhemoglobin, total work, oxygen saturation, and rating of perceived exertion per half of the simulated team-sport running protocol at each altitude are presented in **Figure 2**. The mean ± standard deviation for mean and peak power during all sprint efforts, per level of altitude and each half, is presented in **Figure 3**. The mean ± standard deviation for Vastus lateralis [HHb] during recovery periods and average blood oxygenation saturation per half is presented in **Figure 4**. The magnitude of change in performance and physiological variables, across

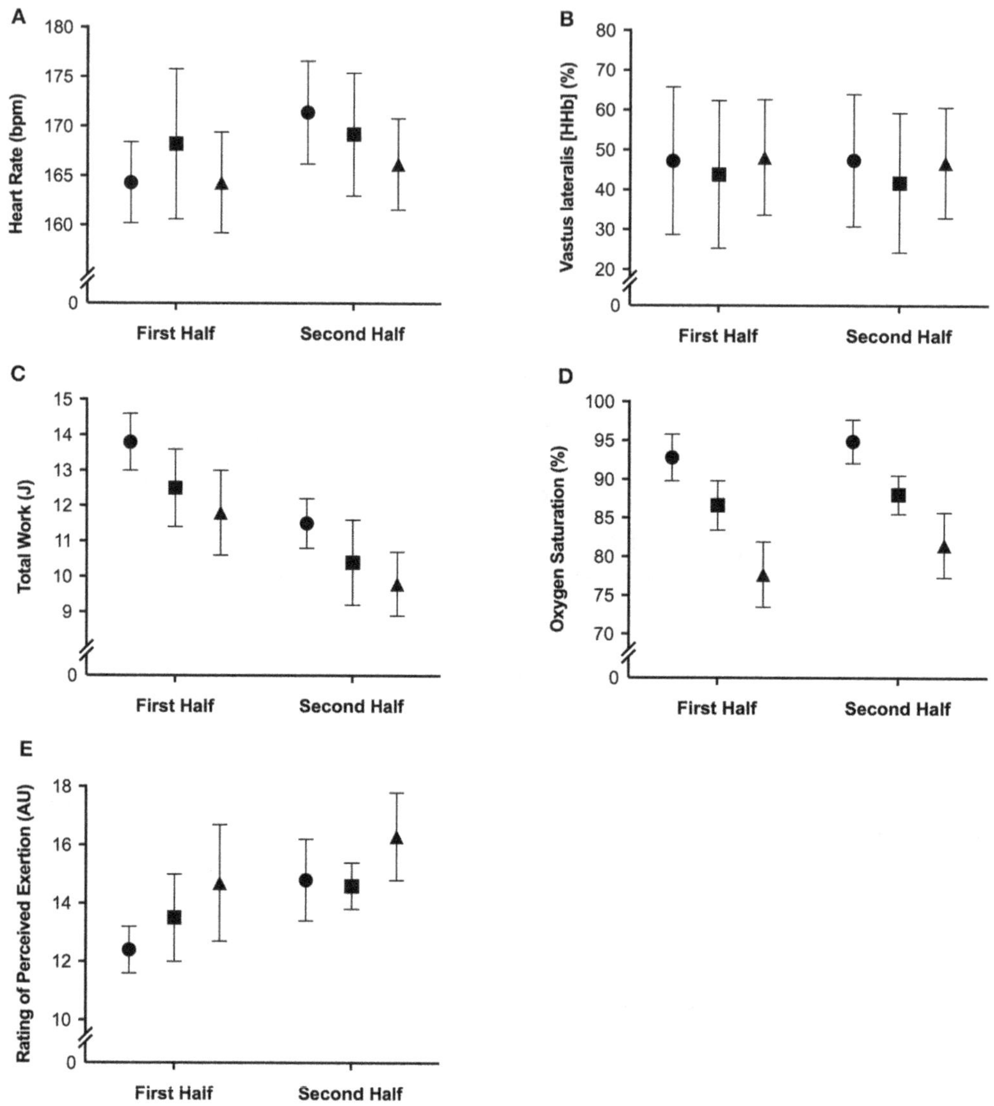

FIGURE 2 | The mean ± standard deviation for (A) heart rate; **(B)** vastus lateralis deoxyhemoglobin; **(C)** total work; **(D)** oxygen saturation, and **(E)** rating of perceived exertion per half of the simulated team-sport running protocol. Circles: 0 m; rectangles: 2,000 m; triangles: 3,000 m.

the entire protocol, per half, and compared across levels of altitude are presented in **Table 1**. The magnitude of change in performance and physiological variables, during repeated sprints, per half, and compared across levels of altitude are presented in **Table 2**. The magnitude of change in performance and physiological variables at altitude, across the second half of the protocol, and during the final trial, are presented in **Table 3**. The magnitude of change in performance and physiological variables at altitude, during repeated-sprints only, across the second half of the protocol, and during the final trial, are presented in **Table 4**.

DISCUSSION

Mean total work was substantially reduced during simulated team-sport movement at 2,000 and 3,000 m compared to sea-level. Mean total work was also most likely reduced in the second half of the protocol compared to the first at sea-level, 2,000 and 3,000 m. During sprint efforts across the simulated running protocol, mean and peak power was reduced at 3,000 m compared to sea-level. During repeated-sprints in the second half of the protocol, mean power was possibly reduced at 3,000 m, with no clear differences at 2,000 m or sea-level. During recovery from repeated-sprint efforts, vastus lateralis [HHb] was possibly reduced at 3,000 m compared to SL. This study is the first to use linear mixed modeling to examine the effect of titrated altitude on muscle oxygenation during simulated team-sport movement. This statistical approach provides detail on the percentage effects of fixed and individual factors, superior to other commonly used statistical methods, that may contribute to a decrement in performance at altitude.

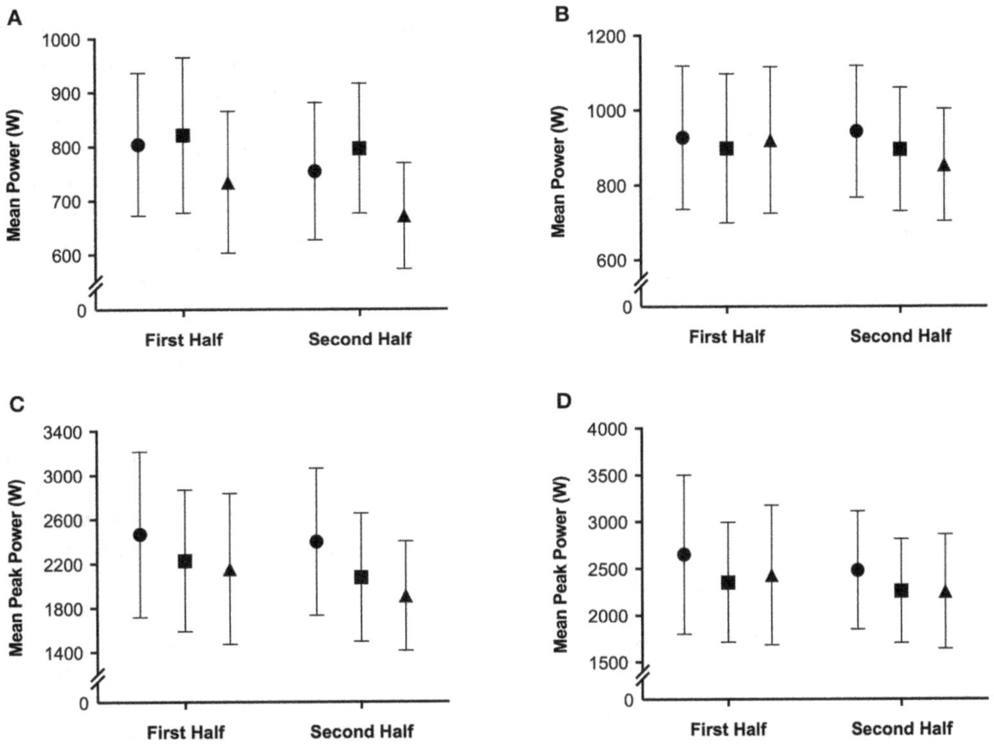

FIGURE 3 | The mean ± standard deviation for (A) mean power during all sprint efforts; **(B)** mean power during repeated sprints only; **(C)** mean peak power during all sprint efforts; **(D)** mean peak power during repeated sprints only per half of the simulated team-sport running protocol. Circles: 0 m; rectangles: 2,000 m; triangles: 3,000 m.

During repeated-sprint efforts, vastus lateralis [HHb] was likely higher in the second half at 2,000 m compared SL. This reoxygenation impairment is in agreement with the increased [HHb] (relative to normoxia) and performance decrement observed during recovery of ten 10 s sprints under 0.13 F_iO_2 Billaut and Buchheit (2013) during occlusion-free conditions, it is still debated whether the primary determinant of muscle post-exercise reoxygenation is muscle O_2 delivery or local utilization (Hamaoka et al., 1998; Kime et al., 2003). In the present study, the incomplete muscle reoxygenation observed in the second half at 3,000 m was likely related to limited muscle O_2 delivery post-sprint (Billaut and Buchheit, 2013). The resynthesis of PCr is derived solely from aerobic sources (Harris et al., 1976). In hypoxia, aerobic capacity is considerably impaired (Gore et al., 1996) and an inverse relationship between O_2 supply and PCr resynthesis rate has been established *in vitro* (Idstrom et al., 1985). In normoxia, PCr stores recovered to only 45% of resting concentrations after five 6 s sprints interspersed with 24-s passive recovery (Dawson et al., 1997). The current study employed 4-s repeated-sprints interspersed with 14-s recovery. Between RS efforts, PCr was likely not fully resynthesized due to a hypoxia-induced decrease in O_2 availability to working musculature, with S_pO_2 7.7 and 14.6% lower across the entire protocol at 2,000 and 3,000 m, respectively. Metabolic recovery and subsequent sprint performance was likely compromised, although the resynthesis of PCr was not measured in the present study. Impaired O_2 transport in hypoxia likely increased the contribution of anaerobic glycolysis to exercise metabolism, (Morales-Alamo et al., 2012) accelerating the development of peripheral muscle fatigue and decreased central motor drive (Amann and Dempsey, 2008). Cerebral oxygenation and electromyography data would provide a detailed understanding of the acute fatigue mechanisms during repeated-sprint sets at titrated altitudes.

Mean total work performed during the simulated team-sport movement was considerably diminished at 2,000 and 3,000 m compared to SL. This is in agreement with the large reduction in total work during three sets of (9 × 4 s) repeated running sprints at 2,000 and 3,000 m simulated altitude (Goods et al., 2014). In the present study, total work was reduced by ~5.1% per 1,000 m rise in altitude, lower than the ~7% per 1,000 m decline during 5 min time-trial performance (Clark et al., 2007), and 14% per 1,000 m decrement in a time-to-exhaustion (total duration of 308 s) test (Wehrlin and Hallen, 2006). The smaller reduction in the present study may be attributed to variation in the length and type of exercise. In contrast with the relatively short-duration, all-out time-trial (Clark et al., 2007), and time-to-exhaustion (Wehrlin and Hallen, 2006) tests, the 26.4 min protocol included lower-intensity movements and recovery, closer to replicating team-sport running. The recovery afforded by these lower-intensity periods (and associated lower energy expenditure) likely assisted the maintenance of repeated-sprint performance.

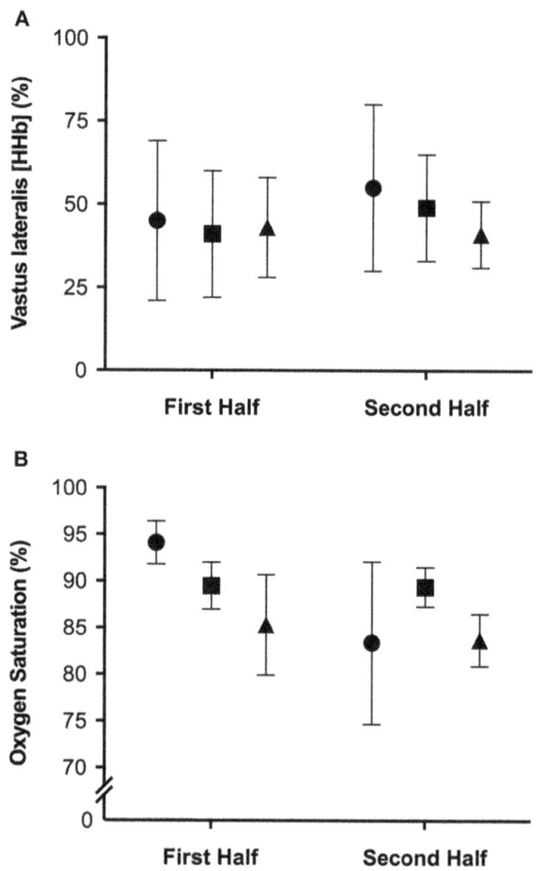

FIGURE 4 | The mean ± standard deviation values for (A) vastus lateralis deoxyhemoglobin during recovery from repeated sprints; **(B)** oxygen saturation during repeated sprints, per half. Circles: 0 m; rectangles: 2,000 m; triangles: 3,000 m.

Although, an active recovery from short repeated cycling sprints may disrupt the resynthesis of PCr (Spencer et al., 2008), our findings are reinforced by data collected during an elite youth soccer match at 1,600 m (Garvican et al., 2013). High-speed running was impaired by 15% and low-speed running plus total distance were reduced by 9 and 8%, respectively (Garvican et al., 2013). During a match at 3,600 m, peak 5 min running distance by elite youth soccer athletes was also reduced by 13–16% (Aughey et al., 2013). Collectively, this data demonstrates the negative impact of altitude on team-sport running performance.

Participants may have paced their effort, via self-selecting a lower intensity under hypoxia, between repeated-sprint sets in an attempt to preserve the ability to perform high-intensity efforts. Whilst the majority of pacing research focuses on continuous events (de Koning et al., 2011), pacing is also evident during repeated-sprint exercise. Knowledge of an exercise end-point can determine athletic performance. During a deception trial (where participants were uninformed on the number of sprints to be completed), less muscle mass was recruited and mechanical work lowered, presumably to avoid excessive metabolic disturbances, and muscle fatigue (Billaut et al., 2011). In the present study, participants were aware of the duration and number of sprints to be completed. Participants were also visually guided on the speed to be performed throughout the entire protocol, including the sprints.Participants may have been slower to reach target velocities or maintain these velocities during sprint efforts embedded in the protocol, in the aim of maintaining repeated-sprints located at the end of the protocol. The preservation of repeated-sprint efforts at 2,000 m are in agreement with the maintenance of repeated-running sprints in hypoxia from 12 to 21% O_2 (Bowtell et al., 2014). Fatigue index (calculated as the percentage decrease in peak speed from fastest to slowest speed) was greater when breathing 12% O_2 (corresponding altitude of 4,345 m; Bowtell et al., 2014). At a simulated altitude of 4,000 m, mean power output was also reduced during the first set of 9 × 4 s running repeated-sprint (Goods et al., 2014). Mean power was also lowered in subsequent sets at 2,000, 3,000, and 4,000 m (Goods et al., 2014), emphasizing the critical role of O_2 in PCr resynthesis and repeated-sprint performance (Harris et al., 1976).

Due to the chaotic nature of competition, athletes are unaware of the number of high-intensity bouts to be completed. Many high-intensity actions are performed when the ball is in possession, dispute or an opportunity to score arises (Faude et al., 2012). Thus, team-sport athletes are less able to modulate lower speed activities to preserve sprint capacity. This is in opposition with laboratory-based repeated-sprint studies, where participants are typically aware of the number of efforts to be completed. In the present study, participants were informed about lower-intensity activities and despite constant visual information on the speed to be maintained, they were unable or chose not to do so in hypoxia. At 3,000 m simulated altitude, the hypoxic stress appears to negatively influence physical output compared to 2,000 m. Coaching and conditioning staff should be aware of the negative impact of 3,000 m altitude upon team-sport running performance. Athletes may need to be interchanged or substituted when competing at 3,000 m, to minimize the detrimental impact of high altitude and allow sufficient recovery from high-speed running. Training at 3,000 m prior to competing at altitude may negate the detrimental effects of hypoxia on team-sport running, although this remains to be investigated. The short protocol duration of 26.4 min, in the present study, was designed to simulate an intensified period of team-sport activity. A 30 min simulated team-sport running protocol is a reliable tool for assessing and monitoring the physiological and performance of team-sport activity (Sirotic and Coutts, 2008). Increasing the protocol duration of the current study to 52.8 or 79.2 min could more closely replicate the duration of a team-sport match although it is unclear what impact this would have on test-retest variation, particularly at hypoxia. Future studies should investigate the impact of hypoxia on a longer simulated running protocol and use a linear-mixed modeling approach to estimate the individual and fixed factors that contribute to performance. Future studies investigating individual responses to simulated altitude should also monitor the training loads, sleep, nutrition, and recovery of participants during performance testing.

TABLE 1 | The difference in magnitude of change between levels of altitude on mean total work, heart rate, vastus lateralis deoxygenation, rating of perceived exertion, blood oxygenation saturation, mean sprint power, and mean sprint peak power across the entire protocol.

	Comparison (m)	Difference across entire protocol	Difference in second half of protocol
Mean total work (%)	2,000–0	−10.3, ±5.5; ↓ ***	0.1, ±4.7
	3,000–0	−14.9, ±5.2; ↓ ****	−0.3, ±4.7
	3,000–2,000	−5.1, ±2.7; ↓ ***	−0.4, ±4.7
Mean HR (bpm)	2,000–0	0.4, ±2.5	−3.6, ±2.3
	3,000–0	−2.7, ±2.4; ↓ **	−3.4, ±2.4; ↓ **
	3,000–2,000	−3.1, ±2.5; ↓ **	0.2, ±2.5
Mean Δ[HHb] (%)	2,000–0	−3.9, ±9.1	−2.2, ±3.3; ↔^{00}
	3,000–0	0.7, ±8.8	−1.5, ±3.3; ↔^{00}
	3,000–2,000	4.5, ±7.3; ↑ *	0.7, ±3.3; ↔^{00}
Mean RPE (AU)	2,000–0	0.1, ±1.6	−1.1, ±0.8; ↓ **
	3,000–0	1.7, ±1.4; ↑ **	−0.5, ±0.8
	3,000–2,000	1.5, ±1.3; ↑ **	0.6, ±0.8; ↑ *
Mean S_pO_2(%)	2,000–0	−7.7, ±2.5; ↓ ****	1.4, ±1.4; ↑ **
	3,000–0	−14.6, ±2.4; ↓ ****	2.3, ±1.3; ↑ ***
	3,000–2,000	−7.0, ±1.7; ↓ ****	0.9, ±1.0; ↑ *
Sprint mean Power (%)	2,000–0	−1.9, ±4.9; ↔^{00}	3.8, ±6.8; ↑ *
	3,000–0 m	−13.8, ±4.3; ↓ ****	−1.9, ±3.6; ↔^{00}
	3,000–2,000	−12.0, ±2.9; ↓ ****	−5.5, ±3.5; ↓ **
Sprint mean peak Power (%)	2,000–0	−10.1, ±6.4; ↓ **	−4.9, ±6.1; ↓ *
	3,000–0	−15.6, ±6.0; ↓ ***	−8.7, ±5.8; ↓ *
	3,000–2,000	−6.1, ±3.7; ↓ *	−4.0, ±6.1; ↔^{00}

*Values are presented as raw or % change in mean, ±90% CI or ±99% CI; Direction of response: positive ↑ negative ↓ trivial ↔; Symbols denote: *possibly, **likely, ***very likely, and ****most likely chance of the true effect exceeding a small (0.2) effect. Trivial changes indicated by ^{0}. m, meters; HR, heart rate; Δ[HHb], change in deoxyhemoglobin; RPE, rating of perceived exertion; S_pO_2, blood oxygenation saturation. Bold text indicates change in the mean at the 99% confidence interval (CI).*

TABLE 2 | The difference in magnitude of change between levels of altitude on mean and peak power, vastus lateralis deoxygenation during recovery periods, and blood oxygenation saturation during repeated sprints only.

	Comparison	Difference across entire protocol	Difference in second half of protocol
Repeated sprint mean power (%)	2,000–0	−4.6, ±3.3; ↓ *	−1.7, ±5.3;↔^{00}
	3,000–0	−5.5, ±3.2; ↓ *	−8.8, ±4.9; ↓ **
	3,000–2,000	−1.0, ±1.8; ↔^{0000}	−7.2, ±5.0; ↓ *
Repeated sprint mean peak power (%)	2,000–0	−7.8, ±7.3; ↓ *	1.3, ±12.6
	3,000–0	−7.5, ±7.2; ↓ *	−2.2, ±12.1
	3,000–2,000	−0.3, ±5.1; ↔^{0000}	−3.5, ±12.0
Mean recovery HHb (%)	2,000–0	−3.5, ±11.6	−1.3, ±12.3
	3,000–0	−6.9, ±10.7; ↓ *	−11.0, ±12.3; ↓ **
	3,000–2,000	−3.4, ±12.2	−9.7, ±12.3; ↓ **
Mean set S_pO_2(%)	2,000–0	−0.4, ±6.8	15.0, ±3.7; ↑ ****
	3,000–0	−5.3, ±6.5; ↓ **	13.1, ±3.6; ↑ ****
	3,000–2,000	−4.9, ±6.4	−1.9, ±3.5

*Values are presented as % change in mean, ± 90% CI or ±99% CI; Direction of response: positive ↑ negative↓ trivial ↔; Symbols denote: *possibly, **likely, ***very likely, and ****most likely chance of the true effect exceeding a small (0.2) effect. Trivial changes indicated by ^{0}. m, meters; Δ[HHb], change in deoxyhemoglobin; S_pO_2, blood oxygenation saturation. Bold text indicates change in the mean at the 99% confidence interval (CI).*

TABLE 3 | The difference in magnitude of change at altitude on mean total work, heart rate, vastus lateralis deoxygenation, rating of perceived exertion, blood oxygenation saturation, mean sprint power, and mean sprint peak power across the second half of the protocol and during the final trial, irrespective of altitude.

	Altitude (m)	Difference in second half of protocol	Difference in final trial
Mean total work (%)	0	**−16.9, ±3.5; ↓ ******	−0.5, ±2.9
	2,000	**−16.8, ±3.5; ↓ ******	
	3,000	**−17.2, ±3.5; ↓ ******	
Mean HR (bpm)	0	**4.5, ±2.7; ↑ ****	−0.2, ±2.4
	2,000	0.7, ±2.5; ↔^{00}	
	3,000	0.9, ±2.6	
Mean Δ[HHb] (%)	0	0.2, ±2.8	−1.1, ±7.2
	2,000	−2.0, ±2.7; ↓ *	
	3,000	−1.3, ±2.7; ↓ *	
Mean RPE (AU)	0	**2.2, ±1.1; ↑ ***	0.2, ±1.3
	2,000	**1.1, ±1.1; ↔^{00}**	
	3,000	**1.7, ±1.1; ↑ ***	
Mean S_pO_2(%)	0	**0.5, ±1.1; ↔^{000}**	−0.6, ±1.7; ↑ *
	2,000	**1.9, ±0.8; ↑ *****	
	3,000	**2.8, ±0.8; ↑ ******	
Sprint mean power (%)	0	**−6.3, ±2.9; ↓ ******	**10.9, ±3.7; ↑ ******
	2,000	−2.8, ±3.0; ↓ **	
	3,000	**−8.1, ±2.8; ↓ ******	
Sprint mean peak power (%)	0	−1.8, ±8.4	−2.3, ±6.2
	2,000	−6.5, ±8.0	
	3,000	−10.3, ±7.6; ↓ ***	

*Values are presented as raw or % change in mean, ±90% CI or ± 99% CI; Direction of response: positive ↑ negative↓ trivial ↔; Symbols denote: *possibly, **likely, ***very likely, and ****most likely chance of the true effect exceeding a small (0.2) effect. Trivial changes indicated by ^{0}. m, meters; HR, heart rate; Δ[HHb], change in deoxyhemoglobin; RPE, rating of perceived exertion; S_pO_2, blood oxygenation saturation. Bold text indicates change in the mean at the 99% confidence interval (CI).*

TABLE 4 | The difference in magnitude of change at altitude on mean and peak power, vastus lateralis deoxygenation during recovery periods, and blood oxygenation saturation during repeated sprints only and during the final trial, irrespective of altitude.

	Altitude (m)	Difference in second half of protocol	Difference in final trial
Repeated sprint mean power (%)	0	2.4, ±8.3	**0.8, ±1.8; ↔^{0000}**
	2,000	0.6, ±8.2	
	3,000	−6.6, ±7.6; ↓ *	
Repeated sprint mean peak power (%)	0	−4.3, ±10.6; ↓ *	**−3.0, ±4.9; ↔^{00}**
	2,000	−3.1, ±10.8	
	3,000	−6.4, ±10.4; ↓ *	
Mean recovery HHb (%)	0	**9.8, ±7.9; ↑ ****	−2.0, ±12.2
	2,000	8.5, ±7.9; ↑ **	
	3,000	−1.3, ±7.9	
Mean set S_pO_2(%)	0	**−14.7, ±2.6; ↓ ******	−2.1, ±6.4
	2,000	0.3, ±2.3	
	3,000	−1.5, ±2.6; ↓ *	

*Values are presented as % change in mean, ±90% CI or ± 99% CI; Direction of response: positive ↑ negative↓ trivial ↔; Symbols denote: *possibly, **likely, ***very likely, and ****most likely chance of the true effect exceeding a small (0.2) effect. Trivial changes indicated by ^{0}. m, meters; Δ[HHb], change in deoxyhemoglobin; S_pO_2, blood oxygenation saturation. Bold text indicates change in the mean at the 99% confidence interval (CI).*

CONCLUSION

During simulated team-sport movement, repeated-sprint and single-sprint efforts are compromised at 3,000 m altitude, possibly due to limited muscle O_2 availability during recovery periods. To overcome this decrement, participants reduced their total work completed despite strong verbal encouragement. Whilst this strategy may have assisted in largely maintaining repeated-sprint and single-sprint efforts at 2,000 m, the elevated physiological demands at 3,000 m may have been overwhelming. Consequently, repeated-sprint and single-sprint performance was subsequently impaired. Under hypoxia, the decrement in work completed during intermittent running is lower than previously reported for time-trial and time-to-exhaustion tests.

AUTHOR CONTRIBUTIONS

Conceived and designed the experiments: FB and RA. Performed experiments: AS, FB, RR, MV, and RA. Analyzed data: AS. Interpreted results of research: AS, RA, RR, MV, FB, WH. Drafted manuscript and prepared tables/figures: AS. Edited, critically revised paper, and approved final version of manuscript: AS, RR, MV, FB, WH, and RA.

ACKNOWLEDGMENTS

The authors wish to thank the study participants for their involvement, plus Ian Fairweather and James Zois for their assistance.

REFERENCES

Aldous, J. W., Chrismas, B. C., Akubat, I., Dascombe, B., Abt, G., and Taylor, L. (2015). Hot and Hypoxic environments inhibit simulated soccer performance and exacerbate performance decrements when combined. *Front. Physiol.* 6:421. doi: 10.3389/fphys.2015.00421

Amann, M., and Dempsey, J. A. (2008). The concept of peripheral locomotor muscle fatigue as a regulated variable. *J. Physiol.* 586, 2029–2030. doi: 10.1113/jphysiol.2008.152496

Aughey, R. J., Goodman, C. A., and McKenna, M. J. (2014). Greater chance of high core temperatures with modified pacing strategy during team sport in the heat. *J. Sci. Med. Sport* 17, 113–118. doi: 10.1016/j.jsams.2013.02.013

Aughey, R. J., Hammond, K., Varley, M. C., Schmidt, W. F., Bourdon, P. C., Buchheit, M., et al. (2013). Soccer activity profile of altitude versus sea-level natives during acclimatisation to 3600 m (ISA3600). *Br. J. Sports Med.* 47, i107–i113. doi: 10.1136/bjsports-2013-092776

Bartsch, P., Saltin, B., and Dvorak, J. (2008). Consensus statement on playing football at different altitude. *Scand. J. Med. Sci. Sports* 18, 96–99. doi: 10.1111/j.1600-0838.2008.00837.x

Billaut, F., Bishop, D. J., Schaerz, S., and Noakes, T. D. (2011). Influence of knowledge of sprint number on pacing during repeated-sprint exercise. *Med. Sci. Sports Exerc.* 43, 665–672. doi: 10.1249/MSS.0b013e3181f6ee3b

Billaut, F., and Buchheit, M. (2013). Repeated-sprint performance and vastus lateralis oxygenation: effect of limited O(2) availability. *Scand. J. Med. Sci. Sports* 23, e185–e193. doi: 10.1111/sms.12052

Billaut, F., Gore, C. J., and Aughey, R. J. (2012). Enhancing team-sport athlete performance is altitude training relevant? *Sports Med.* 42, 751–767. doi: 10.2165/11634050-000000000-00000.

Bowtell, J. L., Cooke, K., Turner, R., Mileva, K. N., and Sumners, D. P. (2014). Acute physiological and performance responses to repeated sprints in varying degrees of hypoxia. *J. Sci. Med. Sport* 17, 399–403. doi: 10.1016/j.jsams.2013.05.016

Buchheit, M., Hammond, K., Bourdon, P. C., Simpson, B. M., Garvican-Lewis, L. A., Schmidt, W. F., et al. (2015). Relative match intensities at high altitude in highly-trained young soccer players (ISA3600). *J. Sports Sci. Med.* 14, 98–102.

Castagna, C., and Abt, G. (2003). Intermatch variation of match activity in elite Italian soccer referees. *J. Strength Cond. Res.* 17, 388–392. doi: 10.1519/00124278-200305000-00029

Clark, S. A., Bourdon, P. C., Schmidt, W., Singh, B., Cable, G., Onus, K. J., et al. (2007). The effect of acute simulated moderate altitude on power, performance and pacing strategies in well-trained cyclists. *Eur. J. Appl. Physiol.* 102, 45–55. doi: 10.1007/s00421-007-0554-0

Dawson, B., Goodman, C., Lawrence, S., Preen, D., Polglaze, T., Fitzsimons, M., et al. (1997). Muscle phosphocreatine repletion following single and repeated short sprint efforts. *Scand. J. Med. Sci. Sports* 7, 206–213. doi: 10.1111/j.1600-0838.1997.tb00141.x

De Blasi, R. A., Cope, M., Elwell, C., Safoue, F., and Ferrari, M. (1993). Noninvasive measurement of human forearm oxygen consumption by near infrared spectroscopy. *Eur. J. Appl. Physiol. Occup. Physiol.* 67, 20–25. doi: 10.1007/BF00377698

de Koning, J. J., Foster, C., Bakkum, A., Kloppenburg, S., Thiel, C., Joseph, T., et al. (2011). Regulation of pacing strategy during athletic competition. *PLoS ONE* 6:e15863. doi: 10.1371/journal.pone.0015863

Faude, O., Koch, T., and Meyer, T. (2012). Straight sprinting is the most frequent action in goal situations in professional football. *J. Sports Sci.* 30, 625–631. doi: 10.1080/02640414.2012.665940

Garvican, L. A., Hammond, K., Varley, M. C., Gore, C. J., Billaut, F., and Aughey, R. J. (2013). Lower running performance and exacerbated fatigue in soccer played at 1600 m. *Int. J. Sports Physiol. Perform.* 9, 397–404. doi: 10.1123/ijspp.2012-0375

Giacomoni, M., Billaut, F., and Falgairette, G. (2006). Effects of the time of day on repeated all-out cycle performance and short-term recovery patterns. *Int. J. Sports Med.* 27, 468–474. doi: 10.1055/s-2005-865822

Goods, P. S., Dawson, B. T., Landers, G. J., Gore, C. J., and Peeling, P. (2014). Effect of different simulated altitudes on repeat sprint performance in team sport athletes. *Int. J. Sports Physiol. Perform.* 9, 857–886. doi: 10.1123/ijspp.2013-0423

Gore, C. J., Hahn, A. G., Scroop, G. C., Watson, D. B., Norton, K. I., Wood, R. J., et al. (1996). Increased arterial desaturation in trained cyclists during maximal exercise at 580 m altitude. *J. Appl. Physiol.* 80, 2204–2210.

Gore, C. J., Little, S. C., Hahn, A. G., Scroop, G. C., Norton, K. I., Bourdon, P. C., et al. (1997). Reduced performance of male and female athletes at 580 m altitude. *Eur. J. Appl. Physiol. Occup. Physiol.* 75, 136–143. doi: 10.1007/s004210050138

Hamaoka, T., Mizuno, M., Katsumura, T., Osada, T., Shimomitsu, T., and Quistoref, B. (1998). Correlation between indicators determined by near infrared spectroscopy and muscle fiber types in humans. *Jpn. J. Appl. Physiol.* 28, 243–248.

Harris, R. C., Edwards, R. H., Hultman, E., Nordesjo, L. O., Nylind, B., and Sahlin, K. (1976). The time course of phosphorylcreatine resynthesis during recovery of the quadriceps muscle in man. *Pflugers Arch.* 367, 137–142. doi: 10.1007/BF00585149

Hopkins, W. G., Marshall, S. W., Batterham, A., and Hanin, J. (2009). Progressive statistics for studies in sports medicine and exercise science. *Med. Sci. Sports Exerc.* 41:3. doi: 10.1249/MSS.0b013e31818cb278

Idstrom, J. P., Subramanian, V. H., Chance, B., Schersten, T., and Bylund-Fellenius, A. C. (1985). Oxygen dependence of energy-metabolism in contracting and recovering rat skeletal-muscle. *Am. J. Physiol.* 248, H40–H48.

Kime, R., Katsumura, T., Hamaoka, T., Osada, T., Sako, T., Murakami, M., et al. (2003). Muscle reoxygenation rate after isometric exercise at various intensities in relation to muscle oxidative capacity. *Adv. Exp. Med. Biol.* 530, 497–507. doi: 10.1007/978-1-4615-0075-9_47

Morales-Alamo, D., Ponce-González, J. G., Guadalupe-Grau, A., Rodríguez-García, L., Santana, A., Cusso, M. R., et al. (2012). Increased oxidative stress and anaerobic energy release, but blunted Thr172-AMPKα phosphorylation, in response to sprint exercise in severe acute hypoxia in humans. *J. Appl. Physiol.* 113, 917–928. doi: 10.1152/japplphysiol.00415.2012

Morrison, J., McLellan, C., and Minahan, C. (2015). A clustered repeated-sprint running protocol for team-sport athletes performed in normobaric hypoxia. *J. Sports Sci. Med.* 14, 857–863.

Robertson, E. Y., Saunders, P. U., Pyne, D. B., Aughey, R. J., Anson, J. M., and Gore, C. J. (2010). Reproducibility of performance changes to simulated live high/train low altitude. *Med. Sci. Sports Exerc.* 42, 394–401. doi: 10.1249/MSS.0b013e3181b34b57

Serpiello, F. R., McKenna, M. J., Stepto, N. K., Bishop, D. J., and Aughey, R. J. (2011). Performance and physiological responses to repeated-sprint exercise: a novel multiple-set approach. *Eur. J. Appl. Physiol.* 111, 669–678. doi: 10.1007/s00421-010-1687-0

Sirotic, A. C., and Coutts, A. J. (2007). Physiological and performance test correlates of prolonged, high-intensity, intermittent running performance in moderately trained women team sport athletes. *J. Strength Cond. Res.* 21, 138–144. doi: 10.1519/00124278-200702000-00025

Sirotic, A. C., and Coutts, A. J. (2008). The reliability of physiological and performance measures during simulated team-sport running on a non-motorised treadmill. *J. Sci. Med. Sport* 11, 500–509. doi: 10.1016/j.jsams.2007.04.008

Spencer, M., Dawson, B., Goodman, C., Dascombe, B., and Bishop, D. (2008). Performance and metabolism in repeated sprint exercise: effect of recovery intensity. *Eur. J. Appl. Physiol.* 103, 545–552. doi: 10.1007/s00421-008-0749-z

Ufland, P., Lapole, T., Ahmaidi, S., and Buchheit, M. (2012). Muscle force recovery in relation to muscle oxygenation. *Clin. Physiol. Funct. Imaging* 32, 380–387. doi: 10.1111/j.1475-097X.2012.01141.x

Wehrlin, J. P., and Hallen, J. (2006). Linear decrease in.VO2max and performance with increasing altitude in endurance athletes. *Eur. J. Appl. Physiol.* 96, 404–412. doi: 10.1007/s00421-005-0081-9

Zois, J., Bishop, D., Fairweather, I., Ball, K., and Aughey, R. J. (2013). High-intensity re-warm-ups enhance soccer performance. *Int. J. Sports Med.* 34, 800–805. doi: 10.1055/s-0032-1331197

20

Nitrate Intake Promotes Shift in Muscle Fiber Type Composition During Sprint Interval Training in Hypoxia

Stefan De Smet[1], Ruud Van Thienen[1], Louise Deldicque[1,2], Ruth James[3], Craig Sale[3], David J. Bishop[4] and Peter Hespel[1,5]*

[1] Exercise Physiology Research Group, Department of Kinesiology, Katholieke Universiteit Leuven, Leuven, Belgium, [2] Institute of Neuroscience, Université Catholique de Louvain, Louvain-la-Neuve, Belgium, [3] Musculoskeletal Physiology Research Group, Sport, Health and Performance Enhancement Research Centre, School of Science and Technology, Nottingham Trent University, Nottingham, UK, [4] Institute of Sport, Exercise and Active Living, Victoria University, Melbourne, VIC, Australia, [5] Department of Kinesiology, Bakala Academy–Athletic Performance Center, KU Leuven, Leuven, Belgium

***Correspondence:**
Peter Hespel
peter.hespel@kuleuven.be

Purpose: We investigated the effect of sprint interval training (SIT) in normoxia, vs. SIT in hypoxia alone or in conjunction with oral nitrate intake, on buffering capacity of homogenized muscle (βhm) and fiber type distribution, as well as on sprint and endurance performance.

Methods: Twenty-seven moderately-trained participants were allocated to one of three experimental groups: SIT in normoxia (20.9% F_iO_2) + placebo (N), SIT in hypoxia (15% F_iO_2) + placebo (H), or SIT in hypoxia + nitrate supplementation (HN). All participated in 5 weeks of SIT on a cycle ergometer (30-s sprints interspersed by 4.5 min recovery-intervals, 3 weekly sessions, 4–6 sprints per session). Nitrate (6.45 mmol $NaNO_3$) or placebo capsules were administered 3 h before each session. Before and after SIT participants performed an incremental VO_{2max}-test, a 30-min simulated cycling time-trial, as well as a 30-s cycling sprint test. Muscle biopsies were taken from *m. vastus lateralis*.

Results: SIT decreased the proportion of type IIx muscle fibers in all groups ($P < 0.05$). The relative number of type IIa fibers increased ($P < 0.05$) in HN ($P < 0.05$ vs. H), but not in the other groups. SIT had no significant effect on βhm. Compared with H, SIT tended to enhance 30-s sprint performance more in HN than in H ($P = 0.085$). VO_{2max} and 30-min time-trial performance increased in all groups to a similar extent.

Conclusion: SIT in hypoxia combined with nitrate supplementation increases the proportion of type IIa fibers in muscle, which may be associated with enhanced performance in short maximal exercise. Compared with normoxic training, hypoxic SIT does not alter βhm or endurance and sprinting exercise performance.

Keywords: sprint interval training, hypoxia, intermittent hypoxic training, nitrate, muscle fiber type composition, muscle buffering capacity, carnosine, citrate synthase

INTRODUCTION

Interest in intermittent hypoxic training (IHT) to boost endurance and high-intensity exercise performance in athletes is growing (Hoppeler et al., 2008; McLean et al., 2014). This might partly be explained by the commercialization of user-friendly, normobaric hypoxicators to simulate altitude within the normal lowland habitat. Well-controlled studies have provided evidence that high-intensity hypoxic endurance training can enhance muscle mitochondrial and capillary density (Geiser et al., 2001; Vogt et al., 2001; Schmutz et al., 2010; Desplanches et al., 2014), as well as stimulate other markers of mitochondrial metabolism and biogenesis (Terrados et al., 1990; Melissa et al., 1997; Green et al., 1999; Zoll et al., 2006). IHT in the form of both endurance training (Vogt et al., 2001; Zoll et al., 2006) and sprint training (Faiss et al., 2013b; Puype et al., 2013) elevated muscle phosphofructokinase (PFK) mRNA and/or activity, as well as other markers of glycolytic metabolism and pH regulation. Nonetheless, research into the effects of IHT on sea-level exercise performance is equivocal, with the current literature suggesting higher training intensities involving anaerobic energy input to be more favorable than predominantly aerobic workouts (Hoppeler et al., 2008; Faiss et al., 2013a; McLean et al., 2014). This might be explained by impaired workload in endurance training due to inhibition of oxidative energy provision, resulting in higher glycolytic energy contribution and premature fatigue development (Weyand and Lee, 1999; Calbet et al., 2003; Wehrlin and Hallén, 2006).

Attention has recently shifted toward IHT in the form of sprint training (Faiss et al., 2013b, 2015; Galvin et al., 2013; Puype et al., 2013), because maximal power (Calbet et al., 2003) and anaerobic capacity (Friedmann et al., 2007) are well-maintained in hypoxia. This may allow for more explicit systemic and muscular adaptations due to elevated hypoxic and oxidative stress in conjunction with pertinent neuromuscular and neuromechanical loading (Morales-Alamo et al., 2012; McGinnis et al., 2014). Support for such a contention comes from recent studies showing that repeated sprint training in hypoxia (RSH), characterized by several short (<30 s) sprints interspersed with incomplete recovery (exercise-to-rest ratio <1:4), increased hypoxia-inducible factor-1α (HIF-1α) mRNA (Faiss et al., 2013b), and repeated-sprint ability (RSA) performance (Faiss et al., 2013b, 2015; Galvin et al., 2013) more than identical repeated sprint training in normoxia. However, the beneficial effect of RSH on exercise performance (Faiss et al., 2015) has been debated (Montero and Lundby, 2015), and needs to be confirmed. HIF-1α is implicated in the regulation of the genes controlling the expression of proteins involved in glycolysis and pH regulation (Porporato et al., 2011). In line with this, RSH has been shown to increase gene transcription of monocarboxylate transporter 4 (MCT-4) and carbonic anhydrase III (CA3) in muscle (Faiss et al., 2013b). We have shown that 6 weeks of sprint interval training (SIT), characterized by 30-s sprints interspersed with long recovery periods of 4–5 min, increases muscle MCT-1, but not MCT-4 protein content, irrespective of whether the training was performed in normoxia or in hypoxia (Puype et al., 2013). SIT in hypoxia but not in normoxia also elevated PFK activity (Puype et al., 2013), presumably due to increased glycolytic ATP turnover to compensate for impaired aerobic energy production during the hypoxic training workouts (Weyand and Lee, 1999; Calbet et al., 2003). Given that post-exercise phosphocreatine (PCr) resynthesis is impaired under hypoxic conditions (Haseler et al., 1999; Holliss et al., 2013; Vanhatalo et al., 2014), long recovery time between sprints is required to allow substantial recovery of PCr prior to each sprint (Bogdanis et al., 1996; Parolin et al., 1999) and may assist maintenance of high power output throughout the training session.

As the contribution of glycolysis to energy provision increases, buffering capacity becomes a pivotal determinant of the capacity to maintain high muscle power outputs. Counter-intuitively, the extent of H^+ accumulation in muscle fibers during training does not seem to be the primary stimulus for the development of higher buffering capacity of homogenized muscle (βhm). Indeed, rat (Thomas et al., 2007) and human (Edge et al., 2006a) studies have shown that bicarbonate-induced myocellular alkalosis during work-matched interval training did not inhibit adaptations in βhm. Furthermore, a large acidic load (pH < 6.8) during training has been reported to reduce βhm, possibly due to cumulative transient decreases in βhm during consecutive training sessions (Bishop et al., 2008). In line with this rationale, performing SIT in hypoxic conditions might even impair βhm compared with similar training in normoxia. Alternatively, however, both "live high–train high" (Mizuno et al., 1990; Saltin et al., 1995) and "live high–train low" experiments (Gore et al., 2001) have shown that "live high" compared to "live low" enhances βhm. However, these findings have also been recently debated (Clark et al., 2004; Nordsborg et al., 2012), and the specific effect of IHT on βhm during "live low" conditions remains unclear.

Oral nitrate supplementation can enhance endurance exercise performance in hypoxia (Vanhatalo et al., 2011; Masschelein et al., 2012; Muggeridge et al., 2014), presumably by enhancing mitochondrial efficiency (Larsen et al., 2011) and/or by reducing the energy cost of muscle contraction (Bailey et al., 2010). It is well-documented that the fraction of aerobic energy provision gradually increases during intermittent sprints due to impaired re-activation of glycolysis (Parolin et al., 1999). Recent data indicate that nitrate intake increases blood flow and contractility to a greater extent in fast-glycolytic than in slow-oxidative whole muscle and muscle fibers (Hernández et al., 2012; Ferguson et al., 2013). This may explain the more explicit effects of nitrate supplementation on performance during high-intensity exercise requiring greater input of type II fibers for production of high power outputs at high contraction velocities (Vanhatalo et al., 2011; Breese et al., 2013; Bailey et al., 2015; Coggan et al., 2015). Higher muscle blood flow during recovery (Alvares et al., 2012) could conceivably facilitate the clearance of waste metabolites during intermittent maximal exercise bouts and could, amongst the other aforementioned mechanism, contribute to increased total work output during resistance training (Mosher et al., 2016). Furthermore, nitrate supplementation in hypoxia was shown to stimulate the rate of post-exercise muscle PCr resynthesis (Vanhatalo et al., 2011, 2014). Taken together, these results suggest that oral nitrate supplementation could enhance performance during SIT in hypoxia and by this means potentiate training adaptations.

We, therefore, aimed to investigate whether SIT performed in hypoxic conditions elicited greater muscular and performance adaptations compared to similar training performed in normoxic conditions. Secondly, we aimed to investigate whether oral nitrate supplementation during training enhanced the effects of SIT in hypoxia.

MATERIALS AND METHODS

Participants

Thirty healthy men were recruited from the student population at the KU Leuven by word of mouth and via announcements on social media. To avoid confounding effects due to prior altitude acclimatization, participants who were exposed to altitudes higher than 1500 m during the 6 months prior to the study were excluded from participation. From the initial sample of 30 eligible participants, one did not complete the study due to SIT intolerance, and two withdrew from the study for reasons unrelated to the study protocol. Twenty-seven participants completed the full study protocol and were included in the final data analyses (for general characteristics see **Table 1**). Participants were recreationally active [2.7 ± 1.6 h (*SD*) exercise participation per week; i.e., soccer, basketball, cycling, running, swimming, strength training], but had not engaged in a consistent training program or any sport at a competitive level. Participants were non-smokers and did not use medication or dietary supplements in the 3 months prior to the study or during the period of the study. They were instructed to maintain their habitual physical activity level and normal diet throughout the study. Participants received a summary table of nitrate-rich foods and were instructed to avoid these foods throughout the study period. The study was approved by the KU Leuven Biomedical Ethics Committee (B322201316517) and was conducted in accordance with the Declaration of Helsinki. All participants provided written informed consent after clearing medical screening and being fully informed about the content of the experiments and the risks involved.

Study Protocol

The study involved a test before (pretest) and after (posttest) a 5-week controlled SIT program. The pretest and posttest consisted of two experimental sessions separated by a 2-day interval. Between 3 and 2 weeks prior to the start of the study, participants completed two sessions of familiarization with the experimental procedures. In the first familiarization session, participants performed a maximal incremental VO_{2max}-test on a cycle ergometer (Avantronic Cyclus II, Leipzig, Germany). The initial workload was set at 70 W and was increased by 30 W per min until volitional exhaustion. Respiratory gas exchange was measured continuously during the test (Cortex MetaLyzer II, Leipzig, Germany), and the highest oxygen uptake measured over a 30-s period was defined as the maximal oxygen uptake rate (VO_{2max}). Participants then cycled for 15 min at 50 W to recover, after which a 30-s modified Wingate test (W_{30s}) was performed. To avoid limitations of power output by co-ordination problems due to excessive cadence increase (cadence > 120 rev·min^{-1}), cadence during W_{30s} was fixed at 100 rev·min^{-1} by using the isokinetic mode setting of the cycle ergometer. In the second familiarization session, participants completed a 30-min simulated time-trial (TT_{30min}). They were instructed to keep their cadence between 80 and 100 rev·min^{-1}, and adjust the resistance to develop the highest possible mean power output (W). Following familiarization, participants were matched into triplets by VO_{2max}, mean power output during TT_{30min}, mean power output during W_{30s}, as well as body mass and height. Thereafter, the triplets were randomly assigned to one of three experimental groups. One group performed the SIT program in normoxia (F_iO_2 = 20.9%, n = 10) and received a placebo supplement (N). All other participants trained in hypoxia (F_iO_2 = 15.0%, ~2750 m), with eight participants receiving a placebo (H) and nine participants receiving a nitrate (HN, n = 9) supplement. Participants were not blinded for the normoxic vs. hypoxic training conditions. Supplements were ingested 3 h prior to each training session so as to produce high plasma nitrite levels during the training in HN(Webb et al., 2008). Nitrate was administered in the form of capsules containing 6.45 mmol $NaNO_3$ (~400 mg molecular NO_3^-). Placebo capsules contained an equivalent amount of sodium (6.45 mmol) in the form of NaCl. All supplements were identical in appearance, and were administered single-blinded in N and double-blinded in H and HN.

TABLE 1 | Participant characteristics.

	N	H	HN
Age (y)	23 ± 3	24 ± 2	25 ± 2
Height (cm)	180 ± 8	180 ± 6	182 ± 6
Body mass (kg)	74.0 ± 10.2	79.5 ± 12.1	78.5 ± 11.7

Data are mean ± SD and represent baseline characteristics of the participants training in normoxia (F_iO_2 = 20.9%) while receiving placebo supplementation (N, n = 10), and participants training in hypoxia (F_iO_2 = 15.0%) while receiving either placebo (H, n = 8) or nitrate supplements (HN, n = 9).

SIT Training Program

All SIT sessions were performed in the same normobaric hypoxic facility (SportingEdge, Sherfield on London, UK) set at either 20.9% F_iO_2 (N), or 15.0% F_iO_2 (~2750 m; H and HN). The ambient O_2 fraction was checked before the start of each training session (MaxO_2^+A Scuba, Maxtec, Utah). Participants cycled on cycle ergometers (Avantronic Cyclus II, Leipzig, Germany) that were calibrated prior to the start of the study. Participants completed three training sessions per week, with each separated by 48-h of recovery. Each session consisted of intermittent 30-s maximal sprints, interspersed by 4.5 min active recovery intervals at 50 W. Cadence during the sprints was fixed at ~100 rev·min^{-1} by using the isokinetic operation mode of the ergometers. The number of sprints was increased from four in weeks 1–2, to five in weeks 3–4, and six in the final week. Including 5-min warm-up and cool-down @50 Watt, the training sessions lasted

30 min in week 1, increasing to 40 min in week 5. During each session participants were given verbal encouragement to perform maximally during each sprint. To evaluate the effect of SIT on arterial oxygenation, arterial oxygen saturation (SpO_2) was monitored in the final week of the training period by pulse oximetry (Nellcor OxiMax N-600x, Mallinckrodt, St. Louis, MO) with a sensor placed 2 cm above the eyebrow.

Pretest and Posttest

All exercise testing was performed in normoxia. Participants were instructed to refrain from any strenuous physical activity for at least 48 h prior to the pretest. In order to minimize potential diet-induced variations in muscle metabolism, participants received a standardized carbohydrate-rich dinner (~1500 kcal; 65% carbohydrate, 15% fat, 20% protein) on the evening before each experimental day. For the first session they reported to the laboratory between 12:00 a.m. and 4:00 p.m. All participants received a standardized breakfast (~750 kcal, 70% carbohydrate, 10% fat, 20% protein) between 7:00 and 10:30 a.m. Participants completing sessions beyond 1:30 p.m. also received a standardized lunch (~650 kcal, 70% carbohydrate, 10% fat, 20% protein), with the last meal consistently being served between 3 and 2.5 h prior to the start of the experiments. Following a 1-h rest in a comfortable chair, a percutaneous needle biopsy (100–200 mg) was taken from the middle portion of the belly of the right *m. vastus lateralis* using a 5-mm Bergström-type needle under suction. Muscle samples were dissected in two parts. One part was rapidly frozen in liquid N_2 and stored at −80°C until subsequent biochemical analyses. The other part was frozen in isopentane on liquid N_2 and stored at −80°C for later histochemical analyses. Following the biopsy, participants warmed up for 20 min at incremental workloads corresponding to 70% (10 min) and then 90% (10 min) of their average power output recorded during the TT_{30min} familiarization session. During TT_{30min} heart rate was monitored continuously (Polar, Kempele, Finland) and blood lactate concentration was measured (Lactate Pro1, Arkray, Japan) at 10-min intervals from an earlobe capillary blood sample. Participants were allowed to drink water *ad libitum* and received on-line feedback about the time remaining to completion. No verbal encouragement was given. At the end of the experimental session, participants were instructed to refrain from any strenuous physical activity, before returning to the laboratory for the second session 2 days later. For this second session they arrived between 6 a.m. and 11 a.m. after an overnight fast. Following a 20-min rest period, they performed a maximal incremental VO_{2max}-test on the cycle ergometer (Avantronic Cyclus II, Leipzig, Germany). Initial workload was set at 70 W and was increased by 30 W every 3 min until volitional exhaustion. Thereafter participants cycled for 15 min at 50 W to recover, whereupon the W_{30s} commenced. The cycle ergometer was set in the isokinetic mode with cadence fixed at 100 rev·min^{-1}. During both tests heart rate was monitored continuously (Polar, Kempele, Finland). Standardized verbal encouragement was given only during W_{30s}. Respiratory gas exchange was continuously measured (Cortex MetaLyzer II, Leipzig, Germany) during the incremental test, VO_{2max} was determined as the highest oxygen uptake rate measured over a 30-s period. Maximal power output (MPO) was calculated by summing the workload during the last full stage, plus 30 W multiplied by the fraction of the final stage completed. Capillary blood samples for lactate determination (Lactate Pro1, Arkray, Japan) were taken from the earlobe at the end of each workload during the incremental test, and power outputs corresponding to 2 and 4 mmol·L^{-1} blood lactate levels were extrapolated on the lactate-power curve. Blood lactate was also determined 1, 2, and 3 min after the W_{30s}. Room temperature (18–20°C), oxygen content (20.9%), air humidity (40%) as well as air ventilation were standardized. Pretests and the posttests were performed on the same days of the week and time of the day within each participant. The posttest commenced 3 or 4 days following the last training session to eliminate acute physiological effects due to the prior training session.

Analysis of Muscle Samples

Citrate Synthase Activity

Enzymatic activity of citrate synthase (CS) was measured by standard colorimetric method. Briefly, 5 mg of wet muscle tissue was dissolved in 400 μL of ice-cold homogenization buffer (5 mM Hepes, 1 mM EGTA, 0.1% Triton X-100, 1 mM Dithiothreitol, pH 8.7). Protein concentration was determined with a DC protein assay (Bio-Rad). After dilution to 0.5 μg·μL^{-1}, samples and standards were loaded on a 96 well plate to perform the assay in triplicate. CS catalyzes the reaction between acetyl coenzyme A and oxaloacetic acid resulting in citric acid and CoA with a thiol group (CoA-SH). Measurement of its activity is based on the binding of CoA-SH to 5,5′-dithio-bis-(2-nitrobenzoic acid) (DTNB) to form 2-nitro-5-thiobenzoate (TNB). The spectrophotometric absorbance intensity of TNB was measured at 412 nm and CS activity was calculated and expressed as μmol·min^{-1}·g^{-1}. The average coefficient of variation (CV) as determined from the triplicate measures was 4.4%.

Buffering Capacity of Homogenized Muscle (βhm)

Details of the titration method for analysis of βhm have been described elsewhere (Edge et al., 2006b). Briefly, freeze-dried muscle samples (1.7–2.5 mg dm) were dissected from blood and connective tissue and homogenized on ice in a sodium fluoride containing buffer (33.3 μl 10 mM NaF per mg dm). The homogenates were warmed in a hot water bath at 37.4°C for 5 min. Basal pH measurement was performed with a glass microelectrode (MI-410, Microelectrodes, Bedford, NH, USA) connected to a pH meter (Lab 850, Schott Instruments GmbH, Mainz, Germany). The homogenates were first adjusted to pH ~7.2 with sodium hydroxide (0.02 M NaOH). Then a serial addition of 2 μL hydrochloric acid (0.01 M HCl) was titrated until a pH of ~6.1 was reached. After each titration, the homogenates were briefly vortexed to ensure a homogeneously mixed solution. The number of moles of H^+ per kg dry muscle required to change pH from 7.1 to 6.5 was interpolated from the fitted titration trend line and expressed as mmol H^+ per kg dm per unit pH as a unit for βhm. Each sample was measured in duplicate from which the mean was taken. The average CV as determined from the duplicate measures was 5.1%.

Muscle Carnosine Concentration

Details of muscle carnosine concentration determination by high performance liquid chromatography (HPLC) have been described elsewhere (Mora et al., 2007). Briefly, about 5 mg of dry muscle was dissected from blood and connective tissue and extracted in a buffer containing perchloric acid (0.5 M PCA) and 1 mM EDTA. After centrifuging the samples for 4 min at 13,000 rev·min^{-1} at 4°C, the supernatant was collected and neutralized with a potassium bicarbonate containing buffer (2.1 M KHCO). Samples were placed on ice for 5 min to allow CO_2 to escape, after which they were centrifuged at 5000 rev·min^{-1} for 4 min at 4°C. The supernatant was then filtered through a 0.22 μm membrane filter where after 20 μL of supernatant was injected into a Perkin-Elmer HPLC system with an Atlantis HILIC Silica column (4.6 × 150 mm, 3 μm). Mobile phase A contained 0.65 mM ammonium acetate in ultrapure water/acetonitrile (25:75 ratio) at a pH of 5.5. Mobile phase B contained 4.55 mM ammonium acetate in ultrapure water/acetonitrile (70:30 ratio) at a pH of 5.5. A linear gradient from 100% phase A to 100% phase B in 13 min at a flow rate of 1.4 mL·min^{-1} was used for separation. Separation was monitored at a wavelength of 214 nm with a UV detector. The average CV as calculated from 12 duplicate injections in the HPLC system was 1.5%.

Muscle Fiber Type Composition

Serial 7-μm-thick cryosections were cut with a cryostat at −20°C. Cryosections were blocked for 60 min in phosphate buffered saline (PBS) containing 1% BSA. Hereafter they were incubated in primary antibodies for myosin heavy chain I (MHCI) (BA-F8, Developmental Studies Hybridoma Bank) and MHCIIa (SC-71, Developmental Studies Hybridoma Bank) dissolved in PBS with 0.5% BSA for 120 min. Dilutions of primary antibodies for MHCI and MHCII were 1:50 and 1:100, respectively. After washing in PBS, cryosections were incubated in appropriate conjugated secondary antibodies (type I: Alexa 647 goat anti-mouse IgG2b, Invitrogen, diluted 1:300 in PBS with 0.5% BSA; type IIa: Alexa 350 goat anti-mouse IgG1, Invitrogen, diluted 1:300 in PBS with 0.5% BSA) for 60 min. Additionally, together with the secondary antibodies, membranes were stained using wheat germ agglutinin (WGA) Texas Red (Life Technologies). Slides were visualized by fluorescence microscopy (Nikon E1000, Nikon, Boerhavedorp, Germany). The epifluorescence signal was recorded using Cy5, DAPI, and Texas Red excitation filters for visualization of type I fibers, type IIa fibers, and cell membranes, respectively. Muscle fibers were classified as type I, type IIa, or type IIx (unstained fibers). Photos of the slides were analyzed with ImageJ software (version 1.41, National Institutes of Health, USA). Only fibers with adequate cross-sections showing no signs of distortion or folding were counted. 225 ± 27 (*SD*) fibers were analyzed per biopsy.

Statistical Analysis

Differences in baseline values between N and H and between H and HN were tested using a Student's *t*-test. Main and interaction effects were evaluated by two-way (group × time) repeated measures ANOVA (SigmaStat and SigmaPlot software, Chicago, IL, USA). We performed two separate ANOVA's to test the two *a priori* hypotheses: N was compared with H to evaluate whether SIT yielded different effects in hypoxia vs. normoxia; H was compared with HN to evaluate whether nitrate administration was able to potentiate the effects of training in hypoxia. Tukey's honestly significant difference *post hoc*-test was run whenever appropriate to identify specific effects. A probability level $P < 0.05$ was considered statistically significant. All data are expressed as mean ± standard error of the mean (*SEM*) unless otherwise stated.

RESULTS

Arterial O_2-Saturation during Training (Figure 1)

Arterial O_2-saturation (SpO_2) was continuously measured during the SIT sessions in week 5. In N, resting SpO_2-values were 98.7 ± 0.4 and 97.6 ± 0.5% at the start and at the end of the sessions (n.s.). Corresponding values in H were lower, both at the start (91.0 ± 0.8%) and at the end of the sessions (89.3 ± 1.4%; $P < 0.05$). Compared with sprint 1, post-exercise SpO_2-values were lower in the latter sprints of the session in both groups. Each sprint also reduced SpO_2 more in H (-6.0 ± 0.6%) than in N (−1.9 ± 0.2%, $P < 0.05$). SpO_2-values were not significantly different between H and HN: average SpO_2 during SIT was 85.0 ± 0.6% in H vs. 86.7 ± 0.3% in HN ($P = 0.20$).

Training Performance (Figure 2)

The number of sprints per session was increased from four in weeks 1–2, to five in weeks 3–4, and to six in week 5. Irrespective of the experimental group, mean power output in sprint 1 on average was 667 ± 31 W, decreasing to 561 ± 25 W in the final sprint of the session. There were no significant differences in power output between experimental groups at any time during training. Average total work done (kJ) per training session per week was similar between the groups from

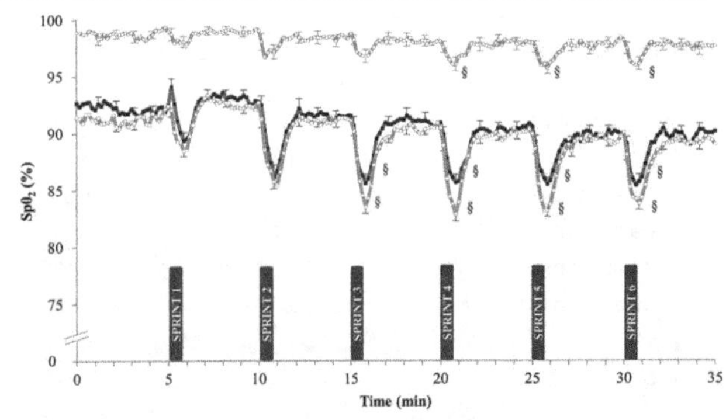

FIGURE 1 | Effect of SIT on arterial oxygen saturation. Data are mean ± SEM and represent arterial oxygen saturation (%SpO_2) during the final week of SIT. Participants performed six 30-s all-out sprints interspersed by 4 min and 30 s of active recovery on a cycle ergometer. One group trained in normoxia (F_iO_2 = 20.9%) while receiving placebo (N, ○). The other groups trained in hypoxia (F_iO_2 = 15.0%) while receiving either placebo (H, □) or nitrate supplements (HN, ■). §, $P < 0.05$ compared to SPRINT 1.

the start to the end of the training period (**Figure 2**). Accordingly, total work output over the 5-week training period was 1340 ± 39 kJ in N, 1311 ± 52 kJ in H, and 1261 ± 51 kJ in HN ($P > 0.50$). Blood lactate concentrations at the end of the training sessions peaked at ~14–15 mmol·L^{-1} on average in all groups.

Exercise Performance (Table 2)

Baseline values of the incremental exercise test, TT_{30min} and W_{30s} were not significantly different between N and H ($P > 0.05$) or H and HN ($P > 0.05$). Compared with the pretest, VO_{2max} in the posttest was increased ($P < 0.05$) by ~16% in N vs. ~11% in both H and HN ($P < 0.05$), but there were no significant differences in VO_{2max} or change in VO_{2max} between N and H ($P = 0.26$) or between H and HN. Similarly, SIT increased ($P < 0.05$) time to exhaustion (10–11%), peak power output (8–10%), and power output corresponding to 4 mmol·L^{-1} blood lactate concentrations (5–11%) in the three experimental groups without significant differences between N and H or H and HN. Mean power output during the TT_{30min} in the pretest was, on average, ~200 W. Training tended to increase mean power output during the TT_{30min} in N (+4%, $P = 0.062$) and significantly increased power output during the TT_{30min} in H and HN (+8%, $P < 0.05$), but there were no significant differences between N and H or H and HN. Blood lactate concentrations during the TT_{30min} were, on average, ~6 mmol·L^{-1} at a heart rate of ~174 b·min^{-1} in each group in both the pretest and the posttest (data not shown). Mean power output during W_{30s} in the pretest also was similar between the groups (660–670 W). SIT increased power output by ~6% in N and H ($P < 0.05$), vs. +12% in HN ($P < 0.05$), yet differences between H and HN were not significant (HN, $P = 0.085$). Accordingly, W_{30s} produced similar peak blood lactate concentrations (~10–12 mmol·L^{-1}) in the three experimental groups in both the pretest and the posttest.

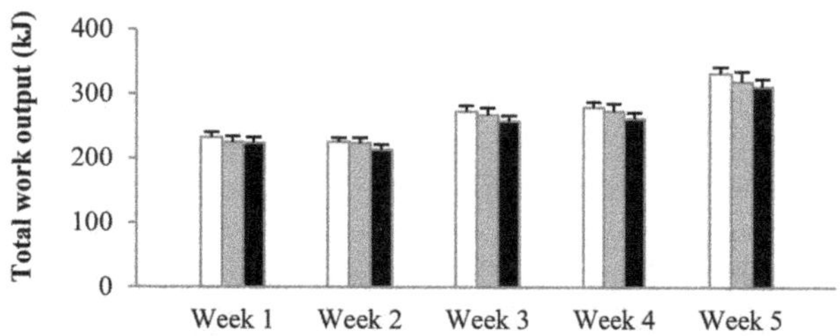

FIGURE 2 | Effect of hypoxia and nitrate intake on training workload. Data are mean ± SEM and represent average total work output (kJ) per training session per week. The number of sprints per session was increased from four in weeks 1–2, to five in weeks 3–4, and six in the final week. One group trained in normoxia ($F_iO_2 = 20.9\%$) while receiving placebo (N, open bars). The other groups trained in hypoxia ($F_iO_2 = 15.0\%$) while receiving either placebo (H, gray bars) or nitrate supplements (HN, black bars).

Muscle Fiber Type Composition (Table 3)

The relative number of type I (~45–50%), type IIa (~40–45%), and type IIx fibers (~10%) in *m. vastus lateralis* in the pretest was similar between N and H ($P > 0.05$ for all fiber types) as well as between H and HN ($P > 0.05$ for all fiber types). SIT reduced the proportion of type IIx fibers in all the groups ($P < 0.05$). In the posttest the proportion of type IIa fibers was higher in HN than in H ($P < 0.05$), with training significantly increasing the proportion of IIa fibers from 45 to 56% in HN ($P < 0.05$), but not in N (main effect of time $P = 0.07$) or H ($P = 0.40$). Similar changes occurred for fiber-specific CSAs, which also were similar

TABLE 2 | Effects of training and nitrate supplementation on physiological parameters and exercise performances.

	N		H		HN	
	Pretest	**Posttest**	**Pretest**	**Posttest**	**Pretest**	**Posttest**
INCREMENTAL VO_{2max} TEST						
VO_{2max} (mL·min^{-1}·kg^{-1})	53.5 ± 2.6	62.3 ± 3.4*	54.3 ± 4.9	60.2 ± 3.5*	51.2 ± 2.2	56.9 ± 2.3*
Time to exhaustion (min)	23.1 ± 1.1	25.5 ± 1.0*	23.8 ± 1.8	26.4 ± 1.7*	22.4 ± 1.1	25.0 ± 1.2*
Peak power (W)	275 ± 12	295 ± 11*	278 ± 18	304 ± 17*	264 ± 11	290 ± 12*
Peak heart rate (beats·min^{-1})	188 ± 3	186 ± 3	188 ± 2	188 ± 3	190 ± 4	191 ± 3
Peak blood lactate (mmol·L^{-1})	11.2 ± 0.7	11.4 ± 0.4	11.0 ± 1.1	11.8 ± 1.0	12.1 ± 0.9	12.5 ± 0.6
Power output at 2 mmol·L^{-1} (W)	175 ± 10	189 ± 13#	161 ± 20	179 ± 14*	148 ± 14.1	172 ± 11*
Power output at 4 mmol·L^{-1} (W)	216 ± 10	227 ± 13*	213 ± 18	230 ± 14*	196 ± 12.0	217 ± 11*
TT_{30min}						
Mean power output (W)	203 ± 10	211 ± 12#	205 ± 16	221 ± 15*	193 ± 13	209 ± 12*
W_{30s}						
Mean power output (W)	662 ± 23	699 ± 21*	677 ± 25	719 ± 34*	663 ± 45	746 ± 41*
Peak blood lactate (mmol·L^{-1})	9.2 ± 0.7	11.1 ± 0.9*	11.5 ± 0.7	12.4 ± 0.5	9.8 ± 0.7	12.4 ± 0.4*

Data are mean ± SEM for the maximal incremental VO_{2max}-test, the 30-min simulated time-trial (TT_{30min}), and the 30-s Wingate test (W_{30s}) in the pretest and in the posttest. One group trained in normoxia ($F_iO_2 = 20.9\%$) while receiving placebo (N, n = 10). The two other groups trained in hypoxia ($F_iO_2 = 15.0\%$) and received either placebo (H, n = 8) or nitrate supplements (HN, n = 9).

**$P < 0.05$ compared to the pretest.*

#$P < 0.10$ compared to the pretest.

TABLE 3 | Effects of training and nitrate intake on muscle fiber composition.

	N		H		HN	
	Pretest	Posttest	Pretest	Posttest	Pretest	Posttest
RELATIVE FIBER NUMBER (%)						
Type I	49 ± 3	49 ± 3	51 ± 5	53 ± 5	45 ± 4	39 ± 2
Type IIa	42 ± 3	49 ± 3	42 ± 4	44 ± 4	45 ± 2	56 ± 2*,†
Type IIx	9 ± 2	2 ± 1*	7 ± 2	3 ± 2*	10 ± 2	5 ± 1*
RELATIVE FIBER CSA (%)						
Type I	48 ± 3	51 ± 2	48 ± 5	50 ± 5	44 ± 4	38 ± 2
Type IIa	44 ± 3	47 ± 2	45 ± 5	47 ± 4	47 ± 2	58 ± 2*
Type IIx	8 ± 2	2 ± 1*	7 ± 2	3 ± 1*	8 ± 2	4 ± 1*
FIBER CSA (μm^2)						
Type I	4769 ± 604	5214 ± 501	5269 ± 204	5843 ± 462	4998 ± 402	5106 ± 434
Type IIa	4952 ± 429	4769 ± 411	5978 ± 281	6554 ± 348	5365 ± 534	5497 ± 573
Type IIx	4507 ± 444	4302 ± 428	4929 ± 664	6078 ± 474*	3976 ± 405	4438 ± 537

Data are mean ± SEM for muscle fiber cross-sectional area (CSA) and fiber number in m. vastus lateralis in the pretest and in the posttest. One group trained in normoxia (F_iO_2 = 20.9%) while receiving placebo (N, n = 10). The other groups trained in hypoxia (F_iO_2 = 15.0%) and received either placebo (H, n = 8) or nitrate supplements (HN, n = 9).
**$P < 0.05$ compared to pretest.*
†$P < 0.05$ group × time interaction.

TABLE 4 | Effects of training and nitrate intake on biochemical measurements in muscle.

	N		H		HN	
	Pretest	Posttest	Pretest	Posttest	Pretest	Posttest
βhm (mmol H^+·kg dm^{-1}·pH^{-1})	136 ± 6	136 ± 6	138 ± 5	137 ± 6	125 ± 6	128 ± 6
Carnosine content (mmol·kg dm^{-1})	33.3 ± 2.3	35.3 ± 2.2	33.8 ± 2.9	38.2 ± 2.9	30.2 ± 2.2	34.0 ± 2.6
Citrate synthase activity (μmol·min^{-1}·g^{-1})	190 ± 19	292 ± 24*	231 ± 10	282 ± 16*	216 ± 17	269 ± 8.2*

Data are mean ± SEM for buffering capacity of homogenized muscle (βhm), carnosine content, and citrate synthase activity in the pretest and the posttest. One group trained in normoxia (F_iO_2 = 20.9%) while receiving placebo (N, n = 10). The other groups trained in hypoxia (F_iO_2 = 15.0%) and received either placebo (H, n = 8) or nitrate supplements (HN, n = 9).
**$P < 0.05$ compared to pretest.*

between N and H or H and HN in the pretest ($P > 0.05$ for all fiber types). SIT reduced the relative CSA of type IIx fibers in all the groups ($P < 0.05$). Conversely, type IIa relative CSA increased in HN (+11%, $P < 0.05$) only and was significantly greater in HN compared to H in the posttest ($P < 0.05$). SIT did not alter mean fiber CSA (μm^2) of the different fiber types, except for type IIx mean fiber CSA in H which increased from the pretest to the posttest ($P < 0.05$). However, type IIx fibers were observed in only half of the participants in H ($n = 4$), in which only few type IIx fibers were observed in the pretest [44 ± 33(*SD*)] and in the posttest [30 ± 28 (*SD*)]. Hence interpretation should be performed with caution. Mean fiber-specific CSAs were not significantly different between N and H or H and HN at any time.

Muscle Biochemistry (Table 4)

Baseline values for muscular buffering capacity, carnosine content, and maximal citrate synthase activity measured in homogenized muscle tissue were not significantly different between N and H or H and HN ($P > 0.05$). Buffering capacity of homogenized muscle was unaffected by SIT irrespective of the experimental condition. SIT on average increased muscle carnosine content by ~13% in H and HN (main effect of time $P < 0.05$, no significant *post hoc* time effects within H ($P = 0.11$) or HN ($P = 0.13$)), but not in N (+6%, $P = 0.072$). Nonetheless, the increase in carnosine content was not significantly different between N and H ($P = 0.48$), and there were no significant differences in muscle carnosine between the groups in either the pretest or the posttest. Maximal citrate synthase activity increased by 54% in N ($P < 0.05$) and by just under half that in H (22%) and HN (25%) ($P < 0.05$), yet changes were not significantly different between N and H ($P = 0.10$).

DISCUSSION

The most striking results from the current study are that (a) 5 weeks of SIT, performed in hypoxic conditions, significantly increased the fraction of type IIa muscle fibers, but only when completed with concomitant dietary nitrate supplementation and (b) SIT performed in hypoxic conditions does not ameliorate physiological adaptations yielding enhanced aerobic or anaerobic endurance exercise performance.

We administered 400 mg of molecular nitrate ~3 h before each SIT session in HN, which has previously been shown to significantly increase the plasma nitrite concentration (Wylie et al., 2013) and improve oxygen-efficiency of the skeletal muscle during exercise (Bailey et al., 2010; Larsen et al., 2011). We postulated that this might delay fatigue development and thereby attenuate the reduced training intensity often shown during hypoxic sprint training (Kelly et al., 2014; Thompson et al., 2015). Training workloads were, however, similar between all groups, regardless of whether the training was performed in normoxia (N) or in hypoxia, either with (HN) or without (H) nitrate supplementation. Thus, the degree of neuromechanical activation during training was similar between all experimental conditions.

Even in the absence of fiber hypertrophy, fiber type transition from IIx to IIa might be expected during short-term SIT involving 30-s sprints in healthy volunteers (for review, see Ross and Leveritt, 2001). In keeping with the published findings (Allemeier et al., 1994), 5 weeks of SIT did not induce muscle fiber hypertrophy in the current study. Consistent with this, SIT in normoxia reduced the relative type IIx fiber number, whilst the proportion of type IIa fibers tended to increase. SIT in hypoxia (H) also reduced type IIx fiber number, but did not alter the fraction of type IIa fibers. Interestingly, when nitrate supplementation was provided during SIT in hypoxic conditions (HN), relative type IIa fiber number increased from 45 to 56%.

Previous evidence indicates that nitric oxide (NO) plays a pivotal role in MHC-based muscle fiber type transition (Smith et al., 2002; Martins et al., 2012; Suwa et al., 2015). NO is suggested to increase inhibitory phosphorylation of glycogen synthase kinase (GSK)-3β in rat fast-twitch muscle, promoting nuclear factor of activated T-cell c1 (NFATc1) dephosphorylation and nuclear accumulation, resulting in a fast-to-slow fiber type transition (Martins et al., 2012). Furthermore, pharmacological inhibition of NO-synthase (NOS) activity by N^G-nitro-L-arginine-methyl-ester (L-NAME) negated overload-induced type II to I fiber type transition (Smith et al., 2002). Results from both rodent (Hernández et al., 2012; Ferguson et al., 2013) and human (Bailey et al., 2015; Coggan et al., 2015) exercise studies indicated that oral nitrate intake exerts its actions primarily in type II muscle fibers by increasing blood flow (Ferguson et al., 2013), by elevating sarcoplasmic reticulum calcium stores and the expression of calcium handling proteins such as calsequestrin 1 and the dihydropyridine receptor (Hernández et al., 2012), as well as by reducing muscle metabolic perturbation (Vanhatalo et al., 2011). Nitrate supplementation also stimulated rate of force development (Hernández et al., 2012) and power output (Bailey et al., 2015; Coggan et al., 2015) during high-intensity and high-velocity muscle contractions. Thus, while endogenous NO production during acute exposure of lowlanders to hypoxia is reduced, due to inhibition of the L-arginine–NOS pathway (Lundberg et al., 2008), exogenous nitrate provides an alternative pathway to stimulate NO production via nitrate to nitrite to NO conversion (Lundberg et al., 2008). Given that NO probably plays an important role in exercise-induced MHC-based adult fiber type transitions, it is plausible that oral nitrate intake during SIT in hypoxia served as an adequate back-up mechanism for NO-induced muscle fiber transformation to compensate for impaired NOS activity. However, in contrast to what could be expected from the current literature, i.e., stimulation of type IIx to IIa and IIa to type I fiber type transition (Smith et al., 2002; Martins et al., 2012; Suwa et al., 2015), nitrate supplementation during hypoxic SIT did not stimulate the transition of type IIa to type I muscle fibers. Follow-up studies are needed to elucidate the cellular mechanisms by which oral nitrate intake can stimulate the conversion to type IIa muscle fibers during SIT in hypoxia.

Despite a decrease in the fraction of IIx muscle fibers in all conditions and an increase in the fraction of IIa muscle fibers in HN, there was no change in βhm with training in any of the three groups. We postulated that SIT in hypoxia, due to an enhanced contribution of glycolysis to ATP production, might impair βhm compared with identical training in normoxia. Contrary to our hypothesis, however, SIT did not alter βhm, regardless of whether the training was completed in normoxia or hypoxia. Our data shows that SIT is not an adequate strategy to improve βhm, at least in healthy recreationally active volunteers during short-term training. Findings from the present and earlier studies support the opinion that high-intensity interval training (HIT) at workloads corresponding to 120–170% of the lactate threshold (Edge et al., 2006a,b) is probably more effective to raise βhm than explicit "glycolytic training" via SIT (Nevill et al., 1989; Harmer et al., 2000; Baguet et al., 2011). Adaptations of βhm during long-term SIT in elite sprinters may be different, given their substantially higher proportion of type II fibers and higher glycolytic capacity.

The physicochemical buffer capacity of muscle (~ βhm) is composed of proteins, inorganic phosphate, bicarbonate, and the histidine-containing dipeptide carnosine. The histidine containing dipeptide content of muscle (carnosine in human muscle) contributes ~7–8% to total βhm (Harris et al., 1990; Mannion et al., 1992; Hill et al., 2007), and elevations through training or dietary supplementation remain a plausible mechanism for increasing βhm. Accordingly, we determined the effect of SIT on muscle carnosine content and observed no significant effect in normoxic conditions. However, a main effect of time (pretest vs. posttest), though without significant *post hoc* effects, was found for the increase in muscle carnosine content following training in hypoxic conditions (H and HN), yet the training-induced changes were not significantly different between N and H. Earlier experiments in our laboratory (Puype et al., 2013) have shown that SIT in hypoxia did not increase muscle carnosine content (unpublished observations), suggesting some equivocality in the findings across our own studies. This would seem in line with the existing literature, given that SIT has previously been shown to substantially increase muscle carnosine content in one study (Suzuki et al., 2004), although no such training-effect has been shown in any other longitudinal intervention study using SIT (Baguet et al., 2011) or resistance training involving either short (~10 s) (Kendrick et al., 2009) or longer (~20–45 s) series of maximal muscle contractions in normoxia (Mannion et al., 1994). Future studies performing single-fiber determination of muscle carnosine are warranted for clear interpretation of training-induced changes in fiber-specific myocellular carnosine content.

Buffering capacity of homogenized muscle, as measured in the present study, is different to muscle buffering capacity *in vivo* and reflects the altered state and chemistry of muscle after homogenization. Assuming that there would be no change in any other source of myocellular buffering, it could be estimated that a 13% increase in muscle carnosine content (i.e., 4 mmol·kg dm^{-1}) would increase homogenized muscle buffering capacity over the titration pH range of 7.1 to 6.5 by 2.21 mmol H^{+}·kg dm^{-1}·pH^{-1}, given that at pH 7.1 and pH 6.5 34.9 and 68.1% of the additional carnosine content is already in the protonated form, respectively (Harris et al., 1990). This represents an increase of ~1.7% of the initial βhm in the present study and falls below the detection limit of the titration assay used. However, as we don't know what muscle buffering capacity *in vivo* is over this range, we cannot calculate the importance of this increase.

We also evaluated the effect of SIT on muscle oxidative capacity by measuring citrate synthase (CS) maximal activity. SIT substantially elevated CS activity (+25–50%), independent of whether the training was performed in normoxia or in hypoxia. These findings are in contrast with reports from single-leg studies reporting greater increases in CS activity following endurance training (30 min at 65–75% maximal work capacity) in hypoxic conditions compared to training at similar absolute workloads in normoxic conditions (Terrados et al., 1990; Melissa et al., 1997; Green et al., 1999). However, if the training workloads are matched for relative intensity, endurance training in hypoxic conditions abolishes rather than augments training-induced changes in muscle oxidative function (Bakkman et al., 2007). Training workloads during SIT in the present study were similar between normoxic and hypoxic conditions in both absolute and relative terms. In line with previous reports, SIT in normoxic conditions increased CS activity (for review see Sloth et al., 2013), but sprint training in hypoxic conditions did not augment adaptations in muscle oxidative capacity (Faiss et al., 2013a; Puype et al., 2013).

The hypothesis driving the current study was underpinned by the notion that performing SIT in hypoxic conditions, alone or in combination with oral nitrate intake, might yield specific physiological adaptations to boost exercise performance. Anaerobic glycolysis accounts for about 50% of the total ATP production during a 30-s maximal exercise bout (Putman et al., 1995). It is therefore reasonable to postulate that a higher proportion of type IIa muscle fibers, providing a higher capacity for glycolytic ATP production, should be ergogenic during a 30-s all-out exercise. As discussed above, hypoxic SIT in conjunction with oral nitrate supplementation increased relative type IIa muscle area compared with hypoxic SIT alone. Interestingly, this also tended to translate into a greater gain in power output during W_{30s} (+12% in HN vs. +6% in H, $P = 0.08$), which indicates that short-term oral nitrate supplementation in conjunction with SIT may be a valid strategy to enhance performance in "glycolytic" exercise events such as a 400-meter dash, by contributing to a beneficial fiber type shift. Future studies should seek to confirm this possibility. It is also important to emphasize that we did not study the effect of nitrate intake during SIT in normoxia, neither did we study exercise performance in hypoxia. Thus, we cannot extrapolate our findings to these conditions. Contrary to 30-s sprint performance, determinants of aerobic exercise capacity were similar between the groups. Five weeks of SIT enhanced cycling power output corresponding to 2 and 4 mmol·L^{-1} blood lactate levels, VO_{2max}, and 30-min cycling time-trial performance, independent of whether the training was performed in normoxia, or in hypoxia with or without oral nitrate supplementation. These findings indicate that short-term SIT in hypoxic compared to normoxic conditions is not an advantageous strategy for enhancing normoxic endurance exercise performance in recreationally active individuals.

In conclusion, the current experiment demonstrated that oral nitrate supplementation during short-term sprint-interval training increased the proportion of type IIa muscle fibers in muscle, which may contribute to enhanced performance in short maximal exercise events requiring a very high glycolytic rate. Compared with SIT in normoxia, SIT in hypoxia did not generate beneficial physiological adaptations yielding enhanced aerobic or anaerobic endurance exercise performance.

AUTHOR CONTRIBUTIONS

Conception and design of the study: PH and SD. All authors contributed to the collection and interpretation of the data, and reviewed and approved the final manuscript written by PH and SD.

ACKNOWLEDGMENTS

We thank all participants for their participation in this study. The authors would also like to acknowledge Monique Ramaekers for skillful technical assistance during the experiments, Cian McGinley for technical assistance during the βhm assay, and Prof. Roger Harris for his insightful comments and interpretation of the data. This work was supported by the Flemish Ministry of Sport, BLOSO—"Leerstoel Topsport Inspanningsfysiologie."

REFERENCES

Allemeier, C. A., Fry, A. C., Johnson, P., Hikida, R. S., Hagerman, F. C., and Staron, R. S. (1994). Effects of sprint cycle training on human skeletal muscle. *J. Appl. Physiol.* 77, 2385–2390.

Alvares, T. S., Conte, C. A., Paschoalin, V. M. F., Silva, J. T., Meirelles, C. D. M., Bhambhani, Y. N., et al. (2012). Acute l-arginine supplementation increases muscle blood volume but not strength performance. *Appl. Physiol. Nutr. Metab.* 37, 115–126. doi: 10.1139/h11-144

Baguet, A., Everaert, I., De Naeyer, H., Reyngoudt, H., Stegen, S., Beeckman, S., et al. (2011). Effects of sprint training combined with vegetarian or mixed diet on muscle carnosine content and buffering capacity. *Eur. J. Appl. Physiol.* 111, 2571–2580. doi: 10.1007/s00421-011-1877-4

Bailey, S. J., Fulford, J., Vanhatalo, A., Winyard, P. G., Blackwell, J. R., DiMenna, F. J., et al. (2010). Dietary nitrate supplementation enhances muscle contractile efficiency during knee-extensor exercise in humans. *J. Appl. Physiol.* 109, 135–148. doi: 10.1152/japplphysiol.00046.2010

Bailey, S. J., Varnham, R. L., DiMenna, F. J., Breese, B. C., Wylie, L. J., and Jones, A. M. (2015). Inorganic nitrate supplementation improves muscle oxygenation, O2 uptake kinetics, and exercise tolerance at high but not low pedal rates. *J. Appl. Physiol.* 118, 1396–1405. doi: 10.1152/japplphysiol.0114 1.2014

Bakkman, L., Sahlin, K., Holmberg, H. C., and Tonkonogi, M. (2007). Quantitative and qualitative adaptation of human skeletal muscle mitochondria to hypoxic compared with normoxic training at the same relative work rate. *Acta Physiol.* 190, 243–251. doi: 10.1111/j.1748-1716.2007.01683.x

Bishop, D., Edge, J., Thomas, C., and Mercier, J. (2008). Effects of high-intensity training on muscle lactate transporters and postexercise recovery of muscle lactate and hydrogen ions in women. *Am. J. Physiol. Regul. Integr. Comp. Physiol.* 295, R1991–R1998. doi: 10.1152/ajpregu.0086 3.2007

Bogdanis, G. C., Nevill, M. E., Boobis, L. H., and Lakomy, H. K. (1996). Contribution of phosphocreatine and aerobic metabolism to energy supply during repeated sprint exercise. *J. Appl. Physiol.* 80, 876–884.

Breese, B. C., McNarry, M. A., Marwood, S., Blackwell, J. R., Bailey, S. J., and Jones, A. M. (2013). Beetroot juice supplementation speeds O_2 uptake kinetics and improves exercise tolerance during severe-intensity exercise initiated from an elevated metabolic rate. *Am. J. Physiol. Regul. Integr. Comp. Physiol.* 305, R1441–R1450. doi: 10.1152/ajpregu.00295.2013

Calbet, J. A. L., De Paz, J. A., Garatachea, N., Cabeza De Vaca, S., and Chavarren, J. (2003). Anaerobic energy provision does not limit Wingate exercise performance in endurance-trained cyclists. *J. Appl. Physiol.* 94, 668–676. doi: 10.1152/japplphysiol.00128.2002

Clark, S. A., Aughey, R. J., Gore, C. J., Hahn, A. G., Townsend, N. E., Kinsman, T. A., et al. (2004). Effects of live high, train low hypoxic exposure on lactate metabolism in trained humans. *J. Appl. Physiol.* 96, 517–525. doi: 10.1152/japplphysiol.00799.2003

Coggan, A. R., Leibowitz, J. L., Kadkhodayan, A., Thomas, D. P., Ramamurthy, S., Spearie, C. A., et al. (2015). Effect of acute dietary nitrate intake on maximal knee extensor speed and power in healthy men and women. *Nitric Oxide* 48, 16–21. doi: 10.1016/j.niox.2014.08.014

Desplanches, D., Amami, M., Dupré-Aucouturier, S., Valdivieso, P., Schmutz, S., Mueller, M., et al. (2014). Hypoxia refines plasticity of mitochondrial respiration to repeated muscle work. *Eur. J. Appl. Physiol.* 114, 405–417. doi: 10.1007/s00421-013-2783-8

Edge, J., Bishop, D., and Goodman, C. (2006a). Effects of chronic NaHCO3 ingestion during interval training on changes to muscle buffer capacity, metabolism, and short-term endurance performance. *J. Appl. Physiol.* 101, 918–925. doi: 10.1152/japplphysiol.01534.2005

Edge, J., Bishop, D., and Goodman, C. (2006b). The effects of training intensity on muscle buffer capacity in females. *Eur. J. Appl. Physiol.* 96, 97–105. doi: 10.1007/s00421-005-0068-6

Faiss, R., Girard, O., and Millet, G. P. (2013a). Advancing hypoxic training in team sports: from intermittent hypoxic training to repeated sprint training in hypoxia. *Br. J. Sports Med.* 47(Suppl. 1), I45–I50. doi: 10.1136/bjsports-2013-092741

Faiss, R., Léger, B., Vesin, J.-M., Fournier, P.-E., Eggel, Y., Dériaz, O., et al. (2013b). Significant molecular and systemic adaptations after repeated sprint training in hypoxia. *PLoS ONE* 8:e56522. doi: 10.1371/journal.pone.0056522

Faiss, R., Willis, S., Born, D. P., Sperlich, B., Vesin, J. M., Holmberg, H. C., et al. (2015). Repeated double-poling sprint training in hypoxia by competitive cross-country skiers. *Med. Sci. Sports Exerc.* 47, 809–817. doi: 10.1249/MSS.0000000000000464

Ferguson, S. K., Hirai, D. M., Copp, S. W., Holdsworth, C. T., Allen, J. D., Jones, A. M., et al. (2013). Impact of dietary nitrate supplementation via beetroot juice on exercising muscle vascular control in rats. *J. Physiol. (Lond).* 591, 547–557. doi: 10.1113/jphysiol.2012.243121

Friedmann, B., Frese, F., Menold, E., and Bärtsch, P. (2007). Effects of acute moderate hypoxia on anaerobic capacity in endurance-trained runners. *Eur. J. Appl. Physiol.* 101, 67–73. doi: 10.1007/s00421-007-0473-0

Galvin, H. M., Cooke, K., Sumners, D. P., Mileva, K. N., and Bowtell, J. L. (2013). Repeated sprint training in normobaric hypoxia. *Br. J. Sports Med.* 47, I74–I79. doi: 10.1136/bjsports-2013-092826

Geiser, J., Vogt, M., Billeter, R., Zuleger, C., Belforti, F., and Hoppeler, H. (2001). Training high-living low: changes of aerobic performance and muscle structure with training at simulated altitude. *Int. J. Sports Med.* 22, 579–585. doi: 10.1055/s-2001-18521

Gore, C. J., Hahn, A. G., Aughey, R. J., Martin, D. T., Ashenden, M. J., Clark, S. A., et al. (2001). Live high: train low increases muscle buffer capacity and submaximal cycling efficiency. *Acta Physiol. Scand.* 173, 275–286. doi: 10.1046/j.1365-201X.2001.00906.x

Green, H., MacDougall, J., Tarnopolsky, M., and Melissa, N. L. (1999). Downregulation of Na+-K+-ATPase pumps in skeletal muscle with training in normobaric hypoxia. *J. Appl. Physiol.* 86, 1745–1748.

Harmer, A. R., McKenna, M. J., Sutton, J. R., Snow, R. J., Ruell, A., Booth, J., et al. (2000). Skeletal muscle metabolic and ionic adaptations during intense exercise following sprint training in humans. *J. Appl. Physiol.* 89, 1793–1803.

Harris, R. C., Marlin, D. J., Dunnett, M., Snow, D. H., and Hultman, E. (1990). Muscle buffering capacity and dipeptide content in the thoroughbred horse, greyhound dog and man. *Comp. Biochem. Physiol. A Physiol.* 97, 249–251. doi: 10.1016/0300-9629(90)90180-Z

Haseler, L. J., Hogan, M. C., and Richardson, R. S. (1999). Skeletal muscle phosphocreatine recovery in exercise-trained humans is dependent on O_2 availability. *J. Appl. Physiol.* 86, 2013–2018.

Hernández, A., Schiffer, T. A., Ivarsson, N., Cheng, A. J., Bruton, J. D., Lundberg, J. O., et al. (2012). Dietary nitrate increases tetanic [Ca2+]i and contractile force in mouse fast-twitch muscle. *J. Physiol. (Lond).* 590, 3575–3583. doi: 10.1113/jphysiol.2012.232777

Hill, C. A., Harris, R. C., Kim, H. J., Harris, B. D., Sale, C., Boobis, L. H., et al. (2007). Influence of B-alanine supplementation on skeletal muscle carnosine concentrations and high intensity cycling capacity. *Amino Acids* 32, 225–233. doi: 10.1007/s00726-006-0364-4

Holliss, B. A., Fulford, J., Vanhatalo, A., Pedlar, C. R., and Jones, A. M. (2013). Influence of intermittent hypoxic training on muscle energetics and exercise tolerance. *J. Appl. Physiol.* 114, 611–619. doi: 10.1152/japplphysiol.01331.2012

Hoppeler, H., Klossner, S., and Vogt, M. (2008). Training in hypoxia and its effects on skeletal muscle tissue. *Scand. J. Med. Sci. Sports* 18, 38–49. doi: 10.1111/j.1600-0838.2008.00831.x

Kelly, J., Vanhatalo, A., Bailey, S. J., Wylie, L. J., Tucker, C., List, S., et al. (2014). Dietary nitrate supplementation: effects on plasma nitrite and pulmonary O_2 uptake dynamics during exercise in hypoxia and normoxia. *Am. J. Physiol. Regul. Integr. Comp. Physiol.* 307, R920–R930. doi: 10.1152/ajpregu.00068.2014

Kendrick, I. P., Kim, H. J., Harris, R. C., Kim, C. K., Dang, V. H., Lam, T. Q., et al. (2009). The effect of 4 weeks B-alanine supplementation and isokinetic training on carnosine concentrations in type I and II human skeletal muscle fibres. *Eur. J. Appl. Physiol.* 106, 131–138. doi: 10.1007/s00421-009-0998-5

Larsen, F. J., Schiffer, T. A., Borniquel, S., Sahlin, K., Ekblom, B., Lundberg, J. O., et al. (2011). Dietary inorganic nitrate improves mitochondrial efficiency in humans. *Cell Metab.* 13, 149–159. doi: 10.1016/j.cmet.2011.01.004

Lundberg, J. O., Weitzberg, E., and Gladwin, M. T. (2008). The nitrate-nitrite-nitric oxide pathway in physiology and therapeutics. *Nat. Rev. Drug Discov.* 7, 156–167. doi: 10.1038/nrd2466

Mannion, A. F., Jakeman, P. M., Dunnett, M., Harris, R. C., and Willan, P. L. T. (1992). Carnosine and anserine concentrations in the quadriceps femoris muscle of healthy humans. *Eur. J. Appl. Physiol. Occup. Physiol.* 64, 47–50. doi: 10.1007/BF00376439

Mannion, A. F., Jakeman, P. M., and Willan, P. L. (1994). Effects of isokinetic training of the knee extensors on high-intensity exercise performance and skeletal muscle buffering. *Eur. J. Appl. Physiol. Occup. Physiol.* 68, 356–361. doi: 10.1007/BF00571457

Martins, K. J. B., St-Louis, M., Murdoch, G. K., MacLean, I. M., McDonald, P., Dixon, W. T., et al. (2012). Nitric oxide synthase inhibition prevents activity-induced calcineurin-NFATc1 signalling and fast-to-slow skeletal muscle fibre type conversions. *J. Physiol. (Lond).* 590, 1427–1442. doi: 10.1113/jphysiol.2011.223370

Masschelein, E., Van Thienen, R., Wang, X., Van Schepdael, A., Thomis, M., and Hespel, P. (2012). Dietary nitrate improves muscle but not cerebral oxygenation status during exercise in hypoxia. *J. Appl. Physiol.* 113, 736–745. doi: 10.1152/japplphysiol.01253.2011

McGinnis, G., Kliszczewiscz, B., Barberio, M., Ballmann, C., Peters, B., Slivka, D., et al. (2014). Acute hypoxia and exercise-induced blood oxidative stress. *Int. J. Sport Nutr. Exerc. Metab.* 24, 684–693. doi: 10.1123/ijsnem.2013-0188

McLean, B. D., Gore, C. J., and Kemp, J. (2014). Application of "live low-train high" for enhancing normoxic exercise performance in team sport athletes. *Sport. Med.* 44, 1275–1287. doi: 10.1007/s40279-014-0204-8

Melissa, L., MacDougall, J. D., Tarnopolsky, M. A., Cipriano, N., and Green, H. J. (1997). Skeletal muscle adaptations to training under normobaric hypoxic versus normoxic conditions. *Med. Sci. Sports Exerc.* 29, 238–243. doi: 10.1097/00005768-199702000-00012

Mizuno, M., Juel, C., Bro-Rasmussen, T., Mygind, E., Schibye, B., Rasmussen, B., et al. (1990). Limb skeletal muscle adaptation in athletes after training at altitude. *J. Appl. Physiol.* 68, 496–502.

Montero, D., and Lundby, C. (2015). Enhanced performance after repeated sprint training in hypoxia: false or reality? *Med. Sci. Sport. Exerc.* 47, 2483. doi: 10.1249/MSS.0000000000000711

Mora, L., Sentandreu, M. A., and Toldrá, F. (2007). Hydrophilic chromatographic determination of carnosine, anserine, balenine, creatine, and creatinine. *J. Agric. Food Chem.* 55, 4664–4669. doi: 10.1021/jf0703809

Morales-Alamo, D., Ponce-Gonzalez, J. G., Guadalupe-Grau, A., Rodriguez-Garcia, L., Santana, A., Cusso, M. R., et al. (2012). Increased oxidative stress and anaerobic energy release, but blunted Thr172-AMPK phosphorylation, in response to sprint exercise in severe acute hypoxia in humans. *J. Appl. Physiol.* 113, 917–928. doi: 10.1152/japplphysiol.00415.2012

Mosher, S. S., Sparks, A. S., Williams, E., Bentley, D. J., and McNaughton, L. R. (2016). Ingestion of a nitric oxide enhancing supplement improves resistance exercise performance. *J. Strength Cond. Res.* doi: 10.1519/jsc.0000000000001437. [Epub ahead of print].

Muggeridge, D. J., Howe, C. C. F., Spendiff, O., Pedlar, C., James, P. E., and Easton, C. (2014). A single dose of beetroot juice enhances cycling performance in simulated altitude. *Med. Sci. Sports Exerc.* 46, 143–150. doi: 10.1249/MSS.0b013e3182a1dc51

Nevill, M. E., Boobis, L. H., Brooks, S., and Williams, C. (1989). Effect of training on muscle metabolism during treadmill sprinting. *J. Appl. Physiol.* 67, 2736–2782.

Nordsborg, N. B., Siebenmann, C., Jacobs, R. A., Rasmussen, P., Diaz, V., Robach, P., et al. (2012). Four weeks of normobaric "live high-train low" do not alter muscular or systemic capacity for maintaining pH and K+ homeostasis during intense exercise. *J. Appl. Physiol.* 112, 2027–2036. doi: 10.1152/japplphysiol.01353.2011

Parolin, M. L., Chesley, A., Matsos, M. P., Spriet, L. L., Jones, N. L., and Heigenhauser, G. J. F. (1999). Regulation of skeletal muscle glycogen phosphorylase and PDH during maximal intermittent exercise. *Am. J. Physiol. Endocrinol. Metab.* 277, 890–900.

Porporato, P. E., Dhup, S., Dadhich, R. K., Copetti, T., and Sonveaux, P. (2011). Anticancer targets in the glycolytic metabolism of tumors: a comprehensive review. *Front. Pharmacol.* 2:49. doi: 10.3389/fphar.2011.00049

Putman, C. T., Jones, N. L., Lands, L. C., Bragg, T. M., Hollidge-Horvat, M. G., and Heigenhauser, G. J. (1995). Skeletal muscle pyruvate dehydrogenase activity during maximal exercise in humans. *Am. J. Physiol.* 269, E458–E468.

Puype, J., Van Proeyen, K., Raymackers, J.-M., Deldicque, L., and Hespel, P. (2013). Sprint interval training in hypoxia stimulates glycolytic enzyme activity. *Med. Sci. Sports Exerc.* 45, 2166–2174. doi: 10.1249/MSS.0b013e31829734ae

Ross, A., and Leveritt, M. (2001). Long-term metabolic and skeletal muscle adaptations to short-sprint training: implications for sprint training and tapering. *Sport. Med.* 31, 1063–1082. doi: 10.2165/00007256-200131150-00003

Saltin, B., Kim, C. K., Terrados, N., Larsen, H., Svedenhag, J., and Rolf, C. J. (1995). Morphology, enzyme activities and buffer capacity in leg muscles of Kenyan and Scandinavian runners. *Scand. J. Med. Sci. Sports* 5, 222–230. doi: 10.1111/j.1600-0838.1995.tb00038.x

Schmutz, S., Däpp, C., Wittwer, M., Durieux, A.-C., Mueller, M., Weinstein, F., et al. (2010). A hypoxia complement differentiates the muscle response to endurance exercise. *Exp. Physiol.* 95, 723–735. doi: 10.1113/expphysiol.2009.051029

Sloth, M., Sloth, D., Overgaard, K., and Dalgas, U. (2013). Effects of sprint interval training on VO2max and aerobic exercise performance: a systematic review and meta-analysis. *Scand. J. Med. Sci. Sports* 23, 341–352. doi: 10.1111/sms.12092

Smith, L. W., Smith, J. D., Criswell, D. S., Smith, L. W., Smith, J. D., Criswell, D. S., et al. (2002). Involvement of nitric oxide synthase in skeletal muscle adaptation to chronic overload. *J Appl Physiol.* 92, 2005–2011. doi: 10.1152/japplphysiol.00950.2001

Suwa, M., Nakano, H., Radak, Z., and Kumagai, S. (2015). Effects of nitric oxide synthase inhibition on fiber-type composition, mitochondrial biogenesis, and SIRT1 expression in rat skeletal muscle. *J. Sport. Sci. Med.* 14, 548–555.

Suzuki, Y., Ito, O., Takahashi, H., and Takamatsu, K. (2004). The effect of sprint training on skeletal muscle carnosine in humans. *Int. J. Sport Heal. Sci.* 2, 105–110. doi: 10.5432/ijshs.2.105

Terrados, N., Jansson, E., Sylven, C., and Kaijser, L. (1990). Is hypoxia a stimulus for synthesis of oxidative enzymes and myoglobin? *J. Appl. Physiol.* 68, 2369–2372.

Thomas, C., Bishop, D., Moore-Morris, T., and Mercier, J. (2007). Effects of high-intensity training on MCT1, MCT4, and NBC expressions in rat skeletal muscles: influence of chronic metabolic alkalosis. *Am. J. Physiol. Endocrinol. Metab.* 293, E916–E922. doi: 10.1152/ajpendo.00164.2007

Thompson, C., Wylie, L. J., Fulford, J., Kelly, J., Black, M. I., McDonagh, S. T. J., et al. (2015). Dietary nitrate improves sprint performance and cognitive function during prolonged intermittent exercise. *Eur. J. Appl. Physiol.* 115, 1825–1834. doi: 10.1007/s00421-015-3166-0

Vanhatalo, A., Fulford, J., Bailey, S. J., Blackwell, J. R., Winyard, P. G., and Jones, A. M. (2011). Dietary nitrate reduces muscle metabolic perturbation and improves exercise tolerance in hypoxia. *J. Physiol. (Lond).* 589, 5517–5528. doi: 10.1113/jphysiol.2011.216341

Vanhatalo, A., Jones, A. M., Blackwell, J. R., Winyard, P. G., and Fulford, J. (2014). Dietary nitrate accelerates post-exercise muscle metabolic recovery and O2 delivery in hypoxia. *J. Appl. Physiol.* 117, 1460–1470. doi: 10.1152/japplphysiol.00096.2014

Vogt, M., Puntschart, A., Geiser, J., Zuleger, C., Billeter, R., and Hoppeler, H. (2001). Molecular adaptations in human skeletal muscle to endurance training under simulated hypoxic conditions. *J. Appl. Physiol.* 91, 173–182.

Webb, A. J., Patel, N., Loukogeorgakis, S., Okorie, M., Aboud, Z., Misra, S., et al. (2008). Acute blood pressure lowering, vasoprotective, and antiplatelet properties of dietary nitrate via bioconversion to nitrite. *Hypertension* 51, 784–790. doi: 10.1161/HYPERTENSIONAHA.107.103523

Wehrlin, J. P., and Hallén, J. (2006). Linear decrease in VO_{2max} and performance with increasing altitude in endurance athletes. *Eur. J. Appl. Physiol.* 96, 404–412. doi: 10.1007/s00421-005-0081-9

Weyand, P., and Lee, C. (1999). High-speed running performance is largely unaffected by hypoxic reductions in aerobic power. *J. Appl. Physiol.* 86, 2059–2064.

Wylie, L. J., Kelly, J., Bailey, S. J., Blackwell, J. R., Skiba, P. F., Winyard, P. G., et al. (2013). Beetroot juice and exercise: pharmacodynamic and dose-response relationships. *J. Appl. Physiol.* 115, 325–336. doi: 10.1152/japplphysiol.00372.2013

Zoll, J., Ponsot, E., Dufour, S., Doutreleau, S., Ventura-Clapier, R., Vogt, M., et al. (2006). Exercise training in normobaric hypoxia in endurance runners. III. Muscular adjustments of selected gene transcripts. *J. Appl. Physiol.* 100, 1258–1266. doi: 10.1152/japplphysiol.00359.2005

21

Hypoxic Repeat Sprint Training Improves Rugby Player's Repeated Sprint but not Endurance Performance

Michael J. Hamlin[1]*, Peter D. Olsen[2], Helen C. Marshall[2], Catherine A. Lizamore[1] and Catherine A. Elliot[1]

[1] Department of Tourism, Sport and Society, Lincoln University, Christchurch, New Zealand, [2] Department of Nursing, Midwifery and Allied Health, Ara Institute of Canterbury, Christchurch, New Zealand

***Correspondence:**
Mike J. Hamlin
mike.hamlin@lincoln.ac.nz

This study aims to investigate the performance changes in 19 well-trained male rugby players after repeat-sprint training (six sessions of four sets of 5 × 5 s sprints with 25 s and 5 min of active recovery between reps and sets, respectively) in either normobaric hypoxia (HYP; $n = 9$; $F_IO_2 = 14.5\%$) or normobaric normoxia (NORM; $n = 10$; $F_IO_2 = 20.9\%$). Three weeks after the intervention, 2 additional repeat-sprint training sessions in hypoxia ($F_IO_2 = 14.5\%$) was investigated in both groups to gauge the efficacy of using "top-up" sessions for previously hypoxic-trained subjects and whether a small hypoxic dose would be beneficial for the previously normoxic-trained group. Repeated sprint (8 × 20 m) and Yo-Yo Intermittent Recovery Level 1 (YYIR1) performances were tested twice at baseline (Pre 1 and Pre 2) and weekly after (Post 1–3) the initial intervention (intervention 1) and again weekly after the second "top-up" intervention (Post 4–5). After each training set, heart rate, oxygen saturation, and rate of perceived exertion were recorded. Compared to baseline (mean of Pre 1 and Pre 2), both the hypoxic and normoxic groups similarly lowered fatigue over the 8 sprints 1 week after the intervention (Post 1: −1.8 ± 1.6%, −1.5 ± 1.4%, mean change ± 90% CI in HYP and NORM groups, respectively). However, from Post 2 onwards, only the hypoxic group maintained the performance improvement compared to baseline (Post 2: −2.1 ± 1.8%, Post 3: −2.3 ± 1.7%, Post 4: −1.9 ± 1.8%, and Post 5: −1.2 ± 1.7%). Compared to the normoxic group, the hypoxic group was likely to have substantially less fatigue at Post 3–5 (−2.0 ± 2.4%, −2.2 ± 2.4%, −1.6 ± 2.4% Post 3, Post 4, Post 5, respectively). YYIR1 performances improved throughout the recovery period in both groups (13–37% compared to baseline) with unclear differences found between groups. The addition of two sessions of "top-up" training after intervention 1, had little effect on either group. Repeat-sprint training in hypoxia for six sessions increases repeat sprint ability but not YYIR1 performance in well-trained rugby players.

Keywords: normobaric hypoxia, Yo-Yo intermittent recovery test, team sports, repeated sprint ability, intermittent hypoxic training

INTRODUCTION

Rugby union is a fast-paced, field-based sport where strength, power, speed, and endurance are essential (Nicholas, 1997). Moreover, because of the game's intermittent nature, the ability to sprint repetitively is also an important fitness component for the modern rugby player and may be crucial to the outcome of the game (Austin et al., 2011a). In team sports, although different playing positions require different anthropometric and physiological characteristics, the ability to perform repeated sprints is associated with improved measures of game performance (Rampinini et al., 2007). Traditionally, repeat-sprint training involved on-feet, repeated running bouts interspersed with appropriate recovery periods (Tønnessen et al., 2011). Such training has been shown to improve oxygen utilization (Bailey et al., 2009) and increase anaerobic metabolism (Dawson et al., 1998), thereby enhancing repeat sprint ability. However, because the aerobic system is heavily involved in regenerating ATP during recovery from repeated sprints (Spencer et al., 2005), it is thought that strategies used to improve aerobic metabolism may also help to improve repeat sprint ability. As a consequence, there has been an increased interest in the ability of altitude or hypoxic training to enhance repeat sprint ability.

Increased anaerobic glycolytic activity (Svedenhag et al., 1991 #2736; Faiss et al., 2013b) and modified acid-base homeostasis (Nummela and Rusko, 2000) have both been signaled as possible mechanisms responsible for the improved repeat sprint ability after altitude/hypoxic training. A lower rate of oxygen delivery to the muscle during hypoxic training probably increases the stress on the anaerobic metabolic pathways thereby resulting in upregulation of anaerobic metabolism (Faiss et al., 2013b).

However, adding hypoxia to repeat-sprint training has not always resulted in improved repeat sprint ability at sea-level. Faiss et al. (2013b) found that two repeat-sprint training sessions per week (3 sets of 5 × 10 s all-out cycle sprinting at ~3000 m) for 4 weeks had little effect on overall power output during a repeat sprint cycling test. Nevertheless, such training increased the number of all-out 10 s cycling sprints able to be completed prior to exhaustion in the hypoxic (3.6) compared to the normoxic (−0.4) trained groups (Faiss et al., 2013b). On the other hand, Goods et al. (2015) found 15 sessions of repeat-sprint training in hypoxia over 5 weeks (3 sets of 7 × 5 s all-out cycle sprints at ~3000 m), had little effect compared to similar exercise in normoxia on running or cycling repeat sprint ability in Australian football players. While Galvin et al. (2013) found repeat-sprint training (12 sessions over 4 weeks of 1 set of 10 × 6 s all-out treadmill sprints at ~3500 m) in hypoxic compared to normoxic conditions had little effect on repeat sprint ability in trained rugby players. Other researchers have reported adding hypoxia to repeat-sprint training can produce trivial (~1.5%) (Brocherie et al., 2015a) to substantial and long-lasting beneficial effects (2.9% immediately and 2.8% 3-weeks post-training) on repeat sprint ability (Brocherie et al., 2015b). In female participants, conflicting results also exist with some researchers reporting beneficial improvements in repeat sprint ability in the hypoxic compared to the normoxic trained group (Kasai et al., 2015), while others found no such change in repeat sprint ability (Jones B. et al., 2015). For a more detailed review of the use of repeat-sprint training in hypoxia see (Faiss et al., 2013a).

Repeat-sprint training under hypoxic conditions to improve endurance performance has also resulted in conflicting results. Galvin et al. (2013) found significantly improved endurance performance (Yo-Yo intermittent recovery test level 1) after repeat-sprint training in rugby players. More recently, Jones B. et al. (2015) reported significantly faster final running velocities in female field hockey players during a 30–15 intermittent field test after repeat-sprint training under hypoxic compared to control conditions, whereas others have found little effect on 20 m shuttle run performance post hypoxic repeat-sprint training (Goods et al., 2015).

Some of the variation in response to repeat-sprint training under hypoxia between studies is probably due to the methodological differences. While most studies use a similar hypoxic training stimulus (F_IO_2 ~14.5% equivalent to ~3000 m), the repeat-sprint training protocols can vary considerably from repetitions of short duration high-intensity repeats (12 sessions of 1 set of 10 × 6 s; Galvin et al., 2013), to longer-duration and subsequently lower-intensity repeats (six sessions of one set of between eight and 12 × 60 s; Jones M. R. et al., 2015). Exercise prescription theory dictates that exercise training prescription should be as specific as possible to facilitate appropriate physiological adaptations (Reilly et al., 2009). Therefore, repeat-sprint training protocols should be based on work-to-rest ratio's of actual repeat sprint ability while playing the sport (adding hypoxia to this training serves to induce a larger metabolic stimulus resulting in greater adaptation). Using GPS technology (MinimaxX, Catapult Innovation, 10 Hz) Jones M. R. et al. (2015) reported the repeat sprint efforts from 33 professional rugby players over the 2012-2013 season. On average, there were ~8 repeated high-intensity bouts (range from 5 to 11) per game, which had 3–4 efforts per bout with ~5 s between efforts and about 6–12 min recovery between bouts (Jones M. R. et al., 2015). Using time-motion analysis of 20 professional rugby players during the 2008-2009 Super 14 international rugby competition (Austin et al., 2011b), others have reported slightly more bouts of repeat sprint efforts during the game (mean 14, range 7–17), but a similar average recovery between bouts of ~6 min. The authors did not include the rest between efforts in each bout, so comparing the average duration of the bout (~30 s) is difficult. To our knowledge, there are few research studies that have based their repeat-sprint training protocols on data from real matches, particularly when adding hypoxia to the training. Therefore, the aim of this study was to examine the effect of using rugby-specific repeat-sprint training with hypoxia on field-based repeat sprint and endurance ability in rugby players during pre-season training.

It has been suggested that after traditional altitude training there is a small period of attenuated performance (due to the re-establishment of sea-level training volume and intensity), followed by a longer period of improved performance (Millet et al., 2010), as adaptations to the altitude training continue to manifest over time. While the post-training performance period requires further research, we have found that anaerobic performance in well-trained athletes started to decline back to baseline levels 9 days post-intermittent hypoxic training (Hamlin et al., 2010). Because of the natural degradation of the hypoxic adaptations over time, some practitioners have suggested using "top-up" sessions (hypoxic sessions of shorter duration than the initial hypoxic training spaced through-out the training year) in an attempt to maintain beneficial adaptations and performance (Saunders et al., 2009). The effect of a hypoxic repeat-sprint training top-up session on subsequent repeat sprint ability has not been researched to date.

Little information also exists on the minimum number of hypoxic exposures required to improve performance, or how long a possible hypoxic-induced performance enhancement remains. Therefore, a secondary aim of this study was to measure performance 3 weeks post-intervention to gain insight into the longevity of performance change, but also to investigate the effect of a 1-week top-up dose on previously hypoxic and normoxic-trained subjects.

MATERIALS AND METHODS

Subjects

Nineteen representative and club rugby players from Canterbury, New Zealand participated in this study. Players were non-professional and played in the senior and under 21 age-group teams in the Canterbury country competition. These players typically complete two rugby-specific and 1–2 strength and conditioning sessions per week during the pre-season and two rugby-specific, one game and one recovery session per week during the regular season. The research was conducted over the whole pre-season training period which typically lasts 8–10 weeks. This study was carried out in accordance with the recommendations of the Lincoln University Human Ethics guidelines with written informed consent from all subjects. All subjects gave their written informed consent in accordance with the Declaration of Helsinki. The protocol was approved by the Lincoln University Human Ethics Committee (reference 2015-46). Participant characteristics are presented in **Table 1**. All participants were healthy, free from injury, lived at sea level and had not resided at altitude within the previous 6 months. Participants were matched for baseline repeat sprint ability (i.e., cumulated time required to complete 8 × 20 m sprints), and then randomly divided into two groups: a hypoxic group (HYP, $n = 9$) and a control group (NORM, $n = 10$). Participants were asked to maintain their usual pre-season fitness and rugby training sessions throughout the study. Due to injury, one control group participant had to withdraw from the study.

Study Design

This study was single blind, placebo-controlled trial whose intervention was based on repeat sprint bouts found in real rugby matches (Austin et al., 2011b; Jones M. R. et al., 2015). Participants performed seven main trials including two baseline and five post-exposure trials. The baseline trials were performed 4–5 days apart and 1 week before beginning the first repeat-sprint

TABLE 1 | Characteristics and baseline test 1 performance measures.

	NORM ($n = 10$)	HYP ($n = 8$)
Age (yr)	22.0 ± 4.1	20.3 ± 2.1
Body mass (kg)	88.3 ± 14.1	77.1 ± 10.2*
Height (cm)	177.9 ± 5.4	173.9 ± 4.9
Weekly training (min.wk^{-1})	248.2 ± 208.9	270.9 ± 155.8
Weekly Trimp	3463 ± 3187	3642 ± 2191
Cumulated sprint time (s)	27.4 ± 3.2	26.9 ± 3.4
Repeated sprint fatigue^1 (%)	5.5 ± 2.3	5.8 ± 3.4
Repeated sprint fatigue^2 (%)	3.5 ± 1.2	3.5 ± 1.3
Yo-Yo level 1 (m)	1100 ± 426	1200 ± 384

*Data are raw means ± SD. Weekly Trimp, weekly training impulse (training duration × intensity); Cumulated sprint time, total time for 8 sprints; Repeated sprint fatigue^1, % fatigue from sprint 1 to sprint 8 using the linear extrapolation method; Repeated sprint fatigue^2, % fatigue decrement score using the % decrement score method (100 × total sprint time/ideal sprint time) − 100; Yo-Yo level 1; distance covered in the Yo-Yo level 1 intermittent recovery test * Substantial differences.*

training block. After 3 weeks of repeat-sprint training, three post-training trials were completed (1 week apart). A second 1-week repeat-sprint training block followed where both groups trained under hypoxia. Two further post-training trials (1-week apart) followed the "top-up" sessions (see **Figure 1**). The main trials involved field-based fitness tests including a repeat sprint ability test (8 × 20 m all-out running sprints timed to go every 20 s) and a Yo-Yo Intermittent Recovery Level 1 test (YYIR1) commonly used on rugby players (Gore, 2000). To aid in the blinding, all participants were under the impression that they would be receiving altitude training (i.e., breathing hypoxic air).

Participant Preparation

The participants were asked to arrive in a fully rested and hydrated state and to refrain from intense exercise for 24 h and caffeine for 12 h prior to each main trial. All testing was performed at the same time of day (±1 h) to minimize diurnal variation. Participants were also asked to record their dietary intake before the first baseline fitness trial to allow for replication of the diet prior to subsequent trials.

Hypoxic and Normoxic Repetitive Sprint Training

Participants were asked to complete repeat-sprint training on a Wattbike (Wattbike Pro, Nottingham, UK) at air brake resistance level 3, magnetic setting three for training sessions 1–2 and 5–8. The settings were increased for training sessions 3 and 4 (air brake level 5, magnetic setting 3) to increase overload and further challenge the participants. Prior to training, the zero was calibrated for each Wattbike according to the manufacturer's recommendations. Bike dimensions for individual athletes (saddle, handlebar heights, and positions) were initially recorded and replicated at each training session. Participants were asked to cycle in an upright, seated position. Training consisted of six sessions of repeat-sprint intervals over an initial 3 week period (two sessions per week), followed 3 weeks later by a further two top-up sessions over 1 week (**Figure 1**). For the two top-up sessions only, all participants received the normobaric

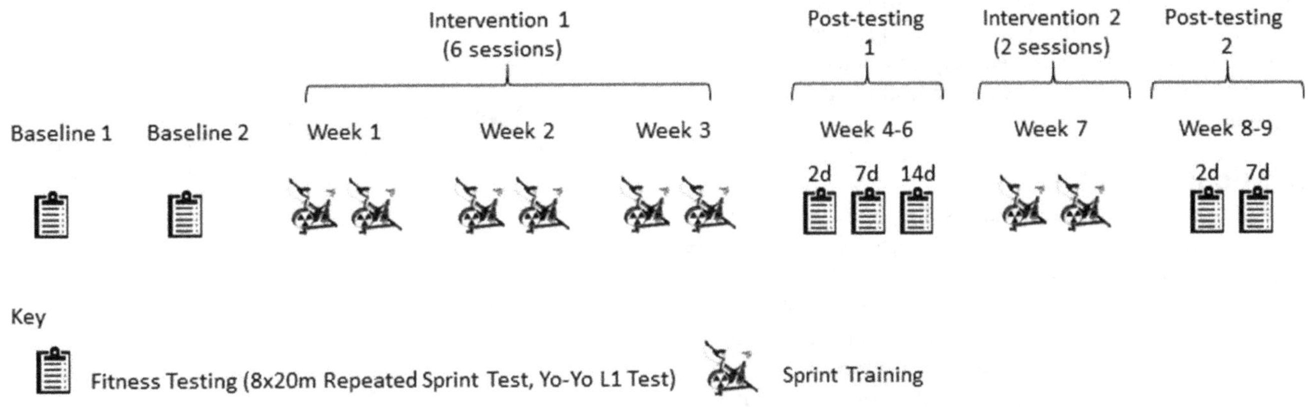

FIGURE 1 | Outline of training and testing schedule.

hypoxic gas (i.e., both the previously hypoxic and normoxic-trained groups). This protocol was to test the effectiveness of a top-up dose on previously hypoxic-trained participants and to test whether a minimum dose of two hypoxic sessions had any beneficial effect on otherwise normally trained participants. Participants maintained their normal pre-season fitness and rugby training routines. As indicated previously, the repeat-sprint interval training programme was designed around GPS data from real match play (Jones M. R. et al., 2015) and consisted of 4 sets of 5 repetitions of 5 s all-out cycling efforts interspersed with 25 s active recovery low cadence cycling (~20–50 W) between efforts and 5 min active recovery low cadence cycling (~20–50 W) between sets. A 5 min warm-up at ~50 W interspersed with a 5 s sprint at the end of each minute was performed prior to the sprint training, making the total exercise time ~35 min per session and 280 min over the total study (i.e., a total of 280 min under hypoxia). All participants were given strong verbal encouragement to maintain effort throughout the training.

During training, subjects received either a normobaric hypoxic (HYP) or a normobaric normoxic gas (NORM) via the GO_2Altitude® hypoxicator system (Biomedtech, Victoria, Australia). After calibrating the equipment at the start of each training session, the hypoxic or placebo (normoxic) gas was sent to two 100L Douglas bags connected in series. Participants breathed from the bags via a leak-free respiratory mask (Hans-Rudolph 8980, Kansas City, Missouri, USA) attached to a one-way non-rebreathing valve (Hans-Rudolph 2700). The fraction of inspired oxygen (F_IO_2) was set at 14.5% (~3000 m) for the HYP group, and 20.9% for the NORM. We selected this hypoxic level based on previous research which suggested an F_IO_2 of between 14.8 and 16.7% (2000–3000 m) increases the physiological stress during repeat-sprint training without exacerbating the speed decline during such training (Bowtell et al., 2014; Goods et al., 2014). Participants were unable to view any oxygen or blood saturation monitors during training and we are confident of the blinding procedure as when asked at the end of intervention one, only a small fraction (i.e., 2 out of 10 controls) thought they might be receiving a higher oxygen dose or not getting hypoxia at all.

Participants recorded their daily training information along with their subjective ratings of stress, fatigue, muscle soreness, quality of sleep, and quality of training performance. Previous research by our group (Hamlin and Hellemans, 2007) and other researchers (Eston and Williams, 1988) indicates that such effort ratings can be used as reliable indicators of exercise intensity. To compare the total training load between groups, training impulse (Trimp) (Banister and Calvert, 1980) was calculated, which was expressed as a product of stress (duration of training) and strain (subjective rating of training intensity). Participants reported their subjective rating with the use of the 15-point (6–20) Borg scale (Borg, 1982).

Performance Tests

Performance testing was composed of a warm-up, a squat jump (not reported here), a repeat sprint ability test, and a Yo-Yo Intermittent Recovery Level 1 test (YYIR1) followed by a warm-down. The order of testing was standardized and participants were rested for 10–15 min between each test. The warm-up consisted of a slow jog for 5 min followed by 5–10 min of dynamic and static stretching. The repeat sprint ability test consisted of eight maximal effort running sprints timed to go every 20 s. Times (to the nearest 0.01 s) for each sprint were recorded using two sets of electronic speed-timing lights (Smartspeed, Fusion Sport Ltd, Australia). Fatigue during the 8 sprints was calculated by two methods; (i) applying a straight line to the data and estimating the predicted time in the first minus the last sprint which was log-transformed to get percent fatigue and (ii) using the percentage decrement score as described by Glaister et al. (2008) (Fatigue = (100 × (total sprint time/ideal sprint time)) − 100). Finally, participants completed a 20-m shuttle run test (Yo-Yo Intermittent Recovery test Level 1, BangsboSport, Denmark, YYIR1). Testing was completed at the same time of day in a covered stadium on slip-free flooring under similar climatic conditions.

Physiological Measures

During the training sessions, heart rate was recorded (FT1; Polar, Kemple, Finland) and arterial oxygen saturation (SpO_2,

Sport-Stat; Nonin Medical, Minneapolis, Minnesota, USA) was monitored manually by the researchers, which was unable to be viewed by the participants. Participant's perceived exertion during sprint training (RPE) was recorded at the end of each set with the Borg scale (6–20).

Statistical Analysis

Changes in the mean of the variables and standard deviations representing the between-and within-subject variability were estimated using a mixed modeling procedure (Proc Mixed) in the Statistical Analysis System (Version 9.3, SAS Institute, Cary North Carolina, USA). We analyzed the natural logarithm of each measure to reduce any effects in non-uniformity of error and to obtain changes in measures and errors as percentages (Hopkins et al., 2009). The fixed effects were test time (the average of baseline 1 and 2, post 1, post 2 etc.), group (HYP, NORM) and their interaction. The random effects were subject and residual variance. Chances that the true effects were substantial were estimated with a spreadsheet (Hopkins, 2006), when a value for the smallest worthwhile effect was entered. We used a value of 1% for performance measures (Paton et al., 2001). For non-performance measures, we chose 0.20 standardized units (change in mean divided by the between-subject *SD* at baseline) as the smallest worthwhile change (Cohen, 1988). To make inferences about the true (population) values of the effect of hypoxia on performance, *P*-values, and statistical significance were not used. Instead, uncertainties in the estimate of changes were presented as 90% confidence intervals and as likelihoods that the true value of the effect was increased, decreased or trivial. The descriptors: increased, trivial or decreased were used to describe the direction of the change. Where the confidence interval spanned all three possibilities (increased, trivial and decreased), the result was deemed unclear. In all other cases, such as no overlap, or an overlap between two possibilities (trivial and increased, or trivial and decreased) a clear result was achieved. Finally, the magnitude or probability of the change was assessed using a qualitative scale defined as: <0.5%: almost certainly not; <5%: very unlikely; <25%: unlikely/probably not; 25–75%: possibly, possibly not; >75%: likely, probably; >95%: very likely; and >99.5%: almost certainly.

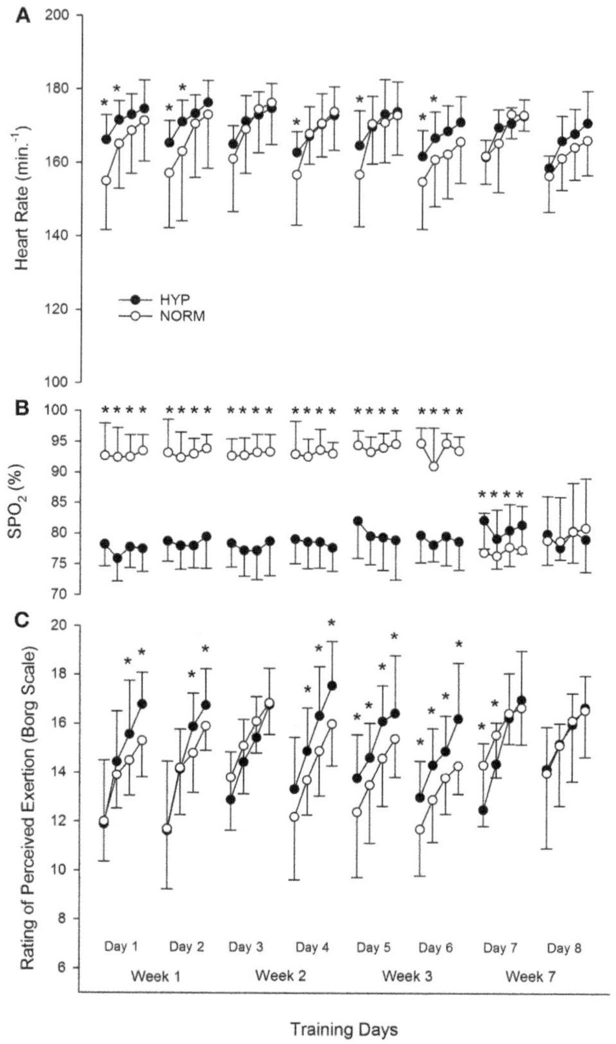

FIGURE 2 | Physiological and perceived exertion data. *Substantially different between groups at each time point. **(A)** Heart rate at the end of each set; **(B)** Arterial oxygen saturation at the end of each set; **(C)** Rating of perceived exertion (Borg 6–20 scale) at the end of each set.

RESULTS

Training Variables

We found no substantial difference in the training volume between groups measured as either training duration or training impulse (Trimp) per week (**Table 1**). The NORM group's mean SpO_2 at the end of each sprint training set remained between 92 and 95% for the first 6 training days, whereas the HYP group's SpO_2 was substantially lower at 77–82%. However, during the last 2 training days where all individuals (HYP and NORM groups) received the hypoxic gas, SpO_2 levels were lower in the NORM group compared to the HYP group initially (training day 7) but was similar in both groups by training day 8 (**Figure 2B**). Relative to the NORM group, the HYP group's heart rate at the end of each sprint training set was consistently elevated, particularly in the first 2 sets throughout the training period, apart from the last 2 training days when both groups received the hypoxic gas during training where heart rates were similar. Ratings of perceived exertion tended to be higher after the last set of each training day. Overall, perceived exertion tended to be higher in participants undertaking repeat sprint training under hypoxic compared to normoxic conditions (**Figure 2C**). Similar to SpO_2 and heart rate, the first day of hypoxic training for the NORM group (training day 7) increased their perceived exertion during training, compared to the HYP group. The average peak power measured in Watts produced during the sprint training (mean of the 20 repeat sprints for each day) was substantially higher in the NORM compared to the HYP group on days 4–6 (**Table 2**), however this difference disappeared once body weight was accounted for (i.e., W kg^{-1}). The average peak power was maintained throughout the 8

TABLE 2 | Peak power output for each training day.

		Intervention 1						Intervention 2	
		Day 1	Day 2	Day 3	Day 4	Day 5	Day 6	Day 7	Day 8
Peak power (W)	HYP	822 ± 217	851 ± 194	821 ± 182	824 ± 181*	811 ± 209*	838 ± 196*	829 ± 220	906 ± 112
	NORM	985 ± 146	996 ± 183	953 ± 195	1012 ± 203	996 ± 203	1029 ± 207	911 ± 237	979 ± 163
Peak power (W kg^{-1})	HYP	10.2 ± 3.0	10.3 ± 3.0	10.2 ± 2.7	10.2 ± 2.5	9.98 ± 2.8	10.4 ± 3.1	10.4 ± 3.0	10.8 ± 2.8
	NORM	11.4 ± 2.3	11.4 ± 2.5	11.3 ± 2.1	11.6 ± 2.5	11.4 ± 2.6	11.8 ± 2.4	10.5 ± 2.9	11.0 ± 2.1

*Data are mean ± SD. HYP, hypoxic group; NORM, normoxic group; Peak power, the average peak power from the WattBike produced during the 20 all out 5-s sprints on each training day. *Substantially different between groups.*

TABLE 3 | Mean changes in performance tests post hypoxic and placebo exposures and the chances that the true differences in changes between groups is substantial.

		Change in mean (%)			Chances that the differences are substantial	
		Within-group, from baseline		Between-group		
Variable	Post-test	HYP ± 90% CL	NORM ± 90% CL	Difference ± 90% CL	%	Qualitative inference
Repeated sprint fatigue[1]	1	−1.8 ± 1.6*	−1.5 ± 1.4*	0.3 ± 2.2	30	Unclear
	2	−2.1 ± 1.8*	−0.9 ± 1.5	1.2 ± 2.4	55	Unclear
	3	−2.3 ± 1.7*	−0.3 ± 1.7	2.0 ± 2.4^	75	Possibly beneficial
	4	−1.9 ± 1.8*	0.4 ± 1.6	2.2 ± 2.4^	81	Likely beneficial
	5	−1.2 ± 1.6*	0.5 ± 1.7	1.6 ± 2.4^	67	Possibly beneficial
Repeated sprint fatigue[2]	1	−0.6 ± 0.9*	−0.1 ± 0.8	0.5 ± 1.2	27	Unclear
	2	−0.9 ± 0.9*	0.1 ± 0.8	1.0 ± 1.3^	50	Possibly beneficial
	3	−1.2 ± 0.9*	−0.3 ± 0.9	0.9 ± 1.4^	46	Possibly beneficial
	4	−0.6 ± 0.8*	0.4 ± 0.9	1.0 ± 1.3^	53	Possibly beneficial
	5	−0.1 ± 0.9	1.1 ± 0.9*	1.2 ± 1.2^	61	Possibly beneficial
Yo-Yo L1	1	15 ± 30	20 ± 26*	6 ± 39	58	Unclear
	2	23 ± 31	26 ± 26*	3 ± 38	53	Unclear
	3	26 ± 31*	13 ± 28	−13 ± 42	68	Unclear
	4	37 ± 31*	26 ± 28*	−11 ± 42	65	Unclear
	5	33 ± 29*	25 ± 31*	−9 ± 42	62	Unclear

Substantially different from mean of baseline tests (see **Table 1); ^Substantially difference between groups. Repeated sprint fatigue[1], % fatigue from sprint 1 to sprint 8 using the linear extrapolation method; Repeated sprint fatigue[2], % fatigue decrement score using the % decrement score method (100 × (total sprint time/ideal sprint time) − 100); Yo-Yo L1 is % change in meters covered in the Yo-Yo intermittent recovery test Level 1.*

training days despite the increased resistance on training days 3 and 4.

Performance

Initially groups were matched for repeat sprint ability using the cumulated sprint time from test 1 (HYP 27.5 ± 3.9, NORM 27.4 ± 3.2) which was altered slightly due to the withdrawal of one participant's data from the hypoxic group (HYP 26.9 ± 3.4). Fatigue during the repeat sprint ability test was similar between groups at the two baseline tests when measured using either the linear extrapolation method (Baseline 1 test, HYP 5.8 ± 3.4%, NORM 5.5 ± 2.3% and Baseline 2 test, HYP 6.1 ± 2.6%, NORM 5.9 ± 1.8%, mean ± *SD*), or the percent decrement method (Baseline 1 test, HYP 3.5 ± 1.3%, NORM 3.5 ± 1.2% and Baseline 2 test, HYP 4.1 ± 1.1%, NORM 3.9 ± 1.4%). Using the linear extrapolation approach to measure fatigue, compared to the mean of the two baseline tests the HYP participants had substantially less fatigue during the repeated sprint tests on all post-test occasions (**Table 3**), however, this was only found in the NORM participants at post-test 1. Compared to the NORM participants, a beneficial effect of adding hypoxia to the repeat sprint training was indicated from post-test 3 onwards. Similar results were found using the percent decrement method to calculate fatigue (**Table 3**). Repeat sprint times for the 2 groups for each test day are presented in **Figure 3**. Test 1 had the lowest times for each sprint in the NORM group, whereas the lowest sprint times were witnessed on test day 5 and 6 (i.e., post-test intervention 3 and 4) for the HYP group. Cumulative times for the 8 sprints were similar between groups for the baseline and early post-intervention tests (post 1 and 2), however

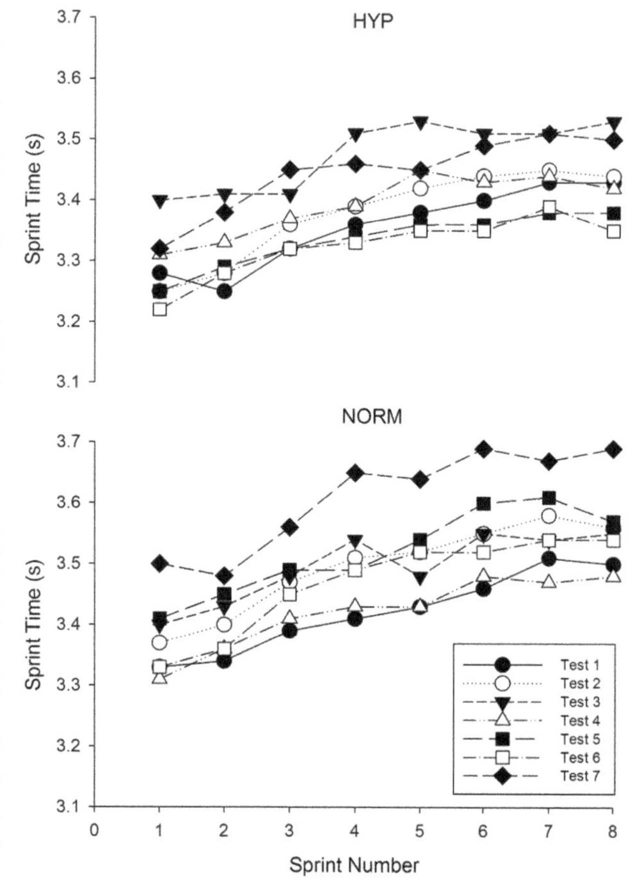

FIGURE 3 | Raw sprint times for the hypoxic (HYP) and normoxic (NORM) groups over the 7 testing periods.

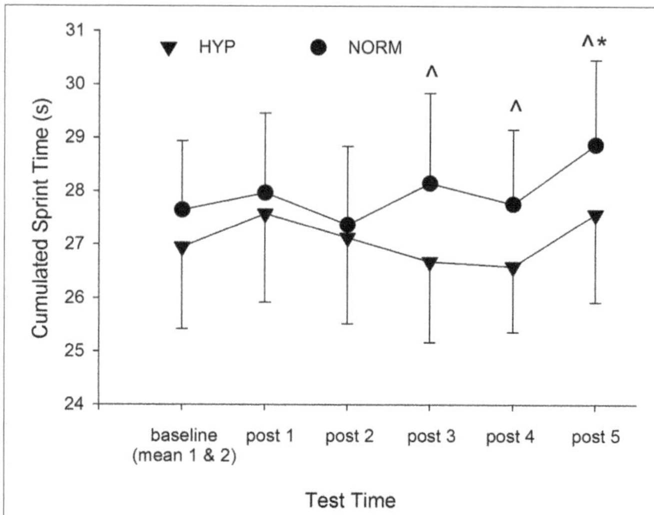

FIGURE 4 | Mean cumulated sprint time at baseline (mean of test 1 and 2) and the 5 post-intervention tests for the hypoxic (HYP) and normoxic (NORM) groups. *Substantially different from baseline. ^Substantially different between groups at each time point.

the HYP group improved cumulative sprint time compared to baseline at post-intervention 3 and 4 (1.0 ± 4.5 and 1.3 ± 4.5%, respectively, mean ± 90% CI, **Figure 4**). In comparison, over the same period the NORM group increased cumulative sprint time compared to baseline (1.7 ± 4.1 and 0.4 ± 4.4% for post-test 3 and 4, respectively). By post-intervention 5, both groups were slower over the 8 sprints compared to baseline (2.2 ± 4.2 and 4.3 ± 4.2% for the HYP and NORM groups, respectively). YYIR1 test performance improved throughout the study for both groups, with the effects of added hypoxia during repeat sprint training being unclear. Adding an extra two top-up sessions at the end of the 3-week post-intervention period had little beneficial effect in terms of further improving repeat sprint ability or YYIR1 performance in the HYP group over the next 2 weeks. Additionally, giving the NORM group two sessions of hypoxic training at the end of the study had little beneficial performance effect over the next 2 weeks (post 4 and 5). Standard deviations representing observed individual responses in performance in the post-exposure trials ranged from 1.7 to 2.8% for the repeat sprint ability test (using linear extrapolation) and 9.4–19.7% for the YYIR1 test. The typical error of the measurement for all participants between the two baseline tests was 0.8% (90% CL = 0.6–1.1%) and 4.7% (90% CL = 3.7–6.6%) for the repeat sprint ability and YYIR1, respectively.

DISCUSSION

The novel findings of this study were that six sessions of repeat-sprint training under hypoxia, simulating rugby match conditions, while otherwise living at sea-level, had long-lasting beneficial effects on sea-level repeat sprint ability in field conditions. In addition, off-feet training (using a cycle ergometer) was beneficial at improving on-feet performance (run-based repeated sprinting) in rugby players. Finally, it seems that six sessions (2 per week for 3 weeks) of hypoxic repeat-sprint training is necessary for improvements in repeat sprint ability and two sessions over 1 week, had little effect at eliciting further enhancement in performance in previously hypoxic trained athletes or athletes new to hypoxic training.

The error of measurement in this study was similar to measures from previous studies ~1–2% for repeat sprints in team-sport athletes (Wood et al., 2006; Hamlin et al., 2012) and indicated good reliability of measures. Individual responses to hypoxia tended to be relatively small for repeat sprint ability and slightly larger for the YYIR1 test.

The hypoxic group in the present study had an ~2% greater improvement in their repeat sprint ability compared to the normoxic group over the last 3 testing trials (**Table 3**), which compares favorably to repeat-sprint training derived improvements in previous hypoxic studies (Jones B. et al., 2015; Brocherie et al., 2015b). In association with less fatigue in the HYP group, these players were also faster over the 8 sprints during this period compared to the NORM group and were ~1% faster at post-testing times three and four compared to baseline. However, not all researchers have found beneficial effects when adding hypoxia to repeat-sprint training

(Galvin et al., 2013; Goods et al., 2015). We suggest the cause of some of the conflicting results are likely to be associated with the mismatch between hypoxic training protocols and subsequent performance testing procedures. For example, Galvin et al. (2013) had rugby players complete 12 sessions of ten 6 s all out sprints with a 30 s recovery on a non-motorized treadmill under hypoxic conditions, but used a performance test that did not match this protocol (i.e., 10 × 20 m running sprints with 30 s rest period). Data derived from the Galvin et al. (2013) study shows that the average time to run 20 m by these athletes was ~3 s. Therefore, to match the training program, these athletes should have been running ~40 m during performance testing. Such details are important, as during training, these athletes would have been stressing and subsequently adapting, more aerobic than anaerobic metabolic processes. But during testing, these athletes would have been relying to a greater extent on anaerobic rather than aerobic metabolic systems. Indeed, these authors reported substantial improvements in endurance (aerobic) performance after training (~15% improvement in hypoxic compared to normoxic group), which suggests the training was more conducive to endurance performance than anaerobic repetitive sprinting performance adaptations.

In contrast, Goods et al. (2015) used similar training and testing procedures to our study but found non-significant changes between normoxic and hypoxic groups post-exposure for repeat sprint running ability. These results conflict with the present study, which showed substantially improved repeat sprint running ability post hypoxic exposure. However, these researchers did not quantify the training loads between groups, which could possibly result in different training stress and therefore adaptation in the groups studied.

The different methods used to quantify the change in repeat sprint ability between studies may also influence results. A recent article suggests using the average or cumulated sprint time overcomes the problem of high variability associated with calculating fatigue scores from the first and last sprints in a set (Oliver, 2009). However, we have found that using a linear function to predict the first and last sprints of the log-transformed data, which can then be subtracted to give a percent fatigue index, can also produce meaningful fatigue values with a low co-efficient of variation (~1%). We acknowledge that using this approach may overestimate the final sprint in a set which can be slightly faster due to participants inadvertently pacing themselves (Glaister et al., 2008), however, we found substituting the predicted 8th sprint with the actual recorded 8th sprint had little effect on the results. Indeed, when we calculated fatigue using the method suggested by Glaister et al. (2008) which can be found in **Table 3** under "Repeated sprint fatigue[2]," we found similar results to the linear extrapolation method.

Performance response to repeat-sprint training under hypoxic conditions is variable and inconsistent. While this study and others (Faiss et al., 2015; Kasai et al., 2015; Brocherie et al., 2015a,b) have shown beneficial changes in repeat sprint ability after repeat-sprint training in hypoxia compared to normoxia, this positive result is not always found (Goods et al., 2015; Montero and Lundby, 2016). Methodological differences including participant characteristics and ability, motivation and encouragement during training and testing, selection, and timing of performance tests and time, degree and frequency of hypoxia may theoretically help explain this variability in performance change. More research investigating these variables may help reduce performance variation with such training.

Postulated mechanisms associated with improved repeat sprint ability after repeat-sprint training in hypoxia include augmented anaerobic glycolytic metabolism (Svedenhag et al., 1991), improved acid-base homeostasis (Nummela and Rusko, 2000) and increased muscle blood perfusion (Faiss et al., 2013b). The increased repeat sprint ability in the hypoxic compared to the normoxic group in this study along with no substantial between group change in the aerobic measure (YYIR1) suggests improvement in the anaerobic rather than the aerobic metabolism is involved. However, this remains speculative since no mechanistic variables were measured in this study.

Generally the addition of hypoxia during exercise results in substantially higher ratings of perceived exertion (Shephard et al., 1992; Buchheit et al., 2012; Goods et al., 2014). It seems that when exercising under hypoxic conditions, even when the workload is reduced to account for the lowered oxygen availability (Buchheit et al., 2012), participants perceive the exercise to be more difficult. Some of this increased effort is probably due to the increased ventilator drive required during hypoxic exercise (Katayama et al., 2001), but increased peripheral muscular sensation via accumulation of hypoxic metabolites (Hogan et al., 1999) is probably also involved. Exercise under hypoxic conditions can also have a negative effect on cerebral oxyhemoglobin levels (Monroe et al., 2016) which may affect sensations directly. The increased perceived effort reported by the athletes in this study when adding normobaric hypoxia to high-intensity exercise (average training RPE increased from 14.7 to 15.6 in the hypoxic group compared to 13.9–15.5, in the normoxic group over the eight training sessions) is similar to previous research (Aliverti et al., 2011), but is in contrast to a recent study (Brocherie et al., 2016). Brocherie et al. (2016) found a slow reduction in the perceived effort reported by elite field hockey athletes as they completed six sessions of repeat-sprint training (four sets of five reps of 5 s running sprints in FIO2 ~14.5%) over 2 weeks (average training RPE decreased from 14.6 to 13.1 in the hypoxic group and increased from 14.4 to 14.8 in the normoxic group over six training sessions). Differences between studies may be due to the exercise mode (cycling compared to running), the caliber of athletes (elite field hockey players compared to well-trained rugby players), or the fact that athletes performed the training while resided at a simulated altitude of ~3000 m (Brocherie et al., 2016). In addition, the current study design with an increased resistance during training days 3 and 4 and a 3-week break between intervention 1 and 2 probably did not allow for such acclimation to be studied as rigorously as Brocherie's study.

A limitation to the current study was the fact that when participants were exercising under hypoxia the training stress was substantially higher compared to participants completing the same exercise under normoxic conditions (as witnessed by the significantly higher training heart rates and perceived exertion,

Figure 2). Therefore, we need to be careful when attributing the benefit of such training to hypoxia, since the performance benefits may simply be due to the harder training load in the hypoxic group. Designing a study that could control for training workload in the hypoxic and control groups would be one way to tease out this effect. A further limitation of this study is that we used well-trained rugby players in this study and therefore the results may not reflect what may occur in elite rugby players. Lastly this study was a field study rather than a lab-based study in order to improve the ecological value of the outcomes, however such studies also increase the risk of elevating variability due to extraneous variables. One such variable was the fact that all the rugby players in this study were required to play a pre-season game of rugby on the Saturday prior to the last testing day, which was probably responsible for the poor repeat sprint ability on the last testing day.

Finally, the present study found that "off-feet" repeat sprint cycling had a substantially beneficial effect on "on-feet" repeat sprint running ability in amateur rugby players. Such cross-over effects in performance enhancement is not always found in such studies (Goods et al., 2015), but indicates a potentially useful training protocol for athletic teams that have heavy on-feet training loads such as running. Currently the professional rugby season in New Zealand spans 9–10 months of the year (early February through to early November) which represents a large training load on players. Any opportunity to relieve on-feet training stress without reducing overall performance would be a useful supplementation to such athletes, however this research was conducted on amateur rugby players and would need to be replicated on professional players before firm recommendations for this group could be made.

AUTHOR CONTRIBUTIONS

MH conceptualized and designed the study, MH, PO, HM, assisted in the planning and acquisition of data, MH, PO, HM, CL, CE helped with the analysis and interpretation of the data, critically revising the manuscript and adding important intellectual content. All authors gave approval for the final version of this manuscript to be published and agree to be accountable for all aspects of the work.

FUNDING

The authors acknowledge the Lincoln University Research Fund (reference 2014-16E/INTF044) and Ara Institute of Canterbury for financial support for this project.

ACKNOWLEDGMENTS

The authors thank the rugby players and their coaches for their assistance. We also acknowledge Dr. Dave Parry, Performance Sport Director, University of Essex for his help with this project.

REFERENCES

Aliverti, A., Kayser, B., Mauro, A. L., Quaranta, M., Pompilio, P., Dellacà, R., et al. (2011). Respiratory and leg muscles perceived exertion during exercise at altitude. *Respir. Physiol. Neurobiol.* 177, 162–168. doi: 10.1016/j.resp.2011.03.014

Austin, D., Gabbett, T., and Jenkins, D. (2011a). The physical demands of Super 14 rugby union. *J. Sci. Med. sport* 14, 259–263. doi: 10.1016/j.jsams.2011.01.003

Austin, D., Gabbett, T., and Jenkins, D. (2011b). Repeated high-intensity exercise in professional rugby union. *J. Sports Sci.* 29, 1105–1112. doi: 10.1080/02640414.2011.582508

Bailey, S. J., Wilkerson, D. P., Dimenna, F. J., and Jones, A. M. (2009). Influence of repeated sprint training on pulmonary O2 uptake and muscle deoxygenation kinetics in humans. *J. Appl. Physiol.* 106, 1875–1887. doi: 10.1152/japplphysiol.00144.2009

Banister, E. W., and Calvert, T. W. (1980). Planning for future performance: implications for long term training. *Can. J. Appl. Sport. Sci.* 5, 170–176.

Borg, G. A. (1982). Psychophysical bases of perceived exertion. *Med. Sci. Sports Exerc.* 14, 377–381. doi: 10.1249/00005768-198205000-00012

Bowtell, J. L., Cooke, K., Turner, R., Mileva, K. N., and Sumners, D. P. (2014). Acute physiological and performance responses to repeated sprints in varying degrees of hypoxia. *J. Sci. Med. Sport.* 17, 399–403. doi: 10.1016/j.jsams.2013.05.016

Brocherie, F., Girard, O., Faiss, R., and Millet, G. (2015a). High-intensity intermittent training in hypoxia: a double-blinded, placebo-controlled field study in youth football players. *J. Strength Cond. Res.* 29, 226–237. doi: 10.1519/JSC.0000000000000590

Brocherie, F., Millet, G., and Girard, O. (2016). Psycho-physiological responses to repeated-sprint training in normobaric hypoxia and normoxia. *Int. J. Sports Physiol. Perform.* doi: 10.1123/ijspp.2016-0052. [Epub ahead of print].

Brocherie, F., Millet, G. P., Hauser, A., Steiner, T., Rysman, J., Wehrlin, J. P., et al. (2015b). "Live high-train low and high" hypoxic training improves team-sport performance. *Med. Sci. Sports Exerc.* 47, 2140–2149. doi: 10.1249/MSS.0000000000000630

Buchheit, M., Kuitunen, S., Voss, S. C., Williams, B. K., Mendez-Villanueva, A., and Bourdon, P. C. (2012). Physiological strain associated with high-intensity hypoxic intervals in highly trained young runners. *J. Strength Cond. Res.* 26, 94–105. doi: 10.1519/JSC.0b013e3182184fcb

Cohen, J. (1988). *Statistical Power for the Behavioural Sciences.* Hilsdale, NJ: Lawrence Erlbaum.

Dawson, B., Fitzsimons, M., Green, S., Goodman, C., Carey, M., and Cole, K. (1998). Changes in performance, muscle metabolites, enzymes and fibre types after short sprint training. *Eur. J. Appl. Physiol. Occup. Physiol.* 78, 163–169. doi: 10.1007/s004210050402

Eston, R. G., and Williams, J. G. (1988). Reliability of ratings of perceived effort regulation of exercise intensity. *Br. J. Sports Med.* 22, 153–155. doi: 10.1136/bjsm.22.4.153

Faiss, R., Girard, O., and Millet, G. P. (2013a). Advancing hypoxic training in team sports: from intermittent hypoxic training to repeated sprint training in hypoxia. *Br. J. Sports Med.* 47, i45–i50. doi: 10.1136/bjsports-2013-092741

Faiss, R., Léger, B., Vesin, J. M., Fournier, P. E., Eggel, Y., Dériaz, O., et al. (2013b). Significant molecular and systemic adaptations after repeated sprint training in hypoxia. *PLoS ONE* 8:e56522. doi: 10.1371/journal.pone.0056522

Faiss, R., Willis, S., Born, D. P., Sperlich, B., Vesin, J. M., Holmberg, H. C., et al. (2015). Repeated double-poling sprint training in hypoxia by competitive cross-country skiers. *Med. Sci. Sports Exerc.* 47, 809–817. doi: 10.1249/MSS.0000000000000464

Galvin, H. M., Cooke, K., Sumners, D. P., Mileva, K. N., and Bowtell, J. L. (2013). Repeated sprint training in normobaric hypoxia. *Br. J. Sports Med.* 47, i74–i79. doi: 10.1136/bjsports-2013-092826

Glaister, M., Howatson, G., Pattison, J. R., and McInnes, G. (2008). The reliability and validity of fatigue measures during multiple-sprint work: an issue revisited. *J. Strength Cond. Res.* 22, 1597–1601. doi: 10.1519/JSC.0b013e31818ab80

Goods, P. S., Dawson, B. T., Landers, G. J., Gore, C. J., and Peeling, P. (2014). Effect of different simulated altitudes on repeat-sprint performance in team-sport athletes. *Int. J. Sports Physiol. Perform.* 9, 857–862. doi: 10.1123/ijspp.2013-0423

Goods, P. S., Dawson, B., Landers, G. J., Gore, C. J., and Pelling, P. (2015). No additional benefit of repeat-sprint training in hypoxia than in normoxia on sea-level repeat-sprint ability. *J.Sports Sci. Med.* 14, 681–688.

Gore, C. J. (ed.). (2000). *Physiological Tests for Elite Athletes.* Champaign, IL: Human Kinetics.

Hamlin, M. J., and Hellemans, J. (2007). Effect of intermittent normobaric hypoxic exposure at rest on haematological, physiological and performance parameters in multi-sport athletes. *J. Sports Sci.* 25, 431–441. doi: 10.1080/02640410600718129

Hamlin, M. J., Marshall, H. C., Hellemans, J., Ainslie, P. N., and Anglem, N. (2010). Effect of intermittent hypoxic training on a 20 km time trial and 30 s anaerobic performance. *Scand. J. Med. Sci. Sports* 20, 651–661. doi: 10.1111/j.1600-0838.2009.00946.x

Hamlin, M. J., Mitchell, C. J., Ward, F. D., Draper, N., Shearman, J. P., and Kimber, N. E. (2012). Effect of compression garments on short-term recovery of repeated sprint and 3-km running performance in rugby union players. *J. Strength Cond. Res.* 26, 2975–2982. doi: 10.1519/JSC.0b013e3182711e0b

Hogan, M. C., Richardson, R. S., and Haseler, L. J. (1999). Human muscle performance and PCr hydrolysis with varied inspired oxygen fractions: a31P-MRS study. *J. Appl. Physiol.* 86, 1367–1373.

Hopkins, W. G. (2006). Spreadsheets for analysis of controlled trials, with adjustment for a subject characteristic. *Sportscience* 10, 46–50. Available online at: http://sportsci.org/2006/wghcontrial.htm

Hopkins, W. G., Marshall, S. W., Batterham, A. M., and Hanin, J. (2009). Progressive statistics for studies in sports medicine and exercise science. *Med. Sci. Sports Exerc.* 41, 3–12. doi: 10.1249/MSS.0b013e31818cb278

Jones, B., Hamilton, D. K., and Cooper, C. E. (2015). Muscle oxygen changes following sprint interval cycling training in elite field hockey players. *PLoS ONE* 10:e0120338. doi: 10.1371/journal.pone.0120338

Jones, M. R., West, D. J., Crewther, B. T., Cook, C. J., and Kilduff, L. P. (2015). Quantifying positional and temporal movement patterns in professional rugby union using global positioning system. *Eur. J. Sport Sci.* 15, 488–496. doi: 10.1080/17461391.2015.1010106

Kasai, N., Mizuno, S., Ishimoto, S., Sakamoto, E., Maruta, M., and Goto, K. (2015). Effect of training in hypoxia on repeated sprint performance in female athletes. *Springerplus* 4, 1. doi: 10.1186/s40064-015-1041-4

Katayama, K., Sato, Y., Morotome, Y., Shima, N., Ishida, K., Mori, S., et al. (2001). Intermittent hypoxia increases ventilation and Sa(O2) during hypoxic exercise and hypoxic chemosensitivity. *J. Appl. Physiol.* 90, 1431–1440.

Millet, G. P., Roels, B., Schmitt, L., Woorons, X., and Richalet, J. P. (2010). Combining hypoxic methods for peak performance. *Sports Med.* 40, 1–25. doi: 10.2165/11317920-000000000-00000

Monroe, D. C., Gist, N. H., Freese, E. C., O'connor, P. J., McCully, K. K., and Dishman, R. K. (2016). Effects of sprint interval cycling on fatigue, energy, and cerebral oxygenation. *Med. Sci. Sports Exerc.* 48, 615–624. doi: 10.1249/MSS.0000000000000809

Montero, D., and Lundby, C. (2016). Repeated sprint training in hypoxia versus normoxia does not improve performance: a double-blind and cross-over study. *Int. J. Sports Physiol. Perform.* doi: 10.1123/ijspp.2015-0691. [Epub ahead of print].

Nicholas, C. W. (1997). Anthropometric and physiological characteristics of rugby union football players. *Sports Med.* 23, 375–396. doi: 10.2165/00007256-199723060-00004

Nummela, A., and Rusko, H. (2000). Acclimitization to altitude and normoxic training improve 400-m running performance at sea level. *J. Sports Sci.* 18, 411–419. doi: 10.1080/02640410050074340

Oliver, J. L. (2009). Is a fatigue index a worthwhile measure of repeated sprint ability? *J. Sci. Med. Sport* 12, 20–23. doi: 10.1016/j.jsams.2007.10.010

Paton, C. D., Hopkins, W. G., and Vollebregt, L. (2001). Little effect of caffeine ingestion on repeated sprints in team-sport athletes. *Med. Sci. Sports Exerc.* 33, 822–825. doi: 10.1097/00005768-200105000-00023

Rampinini, E., Bishop, D., Marcora, S., Bravo, D. F., Sassi, R., and Impellizzeri, F. (2007). Validity of simple field tests as indicators of match-related physical performance in top-level professional soccer players. *Int. J. Sports Med.* 28, 228–235. doi: 10.1055/s-2006-924340

Reilly, T., Morris, T., and Whyte, G. (2009). The specificity of training prescription and physiological assessment: a review. *J. Sports Sci.* 27, 575–589. doi: 10.1080/02640410902729741

Saunders, P. U., Telford, R. D., Pyne, D. D., Gore, C. J., and Hahn, A. G. (2009). Improved race performance in elite middle-distance runners after cumulative altitude exposure. *Int. J. Sports Physiol. Perform.* 4, 134–138. doi: 10.1123/ijspp.4.1.134

Shephard, R. J., Vandewalle, H., Gil, V., Bouhlel, E., and Monod, H. (1992). Respiratory, muscular, and overall perceptions of effort: the influence of hypoxia and muscle mass. *Med. Sci. Sports Exerc.* 24, 556–567. doi: 10.1249/00005768-199205000-00010

Spencer, M., Bishop, D., Dawson, B., and Goodman, C. (2005). Physiological and metabolic responses of repeated-sprint activities. *Sports Med.* 35, 1025–1044. doi: 10.2165/00007256-200535120-00003

Svedenhag, J., Saltin, B., Johansson, C., and Kaiijser, L. (1991). Aerobic and anaerobic exercise capacities of elite middle-distance runners after training at moderate altitude. *Scand. J. Med. Sci. Sports* 1, 205–215. doi: 10.1111/j.1600-0838.1991.tb00297.x

Tønnessen, E., Shalfawi, S. A., Haugen, T., and Enoksen, E. (2011). The effect of 40-m repeated sprint training on maximum sprinting speed, repeated sprint speed endurance, vertical jump, and aerobic capacity in young elite male soccer players. *J. Strength Cond. Res.* 25, 2364–2370. doi: 10.1519/JSC.0b013e3182023a65

Wood, M. R., Dowson, M. N., and Hopkins, W. G. (2006). Running performance after adaptation to acutely intermittent hypoxia. *Eur. J. Sport Sci.* 6, 163–172. doi: 10.1080/17461390600571005

22

Sex-Specific Impact of Ischemic Preconditioning on Tissue Oxygenation and Maximal Concentric Force

Pénélope Paradis-Deschênes[1, 2], *Denis R. Joanisse*[1, 2] *and François Billaut*[1, 2, 3*]

[1] *Département de kinésiologie, Université Laval, Québec, QC, Canada,* [2] *Institut Universitaire de Cardiologie et de Pneumologie de Québec, Québec, QC, Canada,* [3] *Institut National du Sport du Québec, Montréal, QC, Canada*

Correspondence:
François Billaut
francois.billaut@kin.ulaval.ca

Prior peripheral hypoxia induced via remote ischemic preconditioning (IPC) can improve physical performance in male athletes through improved O_2 delivery and utilization. Since females may have an innate protective mechanism against ischemia-reperfusion injury, and since muscle metabolism during contraction differs between sexes, it is relevant to examine the impact of sex in response to IPC to determine whether it is also ergogenic in females. In a randomized, crossover, single-blind study, we investigated muscle performance, hemodynamic and O_2 uptake in strength-trained males ($n = 9$) and females ($n = 8$) performing five sets of 5 maximum voluntary knee extensions on an isokinetic dynamometer, preceded by either IPC (3 × 5-min ischemia/5-min reperfusion cycles at 200 mmHg) or SHAM (20 mmHg). Changes in deoxy-hemoglobin (Δ[HHb], expressed in percentage of arterial occlusion and considered an index of O_2 extraction), and total hemoglobin (Δ[THb]) concentrations of the vastus lateralis muscle were continuously monitored by near-infrared spectroscopy. The metabolic efficiency of the contractions was calculated as the average force/$\Delta[\text{HHb}]_{avg}$ ratio. Cohen's effect sizes (ES) ± 90% confidence limits were used to estimate IPC-induced changes and sex differences. IPC increased total muscular force in males only (13.0%, ES 0.64, 0.37;0.90), and this change was greater than in females (10.4% difference, ES 0.40, 0.10;0.70). Percent force decrement was only attenuated in females (−19.8%, ES −0.38, −0.77;0.01), which was clearly different than males (sex difference: ES 0.45, −0.16;1.07). IPC also induced different changes between sexes for average muscle O_2 uptake in set 2 (males: 6.4% vs. females: −16.7%, ES 0.21, −0.18;0.60), set 3 (males: 7.0% vs. females: −44.4%, ES 0.56, −0.17;1.29), set 4 (males: 9.1% vs. females: −40.2%, ES 0.51, −0.10;1.13), and set 5 (males: 10.2% vs. females: −40.4%, ES 0.52, −0.04;1.09). However, metabolic efficiency was not meaningfully different between conditions and sexes. IPC increased muscle blood volume (↑[THb]) at rest and during recovery between sets, to the same extent in both sexes. Despite a similar IPC-induced initial increase in O_2 delivery in both sexes, males displayed greater peripheral O_2 extraction and greater strength enhancement. This ergogenic effect appears to be mediated in part via an up regulated oxidative function in males. We conclude that strength-trained males might benefit more from IPC than their female counterparts during repeated, maximal efforts.

Keywords: blood flow restriction, muscle function, oxygenation, performance, sex differences, athletes

INTRODUCTION

Ischemic preconditioning of a limb (IPC) is a non-invasive technique inducing transient peripheral hypoxia to subsequently enhance tissue tolerance against ischemia-reperfusion injury. This technique promotes local vasodilation, improves O_2 delivery (Enko et al., 2011; Bailey et al., 2012a), and enhances the efficiency of muscular contraction (Pang et al., 1995; Moses et al., 2005). Higher muscle O_2 utilization was also demonstrated in the quadriceps of strength-trained male athletes after performing IPC compared to placebo compressions (Paradis-Deschenes et al., 2016). It is not surprising, therefore, to observe that IPC can improve maximal physical performance in various exercise modes in male participants (De Groot et al., 2010; Bailey et al., 2012a; Paradis-Deschenes et al., 2016), although this is not a universal finding (Incognito et al., 2015). Before exercise sport performance applications, IPC was originally studied for its potential clinical relevance, and in this context, it is interesting to note that females appeared to display smaller clinical benefits compared with their male counterparts. In a cohort of 382 subjects, a failure to induce preconditioning effects during percutaneous coronary intervention was noted in females (Laskey and Beach, 2003), presumably due to the innate, multiple, protective actions of estrogens (Pitcher et al., 2005). Moreover, since physiological responses to exercise (in particular metabolic pathway utilization and perfusion) may differ between sexes, and that exercise performance data from females is almost inexistent, it is relevant and timely to examine the impact of IPC on females compared to males to more precisely evaluate the potency of this technique for exercise performance applications.

Females have been reported to exhibit less fatigue than males during intense exercise (Parker et al., 2007; Hunter, 2016), but not under conditions of ischemia (Russ and Kent-Braun, 2003), suggesting that muscle perfusion and oxygenation may be involved in the sex-related difference (Russ and Kent-Braun, 2003; Clark et al., 2005; Hunter et al., 2006). Indeed, females exhibit greater vasodilation in the limbs during single knee extensions (Parker et al., 2007), and may have a greater proportional area of type I fibers (Simoneau et al., 1985; Staron et al., 2000) and greater capacity for utilizing oxidative metabolism than males (Kent-Braun et al., 2002). Thus, females exhibit a greater reliance on oxidative metabolism compared with males, which could challenge the ergogenic impact of IPC.

Prior evidence examining sex-related differences in the response to IPC during exercise is limited. Gibson et al. (2015) reported no performance difference between male and female team-sport athletes during five repeated 6-s sprints after performing 3 × 5-min occlusions at 220 mmHg to both legs. However, the IPC procedure used in that study failed to improve performance in either sex, making the sex comparison moot. Another study demonstrated the positive impact of IPC (2 × 3-min at 220-mmHg) on recovery from squat jump test and running sprint performance 24 h after an initial, fatiguing session in males, but the female cohort was too small to draw any firm conclusion (Beaven et al., 2012). Considering the scarcity of studies and that none have attempted to measure relevant physiological responses to provide sex-specific mechanistic insights, any conclusion on the usefulness of IPC for female athletes cannot robustly be drawn.

The aim of the current investigation was therefore to determine the impact of IPC on muscle force and haemodynamics (blood volume and O_2 extraction) derived from near-infrared spectroscopy in males vs. females during repeated maximal efforts separated with incomplete recovery periods. We chose isolated contractions specifically to avoid confounding effects that inspiratory muscle fatigue can have on limb blood flow and O_2 uptake (Kayser et al., 1997).

MATERIALS AND METHODS

Participants

Strength-trained (power and weight lifters, cross-fit and taekwondo athletes) males ($n = 9$, age 25 ± 2 year; height 1.78 ± 0.02 m; weight 86.5 ± 4.9 kg) and females ($n = 8$, age 22 ± 1 year; height 1.66 ± 0.02 m; weight 60.8 ± 2.7 kg) volunteered to take part in this study. All performed 3–5 weight training sessions per week. All participants were non-smokers, free of health problems, did not use any medication, and were asked to avoid vigorous exercise, alcohol and caffeine 24 h before the tests. All but one female (who was amenorrheic) were tested in their follicular phase. Participants provided written informed consent after being informed of experimental procedures, associated risks and potential benefits. The study was approved by the Ethics committee of Université Laval, and adhered to the principles established in the Declaration of Helsinki.

Experimental Design

Participants visited the laboratory for one familiarization and two experimental trials. Resting heart rate and blood pressure (inclusion criteria <140/100 mmHg) were taken prior to every trial. During the first visit, height, weight and thigh circumference were measured. Thigh circumference (males: 61.3 ± 1.9 cm; females: 57.2 ± 1.9 cm) was measured by the same experimenter, 1 cm under the gluteal line. Participants then completed a familiarization session with the experimental set-up, comprising one 3-min compression at a pressure of 200 mmHg, and a standardized warm-up consisting of 5 min of cycling on a Monark ergometer (Ergomedic 828 E) at 100 W. The warm-up was continued with 3–5 right-leg extensions on an isokinetic dynamometer (Kin-Com 500 H, Chattecx Corp., Hixson, TN) at 20°/s, with effort perception progressing from 3 to 9 out of a scale of 10. After 2 min of rest while seated on the dynamometer, participants completed three complete sets of the exercise protocol described below.

Following familiarization, participants were randomized into IPC or SHAM groups in a single-blind, crossover design. In both conditions, participants were seated comfortably on a bed with both legs outstretched, and a non-elastic nylon blood pressure cuff (WelchAllyn, Skaneateles Falls, NY, USA, width: 21 cm) was positioned around the right upper thigh under the gluteal line. In IPC, the cuff was rapidly inflated to 200 mmHg for 5 min, and this was repeated three times with each compression episode separated by 5 min of reperfusion (cuff release) in the same position. A plateau in the NIRS-derived deoxy-hemoglobin concentration signal (see NIRS procedure below) was observed in every subject by 5 min, and taken as a sign of effective occlusion and ischemia. In SHAM, the cuff was inflated to 20 mmHg. To minimize any placebo effect, participants were told that the purpose of the study was to compare the impact of two different cuff pressures that could both alter performance.

The familiarization session and experimental trials were separated by a minimum of 3 days to eliminate the potential effects of the second window of protection caused by IPC (Bolli, 2000), and a maximum of 7 days. All trials were performed at the same time of day for every participant to avoid potentially confounding circadian rhythm effects. The laboratory temperature was controlled and constant (20.31 $\pm$ 0.02°C) throughout all trials.

Exercise Protocol

The exercise protocol started 18.5 $\pm$ 0.1 min after the end of the last cycle of compression. Participants were seated in an upright position on the isokinetic dynamometer, and a strap was secured tightly across the pelvis. The right leg was fixed to the dynamometer with a strap above the ankle external malleoli, and the axis of rotation was aligned to the lateral femoral condyle of the knee joint.

The protocol consisted of five sets of 5 maximum voluntary knee extensions (60° range of motion from 80 to 20°; 0° corresponding to knee fully extended) at 20°/s angular velocity (one extension lasting ~3.0 s). Participants were instructed to contract as hard as they could throughout the extension, and were strongly encouraged during all contractions. Contraction was stopped during flexion when the dynamometer arm automatically returned to 80° at angular velocity of 120°/s (lasting less than 0.5 s), and started immediately after the return of the arm. Subjects rested quietly and relaxed for 30 s between each set and after the last set. After the exercise, participants moved back to the bed to perform an arterial occlusion with the cuff at 200 mmHg (~3–5 min) to obtain a physiological calibration of the NIRS signals. The cuff pressure was released after the deoxy-hemoglobin signal had reached a plateau (see Near-infrared spectroscopy procedure below). Participants were also asked which condition between IPC and SHAM they felt had the greatest impact on their performance, and their verbal answer recorded.

The force produced by participants was measured with a force transducer connected at the end of the level arm of the dynamometer, which was calibrated according to the manufacturer's recommendations before every trial (manufacturer typical error 0.5%). The intra- and inter-day coefficient of variation for force obtained by the main experimenter was 2.4%. Force signals were analyzed in Matlab® between a starting point defined when velocity was $\geq$18°/s, angle was $\geq$80° and force was $\geq$100 N, and an end point when velocity was $\geq$18°/s and angle was $\geq$20°. In every set, peak and average force were calculated. Total force was then calculated as the sum of the average force produced in all sets. Percent force decrement across all sets was calculated as follows: 100 − ([total force output/ideal force output] $\times$ 100), where total and ideal force outputs are the sum of average force values from all sets and the highest average force was multiplied by five, respectively.

Near-Infrared spectroscopy (NIRS)

NIRS is a versatile, non-invasive methodology providing semi-quantitative measures of tissue oxygenation, and is easily applied to study a variety of tissue regions in individuals. NIRS quantifies the changes in hemodynamics from changes in the absorption of near-infrared light by oxyhemoglobin (HbO_2) and deoxyhemoglobin (HHb) (Mccully and Hamaoka, 2000). With this technique, oxygenation can be measured in a discrete region of a tissue in a working physiological setting, which enhances specificity and has distinct advantages as compared to more cumbersome methods. Muscle tissue oxygenation measured by NIRS reflects the balance of O_2 delivery to working muscles and muscle O_2 consumption in capillary beds (De Blasi et al., 1993; Ferrari et al., 2004). Assessment of de- and re-oxygenation kinetics during and after dynamic exercise has become increasingly popular in recent years as a means to non-invasively assess the aerobic function of skeletal muscle. In the current protocol, muscle blood volume and oxygenation were assessed using a portable spatially resolved, dual wavelength NIRS apparatus (PortaMon, Artinis Medical Systems BV, Netherlands). The NIRS device was installed on the distal part of the right vastus lateralis belly (approximately 15 cm above the proximal border of the patella). Skinfold thickness was measured at the site of the application of the NIRS (males: 8.7 $\pm$ 0.9 mm; females: 10.7 $\pm$ 2.0 mm) using a Harpenden skinfold caliper (Harpenden Ltd) during the familiarization session, and was less than half the distance between the emitter and the detector (i.e., 20 mm). This thickness is adequate to let near-infrared light through muscle tissue (Mccully and Hamaoka, 2000). The skin was cleaned with an alcohol swab, and the device was fixed using double-sided stick disks and tape. Black bandages were used to cover the device to eliminate potentially interfering background light. The position of the apparatus was marked with an indelible pen for repositioning during the subsequent visit. The pressure cuff was positioned above the NIRS device, which did not affect the placement of the device during occlusions.

A modified form of the Beer-Lambert law, using two continuous wavelengths (760 and 850 nm) and a differential optical path length factor of 4.95, was used to calculate micromolar changes in tissue oxy-hemoglobin ($\Delta[HbO_2]$), deoxy-hemoglobin (Δ[HHb]) and total hemoglobin ($\Delta[THb] = [HbO_2] + [HHb]$; used as an index of change in regional blood volume). NIRS data were acquired at 10 Hz. At rest, once the signal was stabilized, 1 min of baseline values were analyzed pre IPC and SHAM treatments. Then, NIRS signals were analyzed 2-min post treatment for a duration of 1 min to assess the impact of IPC on resting blood volume ($\Delta[THb]_{rest}$, μM). During exercise, NIRS analysis was limited to Δ[HHb] since this variable is less sensitive than $[HbO_2]$ to perfusion variations and abrupt blood volume changes during contraction and recovery (De Blasi et al., 1993; Ferrari et al., 2004). The [HHb] signal was averaged over the last second of every contraction and over every set to obtain peak ($\Delta[HHb]_{peak}$, % arterial occlusion) and mean ($\Delta[HHb]_{avg}$, % arterial occlusion) O_2 extraction, respectively. These [HHb] data were then normalized to express the magnitude of changes from baseline, and expressed in percentage of the maximal amplitude calculated during an arterial occlusion performed at the end of exercise. Contraction metabolic efficiency was calculated as the average force/Δ[HHb]$_{avg}$ ratio. Finally, during recovery periods between exercise sets, the muscle reoxygenation rate (ΔReoxy, μM.s^{-1}) was calculated as the rate of change in [HHb] from the end of the exercise set to the end of the subsequent recovery period (i.e., the recovery of [HHb]; Billaut and Buchheit, 2013). During this period, the amplitude of change in [THb] (Δ[THb]$_{rec}$) was also analyzed.

Statistical Analysis

All data are reported as means ± standard error (SE) or percentage changes from SHAM. The IPC-SHAM differences within the same group and between sexes were analyzed using Cohen's effect sizes (ES) ± 90% confidence limits (Batterham and Hopkins, 2006; Hopkins et al., 2009). Except for Δ[THb]$_{rest}$ and Δ[THb]$_{rec}$, all variables were log-transformed prior to analysis (Hopkins et al., 2009). Magnitudes of difference between conditions were determined with an effect size of 0.2 set to evaluate the smallest worthwhile change. Standardized effects were classified as small (>0.2), moderate (>0.5) or large (>0.8). The effect was deemed "unclear" if chances of having better/greater or poorer/lower change in performance and physiological variables were both >5% (Batterham and Hopkins, 2006; Hopkins et al., 2009).

RESULTS

All 17 participants met all criteria, completed the entire protocol, and tolerated the IPC procedure without complications. None of the participants could tell what condition produced the greatest change in performance.

Performance

Force parameters for males and females are displayed in **Table 1** and **Figures 1, 2**. After the IPC manoeuver, total force clearly increased in males (13.0%, ES 0.64, 0.37;0.90), but the change was trivial in females (2.3%, ES 0.10, −0.17;0.38). &&&The sex difference for this parameter was clear (ES 0.40, 0.10;0.70; **Figure 1**). Specifically, the IPC-induced increase in average force was greater in males than females in every set of the protocol (set 1–males: 15.2% vs. females: 0.7%, ES 0.53, 0.16;0.90, set 2–males: 15.6% vs. females: 3.6%, ES 0.43, 0.10;0.76, set 3–males: 11.1% vs. females: 2.6%, ES 0.31, 0.02;0.61, set 4–males: 14.5% vs. females: 3.1%, ES 0.41, 0.07;0.76, set 5–males: 8.4% vs. females: 1.7%, ES 0.25, −0.06;0.56; **Figure 2**).

Importantly, although IPC did not increase average force in females, it clearly augmented 1-s peak force in sets 1–3 (**Table 1**), whereas males displayed benefits in sets 1, 2, 4, and 5. This effect was higher in males compared to females in sets 2 and 5.

Percent force decrement was attenuated in females after IPC (−19.8%, ES −0.38, −0.77;0.01), which was clearly different than males (sex difference: ES 0.45, −0.16;1.07).

Muscle Hemodynamics and Oxygenation

Physiological variables are displayed in **Table 2**. No difference was observed between IPC and SHAM in both groups for NIRS variables during baseline before the manoeuver. IPC increased Δ[THb]$_{rest}$ to the same extent in males and females (males: 1.5% vs. females: 1.5%, ES 0.00, −0.80;0.79). After IPC, Δ[THb]$_{rec}$ was increased in males after sets 1 (1.2%, ES 0.33, −0.14;0.80) and 5 (1.5% ES 0.44, 0.17;0.70). In females, Δ[THb]$_{rec}$ was only enhanced after sets 2 (0.7%, ES 0.23, −0.09;0.54) and 3 (1.8% ES 0.54, 0.04;1.04). This change in Δ[THb]$_{rec}$ was higher in males compared to females in set 5 only (sex difference: ES 0.48, 0.10;0.87). There was no change in ΔReoxy within the same group and between sexes.

TABLE 1 | Performance variables in IPC and SHAM conditions for males and females.

	Females			Males			Sex difference
	SHAM	IPC	% difference (ES) 90% CL	SHAM	IPC	% difference (ES) 90% CL	(ES) 90% CL
Peak force S1 (N)	449.1 ± 37.2	481.3 ± 42.1	7.2%, ES 0.24*, −0.07;0.56	627.9 ± 45.1	685.3 ± 35.7	10.2%, ES 0.41*, 0.23;0.59	ES 0.10, −0.24;0.44
Peak force S2 (N)	421.1 ± 32.8	446.3 ± 33.1	6.4%, ES 0.22*, 0.00;0.43	566.3 ± 31.3	648.9 ± 47.6	13.7%, ES 0.54*, 0.32;0.75	ES 0.24*, −0.03;0.50
Peak force S3 (N)	402.5 ± 22.7	429.5 ± 28.3	6.3%, ES 0.22*, 0.05;0.38	558.8 ± 35.7	581.6 ± 41.7	3.8%, ES 0.16, −0.01;0.32	ES −0.09, −0.29;0.12
Peak force S4 (N)	402.5 ± 24.7	422.0 ± 25.0	5.1%, ES 0.18, −0.06;0.41	526.3 ± 29.8	574.6 ± 43.2	8.4%, ES 0.34*, 0.06;0.61	ES 0.11, −0.20;0.42
Peak force S5 (N)	401.8 ± 27.1	397.5 ± 24.5	−0.7%, ES −0.02, −0.17;0.12	506.9 ± 28.3	544.0 ± 39.1	6.7%, ES 0.27*, 0.01;0.54	ES 0.26*, 0.00;0.51
Force decrement (%)	10.4 ± 1.5	8.4 ± 1.4	−19.8%, ES −0.38*, −0.77;0.01	13.7 ± 2.7	15.2 ± 2.2	6.0%, ES0.12, −0.54;0.77	ES 0.45*, −0.16;1.07

Values are mean ± SE.
Asterisks (*) denote "clear" effect sizes (see statistics section).

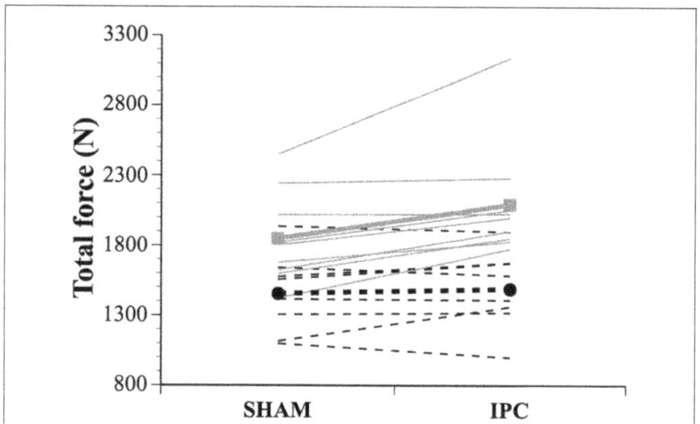

FIGURE 1 | Individual and average total force developed in SHAM and IPC conditions for males (■) and females (•). The IPC-induced change in total force was clearly higher in males than females. Values are mean ± SE.

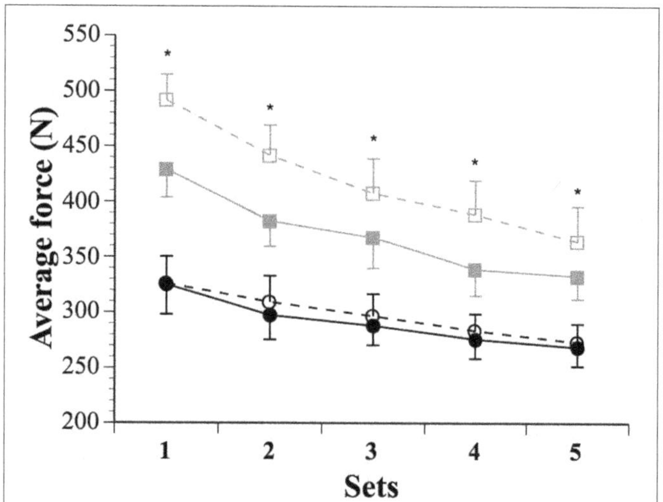

FIGURE 2 | Average force produced during the five sets in males (SHAM: ■ IPC: □) and females (SHAM: ● IPC: ○). Asterisks (*) denote "clear" differences between sexes (see statistics section). Values are mean ± SE.

The IPC maneuver did not alter muscle $\Delta[HHb]_{peak}$ across sets nor between sexes (**Table 2**). However, $\Delta[HHb]_{avg}$ were higher after IPC in males for set 1 (18.1%, ES 0.31, −0.11;0.73), and lower in females for sets 3 (−44.4%, ES −0.25, −0.61;0.11), 4 (−40.2%, ES −0.22, −0.52;0.08), and 5 (−40.4%, ES −0.22, −0.50;0.06). There was a clear sex difference in the impact of IPC on global muscle deoxygenation in sets 2-5 (**Figure 3**). The contraction metabolic efficiency ratio was not altered by IPC during the sets or between sexes (**Table 2**).

DISCUSSION

Summary of Main Findings

This study investigated the impact of sex on performance and vasoactive and oxidative responses to IPC in strength-trained athletes during repeated, maximal contractions. The main findings were that IPC (1) increased muscle force to a greater extent in males than females; (2) increased resting blood volume similarly in both sexes; and (3) increased O_2 extraction in males but decreased it in females. These results challenge the general applicability of IPC on physical performance. While it may be recommended to enhance exercise capacity in males, this preconditioning technique appears less effective in females during maximal efforts.

Muscle Force Parameters

IPC affected muscle force production and the ability to resist neuromuscular fatigue differently between sexes. While male athletes increased peak and average maximal concentric force in every set of the protocol following IPC, the benefits in females were lesser (**Figures 1, 2**). Females only displayed small improvements in peak force in the first three sets, while average force changes were trivial across all sets. Importantly, while IPC yielded acute positive responses in every male, four females out of eight experienced a decrease in performance. Another study did not report any sex difference in repeated-sprint performance, but the IPC protocol employed did not yield any positive effects in either males or females and, therefore, sex-related differences could not be truly assessed (Gibson et al., 2015). Although not studying sex differences *per se*, Gibson and colleagues (Gibson et al., 2013) reported altered 30-m running sprint times after IPC in females, while males displayed no added benefit. Taken together, these results highlight the importance of considering inter-individual responses to IPC in sports, particularly in female athletes. Considering the complex sex modulation of preconditioning mechanisms (such as mitochondrial K_{ATP} channel activation, reactive oxygen species generation, nitric oxide synthase activity, and inflammatory mediator production), as well as robust data documenting that females experience an innate protective mechanism after several forms of acute injury (for review see Pitcher et al., 2005), one could expect a sex-specific impact of remote IPC on physical performance. That said, both sexes are capable of being preconditioned (Pitcher et al., 2005). Hence, it is possible that females in the current study did not reach a sufficient threshold for preconditioning to occur. Thus, contrary to the proposition of a responder vs. non-responder pattern (Beaven et al., 2012; Gibson et al., 2013, 2015), the current data coupled with other clinical studies rather suggest that females may require a greater stimulus for effect. This remains to be elucidated by investigating the influence of varying numbers of IPC cycles and/or the number of limbs occluded at one time.

The sex-specific impact of IPC on fatigability has not been robustly assessed in the literature. The present data demonstrated clear differences between sexes; compared with males, females exhibited a lower force decrement over the five sets of maximal, isokinetic contractions. The lack of change in males is in keeping with previous studies reporting no differences between SHAM and IPC conditions in the measured fatigue index, despite higher peak and mean power outputs during the first repetitions of a series of ten 6 s cycle sprints (Patterson et al., 2015), or higher average force during maximal voluntary knee extensions after IPC (Paradis-Deschenes et al., 2016). This apparent sex

TABLE 2 | Muscle hemodynamic and oxygenation variables in IPC and SHAM conditions for males and females.

	Females			Males			Sex difference
	SHAM	IPC	% difference (ES) 90% CL	SHAM	IPC	% difference (ES) 90% CL	(ES) 90% CL
$[HHb]_{base}$ (μM)	25.3 ± 1.3	25.2 ± 1.1	−0.20%, ES −0.01, −0.35;0.33	37.5 ± 2.7	37.8 ± 2.8	0.85%, ES 0.03, −0.14;0.21	−5.39;7.92
$[THb]_{base}$ (μM)	46.1 ± 3.5	43.8 ± 3.3	−4.80%, ES −0.21, −0.50;0.08	72.2 ± 5.3	72.6 ± 5.6	0.42%, ES 0.02, −0.12;0.15	ES 0.16, −0.06;0.38
$\Delta[THb]_{rest}$ (μM)	0.1 ± 0.4	1.6 ± 0.5	1.5%, ES 1.06*, 0.13;1.99	3.6 ± 0.6	5.1 ± 0.8	1.5%, ES 0.69*, −0.17;1.55	ES 0.00, −0.80;0.79
$\Delta[THb]_{rec}$ S1 (μM)	7.3 ± 1.0	7.8 ± 0.7	0.53%, ES 0.16, −0.27;0.59	9.1 ± 1.1	10.3 ± 1.3	1.16%, ES 0.33*, −0.14;0.80	ES 0.21, −0.46;0.88
$\Delta[THb]_{rec}$ S2 (μM)	5.0 ± 0.8	5.8 ± 0.5	0.75%, ES 0.23*, −0.09;0.54	6.4 ± 0.9	6.5 ± 1.5	0.14%, ES 0.04, −0.50;0.58	ES −0.20, −0.88;0.48
$\Delta[THb]_{rec}$ S3 (μM)	3.7 ± 0.8	5.5 ± 0.8	1.77%, ES 0.54*, 0.04;1.04	6.0 ± 1.0	6.5 ± 1.4	0.57%, ES 0.16, −0.21;0.53	ES −0.40, −1.04;0.25
$\Delta[THb]_{rec}$ S4 (μM)	4.7 ± 1.1	5.2 ± 0.7	0.58%, ES 0.18, −0.24;0.59	5.3 ± 1.1	5.9 ± 1.0	0.64%, ES 0.18, −0.26;0.62	ES 0.02, −0.62;0.66
$\Delta[THb]_{rec}$ S5 (μM)	5.5 ± 0.9	5.6 ± 0.77	0.08%, ES 0.02, −0.23;0.28	3.9 ± 0.9	5.4 ± 1.1	1.54%, ES 0.44*, 0.17;0.70	ES 0.48*, 0.10;0.87
ΔReoxy ($\mu M.s^{-1}$)	0.1 ± 0.0	0.1 ± 0.02	−21.0%,, ES −0.32, −0.89;0.26	0.2 ± 0.1	0.2 ± 0.1	−4.0%,, ES −0.05, −0.38;0.028	ES 0.21, −0.29;0.70
$\Delta[HHb]_{peak}$ S1 (%AO)	59.0 ± 5.5	45.8 ± 13.3	−29.5%, ES −0.97, −2.86;0.92	69.8 ± 5.4	73.9 ± 3.9	7.3%, ES 0.26, −0.38;0.90	ES 1.35, −0.92;3.61
$\Delta[HHb]_{peak}$ S2 (%AO)	72.6 ± 7.3	57.3 ± 11.7	−10.3%, ES −0.30, −0.91;0.31	79.0 ± 5.6	83.9 ± 4.3	7.4%, ES 0.27, −0.35;0.89	ES 0.58, −0.24;1.40
$\Delta[HHb]_{peak}$ S3 (%AO)	75.0 ± 7.8	60.7 ± 11.8	−42.8%, ES −1.55, −4.11;1.01	80.4 ± 5.7	85.5 ± 3.9	7.7%, ES 0.28, −0.36;0.92	ES 2.04, −0.99;5.06
$\Delta[HHb]_{peak}$ S4 (%AO)	71.7 ± 7.3	61.4 ± 11.4	−29.1%, ES −0.95, −2.42;0.51	79.7 ± 6.8	86.3 ± 4.2	10.5%, ES 0.38, −0.24;0.99	ES 1.43, −0.32;3.17
$\Delta[HHb]_{peak}$ S5 (%AO)	68.4 ± 5.7	58.8 ± 11.5	−33.7%, ES −1.14, −2.64;0.36	82.7 ± 7.1	86.2 ± 4.2	6.4%, ES 0.23, −0.40;0.86	ES 1.52, −0.27;3.31
CMER S1	10.5 ± 1.4	5.6 ± 4.3	−4.4%, ES −0.12, −1.84;1.59	13.2 ± 2.5	11.8 ± 1.2	−2.4%, ES −0.04, −0.49;0.41	ES 0.05, −1.42;1.52
CMER S2	5.7 ± 1.3	7.2 ± 9.2	23.3%, ES 0.57, −0.57;1.72	5.6 ± 0.6	6.1 ± 0.8	8.7%, ES 0.14, −0.21;0.49	ES −0.29, −1.29;0.72
CMER S3	5.1 ± 1.1	9.9 ± 5.7	22.2%, ES 0.55, −0.46;1.56	5.1 ± 0.6	5.2 ± 0.6	3.8%, ES 0.06, −0.24;0.37	ES −0.37, −1.26;0.52
CMER S4	4.9 ± 1.0	17.3 ± 8.8	72.4%, ES 1.49, −0.42;3.41	4.7 ± 0.6	4.9 ± 0.5	5.0%, ES 0.08, −0.25;0.41	ES −1.13, −2.75;0.49
CMER S5	4.8 ± 0.9	19.3 ± 11.4	70.5%, ES 1.46, −0.30;3.23	4.6 ± 1.8	4.5 ± 0.5	−1.6%, ES −0.03, −0.36;0.30	ES −1.25, −2.75;0.25

Values are mean ± SE.
Asterisks (*) denote "clear" effect sizes (see statistics section). AO, arterial occlusion; CMER, contraction metabolic efficiency ratio; base, baseline before the IPC manoeuver; ΔReoxy, reoxygenation rate of the muscle; S, sets.

difference in response to IPC could be attributed in part to the fact that males increased their initial and total force leading to greater subsequent metabolic and ionic perturbations (Balsom et al., 1994; Glaister, 2005). However, this cannot be the only explanation, as females clearly improved their resistance to fatigue across the sets by approximately 2%. Sex differences in the availability and use of O_2 could shed some light on these differing responses to IPC.

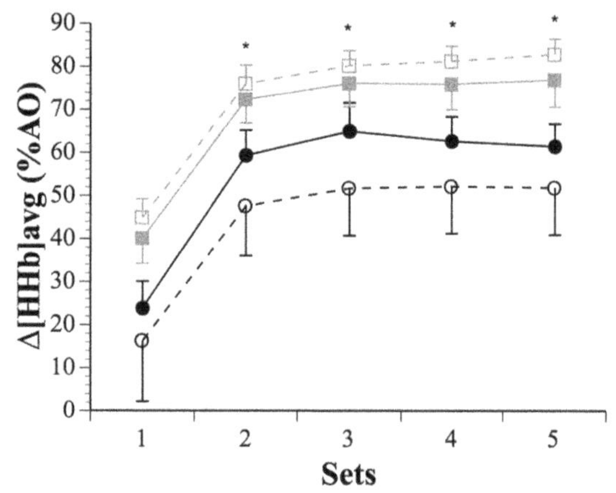

FIGURE 3 | Average changes in (Δ[HHb]$_{avg}$), expressed as a fraction of the maximal values obtained during a transient arterial occlusion (AO) in males (SHAM: ■ IPC: □) and females (SHAM: ● IPC: ○). *Asterisks (*)* denote "clear" differences between sexes (see statistics section). Values are mean ± SE.

Muscle Hemodynamic and Oxygenation

IPC is known to increase blood flow in both ipsilateral (Kraemer et al., 2011) and contralateral limbs (Enko et al., 2011). It also up-regulates endothelial function at rest (Moro et al., 2011), after local transient ischemia (Kharbanda et al., 2001; Loukogeorgakis et al., 2005), and prevents the decline in flow-mediated dilation observed after strenuous exercise (Bailey et al., 2012a) in males. By investigating the NIRS-derived [THb] changes from pre- to post-IPC, we confirmed the acute increase in local blood volume at rest in males, and extended this hyperperfusion finding to females. In fact, these moderate to large hemodynamic changes from baseline were similar in both sexes, of a magnitude of 1.5%. Such data from female participants are very scarce in the literature, and results do vary. While Kharbanda and colleagues reported no sex difference in flow-mediated dilation response during ischaemia-reperfusion after IPC (Kharbanda et al., 2001), the same response was found to be higher in females compared with males immediately post-preconditioning (Moro et al., 2011). There is, however, stronger evidence of a sex difference in vasodilator responsiveness. Females display higher brachial artery flow-mediated dilation (Levenson et al., 2001) and forearm vasodilatory response to acetylcholine and β2-adrenergic receptor stimulation (Dietz, 1999; Kneale et al., 2000) relative to males. At first glance, these sex-based differences in intrinsic physiological responses could explain the differing impact of IPC on performance in males vs. females observed in the current study. Greater effects on endothelial function should improve contractile activity (and/or efficiency) by allowing a better O_2 supply to skeletal muscles during intense exercise. It is not clear why males had a greater increase in muscle force than females for a similar percent increase in $\Delta[THb]_{rest}$, but one could argue that males might benefit more than females from an up-regulated endothelial function since they possess a lower intrinsic vasodilator responsiveness. Nevertheless, NIRS does not offer a robust assessment of blood flow since it does not detect change in blood velocity (Delorey et al., 2003). Studies using Doppler ultrasound are warranted to investigate vasodilation and potential blood flow changes following IPC in males and females.

An augmented blood volume before exercise could facilitate O_2 delivery to active skeletal muscles. While IPC-induced changes in peak muscle O_2 extraction were trivial in males, they displayed meaningful changes in $\Delta[HHb]_{avg}$ across the sets (**Figure 3**). Males extracted more O_2 than females after IPC in sets 2–5, with clearly increased muscle force. IPC has been reported to increase systemic maximal O_2 uptake (De Groot et al., 2010), as well as local tissue deoxygenation at task failure during handgrip exercise at 45% maximal voluntary contraction (Barbosa et al., 2015), and decrease blood lactate accumulation during submaximal running exercise (Bailey et al., 2012b). IPC also accelerates muscle deoxygenation dynamics and enhances performance during whole-body cycling and sustained isometric contraction of the knee in males (Kido et al., 2015; Tanaka et al., 2016). However, despite large $\Delta[THb]_{rest}$, IPC decreased $\Delta[HHb]_{avg}$ in females in the current study. The above studies exclusively recruited males, thus the current study adds to the literature by demonstrating that IPC might not induce similar metabolic responses in female athletes. Although we did not measure blood flow *per se*, the similar $\Delta[THb]_{rest}$ after IPC in both sexes suggest that the sex difference in O_2 extraction might not be directly related to a difference in O_2 availability. Furthermore, intramuscular pressure is positively correlated with contraction intensity, and it is accepted that occlusion of muscle blood flow occurs at 50–60% maximal voluntary contraction (Wigmore et al., 2004), thereby limiting its impact on sex differences observed in O_2 metabolism when contractions are performed maximally as in the current study. In fact, the excessive intramuscular pressures of the contractions made our [THb] data collected during contractions unusable. And along this line of reasoning, it is of note that sex differences in fatigue development and performance disappear when blood flow is occluded (Maughan et al., 1986; Yoon et al., 2007). This could suggest that O_2 availability does not explain the current finding of upregulated O_2 extraction in males only. Caution is of course needed when interpreting NIRS-derived results due to methodological confounding factors such as subcutaneous fat layer thickness (although it was below the recommended emitter-receptor distance in both sexes) and possible NIRS sensor movement on the skin. Finally, muscle re-perfusion and thereby re-oxygenation occurring between maximal efforts is correlated with the recovery of muscle performance mainly via the resynthesis of phosphocreatine and by-products removal (Kime et al., 2003; Billaut and Buchheit, 2013). However, sex differences in $\Delta[THb]_{rec}$ were mostly unclear, as was the case for ΔReoxy. Based on these data, the sex-specific impact of IPC on exercise performance does not appear to be attributed to recovery processes.

There is also the possibility of a preferential impact of IPC on type II muscle fibers. A lower proportional area of type I fibers has been found in the vastus lateralis of males compared with females (Simoneau et al., 1985; Staron et al., 2000). Type II fibers display greater fractional O_2 extraction with faster kinetics and lower microvascular O_2 partial pressure (i.e., better muscle

O_2 diffusion index), despite a lower overall O_2 consumption (Mcdonough et al., 2005). Interestingly, extraneous infusion of adenosine, which is a key acting molecule released during IPC, preferentially enhances vasodilation of arterioles to type II fibers (Wunsch et al., 2000). Therefore, due to the greater O_2 extraction of type II fibers when highly perfused (Wilson et al., 1977), it has been suggested that these fibers might benefit more from an increase in blood perfusion than the more aerobic type I fibers (Faiss et al., 2013; Paradis-Deschenes et al., 2016), which could explain the higher $\Delta[HHb]_{avg}$ in strength-trained males in the present study.

In conclusion, this applied study demonstrated that strength-trained males might benefit more clearly from IPC than their female counterparts during repeated, maximal contractions. This strengthens clinical observations that sex may be a confounder in the response to this stimulus. Despite a similar increase in blood volume ($\uparrow$[THb]) in both sexes immediately after IPC, and thus presumably similar increase in O_2 availability, males displayed greater peripheral O_2 extraction ($\uparrow\Delta$[HHb]). This ergogenic effect therefore appears to be mediated in part via an upregulation of oxidative function in males, possibly within type II muscle fibers.

AUTHOR CONTRIBUTIONS

PPD, DRJ, and FB conceptualized and designed the research project; PPD acquired the data and conducted the statistical analysis; PPD interpreted results with assistance from DRJ and FB; PPD wrote the manuscript with revisions from DRJ and FB. All authors reviewed and agreed upon the final manuscript.

ACKNOWLEDGMENTS

The authors thank the athletes for their participation in the study. We also sincerely thank Pr Normand Teasdale and Mr. Marcel Kaszap for their valuable technical support and assistance.

REFERENCES

Bailey, T. G., Birk, G. K., Cable, N. T., Atkinson, G., Green, D. J., Jones, H., et al. (2012a). Remote ischemic preconditioning prevents reduction in brachial artery flow-mediated dilation after strenuous exercise. *Am. J. Physiol. Heart Circ. Physiol.* 303, H533–H538. doi: 10.1152/ajpheart.00272.2012

Bailey, T. G., Jones, H., Gregson, W., Atkinson, G., Cable, N. T., and Thijssen, D. H. J. (2012b). Effect of ischemic preconditioning on lactate accumulation and running performance. *Med. Sci. Sports Exerc.* 44, 2084–2089. doi: 10.1249/MSS.0b013e318262cb17

Balsom, P. D., Gaitanos, G. C., Ekblom, B., and Sjödin, B. (1994). Reduced oxygen availability during high intensity intermittent exercise impairs performance. *Acta Physiol. Scand.* 152, 279–285. doi: 10.1111/j.1748-1716.1994.tb09807.x

Barbosa, T. C., Machado, A. C., Braz, I. D., Fernandes, I. A., Vianna, L. C., Nobrega, A. C. L., et al. (2015). Remote ischemic preconditioning delays fatigue development during handgrip exercise. *Scand. J. Med. Sci. Sports* 25, 356–364. doi: 10.1111/sms.12229

Batterham, A. M., and Hopkins, W. G. (2006). Making meaningful inferences about magnitudes. *Int. J. Sports Physiol. Perform.* 1, 50–57. doi: 10.1123/ijspp.1.1.50

Beaven, C. M., Cook, C. J., Kilduff, L., Drawer, S., and Gill, N. (2012). Intermittent lower-limb occlusion enhances recovery after strenuous exercise. *Appl. Physiol. Nutr. Metab.* 37, 1132–1139. doi: 10.1139/h2012-101

Billaut, F., and Buchheit, M. (2013). Repeated-sprint performance and vastus lateralis oxygenation: effect of limited O2 availability. *Scand. J. Med. Sci. Sports* 23, e185–e193. doi: 10.1111/sms.12052

Bolli, R. (2000). The late phase of preconditioning. *Circ. Res.* 87, 972–983. doi: 10.1161/01.RES.87.11.972

Clark, B. C., Collier, S. R., Manini, T. M., and Ploutz-Snyder, L. L. (2005). Sex differences in muscle fatigability and activation patterns of the human quadriceps femoris. *Eur. J. Appl. Physiol.* 94, 196–206. doi: 10.1007/s00421-004-1293-0

De Blasi, R. A., Cope, M., Elwell, C., Safoue, F., and Ferrari, M. (1993). Noninvasive measurement of human forearm oxygen consumption by near infrared spectroscopy. *Eur. J. Appl. Physiol.* 67, 20–25. doi: 10.1007/BF00 377698

De Groot, P. C., Thijssen, D. H., Sanchez, M., Ellenkamp, R., and Hopman, M. T. (2010). Ischemic preconditioning improves maximal performance in humans. *Eur. J. Appl. Physiol.* 108, 141–146. doi: 10.1007/s00421-009-1195-2

Delorey, D. S., Kowalchuk, J. M., and Paterson, D. H. (2003). Relationship between pulmonary O2 uptake kinetics and muscle deoxygenation during moderate-intensity exercise. *J. Appl. Physiol.* 95, 113–120. doi: 10.1152/japplphysiol.00956.2002

Dietz, N. M. (1999). Gender and nitric oxide-mediated vasodilation in humans. *Lupus* 8, 402–408. doi: 10.1177/096120339900800515

Enko, K., Nakamura, K., Yunoki, K., Miyoshi, T., Akagi, S., Yoshida, M., et al. (2011). Intermittent arm ischemia induces vasodilatation of the contralateral upper limb. *J. Physiol. Sci.* 61, 507–513. doi: 10.1007/s12576-011-0172-9

Faiss, R., Léger, B., Vesin, J. M., Fournier, P. E., Eggel, Y., Deriaz, O., et al. (2013). Significant molecular and systemic adaptations after repeated sprint training in Hypoxia. *PLoS ONE* 8:e56522. doi: 10.1371/journal.pone.0056522

Ferrari, M., Mottola, L., and Quaresima, V. (2004). Principles, techniques, and limitations of near infrared spectroscopy. *Can. J. Appl. Physiol. Rev.* 29, 463–487. doi: 10.1139/h04-031

Gibson, N., Mahony, B., Tracey, C., Fawkner, S., and Murray, A. (2015). Effect of ischemic preconditioning on repeated sprint ability in team sport athletes. *J. Sports Sci.* 33, 1182–1188. doi: 10.1080/02640414.2014.988741

Gibson, N., White, J., Neish, M., and Murray, A. (2013). Effect of ischemic preconditioning on land-based sprinting in Team-Sport Athletes. *Int. J. Sports Physiol. Perform.* 8, 671–676. doi: 10.1123/ijspp.8.6.671

Glaister, M. (2005). Multiple sprint work - Physiological responses, mechanisms of fatigue and the influence of aerobic fitness. *Sports Med.* 35, 757–777. doi: 10.2165/00007256-200535090-00003

Hopkins, W. G., Marshall, S. W., Batterham, A. M., and Hanin, J. (2009). Progressive statistics for studies in sports medicine and exercise science. *Med. Sci. Sports Exerc.* 41, 3–13. doi: 10.1249/MSS.0b013e31818cb278

Hunter, S. K. (2016). The relevance of sex differences in performance fatigability. *Med. Sci. Sports Exerc.* 48, 2247–2256. doi: 10.1249/MSS.0000000000000928

Hunter, S. K., Schletty, J. M., Schlachter, K. M., Griffith, E. E., Polichnowski, A. J., and Ng, A. V. (2006). Active hyperemia and vascular conductance differ between men and women for an isometric fatiguing contraction. *J. Appl. Physiol.* 101, 140–150. doi: 10.1152/japplphysiol.01567.2005

Incognito, A. V., Burr, J. F., and Millar, P. J. (2015). The effects of ischemic preconditioning on human exercise performance. *Sports Med.* 46, 531–544. doi: 10.1007/s40279-015-0433-5

Kayser, B., Sliwinski, P., Yan, S., Tobiasz, M., and Macklem, P. T. (1997). Respiratory effort sensation during exercise with induced expiratory-flow limitation in healthy humans. *J. Appl. Physiol.* (1985) 83, 936–947.

Kent-Braun, J. A., Ng, A. V., Doyle, J. W., and Towse, T. F. (2002). Human skeletal muscle responses vary with age and gender during fatigue due to incremental isometric exercise. *J. Appl. Physiol.* 93, 1813–1823. doi: 10.1152/japplphysiol.00091.2002

Kharbanda, R. K., Peters, M., Walton, B., Kattenhorn, M., Mullen, M., Klein, N., et al. (2001). Ischemic preconditioning prevents endothelial injury and systemic neutrophil activation during ischemia-reperfusion in humans *in vivo*. *Circulation* 103, 1624–1630. doi: 10.1161/01.CIR.103.12.1624

Kido, K., Suga, T., Tanaka, D., Honjo, T., Homma, T., Fujita, S., et al. (2015). Ischemic preconditioning accelerates muscle deoxygenation dynamics and enhances exercise endurance during the work-to-work test. *Physiol. Rep.* 3:e12395. doi: 10.14814/phy2.12395

Kime, R., Katsumura, T., Hamaoka, T., Osada, T., Sako, T., Murakami, M., et al. (2003). "Muscle reoxygenation rate after isometric exercise at various intensities in relation to muscle oxidative capacity," in *Oxygen Transport to Tissue Xxiv*, eds J. F. Dunn and H. M. Swartz (New York, NY: Springer Science+Business Media), 497–507.

Kneale, B. J., Chowienczyk, P. J., Brett, S. E., Coltart, D. J., and Ritter, J. M. (2000). Gender differences in sensitivity to adrenergic agonists of forearm resistance vasculature. *J. Am. Coll. Cardiol.* 36, 1233–1238. doi: 10.1016/S0735-1097(00)00849-4

Kraemer, R., Lorenzen, J., Kabbani, M., Herold, C., Busche, M., Vogt, P. M., et al. (2011). Acute effects of remote ischemic preconditioning on cutaneous microcirculation–a controlled prospective cohort study. *BMC Surg.* 11:32. doi: 10.1186/1471-2482-11-32

Laskey, W. K., and Beach, D. (2003). Frequency and clinical significance of ischemic preconditioning during percutaneous coronary intervention. *J. Am. Coll. Cardiol.* 42, 998–1003. doi: 10.1016/S0735-1097(03)00909-4

Levenson, J., Pessana, F., Gariepy, J., Armentano, R., and Simon, A. (2001). Gender differences in wall shear-mediated brachial artery vasoconstriction and vasodilation. *J. Am. Coll. Cardiol.* 38, 1668–1674. doi: 10.1016/S0735-1097(01)01604-7

Loukogeorgakis, S. P., Panagiotidou, A. T., Broadhead, M. W., Donald, A., Deanfield, J. E., and Macallister, R. J. (2005). Remote ischemic preconditioning provides early and late protection against endothelial ischemia-reperfusion injury in humans: role of the autonomic nervous system. *J. Am. Coll. Cardiol.* 46, 450–456. doi: 10.1016/j.jacc.2005.04.044

Maughan, R. J., Harmon, M., Leiper, J. B., Sale, D., and Delman, A. (1986). Endurance capacity of untrained males and females in isometric and dynamic muscular contractions. *Eur. J. Appl. Physiol. Occup. Physiol.* 55, 395–400. doi: 10.1007/BF00422739

Mccully, K. K., and Hamaoka, T. (2000). Near-infrared spectroscopy: what can it tell us about oxygen saturation in skeletal muscle? *Exerc. Sport Sci. Rev.* 28, 123–127.

Mcdonough, P., Behnke, B. J., Padilla, D. J., Musch, T. I., and Poole, D. C. (2005). Control of microvascular oxygen pressures in rat muscles comprised of different fibre types. *J. Physiol.* 563, 903–913. doi: 10.1113/jphysiol.2004.079533

Moro, L., Pedone, C., Mondi, A., Nunziata, E., and Antonelli Incalzi, R. (2011). Effect of local and remote ischemic preconditioning on endothelial function in young people and healthy or hypertensive elderly people. *Atherosclerosis* 219, 750–752. doi: 10.1016/j.atherosclerosis.2011.08.046

Moses, M. A., Addison, P. D., Neligan, P. C., Ashrafpour, H., Huang, N., Zair, M., et al. (2005). Mitochondrial K_{ATP} channels in hindlimb remote ischemic preconditioning of skeletal muscle against infarction. *Am. J. Physiol. Heart Circ. Physiol.* 288, H559–H567. doi: 10.1152/ajpheart.00845.2004

Pang, C. Y., Yang, R. Z., Zhong, A. G., Xu, N., Boyd, B., and Forrest, C. R. (1995). Acute ischemic preconditioning protects against skeletal-muscle infarction in the pig. *Cardiovasc. Res.* 29, 782–788. doi: 10.1016/S0008-6363(96)88613-5

Paradis-Deschenes, P., Joanisse, D. R., and Billaut, F. (2016). Ischemic preconditioning increases muscle perfusion, oxygen uptake, and force in strength-trained athletes. *Appl. Physiol. Nutr. Metab.* 41, 938–944. doi: 10.1139/apnm-2015-0561

Parker, B. A., Smithmyer, S. L., Pelberg, J. A., Mishkin, A. D., Herr, M. D., and Proctor, D. N. (2007). Sex differences in leg vasodilation during graded knee extensor exercise in young adults. *J. Appl. Physiol.* 103, 1583–1591. doi: 10.1152/japplphysiol.00662.2007

Patterson, S. D., Bezodis, N. E., Glaister, M., and Pattison, J. R. (2015). The effect of ischemic preconditioning on repeated sprint cycling performance. *Med. Sci. Sports Exerc.* 47, 1652–1658. doi: 10.1249/MSS.0000000000000576

Pitcher, J. M., Wang, M., Tsai, B. M., Kher, A., Turrentine, M. W., Brown, J. W., et al. (2005). Preconditioning: gender effects. *J. Surg. Res.* 129, 202–220. doi: 10.1016/j.jss.2005.04.015

Russ, D. W., and Kent-Braun, J. A. (2003). Sex differences in human skeletal muscle fatigue are eliminated under ischemic conditions. *J. Appl. Physiol.* 94, 2414–2422. doi: 10.1152/japplphysiol.01145.2002

Simoneau, J. A., Lortie, G., Boulay, M. R., Thibault, M. C., Thériault, G., and Bouchard, C. (1985). Skeletal muscle histochemical and biochemical characteristics in sedentary male and female subjects. *Can. J. Physiol. Pharmacol.* 63, 30–35. doi: 10.1139/y85-005

Staron, R. S., Hagerman, F. C., Hikida, R. S., Murray, T. F., Hostler, D. P., Crill, M. T., et al. (2000). Fiber type composition of the vastus lateralis muscle of young men and women. *J. Histochem. Cytochem.* 48, 623–629. doi: 10.1177/002215540004800506

Tanaka, D., Suga, T., Tanaka, T., Kido, K., Honjo, T., Fujita, S., et al. (2016). Ischemic preconditioning enhances muscle endurance during sustained isometric exercise. *Int. J. Sports Med.*. doi: 10.1055/s-0035-1565141

Wigmore, D. M., Damon, B. M., Pober, D. M., and Kent-Braun, J. A. (2004). MRI measures of perfusion-related changes in human skeletal muscle during progressive contractions. *J. Appl. Physiol.* 97, 2385–2394. doi: 10.1152/japplphysiol.01390.2003

Wilson, D. F., Erecinska, M., Drown, C., and Silver, I. A. (1977). Effect of oxygen tension on cellular energetics. *Am. J. Physiol.* 233, C135–C140.

Wunsch, S. A., Muller-Delp, J., and Delp, M. D. (2000). Time course of vasodilatory responses in skeletal muscle arterioles: role in hyperemia at onset of exercise. *Am. J. Physiol. Heart Circ. Physiol.* 279, H1715–H1723.

Yoon, T., Schlinder Delap, B., Griffith, E. E., and Hunter, S. K. (2007). Mechanisms of fatigue differ after low- and high-force fatiguing contractions in men and women. *Muscle Nerve* 36, 515–524. doi: 10.1002/mus.20844

Permissions

All chapters in this book were first published by Frontiers; hereby published with permission under the Creative Commons Attribution License or equivalent. Every chapter published in this book has been scrutinized by our experts. Their significance has been extensively debated. The topics covered herein carry significant findings which will fuel the growth of the discipline. They may even be implemented as practical applications or may be referred to as a beginning point for another development.

The contributors of this book come from diverse backgrounds, making this book a truly international effort. This book will bring forth new frontiers with its revolutionizing research information and detailed analysis of the nascent developments around the world.

We would like to thank all the contributing authors for lending their expertise to make the book truly unique. They have played a crucial role in the development of this book. Without their invaluable contributions this book wouldn't have been possible. They have made vital efforts to compile up to date information on the varied aspects of this subject to make this book a valuable addition to the collection of many professionals and students.

This book was conceptualized with the vision of imparting up-to-date information and advanced data in this field. To ensure the same, a matchless editorial board was set up. Every individual on the board went through rigorous rounds of assessment to prove their worth. After which they invested a large part of their time researching and compiling the most relevant data for our readers.

The editorial board has been involved in producing this book since its inception. They have spent rigorous hours researching and exploring the diverse topics which have resulted in the successful publishing of this book. They have passed on their knowledge of decades through this book. To expedite this challenging task, the publisher supported the team at every step. A small team of assistant editors was also appointed to further simplify the editing procedure and attain best results for the readers.

Apart from the editorial board, the designing team has also invested a significant amount of their time in understanding the subject and creating the most relevant covers. They scrutinized every image to scout for the most suitable representation of the subject and create an appropriate cover for the book.

The publishing team has been an ardent support to the editorial, designing and production team. Their endless efforts to recruit the best for this project, has resulted in the accomplishment of this book. They are a veteran in the field of academics and their pool of knowledge is as vast as their experience in printing. Their expertise and guidance has proved useful at every step. Their uncompromising quality standards have made this book an exceptional effort. Their encouragement from time to time has been an inspiration for everyone.

The publisher and the editorial board hope that this book will prove to be a valuable piece of knowledge for researchers, students, practitioners and scholars across the globe.

List of Contributors

He Huang, Gang Wu, Gang Xu, Bing-Da Sun and Yu-Qi Gao
Institute of Medicine and Hygienic Equipment for High Altitude Region, College of High Altitude Military Medicine, Third Military Medical University, Chongqing, China
Key Laboratory of High Altitude Environmental Medicine, Third Military Medical University, Ministry of Education, Chongqing, China
Key Laboratory of High Altitude Medicine, Chinese People's Liberation Army, Chongqing, China

Bao Liu
Institute of Medicine and Hygienic Equipment for High Altitude Region, College of High Altitude Military Medicine, Third Military Medical University, Chongqing, China
Key Laboratory of High Altitude Environmental Medicine, Third Military Medical University, Ministry of Education, Chongqing, China
Key Laboratory of High Altitude Medicine, Chinese People's Liberation Army, Chongqing, China
The 12th Hospital of Chinese People's Liberation Army, Kashi Xinjiang, China

Ryan L. Sheppard
Department of Submarine Medicine and Survival Systems Groton, Naval Submarine Medical Research Laboratory, Groton, CT, United States
Department of Undersea Medicine, Walter Reed Army Institute of Research and Naval Medical Research Center, Silver Spring, MD, United States

Joshua M. Swift, Aaron Hall and Richard T. Mahon
Department of Undersea Medicine, Walter Reed Army Institute of Research and Naval Medical Research Center, Silver Spring, MD, United States

Erin M. Leonard, Shaima Salman and Colin A. Nurse
Department of Biology, McMaster University, Hamilton, ON, Canada

Julio Brito, Patricia Siques, Raul Romero and Karen Flores
Institute of Health Studies, University Arturo Prat, Iquique, Chile

Rosario López
Department of Preventive Medicine and Public Health, University Autonoma of Madrid, Madrid, Spain

Fabiola León-Velarde
Department of Biological and Physiological Sciences, Facultad de Ciencias y Filosofía/IIA, University Peruana Cayetano Heredia, Lima, Peru

Nicole Lüneburg, Juliane Hannemann and Rainer H. Böger
Institute of Clinical Pharmacology and Toxicology, University Medical Center Hamburg-Eppendorf, Hamburg, Germany

Jiaqi Feng, Ziqian Wei and Hongxiao Yu
Department of Physiology, Hebei Medical University, Shijiazhuang, China

Fang Yuan, Yi Zhang and Sheng Wang
Department of Physiology, Hebei Medical University, Shijiazhuang, China
Hebei Key Laboratory of Vascular Homeostasis and Hebei Collaborative Innovation Center for Cardio-Cerebrovascular Disease, Shijiazhuang, China

Hanqiao Wang
Department of Sleep, Third Hospital of Hebei Medical University, Shijiazhuang, China

Xiangjian Zhang
Hebei Key Laboratory of Vascular Homeostasis and Hebei Collaborative Innovation Center for Cardio-Cerebrovascular Disease, Shijiazhuang, China
Department of Neurology, Second Hospital of Hebei Medical University, Shijiazhuang, China

Sebastián Castillo-Galán and Ismael Hernandez
Unidad de Fisiología y Fisiopatología Perinatal, Programa de Fisiopatología, Instituto de Ciencias Biomédicas, Facultad de Medicina, Universidad de Chile, Santiago, Chile

Roberto V. Reyes, Emilio A. Herrera, Germán Ebensperger and Aníbal J. Llanos
Unidad de Fisiología y Fisiopatología Perinatal, Programa de Fisiopatología, Instituto de Ciencias Biomédicas, Facultad de Medicina, Universidad de Chile, Santiago, Chile
International Center for Andean Studies, Universidad de Chile, Santiago, Chile

Vasthi López and María I. Taborda
Laboratorio de Metabolismo de Aminoácidos e Hipoxia, Departamento de Ciencias Biomédicas, Universidad Católica del Norte, Coquimbo, Chile

Fernando A. Moraga
Laboratorio de Fisiología, Hipoxia y Función Vascular, Departamento de Ciencias Biomedicas, Facultad de Medicina, Universidad Católica del Norte, Coquimbo, Chile

Anibal J. Llanos and German Ebensperger
Laboratorio de Fisiología y Fisiopatología del Desarrollo, Departamento de Ciencias Biomédicas, Universidad de Chile, Santiago, Chile

Elena Uribe
Laboratorio de Enzimología, Departamento de Bioquímica y Biología Molecular, Universidad of Concepción, Concepción, Chile

Andrea Porzionato, Elena Stocco, Diego Guidolin, Veronica Macchi and Raffaele De Caro
Department of Neuroscience, University of Padua, Padua, Italy

Luigi Agnati
Department of Diagnostic, Clinical Medicine and Public Health, University of Modena and Reggio Emilia, Modena, Italy

Patricia Siques, Julio Brito, Karen Flores, Stefany Ordenes, Karem Arriaza and Eduardo Pena
Institute of Health Studies, University Arturo Prat, Iquique, Chile

Ángel L. López de Pablo, M. C. Gonzalez and Silvia Arribas
Department of Physiology, Faculty of Medicine, University Autonoma of Madrid, Madrid, Spain

Esteban A. Moya and Frank L. Powell
Division of Physiology, Department of Medicine, University of California, San Diego, La Jolla, CA, United States

Matiram Pun, Lauren L. Drogos and Sara E. Hartmann
Department of Physiology & Pharmacology, Cumming School of Medicine, University of Calgary, Calgary, AB, Canada
Hotchkiss Brain Institute, Cumming School of Medicine, University of Calgary, Calgary, AB, Canada

Veronica Guadagni
Department of Physiology & Pharmacology, Cumming School of Medicine, University of Calgary, Calgary, AB, Canada
Hotchkiss Brain Institute, Cumming School of Medicine, University of Calgary, Calgary, AB, Canada
Department of Clinical Neuroscience, Cumming School of Medicine, University of Calgary, Calgary, AB, Canada
O'Brien Institute for Public Health, Cumming School of Medicine, University of Calgary, Calgary, AB, Canada

Kaitlyn M. Bettauer
Department of Physiology & Pharmacology, Cumming School of Medicine, University of Calgary, Calgary, AB, Canada
Hotchkiss Brain Institute, Cumming School of Medicine, University of Calgary, Calgary, AB, Canada
Department of Psychology, Faculty of Science, University of British Columbia, Vancouver, BC, Canada

Julie Aitken
Biomedical Engineering Graduate Program, University of Calgary, Calgary, AB, Canada

Michael Furian, Lara Muralt, Mona Lichtblau, Patrick R. Bader, Silvia Ulrich and Konrad E. Bloch
Pulmonary Division, Sleep Disorders Centre and Pulmonary Hypertension Clinic, University Hospital Zürich, Zurich, Switzerland

Jean M. Rawling
Department of Family Medicine, Cumming School of Medicine, University of Calgary, Calgary, AB, Canada

Andrea B. Protzner
Hotchkiss Brain Institute, Cumming School of Medicine, University of Calgary, Calgary, AB, Canada
Department of Psychology, Faculty of Arts, University of Calgary, Calgary, AB, Canada

Barry Giesbrecht
Department of Psychological and Brain Sciences, Institute for Collaborative Biotechnologies, University of California, Santa Barbara, Santa Barbara, CA, United States

Marc J. Poulin
Department of Physiology & Pharmacology, Cumming School of Medicine, University of Calgary, Calgary, AB, Canada
Hotchkiss Brain Institute, Cumming School of Medicine, University of Calgary, Calgary, AB, Canada
Department of Clinical Neuroscience, Cumming School of Medicine, University of Calgary, Calgary, AB, Canada
O'Brien Institute for Public Health, Cumming School of Medicine, University of Calgary, Calgary, AB, Canada
Libin Cardiovascular Institute of Alberta, Cumming School of Medicine, University of Calgary, Calgary, AB, Canada
Faculty of Kinesiology, University of Calgary, Calgary, AB, Canada

Andreas Becke
Institute of Cognitive Neurology and Dementia Research, Otto-von-Guericke-Universität Magdeburg, Magdeburg, Germany
Neuroprotection Laboratory, German Center for Neurodegenerative Diseases (DZNE), Magdeburg, Germany

Paul S. R. Goods
Western Australian Institute of Sport, Perth, WA, Australia

Volkmar Lessmann
Institute of Physiology, Otto-von-Guericke-Universität Magdeburg, Magdeburg, Germany
Center for Behavioral Brain Sciences, Magdeburg, Germany

Notger G. Müller
Neuroprotection Laboratory, German Center for Neurodegenerative Diseases (DZNE), Magdeburg, Germany
Center for Behavioral Brain Sciences, Magdeburg, Germany

Tanja Brigadski
Institute of Physiology, Otto-von-Guericke-Universität Magdeburg, Magdeburg, Germany
Informatics and Microsystem Technology, University of Applied Sciences, Kaiserslautern, Kaiserslautern, Germany

Almaz Akunov and Akpay Sarybaev
Department of Mountain and Sleep Medicine and Pulmonary Hypertension, National Center of Cardiology and Internal Medicine, Bishkek, Kyrgyzstan
Kyrgyz Indian Mountain Biomedical Research Center, Bishkek, Kyrgyzstan

Akylbek Sydykov
Department of Mountain and Sleep Medicine and Pulmonary Hypertension, National Center of Cardiology and Internal Medicine, Bishkek, Kyrgyzstan
Excellence Cluster Cardio-Pulmonary System, Universities of Giessen and Marburg Lung Center, Member of the German Center for Lung Research (DZL), Justus Liebig University Giessen, Giessen, Germany
Chair for Pulmonary Pharmacotherapy, Member of the German Center for Lung Research, Universities of Giessen and Marburg Lung Center, Giessen, Germany

Daniela Salas, Carlos Cespedes and Jessica Diaz-Elizondo
Department of Physiology, Center for Aging and Regeneration CARE UC, Facultad de Ciencias Biológicas, Pontificia Universidad Católica de Chile, Santiago, Chile

Turgun Toktash and Anara Doolotova
Medical Department, Kumtor Gold Company, Bishkek, Kyrgyzstan

Carlos P. Vio
Department of Physiology, Center for Aging and Regeneration CARE UC, Facultad de Ciencias Biológicas, Pontificia Universidad Católica de Chile, Santiago, Chile
Facultad de Medicina y Ciencia, Universidad San Sebastián, Santiago, Chile

Natalia Mendez
Department of Physiology, Center for Aging and Regeneration CARE UC, Facultad de Ciencias Biológicas, Pontificia Universidad Católica de Chile, Santiago, Chile
Institute of Anatomy, Histology, and Pathology, Facultad de Medicina, Universidad Austral de Chile, Valdivia, Chile

Julio Alcayaga
Laboratorio de Fisiología Celular, Departamento de Biología, Facultad de Ciencias, Universidad de Chile, Santiago, Chile

Rodrigo Iturriaga
Laboratorio de Neurobiología, Department of Physiology, Facultad de Ciencias Biológicas, Pontificia Universidad Católica de Chile, Santiago, Chile

Simon Maximilian Platzek, Aleksandar Petrovic, Argen Mamazhakypov, Christina Vroom, Oleg Pak, Norbert Weissmann, Hossein Ardeschir Ghofrani and Ralph Theo Schermuly
Chair for Pulmonary Pharmacotherapy, Member of the German Center for Lung Research, Universities of Giessen and Marburg Lung Center, Giessen, Germany

Djuro Kosanovic
Chair for Pulmonary Pharmacotherapy, Member of the German Center for Lung Research, Universities of Giessen and Marburg Lung Center, Giessen, Germany
Sechenov First Moscow State Medical University (Sechenov University), Moscow, Russia

Abdirashit Maripov, Meerim Sartmyrzaeva, Kubatbek Muratali Uulu, Meerim Cholponbaeva, Aidana Toktosunova, Nazgul Omurzakova and Melis Duishobaev
Kyrgyz National Centre for Cardiology and Internal Medicine, named after Academician Mirsaid Mirrakhimov, Bishkek, Kyrgyzstan

Philip F. Skiba
Department of Sports Medicine, Advocate Lutheran General Hospital, Park Ridge, IL, USA

Torres-Peralta, David Morales-Alamo, José Losa-Reyna, Ismael Pérez-Suárez and José A. L. Calbet
Department of Physical Education, University of Las Palmas de Gran Canaria, Las Palmas de Gran Canaria, Spain
Research Institute of Biomedical and Health Sciences (IUIBS), Las Palmas de Gran Canaria, Spain

Miriam González-Izal and Mikel Izquierdo
Department of Health Sciences, Public University of Navarra, Tudela, Spain

Brendan R. Scott
School of Psychology and Exercise Science, Murdoch University, Perth, WA, Australia

Patrick Müller and Milos Dordevic
Neuroprotection Laboratory, German Center for Neurodegenerative Diseases (DZNE), Magdeburg, Germany

Katie M. Slattery
New South Wales Institute of Sport, Sydney Olympic Park, NSW, Australia

Alice J. Sweeting, Matthew C. Varley, Ramón F. Rodriguez, William G. Hopkins and Robert J. Aughey
Institute of Sport, Exercise and Active Living, Victoria University, Melbourne, VIC, Australia

Stefan De Smet and Ruud Van Thienen
Exercise Physiology Research Group, Department of Kinesiology, Katholieke Universiteit Leuven, Leuven, Belgium

Louise Deldicque
Exercise Physiology Research Group, Department of Kinesiology, Katholieke Universiteit Leuven, Leuven, Belgium
Institute of Neuroscience, Université Catholique de Louvain, Louvain-la-Neuve, Belgium

Ruth James and Craig Sale
Musculoskeletal Physiology Research Group, Sport, Health and Performance Enhancement Research Centre, School of Science and Technology, Nottingham Trent University, Nottingham, UK

Peter Hespel
Exercise Physiology Research Group, Department of Kinesiology, Katholieke Universiteit Leuven, Leuven, Belgium
Department of Kinesiology, Bakala Academy–Athletic Performance Center, KU Leuven, Leuven, Belgium

Nathan E. Townsend, David S. Nichols, Sebastien Racinais and Julien D. Périard
Athlete Health and Performance Centre, Aspetar Orthopaedic and Sports Medicine Hospital, Doha, Qatar

Michael J. Hamlin, Catherine A. Lizamore and Catherine A. Elliot
Department of Tourism, Sport and Society, Lincoln University, Christchurch, New Zealand

Peter D. Olsen and Helen C. Marshall
Department of Nursing, Midwifery and Allied Health, Ara Institute of Canterbury, Christchurch, New Zealand

Pénélope Paradis-Deschênes and Denis R. Joanisse
Département de kinésiologie, Université Laval, Québec, QC, Canada
Institut Universitaire de Cardiologie et de Pneumologie de Québec, Québec, QC, Canada

François Billaut
Département de kinésiologie, Université Laval, Québec, QC, Canada
Institut Universitaire de Cardiologie et de Pneumologie de Québec, Québec, QC, Canada
Institut National du Sport du Québec, Montréal, QC, Canada
Institute of Sport, Exercise and Active Living, Victoria University, Melbourne, VIC, Australia

Index